Handbook of Geriatric Communication Disorders

Handbook of
Geriatric Communication Disorders

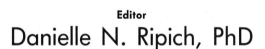

Editor

Danielle N. Ripich, PhD

Co-Editors

Marie R. Haug, PhD
Audrey L. Holland, PhD
Joel C. Kahane, PhD
Craig W. Newman, PhD
Barbara E. Weinstein, PhD
Peter J. Whitehouse, MD, PhD

pro·ed

8700 Shoal Creek Boulevard
Austin, Texas 78757

Printed in the United States of America

Library of Congress Cataloging-in-Publication Data

Handbook of geriatric communication disorders / editor, Danielle
  Ripich : co-editors, Marie Haug . . . [et al.].
     p.   cm.
  Includes bibliographical references and index.
  ISBN 0-89079-423-5
  1. Communicative disorders in old age. I. Ripich, Danielle
Newberry. II. Haug, Marie R.
  [DNLM: 1. Communicative Disorders—in old age. WL 340 H2352]
RC429.H35 1990
618.97′6855—dc20
DMLN/DLC
for Library of Congress   90-14311
                                         CIP

pro·ed

8700 Shoal Creek Boulevard
Austin, Texas 78757

  4   5   6   7   8   9   10   99 98 97 96

This book is dedicated to my grandmother, Marie (Ree) Curtin,
who through her stories gave me a love of language and
through her life gave me a model of successful aging.
She is a remarkable woman.

Contents

Preface

This book grew out of discussions with numerous colleagues about the need to assemble, organize, and examine the current knowledge base in geriatric communication disorders. The purpose of this book is to bring together significant information and to point the way toward future research and clinical intervention in this area. Persons over 65 years of age comprise the fastest growing clinical population, and educational programs are beginning to offer coursework that directly addresses the unique problems of this age group. This text is designed to serve as an advanced undergraduate- and graduate-level text for students in speech-language pathology, audiology, speech and hearing sciences, neurolinguistics, gerontology, geriatric social work, clinical psychology, and neuropsychology. It is also intended to be used as a resource for practicing clinicians in these fields and in medicine.

This book brings together a number of highly respected researchers and clinicians, selected for their competence in the area of geriatric communication disorders. The content and organization of this handbook are consistent with the objective of incorporating information ranging from basic science to clinical care. The text is divided into five sections, each examining a different aspect of geriatric communication disorders.

As the sections and chapters were assembled and edited, three themes emerged. These themes, underlined by authors across various disciplines and perspectives, are interrelated and are critical to the reader's understanding of the literature and integration of clinical implications in aging. First, research and intervention with the elderly often require multiple perspectives. This is a result of the complexity of the problems that are generally encountered with these persons. The value of interdisciplinary approaches to the communication problems of the elderly is reiterated throughout the text. Second, the heterogeneity of the elderly population is pointed out, and the need for considering this factor in the design, interpretation, and generalization of research as well as in clinical decisions is addressed. Third, the need for a comprehensive perspective in examining communication breakdowns is stressed. This broadly based systems approach is recommended in psychosocial, speech production, language, research, and intervention contexts and across a variety of disorders. These three themes suggest that future research in the area of geriatric communication disorders should be interdisciplinary, designed to accommodate a heterogeneous population, and based on a comprehensive model of communication.

This book is grounded in the realization that we have a great deal more to learn about geriatric communication disorders and about communication changes in normal aging. However, the authors wish to gratefully acknowledge the clinicians and researchers whose work provides the basis for this text.

List of Contributors

Rhoda Au, PhD
Research Service (151)
Boston Veterans Administration
    Medical Center
150 South Huntington Avenue
Jamaica Plain, MA 02130

Neal S. Beckford, MD
Department of Otolaryngology
University of Tennessee–Memphis
P.O. Box 18
956 Court Street
Memphis, TN 38163

Fred H. Bess, PhD
Vanderbilt University School of Medicine
Bill Wilkerson Hearing and Speech Center
1114 19th Avenue South
Nashville, TN 37212

Nancy Bowles, PhD
Veterans Administration Outpatient Clinic
Boston Veterans Administration
    Medical Center
17 Court Street
Boston, MA 02108

Sandra B. Chapman, PhD
Program in Communication Disorders
University of Texas at Dallas
Callier Center for Communication Disorders
1966 Inwood Road
Dallas, TX 75235

Richard H. Civil, MD
Department of Neurology
Case Western Reserve University
Cleveland, OH 44106

Lynne W. Clark, PhD
Hunter College of the City University
    of New York
Hunter/Mt. Sinai Geriatric Education Center
261 South Boulevard
Nyack, NY 10960

Susan de Santi, MS
City University of New York
    Graduate Center
Department of Speech and Hearing Science
33 West 42nd Street
New York, NY 10036

Ruth E. Dunkle, PhD
School of Social Work
University of Michigan
1065 Frieze Building
Ann Arbor, MI 48109

Margaret M. Forbes, MA
Department of Psychiatry
University of Pittsburgh School of Medicine
Pittsburgh, PA 15213

Sandra M. Gordon-Salant, PhD
Department of Hearing and Speech Sciences
University of Maryland
College Park, MD 20742

A. Julianna Gulya, MD, FACS
Department of Surgery
George Washington University
2150 Pennsylvania Avenue NW
Washington, DC 20037

Marie R. Haug, PhD
Center on Aging and Health
Allen Memorial Library, Room 101
Case Western Reserve University
Cleveland, OH 44106

Audrey L. Holland, PhD
Department of Speech
University of Pittsburgh
Pittsburgh, PA 15260

Celia R. Hooper, PhD
Division of Speech and Hearing Sciences
Department of Medical Allied
    Health Professions
University of North Carolina–Chapel Hill
76 Wing D Medical School 208H
Chapel Hill, NC 27514

Richard W. Hubbard, PhD
Geriatric Education Center
Case Western Reserve University
12200 Fairhill
Cleveland, OH 44120

Gary P. Jacobson, PhD
Division of Audiology
Henry Ford Hospital
2799 West Grand Boulevard
Detroit, MI 48202

Alex F. Johnson, PhD
Division of Speech-Language Sciences
    and Disorders
Department of Neurology
Henry Ford Hospital
2799 West Grand Boulevard
Detroit, MI 48202

Joel C. Kahane, PhD
Department of Audiology and
    Speech Pathology
Memphis State University
Memphis Speech and Hearing Center
807 Jefferson Avenue
Memphis, TN 38015

Cary S. Kart, PhD
Sociology Department
University of Toledo
Toledo, OH 43606-3390

Patricia B. Kricos, PhD
Department of Speech
University of Florida
335 Dauer Hall
Gainesville, FL 32611

M. Powell Lawton, PhD
Philadelphia Geriatric Center
5301 Old York Road
Philadelphia, PA 19141

Sharon A. Lesner, PhD
University of Akron
West Hall, Room 118
Akron, OH 44325

Michael J. Lichtenstein, MD, MSc
Audie Murphy Veterans Administration
    Hospital
University of Texas Health Science Center
    at San Antonio
7400 Merton Minter Road
San Antonio, TX 78284

Julie M. Liss, PhD
Department of Communicative Disorders
University of Minnesota
Minneapolis, MN 55455

Susan A. Logan, MSc
Vanderbilt University School of Medicine
Bill Wilkerson Hearing and Speech Center
1114 19th Avenue South
Nashville, TN 37212

Craig W. Newman, PhD
Division of Audiology
Henry Ford Hospital
2799 West Grand Boulevard
Detroit, MI 48202

Harvey B. Nudelman, PhD
Department of Neurology
Baylor College of Medicine
One Baylor Plaza
Houston, TX 77030

Loraine K. Obler, PhD
City University of New York
    Graduate Center
Department of Speech and Hearing Sciences
33 West 42nd Street
New York, NY 10036

Danielle N. Ripich, PhD
Department of Communication Sciences
University Center on Aging and Health
Case Western Reserve University
11206 Euclid Avenue
Cleveland, OH 44106

Anne Putnam Rochet, PhD
Department of Speech Pathology
    and Audiology
University of Alberta
400-11044-82 Avenue
Edmonton, Alberta
Canada T6G 0T2

David B. Rosenfield, MD
Baylor College of Medicine
One Baylor Plaza
Houston, TX 77030

James M. Schear, PhD
Gerontology Center
University of Georgia
Athens, GA 30309

Linda L. Skenes, PhD
Speech and Language Services
Veterans Administration Medical
    Center (126)
2460 Wrightsboro Road (10)
Augusta, GA 30910

Barbara C. Sonies, PhD
The Clinical Center
National Institutes of Health
Bethesda, MD 20892

Jacyln B. Spitzer, PhD
Audiology and Speech Pathology
    Section (117)
Veterans Administration Medical Center
West Spring Street
West Haven, CT 06516

Brad A. Stach, PhD
Baylor College of Medicine
The Methodist Hospital
6501 Fannin
Suite NA 200
Houston, TX 77030

W. Renae Stoner, MS
Baylor College of Medicine
6501 Fannin
Suite NA 200
Houston, TX 77030

Hanna K. Ulatowska, PhD
University of Texas at Dallas
4422 Wildwood Road
Dallas, TX 75209

Barbara E. Weinstein, PhD
Lehman College–City University of
    New York
Hunter/Mt. Sinai Geriatric Education Center
Bedford Park Boulevard West
Bronx, NY 10468

Gary Weismer, PhD
Department of Communication Disorders
University of Wisconsin–Madison
1975 Willow Drive
Madison, WI 53706

Peter J. Whitehouse, MD, PhD
Alzheimer Center
University Hospital of Cleveland
Cleveland, OH 44106

Biological and Neurological Aspects of Aging

SECTION

Peter J. Whitehouse, MD, PhD ■

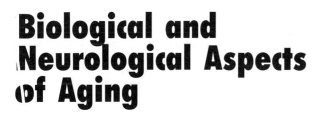

Successful communication is dependent on an intact nervous system. Therefore, professionals attempting to assist older individuals with communication disorders need an understanding of the neural mechanisms involved in communication and how these mechanisms are affected in aging. In the first chapter, neurologists Civil and Whitehouse present an overview of the neurobiology of the aging communication system. They point out that many aspects of brain function are important for successful communication, not only those involved in central language processing. Because of the large number of systems involved in the neurology of communication, the authors stress the importance of interdisciplinary research and clinical assessment.

These authors also point out that our understanding of the normal aging process in the central nervous system is more limited than our knowledge of some of the common age-associated diseases that cause communication failure. After discussing the general changes that occur in the nervous system with age, these authors address age-related changes in specific neural systems. Sensory systems are presented in terms of both general sensations, such as touch, and the special senses, such as hearing and vision. The importance of neurological motor systems is also discussed in relation to successful social communication exchanges. The motor system is divided into voluntary (pyramidal) and involuntary (extrapyramidal) components, with associated age-related changes and age-associated diseases that affect communication function discussed under each topic. In the final section of this chapter, the authors review some of the changes that occur in the so-called higher cognitive functions, focusing specifically on intelligence, language, memory, and additional nonlanguage capabilities that are important for supporting communication. Briefly mentioned are other neurobehavioral syndromes that can affect communication systems in the elderly. Additional specific discussion of these topics is included in later sections of the book, particularly in sections 3 and 4.

Neurolinguists Ulatowska and Chapman build on the discussion of higher brain function and communication by describing the scope of their discipline in the second chapter in this section. They point out that neurolinguistics is a relatively new field with a short but productive history, which has offered important new insights in our understanding of the communication process. Aligning themselves with the authors of the previous chapter, Ulatowska and Chapman lament our lack of understanding of normal age-related changes in neurolinguistic function and, in what will be a recurring theme of importance in this handbook, emphasize the importance of multidisciplinary perspectives in assessment and remediation of the geriatric communication disorders. Several cases of older patients who have suffered from communication disorders are presented to illustrate the novel insights that the neurolinguistic approach can offer. The authors carefully detail important aspects of discourse analysis, emphasizing once again the importance of discipline-specific disease modeling. They contend that regardless of the phonological, syntactic, and semantic impairments that may occur with aging, it is most critical to understand how information can be successfully exchanged between individuals engaged in discourse. Their discussion of discourse analysis also helps communicate to the reader methodological approaches and the conceptual framework of neurolinguistics as an emerging discipline.

The final chapter in this section, by otolaryngologist Gulya, examines in considerable detail age-related changes in the auditory and vestibular systems. After a brief discussion of the cellular mechanisms that have been proposed to underlie the normal aging process, the author focuses on age-related changes in the auditory system, beginning with the ossicular chain, with particular attention given to the organ of Corti. The relevant animal and human research is reviewed and a detailed description of the reported age-related changes that occur in the structure is provided. The author points out the relationship between cellular changes and the resulting functional loss of hearing. Once again, this author reiterates that tremendous gaps exist in our knowledge of the aging process.

The author next discusses age-related changes in the vestibular system, providing, once again, a comprehensive review of the anatomical changes as well as a discussion of the clinical consequences of such age-related pathology, including vestibular ataxia. Gulya concludes by pointing out that additional research will be required to more specifically relate these anatomical changes to the functional impairments that may occur with aging.

Further aspects of biological changes in aging are presented in other sections of the book, particularly those that relate to speech production in section 3. Although the authors in this initial section discuss selected aspects of the functional correlates of anatomical aging changes, the biological, sociological, and psychological ramifications of these anatomical changes are additionally discussed in both sections 2 and 3. The authors of the three chapters in this section have set the stage for the remainder of the book by stressing the importance of both clinical assessment and treatment, as well as of research into communication disorders in the elderly through multidisciplinary approaches.

Neurobiology of the Aging Communication System

CHAPTER

Richard H. Civil, MD, and
Peter J. Whitehouse, MD, PhD ■

One of the most fundamental characteristics of human higher cognitive functioning is the use of sophisticated symbolic communication. The complex acts involved in communication are supported by virtually every aspect of brain function. Afferent sensory stimuli are processed through association regions of increasing complexity and are integrated with stored memories, emotions, and real-time factors relating to attention, arousal, and motivation in order to produce a language or gestural response governed by available behavioral repertoires. When they are functioning properly, these processes result in communication, both symbolic and gestural. Perhaps the best understood functions are those that lie at the extremes of the communication process: the peripheral visual and auditory receptor systems and the motor effector system regulating speech. Only more recently, however, have communication scientists begun exploring the vast and essentially untapped areas of language and nonlanguage behaviors that are integral to the communication process.

Throughout the life-span, the acquisition, development, and maintenance of communication capabilities are dependent on the adequate functioning and appropriate integration of distinct neural networks. Although they are of potentially great importance to our understanding of the human communication system, this chapter will not deal with what may be referred to as the "developmental" disorders of speech and language, which include syndromes such as dyslexia, childhood stuttering, and autism. Instead, the focus will be on changes caused by aging and the age-associated diseases of the central and peripheral nervous systems that may impair selected aspects of the communication system. From the clinical perspective, assessment and treatment of the communication status of an elderly patient requires (a) an understanding of the neurobiological basis of human speech and language systems,

(b) an appreciation of the structural and functional changes that occur in the central nervous system simply as a result of the aging process, and (c) a familiarity with the commonly encountered diseases of the central and peripheral nervous system that affect the communication system in the elderly.

Unfortunately, our understanding of the normal aging process in the nervous system is limited, perhaps more limited than our understanding of the common age-associated disease processes such as stroke and dementia. Even our conception of what constitutes "normal aging" requires clarification. "Normal aging" often refers to the most common or usually encountered functional state of the nervous system in a population of older individuals. Thus, in a tabulation of the "functional status of 'normal' 80 year olds," one textbook of geriatric neurology indicates that fully 48% need help climbing or descending stairs (Wolfson & Katzman, 1983). "Normal aging," in another usage, can also refer to the process of disease-free aging. These terminologic issues raise fundamental questions in aging research. The spectrum of clinical approaches in dealing with these issues can be found in the work of Rowe and Kahn (1987), who distinguished "usual aging" and "successful aging," and in the work of Fries, who emphasized the notion of "compression of morbidity" at the end of a fixed life-span (Fries, 1980).

The diversity of aging theories and their ramifications are of particular importance in the context of geriatric communication disorders (Table 1.1). If, for example, one views aging as inevitable and irreversible, then clinicians should direct their efforts toward those extrinsic factors such as diet, exercise, and personal habits which, when modified, would potentially reduce rather than heighten the disabilities of aging. Using this model, clinicians caring for the elderly can, at best, hope to postpone or compress morbidity into as brief a period as possible prior to death. Alternative theories have been proposed. Based on declining mortality trends in the elderly, the notion

of survival curve derectangularization has been advanced (Schneider & Brody, 1983). This theory suggests that society will soon be faced with a burgeoning number of older individuals, many with chronic illness and disability. Many of these individuals will have communication disorders. The long-term care needs of this population will have profound implications for health care policy makers.

The concept of normality to indicate disease-free or successful aging will be used in this chapter, understanding that in many ways this represents an ideal that is not commonly achieved. The incidence of dementia and stroke, for example, increases exponentially with age. Additionally, it must be acknowledged that there are many unresolved issues concerning the biological basis of the aging process as well as the complex relationships between these age-related changes and age-associated diseases. Indeed, the pathological features seen in certain degenerative neurological diseases such as Alzheimer's disease, Parkinson's disease, and amyotrophic lateral sclerosis may only be quantitatively greater than age-related brain changes. Neuronal loss and grossly observable cerebral atrophy, for example, appear as a consequence of normal aging, but are found to a greater extent in selected brain regions and neuronal subpopulations in the degenerative diseases. In light of these qualitative similarities, one must question whether the degenerative diseases are simply caused by accentuations of normal aging changes. Indeed, a variety of theories based on neurotrophic hormones (Appel, 1981) and environmental factors (Calne, McGeer, Eisen, & Spencer, 1986) have suggested that critical thresholds exist in the nervous system beyond which normal physiological and behavioral functioning is impaired.

Although this chapter will focus on the neurology of the aging communication system, it is clear that many disciplines have been involved in furthering our understanding of geriatric communication disorders. The medical specialties of ophthalmology, otolaryngology, psychi-

TABLE 1.1
Aging Theories and Their Implications

	Inevitability of Mortality	Life-Span Augmentation
Theoretical basis	Life-span fixed	Life-span not fixed
Evidence	Survival curve rectangularization	Survival curve derectangularization
Predictions based on a theoretical model	(a) No increase in elderly due to fixed life-span (b) Chronic disease occupies a smaller proportion of life-span (c) Decreasing needs for health care in late life	(a) increasing survival of elderly (b) No declines in long-term morbidity or disability (c) Increasing needs for long-term care
Goals of care	To extend maximal adult vigor and compress the period of senescence	To better prevent, treat, and manage the common chronic diseases of aging
Health care policy implications	(a) Primary emphasis on improving quality of life (b) Decreasing health care needs of the elderly	(a) Primary emphasis on chronic diseases in the elderly (b) Increasing numbers and care needs of the elderly

atry, and neurology are in especially unique clinical positions to observe communication disorders in the elderly. Additional neuroscience disciplines involved include neuropsychology, neurolinguistics, audiology, and speech-language pathology. Rehabilitation and resource referral needs are frequently addressed by audiologists, speech pathologists, and occupational and physical therapists, as well as by social workers. Thus, it is important for any clinician working in the area of geriatric communication disorders to develop an interdisciplinary and biopsychosocial perspective in order to fully appreciate and manage the spectrum of biological, psychological, and sociological factors associated with communication disorders in the elderly.

This chapter will review some of the general features of the aging neural system before exploring various sensory, motor, and cognitive components of the communication system in greater detail. The input, central processing, and output components will be further dissected into different subsystems. In each of these subsystems, the anatomical changes that occur with aging, and the physiological or functional changes that result from these anatomical changes, will be reviewed. Finally, a brief review of selected communication-related neurobehavioral syndromes resulting from disease of these neural systems will be presented.

General Changes in the Nervous System with Age

The major theme in the aging nervous system is a balance between loss and adaptation or degeneration and regeneration. Classically, the central nervous system has been believed to have little regenerative capacity, although new work demonstrates more potential plasticity than was originally thought (Cotman & Anderson, in press). One of the most characteristic age-related morphological changes is neuronal loss, which is characteristic of many brain regions, including those involved in communication. Sensory neurons in the superior temporal gyrus and bulbar motor neurons clearly diminish as individuals age. Neuronal loss is frequently accompanied by specific pathological features of cellular degeneration including the formation of neuritic plaques and neurofibrillary tangles. In association with this gross cellular loss and degeneration, biochemical and neurotransmitter markers of normal function also diminish with age. The concentrations of neurotransmitters including acetylcholine and noradrenaline as well as their receptor density decrease in later years.

Clinical manifestations and disturbance of either structure or function may not be concordant. Considerable neuronal reserve as well as plastic responses, which probably continue to operate even into the later years, may permit the older individual to maintain communication abilities even in the presence of rather marked anatomical changes. Age-related changes may, in fact, be caused not only by an accelerated or premature degeneration of neurons, but also by an impairment of normally present repair and regenerative mechanisms.

Sensory Systems

General Sensations

The general somatic sensations are mediated by receptors of two types. Cutaneous exteroceptors primarily mediate the modalities of warmth, cold, touch, and pain while deeper proprioceptors convey information concerning position as well as force and direction of movement. Ample evidence exists indicating the importance of intact general somatic sensory function in all forms of purposeful movement. Indeed, sensory and motor functions are best viewed as being interdependent.

Anatomy and Function

Age-related morphological changes in sensory neurons, nerve roots, peripheral axons, and specialized receptors have been demonstrated (see Sabin & Venna, 1984, for review). It has been estimated that in selected spinal regions, 5% to 8% of neurons may be lost per decade (Kawamuara & Dyck, 1977). In addition to this neuronal loss, significant axonal loss and demyelination also occur in the spinal dorsal columns and peripheral nerves, with resulting physiological (sensory and motor nerve conduction abnormalities) and functional (impaired ability to stand on one leg) capabilities.

Diseases

A variety of common medical conditions, including diabetes mellitus and alcoholism, may cause significant sensory or motor neuropathy. Such neuropathies, even when severe, may impair communication only in highly specific instances, such as Braille reading. More centrally located lesions in the sensory system, particularly those in thalamic and parietal regions, may be associated with motor and spatial disorders significant enough to impair written and gestural communication. Diagnostic tests including electromyography and nerve conduction velocity studies can be performed to quantitate the severity and type of damage (either axonal or demyelinating), and to assist in establishing specific diagnoses.

Special Sensory Systems

Hearing

The process of hearing begins by focusing environmental sound on the eardrum. In the cochlea, the process of transduction from sound to electrical signal is completed and the signal is then bilaterally transmitted to temporal cortices through various nuclear relays. Section 5 of this text provides an extensive review of the normal anatomy and specific pathology of otologic disorders in the elderly.

Anatomy

The auditory system may be divided into peripheral and central components, with age-related changes occurring along the entire auditory pathway. Peripherally, bony exostoses can affect the bony structures of the external and internal auditory canal. Degeneration of the hair cells in the organ of Corti, particularly in the basal turn of the cochlea, results in a sensorineural high tone hearing loss. Centrally, neuronal loss has been demonstrated in brainstem auditory nuclei and in the temporal auditory cortex, where more than 50% of the neurons in the superior temporal gyrus are lost by age 80 (Brody, 1955).

Function

Presbycusis has been stated to be an ''inevitable consequence of aging'' (Hayes & Jerger, 1984). The bulk of peripheral sensitivity loss relates to cochlear changes that are associated with progressive loss of high-frequency sensitivity above 1 kHz. Using sophisticated computerized electroencephalographic techniques, auditory-evoked responses, particularly late positive potentials, show latency increases of almost 2 ms per year. Additional changes, particularly those relating to word recognition and sentence identification, have been most intensively investigated, with the former believed to reflect ''peripheral'' changes and the latter reflecting ''central'' changes. The apparent discrepancy between the potential and actual benefits of hearing aid use is commonly attributed to such central changes.

Diseases

Many environmental and pathological processes can affect the different stages of sound transduction and neural processing and exacerbate age-related hearing loss. Chronic infections of the middle and inner ear, bony changes, and ototoxic medications are some of the more common of these processes. Most unilateral diseases of the cerebral hemispheres do not affect hearing because of the bilateral representation in the auditory cortex. Bilateral lesions of the temporal cortex can produce the rare but devastating communication disorder of pure word deafness, as a result of a modality-specific (auditory) disturbance of word recognition.

Vision

The visual system and its communication-related functions are frequently altered by numerous age-related changes and disease states. Pathological processes affecting any component of the axis, including the pupil, lens, retinal receptors, conduction pathways, and brain information processing systems, may significantly alter vision, perception, or symbolic language skills and impair communication.

Anatomy and Function

Age-related changes in pupillary function and lens light transmissibility account for optical changes in the visual system and are frequently cited explanations for age-related presbyopic vision impairment. In addition, however, significant structural and physiological changes occur throughout the retinal and postretinal visual system. Retinal changes include lipofuscin accumulation in ganglion cells and reduced dendritic arborization. Myelin staining of nerve fibers has revealed axonal swelling and axonal loss. A 50% reduction in cortical neurons in the macular projection region has been reported. Electroretinographic changes in retinal A and B waves as well as significantly increased latencies in selected components of the visual evoked response have been observed. These normal age-related structural and functional changes result in clinically diminished visual acuity and impaired night vision, as well as loss of accommodation with resulting near-vision impairment (presbyopia).

Diseases

Diseases affecting vision are legion, and space limitations permit only brief comments. First and foremost, the presence of specific treatable illnesses must be excluded by careful neuro-ophthalmologic examination. Senile cataracts, glaucoma, and presbyopia represent three such conditions occurring commonly in the elderly. Unfortunately, certain disorders remain of unclear etiology, such as senile macular degeneration, an ill-defined term that encompasses the age-related degenerative changes that occur in the posterior pole structures of the aging eye, including photoreceptors, pigment epithelium, and Bruch's membrane. It is important to emphasize that appropriate neuro-ophthalmologic diagnosis often requires a detailed understanding of the complete visual system. In our experience, it is not uncommon to see patients with visual complaints attributable either to the oculomotor disturbance in progressive supranuclear palsy or to the higher visual processing disturbances (Balint's syndrome) in certain Alzheimer's disease variants. Such patients are often unsuccessfully treated with simple refraction correction. Specific neurobehavioral syndromes including alexia without agraphia, pure word blindness, or denial of blindness (Anton's syndrome) may additionally require specific behavioral or neuropsychological assessment.

Motor Systems: Pyramidal and Extrapyramidal

The motor system is organized into several different components, all of which play an important role in communication. A fundamental neurological distinction is made between voluntary and involuntary motor systems. As the name implies, the voluntary (pyramidal) motor system involves the ability of individuals to volitionally move muscles in certain ways, with obvious ramifications on the communication act. Cortical pyramidal neurons (upper motor neurons) send messages to anterior horn cells in the spinal cord (lower motor neu-

rons) which, in turn, communicate with muscles via peripheral motor nerves. The involuntary (extrapyramidal) motor system, which anatomically includes the cerebellum and basal ganglia, coordinates the necessary accompanying motor activity that supports the voluntary motor act, that is, controlling fine motor movements, associated body movements, and posture.

The Pyramidal System

Upper Motor Neurons

Anatomy and Function

In the classic pyramidal motor system, upper motor neurons (UMNs) in the cerebral cortex receive input from various brain regions and send their primary output to the spinal cord via the corticospinal tract. Lesions in this pathway result in a neurological constellation of signs including spasticity, hyperreflexia, weakness, and a positive Babinski sign; this is called the UMN syndrome. Neuroscientists have long since noticed, however, that even after extensive damage to the neocortical motor system with resulting loss of high-resolution movement of the distal extremities, many patients may retain or develop the ability to use proximal musculature. It has been proposed that tiered motor systems exist, and that a "nonpyramidal motor system," innervating proximal musculature bilaterally and mediating postural support, body steering, and orientation of movements, may have considerable value in recovery and rehabilitation in neurological disease (Waxman, 1988). Although a major reduction in pyramidal neurons in the precentral gyrus occurs by the 7th or 8th decade of life, this loss alone should have little impact on functional capabilities.

Diseases

In the elderly, disorders of both UMNs and LMNs (lower motor neurons) frequently coexist. The most common disorder that primarily affects UMNs is hemispheric stroke, which may impair communication simply on the basis of the UMN syndrome with associated dysarthria, spastic or plegic limb, and other symptoms. Depending on the lesion locus, additional disturbances of language, memory, skilled movements, and recognition may occur with obvious communication-related implications.

Lower Motor Neurons and Peripheral Components

The final common pathway for all motor activity is the motor unit, which includes spinal cord motor neurons, their peripheral motor nerves, and their innervated muscle fibers. The clinical manifestations of LMN damage are distinct from UMN damage and include weakness, atrophy, and fasciculations; these make up the LMN syndrome.

Anatomy and Function

Age-related changes include loss of LMNs, reduction of nerve conduction velocity, alterations in the neuromuscular junction, and changes in the muscle fibers themselves. LMNs, both bulbar and spinal, degenerate with age and accumulate lipofuscin. Peripheral motor nerve conduction velocities decrease progressively with age, reflecting morphological changes that include nerve fiber loss and abnormalities of myelination. Muscle wasting or atrophy occurs as a result of the loss of individual muscle fibers. Aging of connective tissue structures may also alter the flexibility of muscles and joints. Structural alterations in the neuromuscular junction and changes in the acetylcholine receptors occur with age. Associated with these structural changes, maximal muscle strength, movement speed, and physiological endurance decrease with age.

Diseases

Numerous diseases occur in the elderly that affect different components of the LMN sys-
tem. The pathology of amyotrophic lateral sclerosis, a fatal neurodegenerative disorder, includes loss of both UMNs and LMNs. UMN and LMN dysfunction, combined with resulting dysarthria, respiratory disturbance, weakness, and spasticity, have devastating effects on all modalities of communication, both verbal and nonverbal. Myopathies can cause profound loss of strength and may impair speech, vision, and the skilled movements required for writing. Myasthenia gravis, an autoimmune disease affecting the neuromuscular junction and neurotransmitter receptors, is associated with a variety of regionally specific neuromuscular symptoms that result from ocular muscle involvement (diplopia, ptosis), bulbar muscle involvement (dysarthria, dysphagia), respiratory muscle involvement (respiratory insufficiency), and more generalized muscular involvement (generalized weakness), all with the capacity to impair communication.

The Extrapyramidal System

When an individual initiates any action or communication using voluntary motor systems, this act is supported by the extrapyramidal motor system. This poorly understood involuntary motor system serves to coordinate the actions of individual muscle groups through a series of feedback loops. On clinical, anatomical, and pharmacological grounds, the extrapyramidal system can be divided into several subsystems that include the cerebellar and basal ganglia systems (including the caudate, putamen, and substantia nigra).

Anatomy

Loss of Purkinje cells in the cerebellum, as well as neuronal loss in the substantia nigra, caudate, and putamen, occur in normal aging. Age-related neurotransmitter abnormalities have also been described. Of particular importance, given the common occurrence of Parkinson's disease, have been demonstrations of age-related reduction in nigrostriatal dopamine and cortical acetylcholine levels.

Function

A number of so-called normal age-related motor findings occur that may relate to the involuntary motor system. For example, fine resting tremors may appear, which are most conveniently classified as being primarily present at rest (resting tremor), maximal with posture maintenance (antigravity or postural tremor), or primarily associated with volitional movements (intention tremor). In addition to tremor, symptoms of extrapyramidal dysfunction include abnormalities of muscle tone, abnormalities of movement initiation (akinesia), disturbance of posture and balance mechanisms, abnormal involuntary movements (chorea, dystonia), and disturbances of gait.

Diseases

The most common disease involving the extrapyramidal motor system is Parkinson's disease, a degenerative disease in which dopaminergic neurons in the substantia nigra are primarily affected. Parkinson's disease is clinically characterized by profound slowing of motor acts (bradykinesia), alterations in muscle tone (rigidity), a resting tremor, and postural instability. Although the basic mechanisms of nigral neuronal death are unknown, significant symptomatic relief can be achieved by replacement of the deficient dopamine. In Parkinson's disease, communication may be significantly impaired by the presence of resting tremor, micrographia, hypophonia, palilalia, stuttering, and akinesia.

Cognitive Functioning

General Intelligence

Perhaps the most intensively studied aspects of normal aging relate to cognitive functioning, particularly intelligence, the speed of cognitive processes, and memory. With respect to general "intelligence," a vast and complicated neuropsychological literature exists. Standardized instruments such as the *Wechsler Adult Intelligence Scale* have demonstrated that certain cognitive abilities including vocabulary, information stores, and comprehension may be relatively insensitive to age-related changes, at least until the age of 75 to 85 (Granick, 1971).

In contrast to these observed domains of verbal IQ preservation, most carefully controlled neuropsychological studies have disclosed a significant age-related decrement of performance IQ function on intelligence testing—a phenomenon known as the "verbal-performance discrepancy" (Albert & Heaton, 1988). Although methodological issues abound, it is generally believed that the performance IQ decrement is a true biological change and not simply a function of either educational effects or cross-sectional study methodology. Numerous theoretical explanations for this phenomenon have been advanced, including the role of time and speed requirements, the notion of general information versus learning and manipulation of unfamiliar materials, "crystallized" versus "fluid" intelligence, and the intriguing notion of selective hemispheric aging.

Reaction Time

Data from both simple reaction time studies and choice reaction time paradigms indicate that the single major component responsible for the slowing of reaction times with age is the time required for central information processing. This apparent slowing of cognitive processes has been referred to as "bradyphrenia" (Rogers, 1986). Using a unique and quite sensitive paradigm developed by Sternberg, slowing of the peripheral and central components of reaction time and central processing speed can be demonstrated to be present even at the age of 50 to 55 (Eriksen, Hamlin, & Daye, 1973).

Using this and additional paradigms, slowing of cognitive processes has been found to occur not only in normal elderly, but in patients with Parkinson's disease as well (Mayeux, Stern, Sano, Cote, & Williams, 1987).

Memory

Based on sophisticated neuropsychological measures, it has been demonstrated that the complex processes involved in learning and memory may not be uniformly affected by the aging process. Memory domains with little age-related decline include primary memory (immediate or working memory), secondary memory (short-term memory), and retrieval of information from long-term storage (long-term memory). At an operational clinical level, neurologists have previously invoked the notion of *benign senescent forgetfulness*, a benign memory disorder, clinically manifested as the transient inability to recall a specific date, time, or name associated with a remote memory the details of which are otherwise accurately remembered (Kral, 1978). A new term, *age-associated memory impairment*, has been recently advanced to describe nondemented elderly individuals with memory complaints who perform one standard deviation less than young adults on selected neuropsychological measures of memory function (Crook et al., 1986).

Language-Related Disorders

Language (the Aphasias)

Based on the pioneering early contributions of Broca and Wernicke, and the later elaborations of both Benson and Geschwind, an extensive literature exists on the hemispheric organization of human language functions. One neurological model, which classifies the aphasic syndromes into eight subtypes based on language performance in tests of fluency, comprehension, and repetition, has been shown to be of great clinical utility (Benson & Geschwind, 1977) (Table 1.2). Extensive data on brain-language relationships have shown that these three cardinal characteristics of aphasia in general correspond anatomically to frontal lobe regions (verbal fluency); posterior perisylvian regions including Wernicke's area, the angular gyrus, and the supramarginal gyrus (comprehension); and a white-matter-connecting pathway known as the arcuate fasciculus (repetition ability). More complete language assessment, however, would be based on a 4x4 stimulus-response matrix (Table 1.3) as proposed by Albert and colleagues (Albert, Goodglass, Helm, Rubens, & Alexander, 1981).

Anatomy

Little is known in great detail about the specific pathology that occurs in language areas with aging. Studies in animals and man have suggested that the language areas do lose neurons. Neurochemical studies have also shown that loss of neurotransmitter markers occurs in these brain regions. However, we have little knowledge of the specific relationships between different neurotransmitters and the functions of these brain regions.

Function

The consequences of these structural changes in the language-related cerebral cortex are unclear. In general, it appears that certain higher-order language processing areas, such as semantics and pragmatics, may be affected in normal aging, whereas phonology and syntax remain relatively intact. Abnormalities in discourse structure including fewer prepositions, impairment of references, and less complicated clause structures have been reported (see chapter 2). Although measures of vocabulary remain intact, generative naming ability has also been shown to be mildly

TABLE 1.2
Neurological Classification of the Aphasias

Type of Aphasia	Type of Speech	Comprehension[a]	Localization
Aphasias with Disordered Repetition			
Broca's	Nonfluent	+	Lower posterior frontal
Wernicke's	Fluent	−	Posterior superior temporal
Conduction	Fluent	+	Usually parietal operculum
Global	Nonfluent	−	Massive perisylvian lesion
Aphasias with Good Repetition			
Transcortical motor	Nonfluent	+	Anterior to Broca's area or supplementary speech area
Transcortical sensory	Fluent	−	Surrounding Wernicke's area posteriorly
Transcortical mixed ("isolation syndrome")	Nonfluent	−	Both of the above
Anomic	Fluent	+	Lesion of angular gyrus or second temporal gyrus

Note. From "Clinical Aspects of Dysphasia" by M. L. Albert, H. Goodglass, N. A. Helm, A. B. Rubens, and M. P. Alexander, 1981. In G. E. Arnold, F. Winkel, and B. D. Wyke (Eds.), *Disorders of Human Communication* (Volume 2). New York: Springer-Verlag. Reprinted by permission.
[a] + = relatively or fully intact, − = definitely impaired.

TABLE 1.3
Stimulus-Response Matrix in Complete Language Assessment

Stimulus	Response			
	Point	Say	Write	Do
See object	Visual matching	Naming	Written naming	Pantomime
Hear words	Word discrimination	Word repetition	Writing from dictation	Following commands
See words	Word-object matching	Oral reading	Copying	Following written commands
Feel objects	Visual-tactile matching	Tactile naming	Tactile-written naming	

Note. From "Clinical Aspects of Dysphasia" by M. L. Albert, H. Goodglass, N. A. Helm, A. B. Rubens, and M. P. Alexander, 1981. In G. E. Arnold, F. Winkel, and B. D. Wyke (Eds.), *Disorders of Human Communication* (Volume 2). New York: Springer-Verlag. Reprinted by permission.

affected with aging. Impairment in semantic processing tasks such as category assignment has also been described. Once again, these impairments tend to be relatively mild and do not significantly affect day-to-day communication abilities.

Diseases

Stroke, one of the most common age-associated neurological diseases, frequently produces aphasia—defined as an acquired disorder of language function resulting from brain damage. Indeed, the Benson-Geschwind aphasia classification system is based primarily on stroke-related language dysfunction; as a result, neurological aphasia classification frequently rests on neuroanatomical and vascular principles rather than on neurolinguistic principles. Communication disorders resulting from stroke-related aphasia will not be considered in any more detail here. The reader is referred to standard texts, such as that of Albert et al. (1981), for additional information.

Language disorders are a common feature in dementia. In most instances, the language deterioration is only part of a more widespread syndrome of cognitive, behavioral, and functional impairment. In early Alzheimer's disease, the language impairment may be a relatively restricted naming disturbance—often associated with the behavioral manifestations of anxiety, frustration, and depression. In the later stages of Alzheimer's disease, the language disturbance may be so severe as to be recognized as one of the standard aphasia subtypes (usually transcortical sensory aphasia or Wernicke's aphasia). Pick's disease is a related degenerative dementia with a preferential frontotemporal distribution of involvement. Although it is difficult to clinically distinguish from Alzheimer's disease, Pick's disease is characterized in the early stages by prominent personality changes and emotional alterations. Later, more specific language-related characteristics include semantic anomia, the use of verbal stereotypes, the so-called gramophone syndrome, and the ultimate emergence of mutism.

Most recently, the clinical syndrome of primary progressive aphasia (Mesulam, 1987) has emerged as an area of clinical and theoretical interest. This language disorder presents as a syndrome of progressively worsening aphasia in the absence of dementia and may have a unique pathology that is distinctive from those of the known degenerative dementias, including Alzheimer's disease and Pick's disease. In addition, a unique pedigree with an autosomally dominantly inherited syndrome of dementia and dysphasia has been described (Morris, Cole, Banker, & Wright, 1984). The relationship of these clinical syndromes with progressive language dysfunction to the more common degenerative dementias remains to be elucidated.

Skilled Movements (the Apraxias)

Commonly associated with the aphasic language disturbances, the apraxias represent disorders of skilled motor movement that are not attributable to elementary disorders of sensation, strength, or coordination. In aphasic disturbances resulting from posterior perisylvian dysfunction, the comprehension disturbance and associated apraxia may be so severe as to make actual delineation of the aphasic and apraxic components virtually impossible. In patients with frontal or callosal lesions, the role of the apraxias is more convincingly demonstrable (Graff-Radford, Welsh, & Godersky, 1987). Such patients, despite normal or near-normal comprehension abilities, may be totally unable to demonstrate the use of objects with the nonplegic left hand. The observation of such a unilateral apraxic syndrome (which involved written communication abilities as well) led Geschwind to ultimately formulate his landmark observations of the human cerebral disconnection syndromes (Geschwind, 1965).

Recognition (the Agnosias)

From the neurological perspective, the agnosias encompass the disorders of recognition, and may be unimodal (modality specific) or multimodal. Prosopagnosia (failure to recognize familiar faces) is one of the more commonly encountered modality-specific agnosias. Patients with prosopagnosia may fail to recognize their spouse's face despite having normal visual acuity functions. When identifying information is supplied in another sensory domain (for instance, when the spouse speaks) appropriate recognition is achieved. Additional modality-specific agnosias include pure word blindness and pure word deafness, rare conditions that are associated with significant ramifications for the communication process.

In Alzheimer's disease, disturbances of naming and recognition may both be present. In such instances, cognitive testing may disclose a variety of error patterns that require careful analysis and interpretation of the data. Failure to name an item on the *Boston Naming Test,* for example, may be the result of educational factors, true anomia, or a disturbance of higher-order visual function. The patient who clearly identifies the dog's muzzle on the *Boston Naming Test* as a "device to keep him from biting people" is clearly demonstrating intact recognition abilities despite naming failure. In contrast to this anomic circumlocution, the agnosic patient may fail to correctly identify the target visual item and may refer to this same target stimulus as either a "lightbulb" or, in severe instances, a "map of a highway interchange."

Additional Nonlanguage Cognitive Systems Involved in Communication

Initiation of Communication

Brain regions outside the perisylvian language zone play vital roles in the initiation of complex cognitive behaviors including communication. In humans, a series of brain structures that are usually midline in location, including the cerebellum, thalamic nuclei, cingulate gyrus, and supplementary motor area, have been shown to play distinct roles in speech initiation. Lesions in these brain regions frequently produce disorders of communication that typically fall on the borderline between pure speech disorders (the dysarthrias) and the aphasic language disturbances. Aphemia is one such condition. Other syndromes may be best viewed as disorders of communication initiation. These are encountered with some regularity by neurologists and neurosurgeons. One need only think of the clinical syndromes of akinetic mutism; transcortical motor aphasia with fluent but sparse speech; and mutism following cerebellar hemispherectomy, corpus callosotomy, or thalamic nuclear ablation to appreciate the occurrence of these syndromes. It is in this area of speech-language pathology that pharmacotherapy has been postulated to be of particular relevance. Patients with transcortical motor aphasia and impaired speech initiation have been successfully treated with dopamine agonists, suggesting a role for specific neurotransmitter abnormalities in the clinical syndromes of speech hypoinitiation (Albert & Helm-Estabrooks, 1988).

Disorders of Affective Components of Language (the Aprosodias)

Patients with lesions of the right or non-language-dominant hemisphere may have disturbed recognition of affective speech intonation and may be unable to impart affective qualities to their speech. The term *aprosodia* has been coined in relation to these "affective disorders of language," and a functional-anatomical organization in the right hemisphere has been defined (Ross, 1981). The significance of prosody and emotional gesturing in communication is succinctly pointed out in one case description of a schoolteacher who, after a right-hemisphere lesion, found herself unable to maintain classroom discipline because of a complete inability to express emotion through speech and action (Ross & Mesulam, 1979).

Communication Impairment in Psychiatric Disorders

Neuroscientists have long since recognized that "language is a vehicle of personality as well as thought" (Sanford, 1942) and that "any considerable aberration of thought or personality will be mirrored in the various levels of articulate speech" (Critchley, 1964). The study of schizophrenic language has been approached using the methodologies of diverse neuroscience disciplines including neurology, psychiatry, linguistics, and aphasiology. Neurologists have emphasized the diagnostic difficulty of distinguishing schizophrenic language from that of a posterior aphasia (Gerson, Benson, & Frazier, 1977). Despite the apparent gross similarity of fluent aphasic and disorganized psychotic verbal output, formal aphasia testing (DiSimoni, Darley, & Aronson, 1977) and neuropsychological measures (Rausch, Prescott, & DeWolfe, 1980) have been reported to adequately discriminate schizophrenic and aphasic language. Although aphasic qualities (impaired auditory comprehension and repetition) are demonstrable components of schizophrenic language dysfunction, discourse analysis has suggested a supramodal disturbance of "discourse planning abilities" (Hoffman, Stopek, & Andreasen, 1986).

Conclusions

In this chapter, we have provided introductory material on the anatomical basis and functional consequences of both the aging process and specific age-associated diseases on communication function in the elderly.

In subsequent chapters in this section, more detailed attention will be focused on speech motor control and auditory systems, as well as on the neurolinguistic aspects of aging.

No discussion of the aging process would be complete without a brief mention of potentially exciting areas of future research and therapeutic interest. The area of neuronal plasticity represents one such issue. The human central nervous system, previously thought to have very little recuperative capacity, has clearly been shown to develop both new synapse formation and axonal sprouting in response to neuronal damage (Cotman & Anderson, in press). What is unfortunately unclear, at present, is whether this apparent lesion-related neuronal plasticity is a generalizable biological phenomenon capable of repairing age-related changes. Similarly, a variety of hormonal and neurotrophic factors are coming under close scrutiny in studies of both aging and a variety of degenerative neurological diseases. The newly emerging field of neural transplantation is also being intensively investigated with obvious implications on the aging process and degenerative central nervous system diseases (Gash, Collier, & Sladek, 1985). Finally, cognitive remediation, defined as a "systematic therapeutic approach designed to improve cognitive functioning after central nervous system insult" (Butler & Namerow, 1988), may be applicable to age-related cognitive changes and selected disease processes. A substantial body of evidence that has accumulated suggests that cognitive training programs may significantly improve the performance of elderly individuals in selected cognitive tasks, particularly those involving memory function (Wilson, 1987). Perhaps the most significant criticism of cognitive rehabilitation in the past has been the failure of generalization of training. Whether cognitive remediation strategies for the elderly are in any way generalizable remains to be determined.

Perhaps one of the most important points to be recognized is the fact that communication function in any specific individual represents the summation of age-related neurobiological changes and age-associated diseases occurring in that individual. Key to the understanding of individual patients is the fact that discipline-specific assessment may focus on isolated components of the communication process but may be unable to adequately assess or treat the communication difficulties of an elderly individual with multiple pathological and age-associated processes. Although neurological methodologies can identify and classify aphasic language disturbances, they have historically been quite insensitive in detecting the neurolinguistic changes that may occur with aging. This only reemphasizes the fact that separate levels of description are necessary for the neurological and psychological aspects of cognition (Marr, 1982). Similarly, even the most precise optical or peripheral auditory enhancement cannot be expected to appreciably influence the central disorders of visual or auditory processing. In light of the widely divergent assessment methodologies, theoretical frameworks for understanding communication, and widespread biological, sociological, and psychological implications of age-related changes and age-associated disease on the communication system, it is of paramount importance that interdisciplinary approaches be utilized.

References

Albert, M. L., & Helm-Estabrooks, N. (1988). Diagnosis and treatment of aphasia. *Journal of the American Medical Association, 259,* 1205–1210.

Albert, M. L., Goodglass, H., Helm, N. A., Rubens, A. B., & Alexander, M. P. (1981). Clinical aspects of dysphasia. In G. E. Arnold, F. Winckel, & B. D. Wyke (Eds.), *Disorders of human communication 2.* New York: Springer-Verlag.

Albert, M. S., & Heaton, R. K. (1988). Intelligence testing. In M. S. Albert & M. B. Moss (Eds.), *Geriatric neuropsychology* (pp. 13–32). New York: Guilford Press.

Appel, S. H. (1981). A unifying hypothesis for the cause of amyotrophic lateral sclerosis,

Parkinsonism, and Alzheimer's disease. *Annals of Neurology, 10,* 499–505.

Benson, D. F., & Geschwind, N. (1977). The aphasias and related disturbances. In A. B. Baker & L. H. Baker (Eds.), *Clinical neurology.* New York: Harper & Row.

Brody, H. (1955). Organization of the cerebral cortex. III: A study of aging in the human cerebral cortex. *Journal of Comparative Neurology, 102,* 511.

Butler, R. W., & Namerow, N. S. (1988). Cognitive retraining in brain-injury rehabilitation: A critical review. *Journal of Neurological Rehabilitation, 2,* 97–101.

Calne, D. B., McGeer, E., Eisen, A., & Spencer, P. (1986). Alzheimer's disease, Parkinson's disease, and motoneurone disease: Abiotropic interaction between aging and environment? *Lancet, 11,* 1067–1070.

Cotman, C. W., & Anderson, K. J. (in press). Synaptic plasticity and functional stabilization in the hippocampal formation: Possible role in Alzheimer's disease. In S. Waxman (Ed.), *Physiologic basis for functional recovery in neurological disease.*

Critchley, M. (1964). The neurology of psychotic speech. *British Journal of Psychiatry, 110,* 353–364.

Crook, T., Bartus, R. T., Ferris, S. H., Whitehouse, P., Cohen, G. D., & Gershon, S. (1986). Age-associated memory impairment: Proposed diagnostic criteria and measures of clinical change—Report of a National Institute of Mental Health work group. In F. J. Pirozzolo (Ed.), *Developmental neuropsychology* (pp. 261–276). Hillsdale, NJ: Lawrence Erlbaum.

DiSimoni, F. G., Darley, F. L., & Aronson, A. E. (1977). Patterns of dysfunction in schizophrenic patients on an aphasia test battery. *Journal of Speech and Hearing Disorders, 42,* 498–513.

Eriksen, C. W., Hamlin, R. M., & Daye, C. (1973). Aging adults and rate of memory scan. *Bulletin of the Psychonomic Society, 1,* 259.

Fries, J. F. (1980). Aging, natural death, and the compression of morbidity. *New England Journal of Medicine, 303,* 130–135.

Gash, D. M., Collier, T. J., & Sladek, J. R. (1985). Neural transplantation: A review of recent developments and potential applications to the aged brain. *Neurobiology of Aging, 6,* 131–150.

Gerson, S. N., Benson, D. F., & Frazier, S. H. (1977). Diagnosis: Schizophrenia versus posterior aphasia. *American Journal of Psychiatry, 134*(9), 966–969.

Geschwind, N. (1965). Disconnexion syndromes in animals and man. *Brain, 88,* 237–284, 585–614.

Graff-Radford, N. R., Welsh, K., & Godersky, J. (1987). Collosal apraxia. *Neurology, 37,* 100–105.

Granick, S. (1971). Psychological test functioning. In S. Granick & R. D. Patterson (Eds.), *Human aging II: An eleven-year followup biomedical and behavioral study.* Rockville, MD: National Institute of Mental Health.

Hayes, D., & Jerger, J. (1984). Neurotology of aging: The auditory system. In M. S. Albert (Ed.), *Clinical neurology of aging* (pp. 362–378). New York: Oxford University Press.

Hoffman, R. E., Stopek, S., & Andreasen, N. C. (1986). A comparative study of manic vs. schizophrenic speech disorganization. *Archives of General Psychiatry, 43,* 831–838.

Kawamuara, Y., & Dyck, P. J. (1977). Lumbar motoneurons of man: III. The number of and diameter distribution of large and intermediate-diameter cytons by nuclear columns. *Journal of Neuropathology and Experimental Neurology, 36,* 861–870.

Kral, V. A. (1978). Benign senescent forgetfulness. In R. Katzman, R. D. Terry, & K. L. Bick (Eds.), *Alzheimer's disease: Senile dementia and related disorders* (Aging Series, Vol. 7, p. 47). New York: Raven Press.

Marr, D. (1982). *Vision: A computational investigation into the human representation and processing of visual information.* New York: W. H. Freeman.

Mayeux, R., Stern, Y., Sano, M., Cote, L., & Williams, J. B. W. (1987). Clinical and biochemical correlates of bradyphrenia in Parkinson's disease. *Neurology, 37,* 1130–1134.

Mesulam, M.-M. (1987). Primary progressive aphasia—Differentiation from Alzheimer's disease. *Annals of Neurology, 22,* 533–534.

Morris, J. C., Cole, M., Banker, B. Q., & Wright, D. (1984). Hereditary dysphasic dementia and the Pick-Alzheimer spectrum. *Annals of Neurology, 16,* 455–466.

Rausch, M. A., Prescott, T. E., & DeWolfe, A. S. (1980). Schizophrenic and aphasic language: Discriminable or not? *Journal of Consulting and Clinical Psychology, 48,* 63–70.

Rogers, D. (1986). Bradyphrenia in Parkinsonism: A historical review. *Psychological Medicine, 16,* 257–265.

Ross, E. D. (1981). The aprosodias: Functional-anatomic organization of the affective components of language in the right hemisphere. *Archives of Neurology, 38,* 561–569.

Ross, E. D., & Mesulam, M.-M. (1979). Dominant language functions of the right hemisphere? Prosody and emotional gesturing. *Archives of Neurology, 36,* 144–148.

Rowe, J. W., & Kahn, R. (1987). Human aging: Usual versus successful. *Science, 237,* 143–149.

Sabin, T. D., & Venna, N. (1984). Peripheral nerve disorders in the elderly. In M. L. Albert (Ed.), *Clinical neurology of aging* (pp. 425–442). New York: Oxford University Press.

Sanford, F. H. (1942). Speech and personality. *Psychological Bulletin, 39,* 811–845.

Schneider, E. L., & Brody, J. A. (1983). Aging, natural death, and the compression of morbidity: Another view. *New England Journal of Medicine, 309,* 854–855.

Waxman, S. G. (1988). Nonpyramidal motor systems and functional recovery after damage to the central nervous system. *Journal of Neurological Rehabilitation, 2,* 1–6.

Wilson, B. A. (1987). *Rehabilitation of memory.* New York: Guilford Press.

Wolfson, L. I., & Katzman, R. (1983). The neurologic consultation at age 80. In R. Katzman & R. D. Terry (Eds.), *The neurology of aging* (pp. 221–224). Philadelphia: F. A. Davis.

Neurolinguistics and Aging

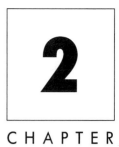

2

CHAPTER

Hanna K. Ulatowska, PhD, and
Sandra B. Chapman, PhD ■

Neurolinguistics is a relatively new and rapidly expanding discipline, which is in its formative stages in terms of both data collection and theory construction. In the early stages, the goal of neurolinguistics was to obtain empirical evidence for the reality of certain linguistic structures and functions in normal language processing. More recently, the trend has been away from studies of narrowly defined linguistic behaviors, which ignore the neurobiological complexity of language, to a broader-based study of language, reflecting an interdisciplinary approach.

In this chapter, our major purpose is to illustrate two principles central to neurolinguistic studies of aging. The first examines language as one cognitive system interdependent on other cognitive and social systems; the second adopts theoretical linguistic constructs for identification of the mechanisms underlying language change and language dissolution. Along with these two themes, current theoretical issues and constructs important to neurolinguistic studies of aging are illustrated with three case studies selected from the literature as well as with a recent study of discourse which we conducted with different geriatric populations. Although some of the concepts presented may change or be redefined with time, it appears likely that the underlying principles described here will remain unchanged.

The Scope of Neurolinguistics

Neurolinguistics is broadly defined as the study of brain-language relationships. The earliest brain-language correlates were described by clinical neurologists within the context of aphasia. The classic cases were those of Broca (1861) and Wernicke (1874), where clinical pathological correlates associated focal brain lesions with impaired language function. These early investigations led to the assumption that certain aspects of language are organized in discrete parts of the brain.

Limitations of early brain-language studies were caused both by the inadequacies of linguistic knowledge in characterizing language performance and by a lack of brain-imaging measures in vivo. Only recently have major advances in both of these areas occurred. In linguistics, early studies used a highly restricted set of descriptive linguistic terms to characterize language symptoms. Advances in specification of linguistic units of analysis have occurred for phonology, syntax, semantics, and pragmatics at word, sentence, and discourse levels of language. These linguistic units have provided a theoretical framework and constructs with which to describe language performance.

Dramatic advances in medical technology have provided a means of viewing not only brain structure but also brain function. Brain structure is measured by computed tomography and magnetic resonance imaging. Functional brain-imaging technology includes ways to measure brain metabolism, cerebral brain blood flow, and brain electrophysiology. These technological advances have allowed more accurate definition of regional brain abnormalities in humans.

Although observations of brain-language relationships have been reported for more than a century now, the field of neurolinguistics emerged less than three decades ago. The combined efforts of neurology and linguistics were motivated by the inadequacies of either discipline in isolation. From a linguistic perspective, language was viewed as a set of constituent systems that could be understood by merely understanding the linguistic units and their systematicity or rule-governed nature. Through such a perspective, the language system was seen more as a product, or sum of its constituents, than as a process. Knowledge of the constituent systems alone did not explain how language was processed or

how it was compromised following injury to the brain. To determine causative links between brain and behavior, one must understand both the language system and the processes involved. For example, syntax may be impaired for various reasons, of which some are linguistic and some cognitive in nature. Linguistically, comprehension of certain syntactic structures, such as embedded clauses, may be more difficult than comprehension of the same information concatenated in simple sentences. It is also possible that comprehension of certain syntactic structures may be reduced by cognitive factors, such as memory impairment, rather than by linguistic deficits.

From a neurological perspective, diseases have been defined using lesion information. This approach has been particularly revealing in aphasia, where consistent associations of lesion sites with behavioral deficits provide the basis for widely accepted "anatomoclinical principles." The brain-language relationships established in aphasia have been supported by both post mortem and ante mortem studies (Basso, Lecours, Moraschini, & Vanier, 1985; Benson & Geschwind, 1971). Despite this consistent relationship, the association between brain and language is incomplete, because different aphasia types often share similar behavioral disturbances.

Recently, the scope of neurolinguistics has expanded to include other disciplines, some firmly grounded in linguistics (e.g., psycholinguistics and sociolinguistics) and others in psychology (e.g., cognitive psychology and neuropsychology). The broadening scope for neurolinguistics reflects the newer view of language as a process rather than a product. When it is viewed as a process, the study of language can take into account variability of linguistic performance attributable to cognitive, psychological, and social factors rather than assuming solely linguistic factors. Language as a process stands in contrast to language viewed as a product in that it reflects the nature of language "in use" by human speakers.

The Biological Basis of Language

At the core of neurolinguistic theory is the belief that language has a prewired biological basis. This is supported by evidence that language is an inherent capacity and that language and the neural basis for language are dynamic processes. Moreover, language is a complex cognitive system, interdependent on other cognitive processes. The strongest evidence for a biological basis for language is the fact that language is inherent and unique to man. For years, researchers have probed the capacity for language in different animal species. The ape has been the main target because of its documented cognitive capacity. The language system of the ape does not even begin to rival the complexity and creativity of language in man. Man appears to be specifically "wired" neurologically for speech and language. The fact that no animal model exists for human language in large part accounts for the relatively slow progress in brain-language research.

Further evidence for the neurobiological basis of language consists of the dynamic changes in language and the brain, in terms of both structure and function, throughout the life-span. Language performance is dynamic, with no performance plateau that is maintained after language has been acquired. Language is capable of change over time; it is acquired early, in adulthood, and even into old age. The fact that changes occur over time makes language a particularly promising cognitive system for investigating brain/behavior relations over the life-span.

Parallel with language changes throughout life are alterations in the human brain, both developmental and pathological. Developmentally, the brain evolves from neural pathways with less specificity yet greater plasticity in the young brain to more specificity with less plasticity in the older brain. The issues of plasticity and specificity are well understood in terms of language. During early life, plasticity is demonstrated by the fact that both hemispheres appear to be able to subserve language. With increasing age, this plasticity decreases as language lateralizes to the left hemisphere. Thus, the left hemisphere becomes more specific for language with increasing age.

The lateralization of language may not be the same for all linguistic components. Some evidence suggests that brain specificity may differ for certain linguistic components, such as phonology, semantics, and syntax. For example, phonological and syntactic functions appear to be more tightly organized in the brain as contrasted with a more diffuse organization of semantic functions. Evidence for a possible differential organization for linguistic components is provided by studies of clinical populations with focal and diffuse lesions. In aphasia, focal lesions to the left inferior frontal cortex are more likely to impair syntax than semantics. In dementing populations with more diffuse cortical lesions, the opposite is true; syntax is relatively spared while semantics is impaired, at least in the early stages of the disease (Kempler, 1988; Schwartz, Marin, & Saffran, 1979).

In addition, neural plasticity in the older brain may be reduced with age as a result of loss of neurons (Brody, 1955). The aging brain does, however, have the ability to maintain and repair itself (Buell & Coleman, 1979; Greenough & Green, 1981). The issues of plasticity and specificity are important for understanding behavioral changes, determining prognoses, and planning treatment in both elderly and pathological populations.

Finally, language is an extremely complex cognitive system with a complicated neurological organization. Language function interacts both behaviorally and neurally with cognitive systems such as memory, perception, and attention. Consequently, deficits in one cognitive system, such as memory, interfere with language performance and vice versa. Similarly, considerable overlap exists in neural organization for different behaviors. For example, the left temporal cortex has been associated with both language and memory function. This behavioral and neurological overlap and actual interdependence of various cognitive systems is reflected in both developmental and pathological states. Awareness of the interdependency of cognitive systems is of particular significance to the study of language in elderly populations.

The Social Aspects of Language

Social factors can affect language in a dramatic way. These factors include number of social partners, purpose of the linguistic exchange, listener's characteristics, and setting of the exchange. Social parameters also include social styles and communicative strategies, both of which change over the life-span. Perhaps the most vivid illustration of the interaction between language and social factors is the story of Genie, a young girl raised in virtual social isolation (Curtiss, Fromkin, Krashen, Rigler, & Rigler, 1974). Genie had essentially no normal social interactions from age 2 until age 13. At the time of her discovery, Genie exhibited severe language deficits for which she received immediate language rehabilitation. Unfortunately, intensive language stimulation did not enable Genie to overcome the negative impact of the environmental factors. Her syntactic ability remained markedly impaired. Although Genie's neurological system was relatively "intact," at age 13 she was beyond a critical period for normal language acquisition.

Recent evidence suggests that social factors affect the language of elderly populations (Lubinski, 1978). The social structure of elderly individuals undergoes dramatic changes as the social network shrinks. Opportunities to interact are reduced by changes in employment status, living environment, and family constellation. Consideration of social factors is mandatory in investigations of language in the elderly because individuals may adopt certain social styles to compensate for the effects of biological changes. For example, there has been speculation that elderly speakers employ different strategies for switching topics than younger speakers and that they may pause longer in narratives and conversations without giving up the floor (Heltrich, 1979).

Goals of Neurolinguistics

In the early developmental stages of neurolinguistics, the primary purpose was to obtain independent empirical support for linguistic hypotheses of normal language processing. This empirical support was derived primarily from correlating information about structure and function of both language and the brain in aphasia. Aphasic individuals provided more insight into brain-language relationships than normals, because language changes could be directly related to changes in the brain. Classical anatomoclinical principles of aphasia indicate that lesions to the left inferior frontal cortex produce nonfluent speech and lesions to the left superior temporal cortex produce comprehension deficits. In contrast, no neurological correlates for language could be established by studying normally functioning individuals. Geschwind (1983), however, warned that conclusions drawn from lesioned patient populations about normal language processes must be interpreted cautiously. During neurological and behavioral recovery, alterations occur in neural pathways and behavior. In some instances, investigators may be deceived by apparent recovered behavior that may, at first glance, appear similar to normal behavior. In actuality, the recovered behavior may reflect compensatory strategies with different underlying processes and different anatomical substrates.

In more recent neurolinguistic studies, a belief has emerged that investigations of linguistic performance alone provide an incomplete model of how language actually works. Rather, the study of language must include examination of linguistic systems as well as evaluation of other cognitive systems. To relegate language to the status of an independent mental system would be to dismiss the important interfaces of various cognitive systems. Arguments can be made for considering aspects of the language system independent of those of other cognitive systems. For example, this is the case when describing dissociations or selective impairments of certain linguistic structures in different types of aphasia. For the most part, however, consideration of language structures isolated from other linguistic and cognitive systems provides an incomplete picture of language processing.

Empirical knowledge of the neural mechanisms underlying language may be investigated in various ways. Additional studies of the specific linguistic and psycholinguistic capacities of individual patients would increase this knowledge in relation to brain-language relationships. With increased understanding of the structure of language and the psychological processes associated with language, documentation of impaired and spared abilities in various neurological patient populations will be possible. At the present stage of neurolinguistics, simply measuring the presence or severity of language impairments is insufficient to demonstrate the neurobiological complexity of language. Systematic examinations of preservations of language functioning as contrasted with clearly evident disturbances in some aspects of language provide an appreciation of that underlying complexity. Furthermore, the losses must be carefully examined to identify any systematic linguistic and psychological principles that may underlie the aberrant performance.

In neurolinguistics, there is a pressing need to develop increasingly more detailed models of language processing. Moreover, suitable methodologies are needed that will relate patterns of acquired language disorders to models of normal cognitive systems. The models should characterize the principal features of certain language abilities and account for the sequence of operations that underlie these behaviors, such as naming, syntax, or producing morphological endings.

Methodological Problems in Studies of the Elderly

Neurolinguistic studies in the elderly are confounded by problems that limit the ability to make generalizations about language change with age. Methodological difficulties relate to defining the population and accounting for performance variability. One of the major issues that must be addressed is how to define "elderly." The well-recognized heterogeneity in this population creates difficulties in defining appropriate comparison groups. While most studies use chronological age as a means of defining "elderly," few differentiate between young-elderly and old-elderly (older than 85 years). Evidence that language changes do occur in old-elderly suggests that grouping all individuals over 65 years of age into one group is inappropriate (Ulatowska, Cannito, Hayashi, & Fleming, 1984; Ulatowska & Chapman, in press). Identifying changes according to chronological age may not be the best way to study aging. A more appropriate way of clustering patients may be to consider their performance on mental status measures or health and social factors.

Another major methodological problem is identification of factors that affect performance. Not only is there considerable heterogeneity in elderly populations, but there is marked variability in performance. Variability is evident both across individuals and within a single individual. In addition, cognitive slowing with age affects performance, especially on timed tasks. Lack of task saliency may also affect performance in the elderly. Metalinguistic tasks, for example, may appear difficult for the elderly not because of impaired linguistic competence but rather because of difficulty relating to the task. Some performance deficits observed in aging may also be attributed to reduced cognitive flexibility—that is, the ability to shift sets.

Information regarding language change through adulthood is sparse, especially for discourse performance. Although a number of deficits have been described, no norms exist on language competence in early adulthood or middle age other than the limited norms measured on adult intelligence scales. A number of studies of language in the elderly have attempted to offer explanations for reported language deficits. For example, comprehension deficits in the elderly have been suggested as arising from both linguistic and cognitive factors, such as syntactic disruptions and attention or memory impairments (Peach, 1987). Cohen (1979) indicated that comprehension deficits in the elderly result from a decreased ability to simultaneously understand the surface meaning while carrying out integrative, constructive, and organizing processes. Hartley (1988) suggested that comprehension for prose is reduced in the elderly because of limitations of processing resources—for example, a reduced working-memory capacity.

In order to understand aging as a factor in language-brain relations, we need to discover patterns of preserved and impaired abilities. Identification of stable and vulnerable abilities in aging has been limited. Furthermore, it is important to document relative rates of development or change and decline among the different language functions—for example, how decline in vocabulary compares to decline in syntactic abilities in progressive disorders. As a result of the major void in normative data, most of the linguistic studies of aging are primarily descriptive as opposed to hypothesis driven.

Perhaps the greatest challenge facing neurolinguistic aging studies is in isolating confounding factors. It is extremely difficult to differentiate the effects of disease processes from the effects of aging on neurophysiological systems. Confounding factors such as environment, concomitant health problems, changes in life-style, and changes in sensory function (vision and hearing) interfere with isolating the language changes that are the consequence of aging alone.

Neurolinguistic Case Studies

In this section, three case studies from the literature are summarized. These particular cases were chosen because they address important methodological issues in neurolinguistic studies of aging populations. The cases reflect the perspectives of different disciplines, such as speech-language pathology, neurology, neuropsychology, and neurolinguistics. Taken as a group, these studies demonstrate the necessity of an interdisciplinary approach for offering explanations of language-brain relations in aging.

These case studies illustrate the disintegration of brain behaviors as reflected in specific dissociations of function. The dissociations described include differential preservations and vulnerabilities between two different systems, for example, between cognition and language, between spoken and written language, between semantics and syntax, and between automatic and volitional processing. Finally, these single-case studies document the fine distinctions that exist between different dementing disorders, such as Pick's disease and dementia of the Alzheimer's type (DAT).

Case One

The first case study described behavioral changes in a patient over 12½ years, from the time of diagnosis until death (Holland, McBurney, Mossy, & Reinmouth, 1985). The behavioral changes followed an atypical course in that language deteriorated early in the disease with more generalized dementia not appearing until late in the disease process. The primary loss of language makes this case of particular relevance to neurolinguistic studies. Furthermore, an autopsy was performed, providing critical neuropathological information. The patient's behavioral profile and neuropathological studies were reportedly consistent with the diagnosis of Pick's disease.

The investigators in this study included representatives from four disciplines: speech-language pathology, psychology, neuropathology, and neurology.

This case illustrates five important methodological issues: (a) patterns of preservations and vulnerabilities, (b) behavioral changes over time, (c) the significance of the patient's ecological profile, (d) premorbid social and psychological characteristics, and (e) neuropathological correlates. Preserved abilities included relative sparing of calculations, reading, and writing. The patient's memory for names and dates was also strikingly more intact than is normally observed in other dementing disorders. Memory loss is typically one of the earliest diagnostic signs of dementia. Generalized cognitive abilities were preserved relative to linguistic abilities as evidenced by the patient's ability to construct a grandfather clock from a kit and to continue to do his own tax returns! Areas of impairment included auditory comprehension, fluency, speech, and appreciation of music. Documentation of preserved and impaired abilities revealed dissociations between cognition and language and between oral and written language modalities.

The second methodological issue addressed by this study is the importance of documenting aging disorders over the course of the disease. Evaluating this patient at any one stage of the disease would have obscured the progressive nature of the disease process. For example, initial behavioral and neurological evaluations were suggestive of an aphasia subsequent to stroke. The continued behavioral deterioration was not consistent, however, with "typical" aphasia. Furthermore, the continued losses could not be attributed to aging factors alone. Some pathological process, identifiable only by a longitudinal study, appeared to be present. In addition, different rates of decline for various abilities were identified over the course of the disease. The patient's comprehension of spoken language disintegrated years before his comprehension of written language was reduced.

The case description also included an ecological profile reflecting the patient's education, professional achievements, premorbid intellect, and social role. Ecological factors interact with language abilities and must be taken into consideration in aging studies where changes are suspected. For example, this man was described as well educated with an extensive vocabulary, but was relatively quiet in group settings. Initial symptoms included substitution of low-frequency words for higher-frequency words. These symptoms were in sharp contrast with the patient's typical vocabulary usage and consequently alerted the family to arising problems. The reduction in speech output was less noticeable because he was a relatively reticent man. Additionally, the patient had always exchanged notes and letters with friends. The relative preservation of written language may be due, in part, to a strong premorbid proficiency in letter writing. The relationship cannot be ascertained at this point, but careful documentation of premorbid ecological profiles may provide insight into which abilities are more likely to be preserved and which are more likely to be impaired.

Finally, the case presented neuropathological information that ties the behavioral findings to localized neurological findings. The abnormalities, described as the presence of Pick's bodies, were localized primarily to the frontal and temporal lobes of the left hemisphere. These regions are classically associated with fluency of speech and auditory comprehension, respectively. Thus, the language losses may be related to the localized abnormalities of the brain. This type of documentation is essential for understanding brain-language relations. The case described here illustrated a different pattern of language dissolution than is normally seen in other dementias. Characterization of the finer distinctions was possible only because of the in-depth, long-term study of a multidisciplinary nature.

Case Two

The second case characterized dissolution of semantic knowledge in dementia

(Schwartz, Martin, & Saffran, 1979). The patient was a 62-year-old female with an eighth-grade education. The patient obtained an IQ score of 95 on the performance scale of the *Wechsler Adult Intelligence Scale*. Memory was poor for both verbal and nonverbal material. The patient's most obvious deficit was severe reduction in lexical function. She performed at a six-year-old level on the *Peabody Picture Vocabulary Test*. The neurological examination suggested bilateral diffuse cerebral involvement and was supported by brain-imaging measures of both structure and function. The patient was diagnosed as having a primary presenile dementia.

Changes in semantic knowledge have frequently been described in dementia. From a methodological point of view, however, this case illustrates a unique, hypothesis-driven approach. The methodology incorporated assessment of various types of knowledge that underlie semantic knowledge, including linguistic, gestural, and cognitive knowledge. This study showed an appreciation for the interdependencies among different knowledge systems. The methodology allowed discovery of a disparity between the linguistic and conceptual knowledge underlying semantic processing. From a theoretical point of view, the study showed how specific linguistic components such as semantic features can be used to identify systematic changes in semantic knowledge.

In terms of methodology, linguistic knowledge was tapped through naming of common objects, and gestural knowledge through demonstrating functions of common objects. Linguistically, the patient exhibited a severe disturbance in semantic ability as manifested by a failure to name common items. However, more intact semantic knowledge was observed through the gestural system, as the patient was able to gesture common functions of objects.

An interesting disparity in performance was evident between linguistic and cognitive tests. The linguistic test involved labeling animals and the cognitive measure involved categorizing animals. The patient tended to inappropriately label cats as dogs on the linguistic measure. The reverse behavior was observed on the cognitive measure, with dogs miscategorized as cats. This evidence suggested that the patient did not possess the conceptual or cognitive basis for correct animal naming. Thus, the naming deficit appeared to be secondary to a cognitive impairment.

From a theoretical perspective, the use of semantic features to characterize this demented patient provided a means of evaluating patterns of semantic breakdown. The disruption in semantic ability appeared to be systematic, as evidenced by the loss of more specific features before more general ones. For example, the category of dogs was collapsed to include cats but not to include birds, fish, or larger animals such as horses, cows, or elephants. From a neurolinguistic perspective, this evidence documented the power of using linguistic features to capture the rule-governed nature of semantic disruption.

Neurological evidence from a clinical neurological examination, electroencephalogram, and computerized brain tomography studies supported bilateral, diffuse brain involvement. The researchers suggested that semantic knowledge may be selectively vulnerable to the effects of diffuse cerebral pathology. In contrast, syntax and phonology may be selectively vulnerable to focal pathology as seen in aphasia. This finding has important implications for normal aging because diffuse loss of neurons is reported. Perhaps early manifestations of naming problems in aging may have a neural basis.

Case Three

This final case is of theoretical significance because it is the first case in which language dissolution was tested within a neurolinguistic framework (Whitaker, 1976). The patient was a 59-year-old female diagnosed as having presenile dementia on the basis of neurological, neuroradiological, neuropsychological, and language evaluations. She was disoriented for time, place, and person and did not follow simple commands. She had no spontaneous speech, but rather her responses were echolalic with some perseverative responses. All measured aspects of cognitive functions were severely impaired. Neurological and neuroradiological examinations were consistent with diffuse central nervous system disease. The neurolinguistic approach used linguistic stimuli, carefully manipulated to tap "knowledge" of different language components and to demonstrate a dissociation between automatic, overlearned aspects of language and its more volitional, creative aspects.

The ingenuity of this experimental paradigm is in the type of stimuli used to assess a patient with severely limited linguistic abilities. Careful linguistic evaluation revealed a relatively more intact syntactic system as compared to a more impaired semantic system. The investigator had to devise a particularly creative experimental paradigm because the patient's output consisted primarily of echolalic responses. Furthermore, marked comprehension deficits were present, preventing the patient from following even very simple commands. The patient was unable to write, but she could read or at least "call out" words. Therefore, reading and verbal repetition were used to evaluate her performance. Linguistic stimuli included lists of printed words from a variety of word classes. The repetition tasks used syntactically and semantically ambiguous and anomalous sentences.

The results demonstrated that the patient did not simply read or echo the exact stimuli; instead, modifications of the stimuli were observed in her response pattern. These modifications suggested some kind of grammatical processor that filtered incoming language. Evidence of a filtering mechanism was evident in the patient's differential reading of words and repetition of sentences. On reading tasks, the patient could easily read concrete and abstract nouns, verbs, and adjectives. However, some words were syntactically altered to become different syntactic categories, but the derivation was related to the stimulus word. For example, derived nouns were sometimes read as verbs (*fulfillment* became *fulfill*) and sometimes as adjectives (*information* became *informative*). Verbs were sometimes read as nouns (*apprehend* became *apprehension*) and sometimes as adjectives (*excite* became *exciting*). On repetition tasks, the patient spontaneously corrected syntactically anomalous sentences, which resulted in agreement of number, verb tense, and case. She also spontaneously corrected the word order and stress of noun compounds when repeating stimuli. In addition to syntactic correction, she demonstrated sensitivity to phonemic errors (*gold ling* for *gold ring*). She did not attempt to echo sentences from a foreign language, although she did echo nonsense words. If the nonsense word resembled a real English word, she would substitute the English word. The patient completed sentences having nonfinal intonation contours with grammatically correct responses. In contrast, she did not correct semantically anomalous sentences; rather, she simply repeated the sentences without any alteration.

This systematic linguistic evaluation revealed that syntax was more intact than semantics. The explanation offered was that syntax appeared to be a more automatic aspect of language compared to semantics, particularly in reference to tense, number, case, and gender agreement. The fact that this patient modified input and did not simply echo a response indicates that the incoming language was filtered by some kind of grammatical processor and was not simply a reflexive response. The selective echoic behavior exhibited by this case suggests that linguistic function may be accessible even in patients with severely limited linguistic abilities if appropriate theoretical constructs are adopted.

The neuropathological findings provide additional explanatory power for the interesting behavioral findings in this case. The autopsy report revealed diffuse cerebral atrophy with cortical neuronal degeneration involving the cortex and underlying white matter. The investigator suggested that the left perisylvian region might have been relatively spared. If syntax is locally organized in the left perisylvian regions as focal lesioned studies of aphasia suggest, syntax might have been relatively spared in this demented patient, because this region is felt to be intact.

Summary

The three case studies described here are significant from a historical perspective because they demonstrate the early developmental stages and growth of neurolinguistics. The selected studies clearly illustrate the importance of expanding the interdisciplinary scope of neurolinguistics to include a number of disciplines other than pure linguistic and neurological perspectives. Language changes are now considered in the context of linguistic, cognitive, and neuropathological factors. The scientific benefit consists of improved procedures, increased empirical findings, and greater explanatory power for the language changes seen in elderly patients with dementia.

Discourse in Aging Populations

Recently, the scope of neurolinguistics has expanded beyond studies of word- and sentential-level language to the discourse level. Whereas it is frequently described as a series of connected sentences, discourse may be a single word, a phrase, a sentence, or a combination of all these forms. Its length is specified in terms of its communicative function, which is to convey a message. Formulation of the message entails a complex interaction of linguistic, cognitive, and social factors. The message may serve various functions and represent different discourse types (e.g., narrative, procedural, expository, or conversational). In each discourse type, the communicative function and global structure differ. For example, a primary function of narrative discourse is to share everyday experiences, whereas procedural discourse informs or instructs.

This expansion of neurolinguistic studies to include discourse was a natural evolution of insights gained from early neurolinguistic studies. The primary insight was the inadequacy of lower-level language (the word and sentential levels) in accounting for influences such as social and cognitive factors on language performance. Discourse provides an optimal, measurable behavior for conducting interdisciplinary studies, because the inherent nature of discourse interfaces language, cognition, and social aspects. Discourse assessment incorporates the content and form of language; its social context; the organization of information; and the role of memory, attention, perception, and other mental processes involved in the production and comprehension of discourse (Chafe, 1980). Various disciplines have been interested in discourse performance, much more so than in lower levels of language. This is probably so because these lower-level language components were considered to be the expertise of linguists. In contrast, units for discourse description have been proposed by a number of disciplines. One example is the proposition, which is a unit of meaning rather than a grammatical structure. The proposition has been described by both linguists and psychologists. Thus, discourse provides a vast resource of behavioral information that is accessible to multiple disciplines, all of which are interested in elucidating brain-behavior relations.

The second major reason for extension to discourse is to explain the contradictory results reported across studies using word and sentence levels of language. This inconsistency is particularly evident for language studies in geriatric populations. In regard to syntax, some studies indicate preserved syntactic abilities (Cannito, Hayashi, & Ulatowska, 1988; Obler & Albert, 1983), whereas others report impaired abilities (Cohen & Faulkner, 1981; Emery, 1986; Kynette & Kemper, 1986). Described syntactic impairments in the elderly include the absence or misuse of certain grammatical structures in production and impaired comprehension of more complex syntactic structures. This incongruity in the findings may be caused by the artificiality of focusing on sentences out of context. Sentences out of context are those occurring in isolation as well as those viewed in isolation that were extracted from connected language. Describing syntactic errors in isolated sentences without regard to the context may be misleading. Syntactic changes may not be linguistic deficits at all. The differences may merely reflect *cognitive changes*, such as attention deficits, or *stylistic changes*, such as use of the more telegraphic style that is sometimes exhibited in writing. In contrast to inconsistencies at lower language levels, findings of discourse abilities in elderly populations are more consistent. Discourse is more stable because it is less artificial and is the natural form of language used in everyday life. Moreover, discourse subsumes both linguistic and cognitive factors.

An Investigation of Discourse

The final part of this chapter summarizes a recent investigation conducted on narrative discourse in different aging populations (Ulatowska & Chapman, in press). This study illustrates important considerations for neurolinguistic investigations of aging. In discussing populations to be studied, we want to show that carefully selected contrastive populations can illuminate differences and similarities between normal aging adults and aging adults with pathology disorders. Constructs are described for evaluating language as a process by manipulating the linguistic and cognitive aspects of discourse. Finally, findings relevant to language-brain studies in aging populations are presented.

Contrastive Populations

In understanding changes in language as a function of age, important contrasts

between different aging populations are essential. Characteristic features of a particular population become more apparent when they are contrasted with the diagnostic features of other populations. The confounding factors that affect performance throughout the life-span are best illuminated by studying different healthy age groups along the age continuum and pathological groups with disorders common to elderly populations. Contrastive studies provide a way of determining language change as opposed to language dissolution. In addition, contrastive approaches provide insight into the neurological correlates of language and the underlying mechanisms of the disorders.

Although a number of different populations might have been selected for study, four populations were chosen: two healthy and two pathological. The two healthy groups included elderly adults in two age brackets, a younger-elderly group (60 to 75 years of age) and an older-elderly group (older than 85 years of age). The other two groups were neurologically impaired, one with focal brain involvement and the other with diffuse involvement. The focal-brain-lesioned group represented aphasic patients with single cerebral vascular insults, and the group with diffuse brain involvement included patients who had dementia of the Alzheimer's type. These four populations were chosen to explore the similarities and differences commonly reported across these four groups and to elucidate whether different mechanisms underlie the patients' performances.

The contrast of old-elderly and demented populations is of interest because of commonly shared linguistic difficulties in naming and verbosity as well as similar cognitive deficits in memory. The major difference appears to be in the rate of decline and adaptive strategies, with the old-elderly demonstrating a slower rate of decline and more intact compensatory strategies. The contrastive comparisons between demented and old-elderly adults address the differences between normal and pathological aging processes and, in particular, the issue of dementia as an accelerated aging process. The contrasts between younger-elderly and older-elderly contribute to normative data for discourse abilities across the life-span. These normative data are critical, especially because a number of studies have reported language changes in the older-elderly as compared to younger-elderly (Ulatowska, Hayashi, Cannito, & Fleming, 1986; Ulatowska et al., 1985).

Tasks and Procedures

In order to investigate language-brain relations, the methodology should reflect the expanded scope of language as a process. Methods for evaluating language as a product are more advanced than those available for evaluating language as a process. A set of strictly linguistic constituents has been used for evaluating language as a product. Language analysis using these constituents, however, is limited and fails to acknowledge the interdependency of the language system on other cognitive systems, such as memory and attention, as well as the interaction between language and social factors. Methods for evaluating language as a process have emerged only recently.

In the following discussion, a synopsis of one experimental paradigm for measuring language as a process is presented. Although there are a number of ways to measure information processing, certain methodological choices will be highlighted that illustrate important principles central to neurolinguistic studies of aging.

Theoretical Constructs

Methods for describing language as a process have used an expanded set of abstract linguistic constructs, which have been proposed by linguists and cognitive psychologists. The units of analysis most critical to the study described here include *propositions*, *macrostructures*, and *microstructures*. A proposition is the most basic unit of information. Whereas number of words and sentences provide measures of the amount of *language*, propositional analysis measures the amount of *information*. A proposition is defined as an idea unit consisting of one predicate and one or more arguments associated with it. This measure of information is experimentally valuable because it measures information expressed in any form—verbal as well as visual.

The most important construct used to measure language as a process is the macrostructure, which is the global semantic structure of a given discourse. Manipulation of the macrostructure involves selectively reducing information while preserving the central meaning. Discourse tasks that manipulate the macrostructure include producing titles or topics, outlining, summarizing, and providing morals. Macrostructure constructs provide a way of distinguishing linguistic deficits from information-processing deficits. Macroprocessing impairments may produce a number of behavioral deficits. For example, one of the hypotheses in this investigation was that logorrhea may be due to impairment of macroplanning. Without macrolevel processing, propositions do not follow an organizational schema and therefore interfere with communication. In contrast to logorrheic language, truly elaborative language is profuse verbal output that supports a global theme and organization. By adopting macrostructures to evaluate discourse, the ability to manipulate information using language can be measured.

In contrast to the macrostructure, the microstructure consists of sequences of propositions and the methods by which information is connected across propositions. One construct relevant to both the macrostructure and microstructure is the construct of reference, as it reflects the interactive nature of these two levels of processing. Reference within a narrative signals the participants and propositions. At a macrolevel of processing, reference serves to identify the important participants and propositions. These participants and propositions represent important setting information central to the global story. At a microlevel of processing, reference involves repetition of participants and propositions connecting ongoing information throughout a story, so that the sequence of propositions provides a continuous chain of information. Discontinuity of information results from ambiguous reference where identification of the referent is not recoverable. For example, excessive use of pronouns or an extended distance between the noun referent and pronoun may produce ambiguity.

Stimuli

Pictorial stimuli, composed of Norman Rockwell prints, were selected to elicit narrative discourse. These stimuli were selected because they provide some control over the information in the form of response predictability. At the same time, this type of stimulus allows response individuality and creativity. Measuring discourse performance in normally functioning populations, such as healthy elderly adults, requires tasks that incorporate both creativity and control of information. It is possible that response creativity may distinguish healthy old-elderly individuals from patients with early-stage dementia. In addition to providing information control and creativity, pictorial stimuli can eliminate certain processing demands, such as auditory memory and comprehension, that may be impaired in elderly populations. The effects of both auditory memory and comprehension deficits are minimized because neither process is inherent to generating a story from a picture. In addition, pictorial stimuli can be manipulated to evaluate memory for visual stimuli. In this study, subjects' narratives were compared in two conditions, one with the picture present and one with the picture withdrawn. As a result, it was possible to compare story organization produced from stimuli and from memory.

Amount of information was measured in two ways by adopting the construct of proposition, defined previously. First, the total amount of information produced was measured by the number of propositions it contained. Second, the amount of information produced was measured against a set of a priori propositions based upon information depicted in the visual stimuli. This set of a priori information was agreed upon by five judges. The propositions contained in the stimuli provided a core of information against which the patient's propositions could be compared. Amount of language was measured by the number of words and sentences expressed.

In addition to measuring amount of information and language, this study evaluated macrostructure processing in terms of the subject's ability to (a) select essential information instrumental to the communicative goal of telling a narrative, (b) isolate information, and (c) selectively reduce information. Selection of appropriate information was evaluated using narrative components defined by discourse grammars. The essential components of narrative discourse are setting, action, and resolution. Isolation of information was measured by probe questions designed to elicit specific setting information, such as locale and time. Reduction of information was tapped in two ways, one by producing story titles and the second by sorting information according to the importance of items to the global story meaning. Reference was used to measure macro- and microlevel processing.

Findings Relevant to Neurolinguistic Studies of Aging

Theoretical linguistic constructs of proposition, macrostructures, and microstructures and reference were adopted to analyze discourse and to identify similarities and differences across the four populations: younger-elderly, older-elderly, aphasic, and DAT adults. In terms of information processing, older-elderly adults were similar to the mildly impaired DAT adults who were 20 years younger. Severity level for the demented patients was determined using the *Global Deterioration Scale* of Reisberg, Ferris, DeLeon, and Crook (1982). Mild aphasic patients were able to manipulate information better than either the older-elderly or DAT groups at both mild and moderate disease stages. Severity for aphasic patients was determined by the severity rating on the *Boston Diagnostic Aphasia Examination* (Goodglass & Kaplan, 1983). As expected, the younger-elderly were superior on all measures of organization of information.

The information produced by the adult subjects was objectively and systematically measured by using the construct of proposition. Older-elderly and DAT subjects produced less *information* than either aphasic or younger-elderly subjects. In sharp contrast, the older-elderly and DAT subjects produced more *language* than the other two groups as measured by number of words and sentences. Aphasic subjects produced the least amount of language. Comparison between number of propositions and number of sentences revealed a dissociation between these two levels—that is, between amount of information and amount of language. The dissociation was exhibited by the older-elderly, DAT, and aphasic subjects, with the aphasic subjects showing the converse dissociation of information near normal with severe reduction of language.

The older-elderly exhibited reduced syntactic complexity (measured by amount of clausal embedding) as compared to younger-elderly subjects. This finding documents subtle changes in syntactic complexity in aging. A similar reduction in syntactic complexity was also found in the DAT group. It is of interest to note that sentential length was not reduced for older-elderly subjects as compared to younger-elderly subjects. Thus, syntactic complexity in healthy older-elderly and DAT adults was reduced without altering the length of the basic syntactic unit of sentence.

Another finding that emerged from the study consisted of differentiation among the diagnostic subgroups according to distribution of information within the macrostructure organization. Older-elederly and DAT subjects exhibited greater quantities of setting information than did younger-elderly

and aphasic subjects. Setting information sets the stage for the story by identifying the characters, propositions, time, and locale central to the narrative. Setting information may be more prevalent in the language of these two populations for cognitive and/or linguistic reasons. Setting information is conceptually simpler than other narrative components such as resolution, and it can be expressed linguistically in simpler grammatical structures.

Differences between types of setting information (e.g., locative and temporal information) were also found across the populations studied. DAT and older-elderly subjects exhibited more difficulty with temporal information than with locative information, both in spontaneous story productions and in response to probe questions. These two types of information represent conceptually different levels. Temporal information is inferentially derived from the pictures, whereas locative information is explicitly depicted, making temporal information conceptually more difficult.

In regard to discourse genre, similarities were again observed between older-elderly and DAT subjects that were distinct from those of aphasic and younger-elderly subjects. Both older-elderly and DAT subjects produced more descriptive genre types, whereas the latter two groups produced more narrative genres, which is the more appropriate type according to task demands. Conceptually, descriptive genre is simpler because all information is equally weighted and can be expressed without providing a conceptual linkage across propositions. With narrative discourse, on the other hand, the story unfolds in a chronological sequence where one event logically follows another.

Disruption of reference was found in both older-elderly and DAT subjects. This disruption altered the quality of the stories produced by these two groups. Referential errors were manifested by occurrences of indefinite reference and ambiguous reference. This finding has been previously reported and was confirmed in this study

(Ulatowska & Chapman, in press; Ulatowska et al., 1986).

One final diagnostically important finding was the interface between language and memory. Older-elderly and DAT subjects were inferior to aphasic and younger-elderly subjects on memory for pictured objects and repetition of stories from memory. The differences were dramatic when subjects' performances were compared to their ability to name objects and produce stories when the stimulus was present. In some cases, the moderately impaired DAT subjects could not retrieve any of the story or the pictured items when the picture was removed even though they produced a story and named objects with the picture present. This finding exemplifies the profound effect memory impairment can have on language performance.

This study has been described in order to illustrate the importance of a hypothesis-driven methodology in research on language of the elderly. Certain hypotheses based on empirical data motivated (a) selection of comparison populations, (b) choice of theoretical constructs, and (c) task design. First, DAT subjects were compared with older-elderly as well as age-matched controls to test the hypothesis that discourse changes in dementia reflect an acceleration of normal aging. The results revealed a clustering of subgroups, with the older-elderly similar to the DAT subjects and the aphasic similar to the younger-elderly subjects. This evidence suggests that DAT may well represent an early aging process, at least behaviorally. Second, theoretical constructs were selected that were capable of distinguishing between impairment of language and impairment of information processing. Our hypothesis was that communicative deficits in dementia are the result of difficulty manipulating information as well as of linguistic problems. The results showed that DAT and older-elderly subjects were distinguishable from younger-elderly on measures of information structure (propositions, microstructure, and macrostructure) but not necessarily on purely linguistic measures. The finding that amount of language did not correspond with amount of information signifies that language measures should not be equated with information measures. Finally, the task design for the experiment reflected different components that were hypothesized to be impaired in elderly populations—for example, memory (labeling and retelling a story from memory) and information processing (selecting ideas according to their importance). These components showed clear differences between older-elderly and younger-elderly, but not to the same extent as between DAT and younger-elderly. A hypothesis-driven study is critical to neurolinguistic examination of aging in order to derive interpretations for empirical findings.

Conclusions

It was not feasible in a chapter of this scope to provide a comprehensive review of all the issues. For clarity, a summary follows of the major points regarding issues in neurolinguistic studies of aging.

First, neurolinguistic studies of aging should represent the extended scope of language viewed as a complex cognitive ability that is interdependent on other cognitive systems. Moreover, the nature of language change can best be understood if language is investigated as a process. To this end, the study of discourse, by its inherent nature, provides an optimal context for neurolinguistic studies, because discourse incorporates language both as an interdependent cognitive system and as a process. Furthermore, within the scope of discourse, linguistic constructs of an abstract nature should be adopted for describing language, because these constructs are essential to identification of the potential mechanisms underlying changes in language. Adopting theoretical constructs is not enough, however. Studies of language should be hypothesis driven and not merely descriptive. The hypotheses should be reflected in the task choice. That is, tasks should be designed to address performance concerns for particular groups studied. Furthermore, multiple interrelated tasks should be used as opposed to a battery of tests that tap unrelated behaviors. Tasks should tap both preserved and impaired abilities, to allow documentation of dissociation phenomena. Finally, neurolinguistic studies of both a longitudinal and contrastive nature are essential to elucidate the principles underlying brain-language relations. Longitudinal single-case studies are necessary for in-depth exploration of language changes over the life-span.

As an epilogue, the significance of social, cultural, and neurological factors is reemphasized as they pertain to language change in aging. The fact that societal factors impinge on language in the elderly is exemplified by marked differences in language behavior across cultures. Culture most definitely imposes certain constraints on language. This is illustrated by the Paliyan people of South India, who exhibit limited communication throughout life and become almost mute by the age of 40 (Gardner, 1966). These people repress their language not because of cognitive, linguistic, or neurological deficits, but because of the influence of social values on language. Conversely, some cultures attach great importance to language as essential to self-identity. This is evident in the verbal style of an elderly Jewish culture in California where the people pride themselves in use of language. In reference to this Jewish community, Myerhoff (1978) commented that the "very old" can remain in command of the basic human faculties of insight and creativity until the very end, articulating their long experience of living in splendidly rich language. These reports illustrate the profound effects of culture on language and are particularly relevant to neurolinguistic studies of aging, where cultural constraints change as the living environment changes.

A powerful example of the neurological influences on language is the story of the few elderly survivors of the great sleeping sickness epidemic in the 1920s who later developed Parkinsonism. In a fascinating collection of single-case studies, Sacks (1973) describes the state of mind and the nature of illness of these patients. The patients became "awakened" from complete mutism after many decades and actually began speaking again as a result of the drug L-Dopa. The return of language in these patients with medication after half a century of profound mutism and devastation by the disease is a remarkable testimony to the power and resilience of language—the most complex and inherent ability of the human brain.

References

Basso, A., Lecours, A. R., Moraschini, S., & Vanier, M. (1985). Anatomoclinical correlations of the aphasias as defined through computerized tomography: Exceptions. *Brain and Language, 26,* 201–229.

Benson, D. F., & Geschwind, N. (1971). Aphasic and related cortical disturbances. In A. B. Baker & L. H. Baker (Eds.), *Clinical neurology.* New York: Harper & Row.

Broca, P. (1861). Nouvelle observation d'aphémie produite par une lesion de la partie postérieure des deuxième et troisième circonvolutions. *Bulletin Society Anatomy Paris, 6,* 398–407.

Brody, H. (1955). Organization of the cerebral cortex: A study of aging in the human cerebral cortex. *Journal of Comparative Neurology, 102,* 511–556.

Buell, S. J., & Coleman, P. D. (1979). Dendritic growth in the aged human brain and failure of growth in senile dementia. *Science, 206,* 854–856.

Cannito, M. P., Hayashi, M., & Ulatowska, H. K. (1988). Discourse in normal and pathologic aging: Background and assessment strategies. In H. K. Ulatowska (Ed.), *Aging and Communication Seminars in Speech, Language and Learning, 9*(2), 117–133.

Chafe, W. (Ed.). (1980). *The pear stories. Cognitive, cultural and linguistic aspects of narrative production.* Norwood, NJ: Ablex.

Cohen, G. (1979). Language comprehension in old age. *Cognitive Psychology, 11,* 412–429.

Cohen, G., & Faulkner, D. (1981). Memory for discourse in old age. *Discourse Processes, 4,* 253–265.

Curtiss, S., Fromkin, V., Krashen, S., Rigler, D., & Rigler, M. (1974). The linguistic development of Genie. *Language, 50,* 528–554.

Emery, O. B. (1986). Linguistic decrement in normal aging. *Language and Communication, 6,* 47–64.

Gardner, P. M. (1966). Symmetric respect and memorate knowledge: The structure and ecology of individualistic culture. *Southwestern Journal of Anthropology, 22,* 389–415.

Geschwind, N. (1983). Biological foundations of language and hemispheric dominance. In M. Studdert-Kennedy (Ed.), *Psychobiology of language.* Cambridge, MA: MIT Press.

Goodglass, H., & Kaplan, E. (1983). *The assessment of aphasia and related disorders* (2nd ed., pp. 19–31). Philadelphia: Lea & Febiger.

Greenough, W. T., & Green, E. J. (1981). Experience and changing brain. In J. McGaugh and S. Kiesler (Eds.), *Aging: Biology and behavior.* New York: Academic Press.

Hartley, J. T. (1988). Aging and individual differences in memory for written discourse. *Language, Memory, and Aging, 3,* 36–57.

Heltrich, H. (1979). Age markers in speech. In R. Klaus, H. Scherer, and H. Glides (Eds.), *Social markers in speech.* Cambridge, England: Cambridge University Press.

Holland, L. A., McBurney, D. H., Mossy, J., & Reinmouth, O. M. (1985). The dissolution of language in Pick's disease with neurofibrillary tangles: A case study. *Brain and Language, 24,* 20–35.

Kempler, S. (1988). Geriatric psycholinguistics: Syntactic limitations of oral and written language. In L. L. Light & D. M. Burke (Eds.), *Language, memory, and aging.* Cambridge, England: Cambridge University Press.

Kynnette, D., & Kemper, S. (1986). Aging and the loss of grammatical forms: A cross-sectional study of language performance. *Language and Communication, 6,* 65–72.

Lubinski, R. (1978). Why so little interest in whether or not old people talk: A review of recent research on verbal communication among the elderly. *International Journal of Aging and Human Development, 9,* 237–245.

Myerhoff, B. (1978). *Number our days.* New York: Simon & Schuster.

Obler, L., & Albert, M. (1983). Language and aging: A neurobehavioral analysis. In D. Beasley & G. Davis (Eds.), *Aging: Communication processes and disorders.* New York: Grune & Stratton.

Peach, R. (1987). Language functioning. In H. Mueller and V. Geoffrey (Eds.), *Communication disorders in aging.* Washington, DC: Gallaudet University Press.

Reisberg, B., Ferris, S. H., DeLeon, J. J., & Crook, T. (1982). The global deterioration scale (GDS): An instrument for the assessment of primary degenerative dementia (PDD). *American Journal of Psychiatry, 139,* 1136–1139.

Sacks, O. (1973). *Awakenings.* New York: Dutton.

Schwartz, M., Marin, O., & Saffran, E. (1979). Dissociation of the language function in dementia: A case study. *Brain and Language, 7,* 277–306.

Ulatowska, H. K., Cannito, M. P., Hayashi, M. M., & Fleming, S. G. (1985). Language abilities in the elderly. In H. K. Ulatowska (Ed.), *The aging brain* (pp. 125–140). Austin, TX: PRO-ED.

Ulatowska, H. K., & Chapman, S. (in press). Discourse changes in dementia. In R. Lubinski (Ed.), *Dementia and communication: Research and clinical implications.* Toronto: B. C. Decker.

Ulatowska, H. K., Hayashi, M. M., Cannito, M. P., & Fleming, S. G. (1986). Disruption of reference in aging. *Brain and Language, 28,* 24–41.

Wernicke, C. (1874). Der apasische Symptom encomplex. Breslau: Cohn & Weigert.

Whitaker, H. A. (1976). A case of isolation of the language function. In H. Whitaker & H. A. Whitaker (Eds.), *Studies in neurolinguistics* (Vol. 2, pp. 1–58). New York: Academic Press.

Structural and Physiological Changes of the Auditory and Vestibular Mechanisms with Aging

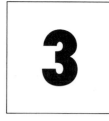

3

C H A P T E R

A. Julianna Gulya, MD, FACS ■

Despite humanity's tremendous strides in advancing knowledge regarding the process of aging, it has thus far eluded attempts at its definition and reversal. Although hopes of foiling the effects of time are probably farfetched, a better understanding of the processes involved in the phenomenon of aging may enable those in the health care professions to mitigate the effects of aging upon their elderly patients and may provide clues to help the young avoid some of those consequences of aging.

This chapter will review what is currently known about the ways in which aging affects the auditory and vestibular systems as well as the physiological (functional) effects these changes have in the aged human.

Aging: General Considerations

Like the neurons of their central pathways, the sensory and neural elements of the auditory and vestibular systems are classified as fixed, postmitotic cells (Nadol, 1980). Cells in this category are incapable of further division and their life-spans are determined by the rate at which they progress to senescence and cell death (Kenney, 1982).

A variety of cellular mechanisms have been proposed to lead to the overall phenomenon of aging including the following (Kenney, 1982):

1. Errors in the repair of DNA or the translation of RNA which in aggregate prove incompatible with cell survival

2. Formation of free radicals (elements that have an unpaired electron), which in turn leads to disruption of membranes and enzyme function, interferes with the intracellular transfer of information, and results in the formation of the aging pigment (lipofuscin)

3. The presence of "death genes," which, as they sequentially terminate specific

cellular processes, produce the phenomenon of aging

4. The production of a pituitary "killer" hormone

The term *presbycusis* describes the physiological result of aging of the auditory system, while "dysequilibrium of aging" to date has been used to encompass the gamut of vestibular manifestations of senescence. Over the life-span of a living organism, not only time, but also genetic factors, climate, diet, toxins, disease, and noise exposure take their toll; because these variables are uncontrolled in the human, it is more difficult to decide through temporal bone evaluation which of the visualized changes are solely the result of the aging process. In addition, patterns of degeneration are variable and are present to varying degrees in each individual. Despite these difficulties, the careful histopathological examination of the geriatric human temporal bone is a prerequisite step in the evolution of testable theories regarding the manifestations of aging in the cochlear and vestibular systems.

The Auditory System

Although there are changes of the ossicular chain associated with aging (Gussen, 1971), they do not seem to precipitate any significant conductive component (Etholm & Belal, 1974); thus they will not be considered further.

It is the cochlear and retrocochlear structures that have been implicated in presbycusis. Cochlear morphological alterations have been sought in the organ of Corti, particularly the hair cells, the spiral ganglion cells and their dendrites, the stria vascularis, and the basilar membrane. Specific histopathological patterns (Schuknecht, 1955, 1964, 1974) have, with some success, been correlated with specific audiometric patterns.

Sensory Presbycusis

In comparison to the normal organ of Corti (Figure 3.1), there seems to be a gradually progressive depletion of the hair cell population with aging, especially of the outer hair cells (Figure 3.2). Degeneration in the organ of Corti begins as early as infancy (Johnsson & Hawkins, 1972) but is more noticeable by middle age (Schuknecht, 1964); nonetheless, because the process progresses so slowly, even in the elderly only a few millimeters of the basal cochlea are affected (Schuknecht, 1974). In early stages of degeneration, light microscopic examination shows distortion and flattening of the organ of Corti (Schuknecht, 1974). Evaluation by means of surface preparation techniques (Bredberg, 1968; Johnsson & Hawkins, 1972, 1977) has shown outer hair cell loss to be most severe in the outermost, third row, and to be the least severe in the first row. Deiters cells produce phalangeal scars that obliterate the breaks in the reticular lamina. As the degeneration progresses, it encompasses the inner hair cells and supporting cells, and it can culminate in the total disappearance of the organ of Corti, which leaves behind only a mound of epithelial cells (Schuknecht, 1974). Neuronal degeneration occurs as a secondary event, possibly related to supporting cell loss, damage to distal neural processes, or inner hair cell loss. If the degeneration in the organ of Corti is restricted to the lower one third of the basal turn, even though radial fibers degenerate, spiral fibers remain (Johnsson & Hawkins, 1972). Apical outer hair cell loss has been observed as well (Bredberg, 1968; Johnsson & Hawkins, 1972, 1977), but it does not seem to be associated with significant neuronal degeneration.

Animal studies (Bhattacharyya & Dayal, 1985; Dayal & Bhattacharyya, 1986a, 1986b) have yielded somewhat contradictory findings, suggesting that although hair cell loss occurs with aging in a number of species, the process appears to proceed from a starting point in the apex of the cochlea.

NORMAL

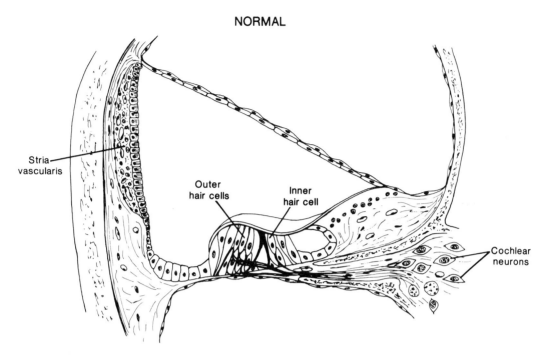

FIGURE 3.1. Line drawing of the normal organ of Corti. *Note.* From ''Aging: Structural and Physiological Changes of the Auditory and Vestibular Mechanisms'' by A. J. Gulya, in *Proceedings of the Research Symposium on Communication Sciences and Disorders and Aging, ASHA Reports No. 19,* Rockville, MD: American Speech-Language-Hearing Association. Copyright 1990 by ASHA. Reprinted by permission.

Lipofuscin accumulation and giant cilia formation (Soucek, Michaels, & Frohlich, 1987) are two ultrastructural changes that have been thought to precede cellular destruction. Lipofuscin, which seems to accumulate progressively in a variety of aging cells, including hair cells (Schuknecht, 1974) and neurons (Ishii, Murakami, Kimura, & Balogh, 1967; Sun et al., 1988), is a strongly autofluorescent, granular, golden-brown pigment. It is theorized to represent the insoluble end products of metabolism that gradually accumulate in the lysosomal fraction (Ishii et al., 1967); with age, lipofuscin accumulates progressively, especially in the subcuticular region of the hair cell, the apical areas of Hensen's, Claudius's and the pillar cells, and the spiral ganglion cells (Ishii et al., 1967; Raafat, Linthicum, & Terr, 1987). The apical region of the vestibular sensory and supporting cells, as well as the neurons of Scarpa's ganglion, also manifest lipofuscin accumulation (Ishii et al., 1967; Raafat et al., 1987). Increasing lipofuscin accumulation has been correlated with the degree of manifested hearing loss (Raafat et al., 1987) and a greater tendency for autolysis (Gleeson & Felix, 1987). Thus it appears that the lipofuscin-laden cells have a physiological handicap and may be similarly functionally handicapped.

The term *sensory presbycusis* has been used by Schuknecht (Schuknecht, 1955, 1964, 1974) to denote the form of presbycusis characterized by hair cell depletion in the basal cochlea. The hearing loss typically begins in middle age, and audiometric evaluation (Figure 3.3) shows bilaterally symmetrical, abruptly dropping threshold curves associated with good speech discrimination scores.

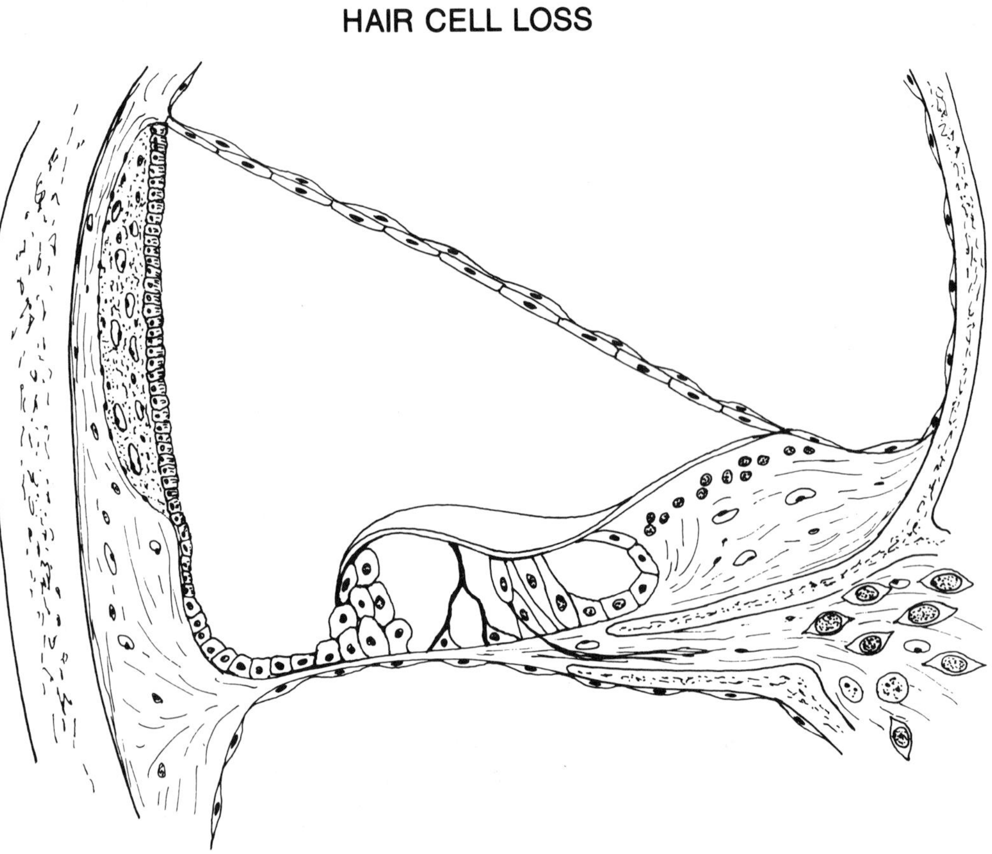

HAIR CELL LOSS

FIGURE 3.2. Artist's depiction of an organ of Corti that has sustained loss of the outer hair cells. *Note.* From "Aging: Structural and Physiological Changes of the Auditory and Vestibular Mechanisms" by A. J. Gulya, in *Proceedings of the Research Symposium on Communication Sciences and Disorders and Aging, ASHA Reports No. 19*, Rockville, MD: American Speech-Language-Hearing Association. Copyright 1990 by ASHA. Reprinted by permission.

Neural Presbycusis

Another form of presbycusis has been correlated with a loss of neurons and nerve fibers out of proportion to degeneration of the organ of Corti (Jorgensen, 1961; Schuknecht, 1955, 1964; Suga & Lindsay, 1976). The greatest losses are seen in the basal cochlea, but the neuronal population often is decreased throughout the cochlea (Figure 3.4) (Schuknecht, 1974). With the surface preparation technique, even though the neuronal bodies cannot be counted, the degree of afferent nerve fiber loss can be visualized well (Bredberg, 1968; Johnsson & Hawkins, 1972, 1977). A theory involv-

ing compressive effects exerted by "hyperostotic" formations at the cribrose area of the modiolar base has been proposed, but not widely accepted, as leading to the neural changes (Stern-Padovan & Vukičevic, 1980). Instead, the depletion of the spiral ganglion is believed (Hansen & Reske-Neilsen, 1965; Jorgensen, 1961; Schuknecht, 1974; Suga & Lindsay, 1976) to be a manifestation of the same process of senescence and death that affects neurons in the central auditory pathways.

Despite the documentation of lipofuscin accumulation (Raafat et al., 1987), the exact mechanism of neuronal loss remains unclear. Studies of aging mice have sug-

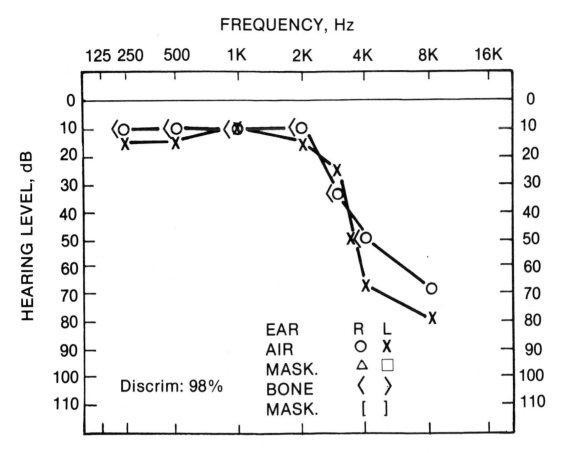

FIGURE 3.3. Audiogram typical of sensory presbycusis. *Note.* From *Quick Reference to Ear, Nose, and Throat Disorders* (pp. 38–39) by W. R. Wilson and J. B. Nadol, Jr., 1983, Philadelphia: J. B. Lippincott. Copyright 1983 by J. B. Lippincott. Adapted by permission.

gested four stages of spiral ganglion cell degeneration (Cohen & Grasso, 1987): (a) beginning demyelinization, (b) contact and fusion, (c) clumping, and (d) resorption with consequent development of fluid-filled spaces.

Pauler and associates (Pauler, Schuknecht, & Thornton, 1986) directly correlated the innervation density of the 15- to 22-mm region of the cochlea, as determined by light microscopic examination, to speech discrimination ability; consideration of other influential factors, such as ultrastructural changes (Nadol, 1979), proved necessary because of the variability of the effect of neuronal depletion on speech discrimination.

Using electron microscopy, Nadol (1979) studied two temporal bones with neural presbycusis. The hair cells were normal, but neural fibers, especially those in the basal turn, demonstrated a variety of degenerative changes, including fewer synapses at the bases of hair cells, "accumulation of cellular debris in the spiral bundles, abnormalities of dendritic fibers and their sheaths in the osseous spiral lamina, and degenerative changes in the spiral ganglion cells and axons" (Nadol, 1979). Vacuoles filled with pleomorphic vesicles and granules were found in the supporting cells that surrounded dendritic twigs. "Myelin figures" were demonstrated in unmyelinated afferent dendritic fibers as well as in the spiral ganglion cells and their supporting cells. Disorganization of the myelin sheath was noted in both dendritic and axonal fibers, especially at paranodal areas and the

NEURAL LOSS

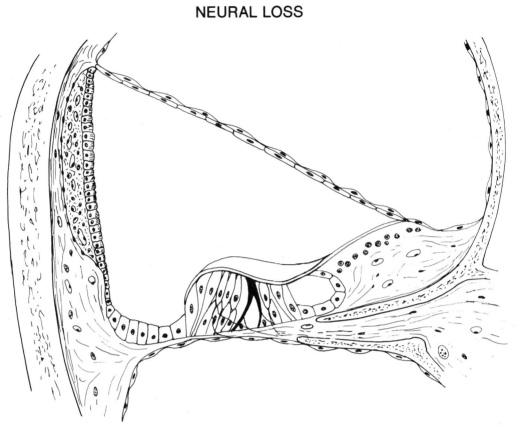

FIGURE 3.4. Although the hair cell population is intact, there is significant neural degeneration, consistent with neural presbycusis. *Note.* From "Aging: Structural and Physiological Changes of the Auditory and Vestibular Mechanisms" by A. J. Gulya, in *Proceedings of the Research Symposium on Communication Sciences and Disorders and Aging, ASHA Reports No. 19*, Rockville, MD: American Speech-Language-Hearing Association. Copyright 1990 by ASHA. Reprinted by permission.

areas near the clefts of Schmidt-Lanterman. Myelin sheath alteration of such magnitude would be expected to disrupt normal saltatory conduction and would cause delay and loss of energy as conduction instead occurs through the cell body.

Neural presbycusis (Schuknecht, 1974) is typified by neural degeneration and upon audiometric evaluation (Figure 3.5) shows loss of speech discrimination out of proportion to the elevation of pure tone thresholds. Genetic factors (Schuknecht, 1974) seem to have an important role in determining its onset, and it becomes manifest usually in late life, when the remaining neural elements can no longer effectively encode and transmit acoustic stimuli.

Metabolic Presbycusis

Another form of presbycusis relates to patchy atrophy of the stria vascularis, especially in the middle and apical turns (Johnsson & Hawkins, 1977) (Figure 3.6). The stria vascularis is believed to function as (a) the site of endolymph formation, (b) the source of the positive 80-mV endocochlear potential, (c) the regulator of the ionic gradients of the inner ear fluids, and (d) the site of the oxidative metabolism that produces the energy essential for cochlear function (Schuknecht, 1974). Logically, a hearing loss would be an expected consequence of disruption of any of these functions.

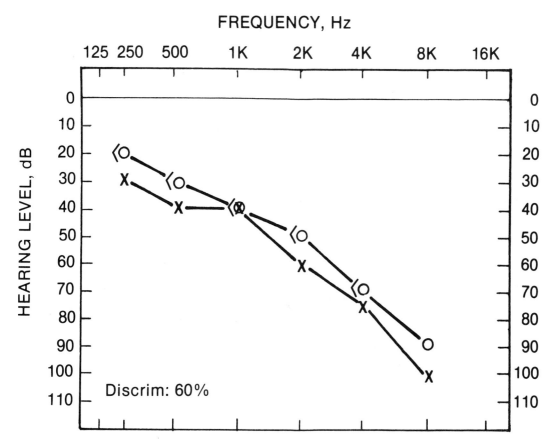

FIGURE 3.5. Audiogram consistent with presbycusis of the neural type. *Note.* From *Quick Reference to Ear, Nose, and Throat Disorders* (pp. 38–39) by W. R. Wilson and J. B. Nadol, Jr., 1983, Philadelphia: J. B. Lippincott. Copyright 1983 by J. B. Lippincott. Adapted by permission.

The cause of strial degeneration remains unclear, although its atrophy was proposed by Jorgensen (1961) to be related to thickening of the walls of the capillaries located in the stria. Alternatively, by phase-contrast microscopy, Johnsson and Hawkins (1977) noted a "devascularization" of the lateral cochlear wall with aging and related this change to the atrophy of the stria vascularis and spiral ligament. More recently, Pauler and associates (Pauler, Schuknecht, & White, 1988) have suggested a genetically determined predisposition for early cellular decay.

Examination with the electron microscope (Schuknecht, 1964) shows that the marginal cells are most severely affected, even though all three layers can be involved. A mere strip of basal cells along the endolymphatic space may be all that remains of the stria in some cases (Kimura & Schuknecht, 1970). Whether hair cell loss occurs as a phenomenon secondary to strial atrophy remains a matter of dispute (Johnsson & Hawkins, 1977; Pauler, Schuknecht, & White, 1988). Using computer-aided morphometric techniques, Pauler and associates (Pauler, Schuknecht, & White, 1988) showed a statistically significant relationship between the extent of strial atrophy and the degree of manifested hearing loss.

Metabolic presbycusis (Hashimoto & Schuknecht, 1987; Schuknecht, 1964, 1974; Schuknecht & Ishii, 1966) describes the flat audiometric configuration associated with strial atrophy (Figure 3.7). The atrophy

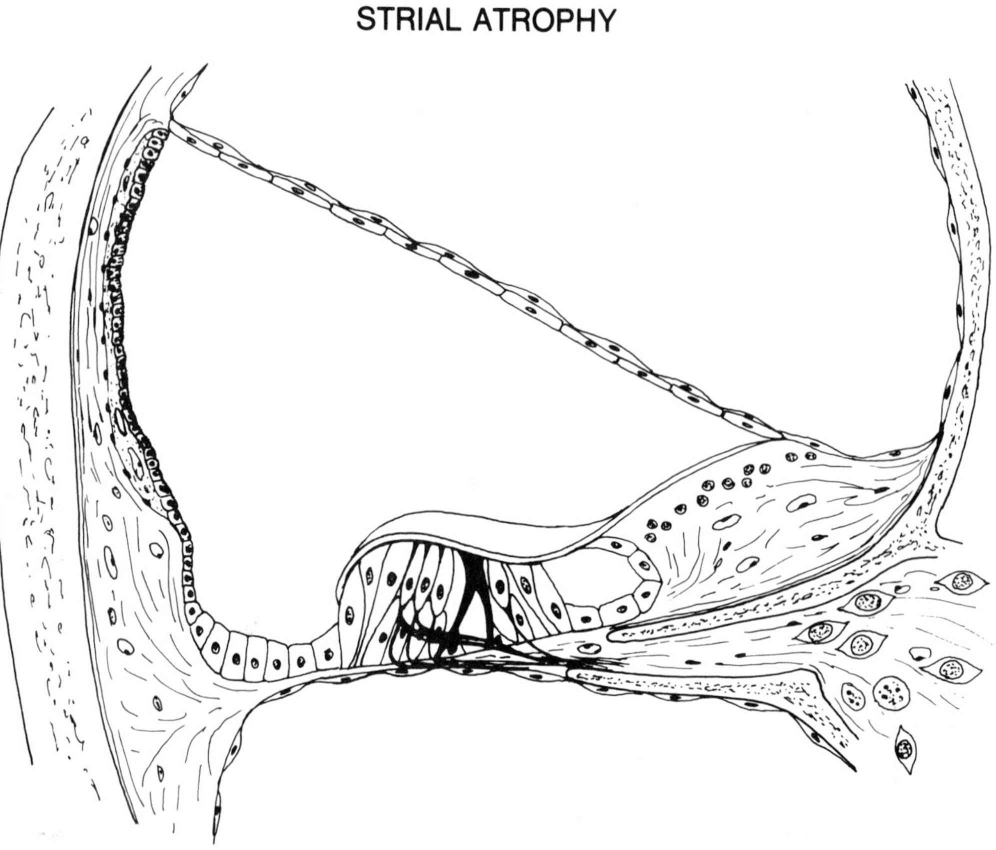

STRIAL ATROPHY

FIGURE 3.6. The only discernible change in this cochlea is the atrophy of the stria vascularis. *Note.* From ''Aging: Structural and Physiological Changes of the Auditory and Vestibular Mechanisms'' by A. J. Gulya, in *Proceedings of the Research Symposium on Communication Sciences and Disorders and Aging, ASHA Reports No. 19*, Rockville, MD: American Speech-Language-Hearing Association. Copyright 1990 by ASHA. Reprinted by permission.

begins its slowly progressive course in the 3rd to 6th decades of life, and upon audiometric evaluation is characterized by excellent speech discrimination scores, often remaining normal until the hearing loss exceeds 50 dB.

Mechanical Presbycusis

One type of presbycusis, characterized by a paucity of significant cochlear histopathological findings, has been explained by hypothesizing a disruption of the motion mechanics of the cochlear duct (Schuknecht, 1964). Structural changes, especially in the basilar membrane as well as the spiral ligament, have been reported and may underlie some hearing loss. Calcification of the basilar membrane was documented by Mayer (1919–1920), whereas the features of hyalinization and calcification were described by Crowe and associates (Crowe, Guild, & Polvogt, 1934). A ''lipidosis'' (deposition of neutral fat and cholesterol in the pars pectinata) of the basilar membrane was reported by Nomura (1970). Most recently, Nadol (1979) demonstrated a marked thickening of the basilar membrane in the basal 10 mm of the cochlea, which could be attributed to an increased number of fibrillar layers in the basilar membrane.

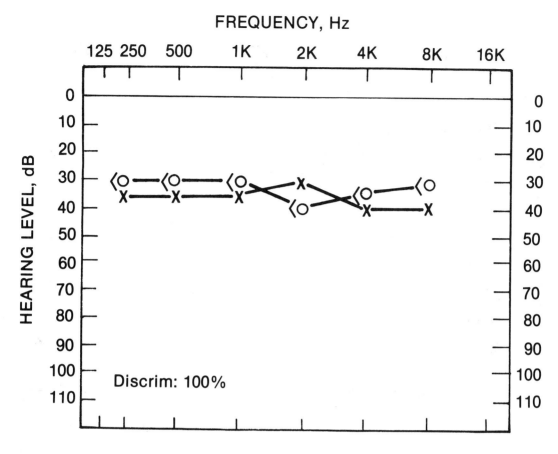

FIGURE 3.7. This flat audiometric curve with excellent discrimination is typical for the hearing loss of metabolic presbycusis. *Note.* From *Quick Reference to Ear, Nose, and Throat Disorders* (pp. 38–39) by W. R. Wilson and J. B. Nadol, Jr., 1983, Philadelphia: J. B. Lippincott. Copyright 1983 by J. B. Lippincott. Adapted by permission.

The type of presbycusis that is believed to be related to these changes in the basilar membrane has been labeled either "mechanical" (Schuknecht, 1964) or "cochlear conductive" (Schuknecht, 1974) presbycusis. The audiogram typically shows a downward-sloping threshold curve (Figure 3.8) with speech discrimination scores varying inversely with the steepness of the slope.

Although "pure" forms of the types of presbycusis have been presented and may occur, it is also possible to see varying combinations of the various types with associated variable audiometric patterns.

Central Auditory Structures

The central auditory pathways are assumed to be subject to alterations by the aging process as well. The spiral ganglion cell depletion of neural presbycusis was related to similar changes in the central nervous system by Schuknecht (1955, 1964, 1974), but evidence to corroborate such speculation has been difficult to accumulate.

In a study encompassing subjects ranging in age from birth to 95 years, Brody (1955) demonstrated a progressive depletion in the cellular population that was not uniformly distributed throughout the cerebral

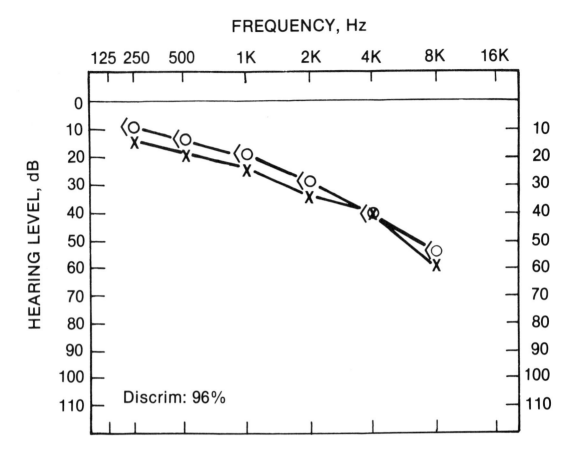

FIGURE 3.8. Cochlear conductive presbycusis is characterized by a downward-sloping threshold curve, with speech discrimination scores that vary inversely with the steepness of the slope. *Note.* From *Quick Reference to Ear, Nose, and Throat Disorders* (pp. 38–39) by W. R. Wilson and J. B. Nadol, Jr., 1983, Philadelphia: J. B. Lippincott. Copyright 1983 by J. B. Lippincott. Adapted by permission.

cortex. Rather, of all the areas assessed, the superior temporal gyrus displayed the greatest drop in cell number, decreasing from an average population of nearly 4,000 cells in the newborn to only 1,100 cells in the 70- to 95-year-old age bracket.

Studies investigating the loss of brain-stem elements have yielded contradictory results. Some investigators (Brody, 1985; Kenney, 1982) have reported that there is no apparent loss of cells except in the locus ceruleus (a region known for its high neuronal epinephrine concentration and its extensive arborization to the cerebral cortex, cerebellum, brainstem, and spinal cord). Other reports have suggested alterations in the central auditory structures with aging, such as the following changes:

1. Atrophy and degeneration of ganglion cells in the ventral cochlear nucleus (Arnesen, 1982; Dublin, 1986; Kirikae, Sato, & Shitara, 1964) as well as of the medial geniculate body with degenerative cells scattered among relatively normal cells in both the superior olivary nucleus and the inferior colliculus (Kirikae et al., 1964)

2. Degeneration of the dorsal cochlear nucleus (Arnesen, 1964; Hansen & Reske-Neilsen, 1965) and accumulation

of corpora amylacea in the inferior colliculus (Hansen & Reske-Neilsen, 1965)

3. Myelin changes throughout the auditory system, including edema, fragmentation, and degeneration (Dublin, 1986; Hansen & Reske-Neilsen, 1965)

4. Accumulation of lipofuscin (Hansen & Reske-Neilsen, 1965; Kirikae et al., 1964; Konigsmark & Murphy, 1972)

Contrasting data have been reported by Konigsmark and Murphy (1972) suggesting that there is no neuronal loss in the ventral cochlear nucleus with aging; rather, there is an increase in its volume in the early decades of life followed by a decrease after the 5th decade. The secondary volume loss was related to parenchymal changes, such as depletion of extracellular space, axon cylinders, myelin, blood vessels, or glial cells, but not to neural loss (Konigsmark & Murphy, 1972). Similarly, studies of the cochlear nucleus of the aging rat have not demonstrated any loss of cells, although examination with electron microscopy occasionally reveals degenerative changes (Feldman & Vaughan, 1977); in the medial nucleus of the trapezoid body, cellular loss has been detected in association with a loss of calycine terminals (Casey, 1986).

Other than for gross lesions, it has been exceedingly difficult to correlate specific functional deficits with specific pathological changes in the central auditory pathways; peripheral hearing loss often is a confounding factor in the evaluation of central auditory dysfunction. Such tests as the competing sentence test (Welsh, Welsh, & Healy, 1985), the binaural fusion test (Welsh et al., 1985), the compressed speech test (Welsh et al., 1985), and the low-pass filtered speech test (Kirikae et al., 1964; Welsh et al., 1985) have been shown to be difficult for the elderly population, but the neuroanatomical correlates remain to be determined.

The Vestibular System

Assessing the effects of aging upon the vestibular system is complicated by its num-erous interconnections in the central nervous system. The five components of the peripheral vestibular system are not equally affected by age-related changes; the cristae ampullares and the saccular macula seem to be particularly affected, whereas the utricular macula manifests relatively fewer alterations. As with the senescent changes seen in cochlear structures, the vestibular structures that undergo morphological alteration are the sensory cells, the supporting cells, the first-order neurons, and the afferent nerve fibers. The otoconia are another element in the vestibular system that undergo functionally significant, age-related changes.

The Cristae Ampullares

Modification of the surface preparation technique has enabled its application to the study of changes in the hair cell populations of the cristae and maculae (Rosenhall, 1972a, 1972b, 1973; Rosenhall & Rubin, 1975). The hair cell population of the cristae remains stable until the age of 40; after this age (Rosenhall, 1972a) there is a significant drop in numbers, which is relatively evenly distributed among the cristae and which eventually results in an average loss of 40% of the total hair cell population of the cristae in the over-70 population. Some specimens show as much as a 60% loss. The periphery of the cristae is much less affected than the summit (Rosenhall, 1973). Unfortunately, the surface preparation technique does not allow for reliable discrimination between type I and type II hair cells (Rosenhall, 1973).

The findings of electron microscopy studies (Engstrom, Bergstrom, & Rosenhall, 1974; Ishii et al., 1967; Rosenhall & Rubin, 1975) essentially recapitulate those provided by evaluation of the cochlear system. Lipofuscin accumulation has been documented in both the sensory and supporting cells of the aged vestibular labyrinth, especially in the type I hair cell. Cilial changes, such as disarrangement, fusion, and the formation of blebs or giant cilia, have been noted

(Engstrom, Ades, Engstrom, Gilchrist, & Bourne, 1977; Rosenhall & Rubin, 1975). The sensory hair loss seen in specimens from the elderly has been related to chemical changes in the aging cupula that result in the cilia becoming tethered in the cupular canals or to a preparation artifact arising from an increased fragility of the stereocilial attachment to the cuticular plate (Rosenhall & Rubin, 1975). Increasing numbers of laminated structures (Engstrom et al., 1977) appear with age in sensory and supporting cells and have a direct relationship to the cuticle and reticular membrane. Similarly, a growing population of vesicular bodies appears, more so in the supporting cells, but also in the sensory cells (Engstrom et al., 1977). Luse bodies (long-spaced collagen) can be found in the loose tissue beneath the sensory epithelium (Engstrom et al., 1977; Gleeson & Felix, 1987; Spoendlin, 1970).

Ampullary dysequilibrium of aging may reflect the functional consequences of such documented changes in the cristae (Schuknecht, 1974). Typically, the patient complains of a persistent sensation of rotation following rapid turns of the head; the unsteadiness following this transient hallucination may linger for hours (Schuknecht, 1974). Studies (Bruner & Norris, 1971; Karlsen, Hassanein, & Goetzinger, 1981; Peterka, Black, Newell, & Schoenhoff, 1987; Wall, Black, & Hunt, 1984) have provided evidence suggesting that the healthy aged population shows a decreased response to caloric and rotational stimuli, thus providing indirect support for the theory that the changes documented in ampullary structures underlie this type of dysequilibrium.

The Saccular Maculae

The modified surface preparation technique (Rosenhall, 1972b, 1973; Rosenhall & Rubin, 1975) has enabled visualization of changes of the sensory cell population of the maculae. A drop in the hair cell population becomes noticeable in individuals over 40 years of age, culminating in an average loss of 20% to 30% in both the saccule and the utricle from individuals 70 years of age and older (Rosenhall, 1973; Rosenhall & Rubin, 1975). The entire macula appears to be uniformly affected (Rosenhall, 1973). Using electron microscopy, investigators have observed apical osmiophilic inclusions in the maculae, especially in the type I hair cells (Rosenhall & Rubin, 1975). Because of these inclusions, the striola in the elderly appear as dark stripes (Rosenhall & Rubin, 1975). Loss of cilia affects the hair cells of the cristae to a greater degree than those of the maculae (Rosenhall & Rubin, 1975).

The Otoconia

Aging is associated with a progressive degeneration of the otoconia as well. In middle and advanced age, the population of otoconia dwindles, more noticeably in the saccule than in the utricle (Ross, Peacor, Johnsson, & Allard, 1976). Proceeding anteriorly from the posterior aspect of the macula, otoconia progress from pit formation to the assumption of a fibrous appearance. Subsequently, the midportion disappears, and finally the otoconia are fragmented (Ross et al., 1976).

Degenerative changes in the otolithic organs have been implicated in macular dysequilibrium of aging (Schuknecht, 1974). Changes of head position relative to gravity precipitate vertigo in affected individuals (Schuknecht, 1974); thus, upon arising in the morning, they find that they must rest on the edge of the bed for a few moments to allow the vertigo to pass before continuing to move about (Schuknecht, 1974). Cochlear changes have been seen in association with saccular degeneration (Schuknecht, Igarashi, & Gacek, 1965).

Deposits of material, presumably of a specific gravity greater than that of endolymph, have been observed on the cupula of the posterior semicircular canal and may represent the insoluble products of the degeneration of aging in the semicircular canals and/or the utricle. With the assumption of particular head positions, affected individuals experience severe, transient vertigo; the disorder is usually self-limiting, but in some individuals it may plague them for the remainder of their lives (Schuknecht, 1974).

The Neural Networks

Aging appears also to be associated with depletion of the vestibular ganglion cells and nerve fibers. A significant drop in the average number of ganglion cells in individuals older than 60 years was noted by Richter (1980). Johnsson (1971), using a microdissection technique, observed a marked degeneration of the saccular nerve network; however, the utricular network was only mildly affected. The loss of vestibular nerve fibers seems to begin around age 40 and eventuates in an average loss of 37% in the geriatric population (Bergstrom, 1973a). The fibers that do remain tend to have a thinner diameter (Bergstrom, 1973b), which is especially obvious in ampullary nerve branches. Slower nerve conduction velocities would presumably result from such changes.

Vestibular ataxia of aging may be at least partially attributed to the changes noted in the vestibular nerves and their networks (Schuknecht, 1974). In support of such a hypothesis are studies showing decreasing vestibulospinal function with increasing age (Peterka et al., 1987). Individuals, particularly those in their 7th and 8th decades, can sit and stand without difficulty but, as a manifestation of the loss of vestibular control over the lower limbs, experience constant dysequilibrium with ambulation (Schuknecht, 1974). Such individuals have caloric responses that are normal for their age (Schuknecht, 1974). A demonstrated deterioration in adaptive capabilities (an active, central process) for the vestibulospinal reflex with age (Norre, Forrez, & Beckers, 1987) suggests that alterations in central structures may also be relevant. To date, the histopathology of the aging human central vestibular system has not been studied systematically.

Vascular Supply

The role of vascular insufficiency in the appearance of degenerative changes of the cochlea and vestibular labyrinth is difficult to distinguish from its role in any primary degenerative process (Babin & Harker, 1982). Jorgensen (1961) observed an increased incidence of PAS-positive thickening of the capillary walls of the stria vascularis with age, but he could not detect any remarkable changes in the capillary network of the spiral ligament and could not relate the changes in the strial vessels to the degree of atrophy of the organ of Corti.

Using microdissection and surface preparation techniques, Johnsson (1973) and Johnsson and Hawkins (1972, 1977) showed strial atrophy accompanied by atrophy and devascularization of the spiral ligament in the osmium-tetroxide-treated labyrinth. The age-related manifestations were most noticeable in the capillary network, with the capillaries of the scala vestibuli manifesting more severe changes than those of the scala tympani (Johnsson, 1973). The radiating arterioles of the spiral ligament of the scala vestibuli also showed narrowing, thickening of the wall, and atrophy, but to a lesser extent (Johnsson, 1973). The arterioles of the scala tympani seemed to be much less affected (Johnsson, 1973).

A series of changes is frequently observed in the outer and inner spiral vessels of the basal cochlea in elderly persons (Johnsson, 1973). Vessel walls thicken, a widened perivascular space is filled with a hyaline substance, and the lumen is obliterated, with only an avascular channel remaining basally (Johnsson, 1973).

Apparently, aging takes much less of a toll on the vessels of the vestibular labyrinth (Johnsson, 1973; Johnsson & Hawkins, 1972; Jorgensen, 1961). The canals show the most obvious changes, with atrophy of the capillaries crossing their perilymphatic spaces (Johnsson, 1973).

In the internal auditory canal, the arterial vessels progressively degenerate with age, most markedly in the tunica adventitia; hyalinization is preceded by thickening and an increase in the compactness of adventitial tissue as well as a progressive loss of fibroblasts (Fisch, Dobozi, & Grieg, 1972). The vasa nervorum, the smallest vessels studied, manifested such alterations the earliest and to the greatest extent, eventually resulting in a narrowed lumen. The larger cochlear, vestibular, and labyrinthine arteries showed no stenosis up to the 9th decade of life (Fisch et al., 1972).

Conclusions

The preceding summary has served to catalog what we seem to know about the aging process and how it affects the cochlea and vestibular labyrinth, as well as their vascular supply. It has also served to point out the significant gaps that currently exist in our database; hopefully, future research endeavors will fill in these gaps and provide us with the necessary knowledge to successfully treat and avoid many auditory and vestibular afflictions in our growing geriatric population.

References

Arnesen, A. R. (1982). Presbyacusis—Loss of neurons in the human cochlear nuclei. *Journal of Laryngology and Otolaryngology, 96,* 503–511.

Babin, R. W., & Harker, L. A. (1982). The vestibular system in the elderly. *Otolaryngol Clin North Am, 15,* 387–393.

Bergstrom, B. (1973a). Morphology of the vestibular nerve. II. The number of myelinated vestibular nerve fibers in man at various ages. *Acta Otolaryngologica* (Stockholm), *76,* 173–179.

Bergstrom, B. (1973b). Morphology of the vestibular nerve. III. Analysis of the calibers of the myelinated vestibular nerve fibers in man at various ages. *Acta Otolaryngologica* (Stockholm), *76,* 331–338.

Bhattacharyya, T. K., & Dayal, V. S. (1985). Age-related cochlear hair cell loss in the chinchilla. *Annals of Otology, Rhinology and Laryngology, 94,* 75–80.

Bredberg, G. (1968). Cellular pattern and nerve supply of the human organ of Corti. *Acta Otolaryngologica* (Stockholm), *236,* (Suppl.), 1–135.

Brody, H. (1955). Organization of the cerebral cortex. III. A study of aging in the human cerebral cortex. *Journal of Comparative Neurology, 102,* 511–556.

Brody, H. (1985). Neuronal changes with increasing age. In H. K. Ulatowska (Ed.), *The aging brain: Communication in the elderly* (pp. 23–31). Austin, TX: PRO-ED.

Bruner, A., & Norris, T. W. (1971). Age-related changes in caloric nystagmus. *Acta Otolaryngology* (Stockholm), *282* (Suppl.), 1–24.

Casey, M. A. (1986). Age-related loss of synaptic terminals in the medial nucleus of the trapezoid body. *Association for Research in Otolaryngology Abstracts, 9,* 146.

Cohen, G. M., & Grasso, J. S. (1987). Further observations on the degeneration of spiral ganglia in aging C57BL/6 mice. *Association for Research in Otolaryngology Abstracts, 10,* 120.

Crowe, S. J., Guild, S. T., & Polvogt, L. M. (1934). Observations on the pathology of high tone deafness. *Bulletin of Johns Hopkins Hospital, 54,* 315–379.

Dayal, V. S., & Bhattacharyya, T. K. (1986a). Cochlear hair cell damage from intermittent noise exposure in young and adult guinea pigs. *American Journal of Otolaryngology, 7,* 294–297.

Dayal, V. S., & Bhattacharyya, T. K. (1986b). Comparative study of age-related cochlear hair cell loss. *Annals of Otology, Rhinology and Laryngology, 95,* 510–513.

Dublin, W. B. (1986). Central auditory pathology. *Otolaryngol Head Neck Surg, 95,* (Suppl.), 363–424.

Engstrom, H., Ades, H. W., Engstrom, B., Gilchrist, D., & Bourne, G. (1977). Structural changes in the vestibular epithelia in elderly monkeys and humans. *Adv Oto-Rhino-Laryng, 22,* 93–110.

Engstrom, H., Bergstrom, B., & Rosenhall, U. (1974). Vestibular sensory epithelia. *Archives of Otolaryngology, 100,* 411–418.

Etholm, B., & Belal, A., Jr. (1974). Senile changes in the middle ear joints. *Annals of Otology, Rhinology and Laryngology, 83,* 49–54.

Feldman, M. L., & Vaughan, D. W. (1977). Changes in the auditory pathway with age. In S. S. Han & D. H. Coons (Eds.), *Special senses in aging: A current biological assessment* (pp. 143–162). Ann Arbor: University of Michigan Press.

Fisch, U., Dobozi, M., & Grieg, D. (1972). Degenerative changes of the arterial vessels of the internal auditory meatus during the process of aging: A histological study. *Acta Otolaryngologica* (Stockholm), *73*, 259–266.

Gleeson, M., & Felix, H. (1987). A comparative study of the effect of age on the human cochlear and vestibular neuroepithelia. *Acta Otolaryngologica* (Stockholm), *436* (Suppl.), 103–109.

Gussen, R. (1971). The human incudomalleal joint: Chondroid articular cartilage and degenerative arthritis. *Arthritis and Rheumatism*, *14* (new series), 465–474.

Hansen, C. C., & Reske-Neilsen, E. (1965). Pathological studies in presbycusis: Cochlear and central findings in 12 aged patients. *Archives of Otolaryngology*, *82*, 115–132.

Hashimoto, S., & Schuknecht, H. F. (1987). Progressive hearing loss from strial dysplasia. *Annals of Otology, Rhinology and Laryngology*, *96*, 229–231.

Ishii, T., Murakami, Y., Kimura, R. S., & Balogh, K., Jr. (1967). Electron microscopic and histochemical identification of lipofuscin in the human inner ear. *Acta Otolaryngologica* (Stockholm), *64*, 17–29.

Johnsson, L. G. (1971). Degenerative changes and anomalies of the vestibular system in man. *Laryngoscope*, *81*, 1682–1694.

Johnsson, L. G. (1973). Vascular pathology in the human inner ear. *Adv Oto-Rhino-Laryng*, *20*, 197–220.

Johnsson, L. G., & Hawkins, J. E., Jr. (1972). Sensory and neural degeneration with aging, as seen in microdissections of the human inner ear. *Annals of Otology, Rhinology and Laryngology*, *81*, 179–193.

Johnsson, L. G., & Hawkins, J. E., Jr. (1977). Age-related degeneration of the inner ear. In S. S. Han & D. H. Coons (Eds.), *Special senses in aging: A current biological assessment* (pp. 119–135). Ann Arbor: University of Michigan Press.

Jorgensen, M. B. (1961). Changes of aging in the inner ear. *Archives of Otolaryngology*, *74*, 164–170.

Karlsen, E. A., Hassanein, R. M., & Goetzinger, C. P. (1981). The effects of age, sex, hearing loss and water temperature on caloric nystagmus. *Laryngoscope*, *91*, 620–627.

Kenney, R. A. (1982). *Physiology of aging: A synopsis* (pp. 65–79). Chicago: Year Book Medical Publishers.

Kimura, R. S., & Schuknecht, H. F. (1970). The ultrastructure of the human stria vascularis. II. *Acta Otolaryngologica* (Stockholm), *70*, 301–318.

Kirikae, I., Sato, T., & Shitara, T. (1964). A study of hearing in advanced age. *Laryngoscope*, *74*, 205–220.

Konigsmark, B. W., & Murphy, E. A. (1972). Volume of the ventral cochlear nucleus in man: Its relationship to neuronal population and age. *Journal of Neuropathology and Experimental Neurology*, *31*, 304–316.

Mayer, P. (1919–1920). Das anatomische Substrat der Altersschwerhorigkeit. *Arch Ohren Nasen Kehlkopfheilkd*, *105*, 1–13.

Nadol, J. B., Jr. (1979). Electron microscopic findings in presbycusic degeneration of the basal turn of the human cochlea. *Otolaryngol Head Neck Surgery*, *87*, 818–836.

Nadol, J. B., Jr. (1980). The aging peripheral hearing mechanisms. In D. S. Beasley & G. A. Davis (Eds.), *Aging communication processes and disorders* (pp. 63–85). New York: Grune & Stratton.

Nomura, Y. (1970). Lipidosis of the basilar membrane. *Acta Otolaryngologica* (Stockholm), *69*, 352–357.

Norre, M. E., Forrez, G., & Beckers, A. (1987). Vestibular dysfunction causing instability in aged patients. *Acta Otolaryngologica* (Stockholm), *104*, 50–55.

Pauler, M., Schuknecht, H. F., & Thornton, A. R. (1986). Correlative studies of cochlear neuronal loss with speech discrimination and pure-tone thresholds. *Archives of Otorhinolaryngology*, *243*, 200–206.

Pauler, M., Schuknecht, H. F., & White, J. A. (1988). Atrophy of the stria vascularis as a cause of sensorineural hearing loss. *Laryngoscope 98*, 754–759.

Peterka, R. J., Black, F. O., Newell, C. D., & Schoenhoff, M. B. (1987). Age-related changes in human vestibulocular and vestibulospinal reflex. *Association for Research in Otolaryngology Abstracts*, *10*, 112.

Raafat, S. A., Linthicum, F. H., Jr., & Terr, L. I. (1987). Quantitative study of lipofuscin accumulation in ganglion cells of the cochlea. *Association for Research in Otolaryngology Abstracts*, *10*, 205.

Richter, E. (1980). Quantitative study of human Scarpa's ganglion and vestibular sensory epithelia. *Acta Otolaryngologica* (Stockholm), *90*, 199–208.

Rosenhall, U. (1972a). Mapping of the cristae ampullares in man. *Annals of Otology, Rhinology and Laryngology, 81*, 882–889.

Rosenhall, U. (1972b). Vestibular macular mapping in man. *Annals of Otology, Rhinology and Laryngology, 81*, 339–351.

Rosenhall, U. (1973). Degenerative patterns in the aging human vestibular neuro-epithelia. *Acta Otolaryngologica* (Stockholm), *79*, 208–220.

Rosenhall, U., & Rubin, W. (1975). Degenerative changes in the human vestibular sensory epithelia. *Acta Orolaryngologica* (Stockholm), *79*, 67–80.

Ross, M. D., Peacor, D., Johnsson, L. G., & Allard, L. F. (1976). Observations on normal and degenerating human otoconia. *Annals of Otology, Rhinology and Laryngology, 85*, 310–326.

Schuknecht, H. F. (1955). Presbycusis. *Laryngoscope, 65*, 402–419.

Schuknecht, H. F. (1964). Further observations on the pathology of presbycusis. *Archives of Otolaryngology, 80*, 369–382.

Schuknecht, H. F. (1974). *Pathology of the ear.* Cambridge, MA: Harvard University Press.

Schuknecht, H. F., Igarashi, M., & Gacek, R. R. (1965). The pathological types of cochleo-saccular degeneration. *Acta Otolaryngologica* (Stockholm), *59*, 154–170.

Schuknecht, H. F., & Ishii, T. (1966). Hearing loss caused by atrophy of the stria vascularis. *Japanese Journal of Otology* (Tokyo), *69*, 1825–1833.

Soucek, S., Michaels, L., & Frohlich, A. (1987). Pathological changes in the organ of Corti in presbycusis as revealed by microslicing and staining. *Acta Otolaryngologica* (Stockholm), *436* (Suppl.), 93–102.

Spoendlin, H. (1970). Auditory, vestibular, olfactory and gustatory organs. In A. Bischoff (Ed.), *Ultrastructure of the peripheral nervous system and sense organs: Atlas of normal and pathologic anatomy* (pp. 173–337). St. Louis, MO: Mosby.

Stern-Padovan, R., & Vukičevic, S. (1980). Histologic changes in the aging spiral tract. *Journal of Laryngology and Otology, 94*, 255–262.

Suga, F., & Lindsay, J. R. (1976). Histopathological observations of presbycusis. *Annals of Otology, Rhinology and Laryngology, 85*, 169–184.

Sun, G. Y., Schroeder, F., Williamson, L. S., Gorka, C., Sun, A. Y., & Wood, W. G. (1988). Dolichols: Their role in neuronal membrane aging. In R. Strong, W. G. Wood, & W. J. Burke (Eds.), *Central nervous system disorders of aging: Clinical intervention and research* (pp. 223–234). New York: Raven Press.

Wall III, C., Black, F. O., & Hunt, A. E. (1984). Effects of age, sex and stimulus parameters upon vestibulo-ocular responses to sinusoidal rotation. *Acta Otolaryngologica* (Stockholm), *98*, 270–278.

Welsh, L. W., Welsh, J. J., & Healy, M. P. (1985). Central presbycusis. *Laryngoscope, 95*, 128–136.

Psychological and Social Aspects of Aging

SECTION

Marie R. Haug, PhD ■

Communication is a social process, involving at least two parties in some type of interaction. Thus, a set of chapters on the contributions of social science to understanding the process, with implications for the treatment of communication disabilities, is particularly appropriate. Represented are various specialties in psychology, as well as sociology, social work, and speech-language pathology.

The chapter by Schear, a clinical neuropsychologist, and Skenes, a speech-language pathologist, comes first in this section because it clarifies for the reader just what is involved in treating elderly persons whose communication abilities are impaired. Discussing in detail the similarities and differences between the training, roles, and responsibilities of the disciplines represented by the authors sets the stage for understanding the issues that arise when the patient is elderly. A major cross-cutting consideration is the distinction as well as the link between diagnosis and treatment, concerning which the convergences and divergences between the skills of the two disciplines are graphically outlined.

With respect to both diagnosis and planning of treatment, assessment is a critical step. While the chapter shows that evaluation procedures in each of the professions are similar in using a multidimensional approach, assessment practices vary between them. Selection of test batteries depends on the investigator's domain of interest, but as the conceptual models in the chapter show, there is much overlap along with distinct areas of expertise. The focus of the discussion of assessment is on the communication problems of geriatric patients with dementia.

The succeeding chapter by Dunkle, a social worker, and Kart, a sociologist, expands on the social characteristics of the elderly patient that affect both identification of problems and rehabilitation efforts. It provides in rich detail basic demographic data relevant to care. Among significant issues that Dunkle and Kart elaborate are living arrangements, marital situations, economic resources, and the general health status of the aged patient. Transitions between roles, such as those between worker and retiree or married person and widow or widower, are among the sources of stress that affect communication rehabilitation, particularly if the changes are unexpected or "off-time." These transitions may produce modifications in the availability of social support, which is often essential to successful therapy.

Dunkle and Kart also address assessment, but in their context they discuss evaluation in terms of the social assets and deficits of the patient. They propose use of an "eco-map," which identifies and diagrams the people and resources in the older person's environment. The very preparation of such an eco-map can be a therapeutic experience for the patient as well as a source of information leading to successful professional treatment.

In Hubbard's chapter on mental health and aging, he highlights areas of mental health, emotional well-being, and functional psychological problems in old age that are also critical for successful clinical practice. A major contribution of his chapter is his explanation of the concept of age-cohort; this is a factor that is often overlooked in references to "the elderly," a term which implies that all persons of advanced years are alike. In fact, as Hubbard shows, old people who were born in different historical periods vary in experiences and attitudes and attribute varying meanings both to their communication deficits and to professional therapies.

Although he raises questions about the validity of the notion of "normal aging," Hubbard delineates various conceptual schemes that have been advanced concerning satisfactory psychological adjustment in later years, with special attention to the "Five R's": review, reconciliation, relevance, respect, and release. A set of guidelines for clinicians working with older adults who are experiencing emotional problems provides useful clues to successful treatment, particularly with respect to age-cohort differences. A companion chart outlines psychological themes related to an illness experience, focusing on the fear of loss of autonomy and control over the environment. A final group of recommendations suggests methods of motivating geriatric patients to carry out the learning tasks required by communication rehabilitation. The chapter concludes with a review of the implications for practice of the stresses often experienced by the elderly in connection with two common mental health conditions, depression and anxiety. The problem of differentiating depression from dementia is only one of the challenges to clinicians. Another is disentangling somatization of the anxious from actual physical problems, differentiating overreporting from underreporting.

Lawton, in his chapter, picks up the theme of the elder's desire for autonomy and control, but he notes that there is a dialectic between the need for control and the need for support. Support comes essentially from transactions between persons and their environments, the topic of the chapter. He introduces two concepts, *proxemics*, or spatial behavior as a form of communication, and *kinesics*, or the use of body movement to send messages to another.

Focusing on the ways in which the environment is involved in these communication processes, Lawton emphasizes the importance of cohort rather than age differences and stresses the central role played by familiarity with the environment. Sensory losses also impinge on the encoding and decoding of the environment by the older individual, as when the individual misreads the meaning of another's physical proximity in a social or treatment situation. Sensory deprivation caused by failing eyesight and hearing may also alter the symbolic meanings of kinesics. For instance, the therapeutic significance of touch may be enhanced by the diminution of other senses. Environmental psychology also emphasizes behavioral design, with reference to both privacy and territoriality. The way in which people personalize their dwellings and exhibit treasured possessions sends messages to others in the environment. The implication of these issues for successful therapy is outlined not only in terms of proxemic and kinesic perspectives, but also in terms of the structure of the physical environment, such as the clinical setting or the elder's living space.

In the final chapter of this section, Clark, a speech-language pathologist (SLP), builds a case for provision of services by SLPs to families of communicatively impaired Alzheimer's patients. Through profiling the variety of caregivers of Alzheimer's patients and discussing the multiple effects of this disease, she points out the complexity of intervention issues with this population. A review of the literature addressing the effects of communication problems on caregiver burden further supports the need for family education and intervention in this area. The final section of this chapter focuses on an approach to education, communication, stress management, and counseling for caregivers. Traditional speech-language therapy has dealt directly with the patient. However, in the case of Alzheimer's patients, providing indirect intervention with the caregiver may improve the quality of life for both the family and the patient.

The message transmitted by these five chapters, in a richness of detail that cannot be adequately captured in this brief introduction, is the heterogeneity of older adults. Those who overlook cohort distinctions, sensory variations, social situation differences, emotional dissimilarities, or environmental issues run the risk of therapeutic ineffectiveness.

The Interface Between Clinical Neuropsychology and Speech-Language Pathology in the Assessment of the Geriatric Patient

James M. Schear, PhD, and Linda L. Skenes, PhD ■

The bedrock of professional services offered by clinical neuropsychologists and speech-language pathologists is the rich array of assessment procedures developed by both disciplines. Indeed, several of the tests used in both areas have been authored by both clinical neuropsychologists and speech-language pathologists. Yet the professional literature has not devoted much attention to the working relationship between the two disciplines. Although introductory texts used in both fields sometimes give definitions of what each discipline offers (see Brookshire, 1986; Darby, 1985; Kolb & Wishaw, 1985; Lezak, 1983), these presentations are often too brief (if they are presented at all) or are limited in imparting practical information about the interrelationship between the disciplines. One noteworthy exception is a chapter by Porch and Haaland (1984) in which they discussed assessment and treatment of the adult aphasic patient. These authors (one a speech-language pathologist and the other a clinical neuropsychologist) provided an approach to assessment based on their own experience, expertise, and clinical setting. They suggested that both disciplines are generally ill prepared for interprofessional work and often tend to duplicate efforts, adopt a competitive stance, and, as a result, end up neglecting important information that could benefit their patients' rehabilitation. Porch and Haaland (1984) suggested that clinical neuropsychologists and speech-language pathologists can form a gratifying

This chapter is supported, in part, by a Veterans Administration Medical Research Service Grant awarded to the first author.

The authors wish to express their appreciation to Christopher Hertzog for his helpful comments on an earlier draft of the chapter.

Correspondence to the first author should be addressed to Suite A, Building C, 3515 Wheeler Road, Augusta, GA 30909.

partnership in their work serving brain-impaired patients.

The present chapter will discuss the interdisciplinary relationship between clinical neuropsychologists and speech-language pathologists in assessment of the geriatric patient. Some of the notions espoused by Porch and Haaland (1984) will be expanded upon, and information will be provided about the ways in which these two disciplines can bring unique expertise to the problems of elderly patients who suffer from brain disorders that require both neuropsychological and speech-language pathology services. First, the education and training of clinical neuropsychologists and speech-language pathologists will be discussed. Assessment approaches in each discipline will be addressed to provide an understanding of the convergences and divergences of each discipline in assessment. A discussion of issues in assessment of the elderly patient, with a focus on dementia, will be offered as an illustration of how each discipline may participate in diagnosis and intervention with patients, families, and caregivers. Two conceptual models of assessment and of professional functions or roles will then be provided, followed by a brief discussion of psychometric issues in tests and measurement in the two disciplines. A final section will be devoted to special considerations for testing the geriatric patient.

Education and Clinical Training

The Clinical Neuropsychologist

Over the past 15 years, clinical neuropsychologists have attempted to delineate the basic education, training, and experience necessary for them to hold themselves out to the public as a profession. Meier (1974, 1981, 1983) has been one of the most consistent spokespersons for this initiative. In 1979, the International Neuropsychological

Society (INS) and the Division of Clinical Neuropsychology (Division 40) of the American Psychological Association (APA) Task Force was formed and charged to develop guidelines for education, accreditation, and credentialing of clinical neuropsychologists. This group eventually published guidelines for the training and experience of clinical neuropsychologists (Meier, 1981). Present standards for defining such education and training, at the doctoral, internship, and postdoctoral levels, have been described as "guidelines" and are included in the Reports of the INS–Division 40 Task Force on Education, Accreditation, and Credentialing (INS/APA, 1987).

In August 1988, the executive committee of Division 40 provided a definition of a clinical neuropsychologist as

> [a] professional psychologist who applies principles of assessment and intervention based upon scientific study of human behavior as it relates to normal and abnormal functioning of the central nervous system. The Clinical Neuropsychologist is a doctoral-level psychology provider of diagnostic and intervention services who has demonstrated competence in the application of such principles for human welfare following:
>
> A. Successful completion of systematic didactic and experiential training in neuropsychology and neuroscience at a regionally accredited university;
>
> B. Two or more years of appropriate supervised training applying neuropsychological services in a clinical setting;
>
> C. Licensing and certification to provide psychological services to the public by the laws of the state or province in which he or she practices;
>
> D. Review by one's peers as a test of these competencies. (Statement of Executive Committee of Division 40, 1989)

An official statement of the executive committee of Division 40 also indicates that the attainment of the diploma offered jointly by the American Board of Clinical Neuropsychology (ABCN) and the American Board of Professional Psychology (ABPP) represents the clearest evidence of competence. At the present time, however, the vast majority of practicing clinical neuropsychologists do not hold such an ABCN/ABPP diploma; this is also true for the other specialty boards of the ABPP (clinical, counseling, school, and industrial-organizational). At this time, specialization in the practice of psychology is still a matter of considerable discussion—some believe that there are today *no* bona fide specialties but rather ''unique proficiencies'' in the practice of applied psychology (Matarazzo, 1988).

The Speech-Language Pathologist

Speech-language pathology has its roots in many professions, including neurology, psychology, education, and linguistics. The first national organization of people interested in speech disorders was formed in 1925. After several name changes, the group adopted the title of The American Speech-Language-Hearing Association (ASHA) in 1978.

A speech-language pathologist is a trained professional who evaluates and treats communication disorders. Most speech-language pathologists either hold the Certificate of Clinical Competence (CCC-Sp) or are working to obtain it. The CCC-Sp is awarded by ASHA to those individuals who meet certain standards. The following revised standards become effective for applications for certification postmarked on January 1, 1993, and thereafter:

1. A master's or doctoral degree. Effective January 1, 1994, all graduate coursework and clinical practicum must have been completed at an institution accredited in speech-language pathology by ASHA's Educational Standards Board.

2. Seventy-five credit hours reflecting a well-integrated program of study pertaining to (a) the biological, physical, and mathematical sciences; (b) the normal aspects of human behavior and communication; and (c) the nature, evaluation, and treatment of speech, language, and hearing disorders.

3. Three hundred seventy-five clock hours of supervised clinical observation and clinical practicum.

4. A passing score on the National Examination in Speech-Language Pathology.

5. A clinical fellowship that consists of at least 36 weeks of full-time professional experience or its part-time equivalent and that must be completed under the supervision of an individual who holds the CCC-Sp (American Speech-Language-Hearing Association, 1989a).

While the master's degree is recognized as the minimum clinical standard by ASHA, there has been considerable discussion in the field about the clinical doctorate becoming the minimum standard for clinical practice. The issue is complex and there are many pros and cons on each side of the argument. It is not the purpose of this chapter to debate this complex issue. The interested reader can find a discussion of the issues in regard to the clinical doctorate in Aronson (1987) and Spriestersbach (1989).

The different levels of training can and do have an impact on the relationship between clinical neuropsychologists and speech-language pathologists. Yet the actual working partnership in patient care is ultimately borne by the individual professionals and is based upon their academic training and clinical experience. Some clinical neuropsychologists receive extensive training and experience in speech-language disorders while others receive much less training and supervised clinical experience. Similarly, speech-language pathologists vary in academic and clinical exposure to neuropsychology as a discipline, as well as to clinical neuropsychologists.

For clinical neuropsychologists the APA *Ethical Principles of Psychologists* (American Psychological Association, 1981a) indicate that competence is critical when holding oneself out to the public as a psychologist practitioner. There are a number of APA publications dealing with these ethical guidelines (American Psychological Association, 1981a) and guidelines for delivery of psychological services (American Psychological Association, 1981b, 1987). Speech-language pathologists are similarly bound by a code of ethics (American Speech-Language-Hearing Association, 1989a).

Ultimately, it remains the responsibility of each practitioner to arrive at the best understanding of the division of duties in assessment and treatment based on his or her own competence and clinical setting. Recently, representatives of Division 40 of the American Psychological Association and an ad hoc committee on interpersonal relationships with neuropsychology of the American Speech-Language-Hearing Association drafted a statement regarding usage of the term *neuropsychology* as applied to each discipline. The following statement was adopted by both Division 40 and the American Speech-Language-Hearing Association:

> Neuropsychology is the scientific study of the relationship between brain function and behavior. As such, neuropsychology, in the generic sense, is an interdisciplinary knowledge area embracing many contributing disciplines and professions. Therefore, it is inappropriate that the knowledge base of neuropsychology be regarded as proprietary by any given discipline or profession.
>
> It is acknowledged that this knowledge base may be applied for the betterment of human welfare by different disciplines and professions with different training emphases. It is assumed that such practice will include techniques and procedures included in discipline-specific training and exclude those for which competence has not been established through such training criteria. Individual practice may also be limited by laws or even ethical considerations in a given instance. It is also recognized that clin-

ical practice with individuals who demonstrate impairment of the central nervous system is frequently an interdisciplinary effort which employs the particular strengths and expertise of various professions and disciplines. Cooperation and mutual respect between professions and disciplines which employ the knowledge base of neuropsychology is encouraged in patient treatment. This is the most appropriate way to ensure the welfare of the patient, which is always the first priority.

> Various techniques and applications of neuropsychology may not be mutually exclusive between professions. However, it is also recognized that different legal jurisdictions impose different limits on the scope of practice of the professions. These limits include educational requirements, training experience, and the designation and description of professional practice.

> All relevant disciplines and professions should contribute to the expanding knowledge base of neuropsychology and to its appropriate applications in patient care. Given the interdisciplinary history of the development of neuropsychology, mutual respect and cooperation between disciplines and professions is an ongoing necessity. (American Psychological Association, 1990; American Speech-Language-Hearing Association, 1990)

In the next section, an attempt is made to clarify some of the areas where clinical neuropsychologists and speech-language pathologists converge and diverge in assessment of the geriatric patient.

Assessment Approaches: Convergences and Divergences

It is probably safe to say that clinical neuropsychologists have been more concerned with diagnostic issues (Alfano & Finlayson, 1987; Diller & Gordon, 1981b), whereas speech-language pathologists have concentrated more on treatment (Brookshire, 1986). This trend has changed in the past several years with clinical neuropsychologists becoming more active in rehabilitation (Meier, Benton, & Diller, 1987), even though some neuropsychologists have engaged in rehabilitation service delivery and research for many years (e.g., Diller & Gordon, 1981a, 1981b). Similarly, speech-language pathologists have actively attempted to advance their work by refining and expanding speech and language assessment procedures (Goodglass & Kaplan, 1972, 1983; Porch, 1967; Schuell, 1965, 1972). Attempts also have been made to make tests of communication ecologically valid by assessing patients' competencies in performing common everyday living tasks (e.g., Holland, 1980; Sarno, 1969).

While clinical neuropsychologists assess overall language skills, a speech-language evaluation usually involves more extensive investigation of communication abilities. A clinical neuropsychologist may administer the *Boston Diagnostic Aphasia Examination* (Goodglass & Kaplan, 1972, 1983), for example, and may even diagnose the type of aphasia, but it is usually the speech-language pathologist who comprehensively describes the communication disorder and sets up a rehabilitation plan aimed at improving communication. This is especially true in the case where the primary deficit is a receptive or expressive speech/language disorder. Clinical neuropsychologists often gather information about anomia, verbal fluency, memory, and paraphasic errors, as does a speech-language pathologist. However, a speech-language pathologist may perform more extensive assessment of expressive language by observing and defining the extent of the aphasic, dysarthric, or apraxic (verbal) impairment. Thus, in the case of the patient with a primary speech and language disorder, both the clinical neuropsychologist and the speech-language pathologist offer diagnostic and treatment data. The clinical neuropsychologist may offer the overall neurobehavioral profile and assess the impact of cognitive and higher adaptive functions on speech and/or language abilities. The speech-language pathologist provides detailed data about the primary speech-language disorders, which may offer important information about their impact on other cognitive and higher adaptive functions, as well as suggesting effective ways to enhance communication with the patient. It is in this context that both sets of data can enrich the clinically useful information about the patient's functional strengths and weaknesses that must be considered in formulating and instituting a rehabilitation plan.

The information gathered by the clinical neuropsychologist may be used by the speech-language pathologist and vice versa. For example, a clinical neuropsychological assessment may determine that in addition to speech-language deficits, the patient also exhibits other higher cognitive and emotional deficits. These additional deficits may adversely affect progress in treatment. Depression can significantly disrupt the therapeutic alliance and represent an obstacle to performing within and outside the treatment or rehabilitation session. Similarly, performance on neuropsychological test batteries can be affected by communication deficits. Impaired language skills can and do decrease performance on verbal mediated tests of cognitive and emotional abilities.

In the same way, speech and language skills must be interpreted in light of cognitive skills. An acquired general cerebral dysfunction can adversely affect the speed and agility of speech and language functions. Similarly, if a patient has a fourth-grade education and a lower level of premorbid intellectual functioning, speech and language abilities must be interpreted accordingly. Thus, decreased performance on difficult receptive and expressive language tasks may have been present premorbidly and may not represent a decline in language skills. The speech-language pathologist will compare responses on communication tests to premorbid functioning by gathering reports and samples of prior communication abilities from family members to determine if, in fact, a change in communication skills has occurred as well as to determine whether the decline was sudden or gradual.

Assessment Practices Shared by Both Disciplines

Assessment practices shared by both disciplines include acquiring in-depth information along a number of dimensions. In the geropsychology and neuropsychology assessment literature, this approach has been referred to as "multidimensional" (Gallagher, Thompson, & Levy, 1980; Hertzog & Schear, 1989; Lezak, 1984; Schear, 1984). A multidimensional approach to assessment simply means that the professionals systematically obtain information about the patient from a number of sources in order to become fully acquainted with the case. This information is obtained by examining the medical history, gathering information about the patient's educational and work experience, interviewing family members and/or caregivers, studying the patient's current treatment including chemotherapy regimens, and obtaining information about the findings of other allied health service providers who have been consulted about the patient's status, such as professionals in audiology, occupational therapy, physical therapy, and neurology. Information gathering of this type is accomplished by reviewing the patient's medical records as well as by conducting interviews with the patient and family. There are several excellent articles, chapters, and edited books in the neuropsychology and speech-language pathology literature that have addressed these issues in regard to the geriatric patient (see Albert, 1981, 1988a, 1988b; Albert & Kaplan, 1980; Albert & Moss, 1988; Beasley & Davis, 1981; Kaszniak, 1987a, 1987b; Obler & Albert, 1980; Schear, 1984). Some comprehensive tests of language function are administered by both clinical neuropsychologists and speech-language pathologists. Based on the constraints of this chapter, we will not discuss these test batteries in detail; instead, we recommend that the interested reader obtain the primary source material (see Brookshire, 1986; Davis, 1983; Emerick & Hatten, 1979; Goodglass & Kaplan, 1983; Porch, 1967; Schuell, 1965).

Assessment Practices in Speech-Language Pathology

Speech-language pathologists assess a patient's communicative skills at a given point in time. Assessment includes delineating the communication impairment in regard to the nature, extent, and type of disorder. A profile of strengths and weaknesses is included along with pragmatic information about how the speech-language impairment will affect communication with others. In addition, the test results serve as a baseline for developing a treatment plan. Family members, significant others, and health care staff are often counseled about ways to improve communication with the patient. Language skills represent one domain in a comprehensive set of behaviors that can disrupt the patient's overall functioning. Interaction may exist between the various domains affected by cerebral dysfunction depending, for example, upon whether symptoms accompany a cerebral vascular accident or represent symptoms of a progressive dementing illness.

Assessment protocols in speech-language pathology vary according to the etiology of the communication deficit and the patient's level of cognitive and speech-language abilities. Most speech and language test batteries for adult geriatric patients are designed to comprehensively explore the four language areas assessed more generally by clinical neuropsychologists and discussed in the next section of this chapter. These four language domains are phonology, lexicon, semantics, and syntax (Albert, 1988b). Most speech and language tests include combinations of the following tasks: automatic speech (e.g., reciting the days of the week, months of the year), object naming, picture naming, matching pictures to printed words, word and phrase repetition, answering printed and spoken questions, pointing to objects and/or pictures, following written and verbal commands, reading aloud, reading and answering questions, writing, and performing simple arithmetic problems (Brookshire,

1986). A spontaneous language sample is essential.

Of utmost importance to geriatric patients is assessment and description of functional communication. Functional communication can be assessed formally with test batteries such as the *Functional Communication Profile* (*FCP*) (Sarno, 1969) or by the more recently developed *Communicative Abilities in Daily Living* (*CADL*) (Holland, 1980). While most tests are laboratory procedures that geriatric patients frequently find offensive, the *FCP* allows the patient to be tested in a familiar environment. Similarly, the *CADL* battery attempts to evaluate communication skills by structuring typical daily tasks and assessing the functional adequacy of responses. Functional communication skills can also be assessed informally by an experienced clinician who studies the patient's orientation, comprehension, verbal expression, speech intelligibility, reading, and writing in a less structured, more flexible atmosphere.

The difference between functional communication and linguistic performance on a standardized test of speech-language skills can be significant. By design, most aphasia tests attempt to minimize social and environmental cues and to elicit a response in a specific modality of communication, such as speech or writing. Communicatively impaired patients may communicate quite well in a less structured environment where social and environmental cues are present and where they can respond in the communication modalities in which they are most able.

Assessment Practices in Clinical Neuropsychology

There are a wide variety of approaches to assessment in clinical neuropsychology that differ primarily on the basis of the tests selected for use in assessment (for a discussion of some of the differences in these neuropsychological assessment approaches see Grant & Adams, 1986; Incagnoli, Goldstein, & Golden, 1986; Logue & Schear, 1984). The various assessment methods in clinical neuropsychology are not only related to the specific test procedures adopted by the clinical neuropsychologists; the inferential process for interpreting the data in case formulation also may differ (see Christensen, 1984; Lezak, 1984; Milberg, Hebben, & Kaplan, 1986; Reitan & Wolfson, 1985; and Schear, 1984, for illustrations of these varied inferential methods). In general, most clinical neuropsychologists are interested in sampling such neurobehavioral domains as attention and concentration; learning and memory; sensory-perceptual abilities; motor functioning; visuospatial ability; constructional abilities; speech and language abilities; mood and affect; personality; and higher-order executive functions including abstract reasoning, conceptualization, and mental flexibility. In assessing the elderly patient, clinical neuropsychologists conduct both screening and comprehensive evaluations depending upon whether the assessment is going to be used to respond to general or specific diagnostic questions; provide a baseline for longitudinal surveillance; and make recommendations for treatment, rehabilitation, and/or management of the patient.

Albert (1988b), for example, represents an approach in geriatric neuropsychology that examines language functions in a comprehensive manner. Language functions are considered to encompass at least four domains—phonology, lexicon, syntax, and semantic knowledge. The literature suggests that each of these four domains can be adversely affected by a dementing illness. In normal aging, phonological knowledge, lexical ability, and syntax are well preserved, although when the task imposes a significant memory demand on syntax, age-related decrements are found. Also, verbal fluency and performance on confrontation naming decrease with increasing age, but usually not until after the age of 70 (see Albert, 1988b, and Bayles & Kaszniak, 1987, for a good review and detailed discussion of these studies).

In clinical neuropsychological assessment, speech and language abilities are one of many domains assessed in the testing session. The interaction of deficits in speech and language with other domains must be understood in order to achieve diagnostic accuracy. In other words, if an elderly patient is exhibiting problems in comprehending speech secondary to an aphasic disorder associated with a recent cerebral vascular accident, then the tests in the neuropsychological battery that rely upon intact verbal functions will need to be either abandoned, postponed, or interpreted differently. Thus, many of the verbal mediated tests that are used to assess conceptualization, for example, will be significantly affected by the aphasic patient's deficits in the speech and language system as a function of both auditory comprehension and oral production deficits. On a practical level, Porch and Haaland (1984) suggest that it is inappropriate for either speech-language pathologists or clinical neuropsychologists to address the areas covered by the other discipline. The difficulty lies in achieving the proper balance based on the individual professionals involved and the clinical setting. The professional environment is quite variable depending upon whether the clinical neuropsychologists and speech-language pathologists are working in an institutional setting or in independent practice in the community.

Conceptual Models for Assessment and Professional Functions

The models presented in this section are *working* models that can and should be modified depending on factors addressed earlier in this chapter that pertain to the clinical competence of the individual professionals involved, the clinical setting, and the needs of the individual patient. These models, therefore, are *one* conceptualization of a working alliance between clinical neuropsychology and speech-language pathology in regard to assessment and professional

functions. In the final analysis, the individual practitioners themselves must consider how they should modify the model to optimize patient care.

Model of Assessment Domains by Discipline

In Figure 4.1, we propose that the individual assessment domains in clinical neuropsychology and speech-language pathology be seen as both overlapping and unique to each discipline.

The primary assessment domains shown in the figure are connected by boldface lines with the discipline. However, some domains are assessed by both disciplines. It should be noted that it is very often the case that the clinical neuropsychologist will assess speech and language functions in a general way, whereas assessment of speech and language functions by the speech-language pathologist usually will be more comprehensive, allowing for a greater in-depth analysis of the patient's communication strengths and weaknesses. Similarly, the speech-language pathologist may examine mental status, including attention, concentration, and orientation, whereas the clinical neuropsychologist will gather considerable information about the integrity of attention by determining whether the deficits are caused by various components such as sustained attention, selective attention, or attentional capacity (Albert, 1988b). Thus, although there is overlap in a variety of areas, the depth of the assessment varies according to the discipline conducting the assessment. In the case where the speech-language pathologist identifies problems in mental status and suspects compromised intellectual functioning, the clinical neuropsychologist will comprehensively assess these areas. In the same way, where the clinical neuropsychologist may identify aphasia, the speech-language pathologist will comprehensively assess speech and language functions and precisely describe the aphasic disturbance. Assessment domains in Figure 4.1 that are connected by fine lines

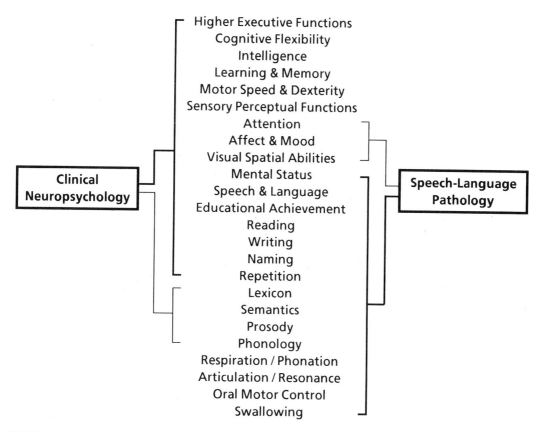

FIGURE 4.1. Conceptual model of assessment domains by discipline.

to the disciplines are possible areas of competence for individual professionals based on their academic training and clinical experience.

Model of Professional Functions by Discipline

It is also important to consider assessment in the context of the role or function each discipline plays in providing services to the patient. In the case of clinical neuropsychology and speech-language pathology, we suggest certain professional functions or roles, shown in Figure 4.2, which again can be seen as overlapping and unique and which depend on the factors noted previously.

In Figure 4.2, the professional functions of each discipline are again separated by

their primary responsibilities in assessment and intervention. There is, of course, overlap in regard to treatment and intervention, especially in regard to the family and attending staff. The speech-language pathologist is always concerned with optimizing the quality of the communication interaction between the patient and others. An important role, then, for the speech-language pathologist is to interpret the results of the speech-language evaluation for the patient, family, and staff. Here the intervention involves describing the patient's strengths and weaknesses in an effort not only to improve communication, but also to contribute to the intervention that is aimed at improving speech and language functions in the patient. The clinical neuropsychologist is involved with the patient, family, and attending staff in a similar way. He or she explains the results of

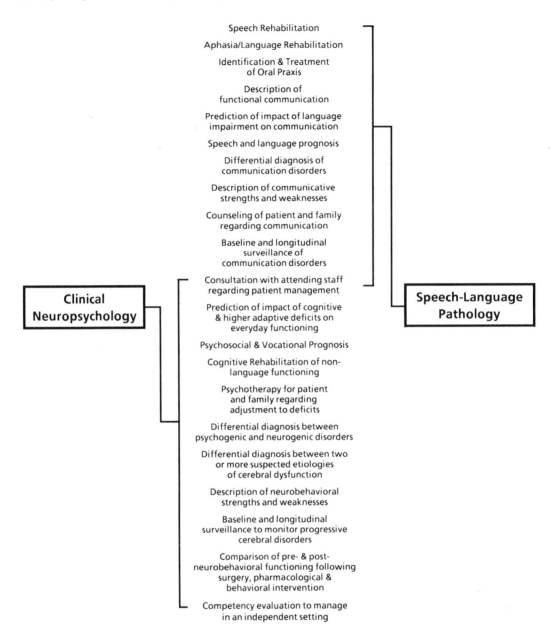

Speech Rehabilitation

Aphasia/Language Rehabilitation

Identification & Treatment
of Oral Praxis

Description of
functional communication

Prediction of impact of language
impairment on communication

Speech and language prognosis

Differential diagnosis of
communication disorders

Description of communicative
strengths and weaknesses

Counseling of patient and family
regarding communication

Baseline and longitudinal
surveillance of
communication disorders

Consultation with attending staff
regarding patient management

Prediction of impact of cognitive
& higher adaptive deficits on
everyday functioning

Psychosocial & Vocational Prognosis

Cognitive Rehabilitation of nonlanguage functioning

Psychotherapy for patient
and family regarding
adjustment to deficits

Differential diagnosis between
psychogenic and neurogenic disorders

Differential diagnosis between two
or more suspected etiologies
of cerebral dysfunction

Description of neurobehavioral
strengths and weaknesses

Baseline and longitudinal
surveillance to monitor progressive
cerebral disorders

Comparison of pre- & post-
neurobehavioral functioning following
surgery, pharmacological &
behavioral intervention

Competency evaluation to manage
in an independent setting

**Clinical
Neuropsychology**

**Speech-Language
Pathology**

FIGURE 4.2. Conceptual model of professional functions by discipline.

the neuropsychological assessment in terms of the patient's neurobehavioral strengths and weaknesses and describes the nature of the deficits and the suspected course of the disorder. It is often the case that the family and attending staff must know how certain behaviors are related to the brain disorder and how these behaviors will affect adjustment and adaptation. Family members need factual information about the patient's neurobehavioral profile in language that is understandable and devoid of professional jargon. They also frequently need time to adjust and accommodate to changes; short-term interventions can have a significant impact on adjustment and management. Both the speech-language pathologist and the clinical neuropsychologist provide important data about the nature, extent, type, and prognosis of the brain disorder and its impact on communication and neuropsychological functions.

Interrelationships Between the Disciplines

The interrelationship between clinical neuropsychologists and speech-language pathologists in the clinical setting can be fostered by specific actions by members of each discipline. Porch and Haaland (1984) have suggested ways to achieve good working relationships. First, they suggest that clinical neuropsychologists and speech-language pathologists learn about each other by contacting each other and *actively* discussing what they do, how they do it, what their skill level is, and what their knowledge is about the other discipline. Second, Porch and Haaland suggest that once contact is established, such an exchange should be ongoing, preferably on a regular basis. Case conferences can be an effective way to foster communication and result in a practical outcome. Third, it is important to establish the responsibilities and domains for each discipline, depending upon the skill and training of the parties involved. Fourth, improvement of relations between the two disciplines should begin at the graduate training level, where coursework should be offered in each discipline's training program that outlines their convergences and divergences. It is also important in establishing working relationships for clinical neuropsychologists and speech-language pathologists to learn each others' "professional vocabulary" so that they can enhance cooperation and consultation in clinical practice.

Assessment of the Geriatric Patient

Clinical neuropsychologists and speech-language pathologists overlap in assessment of the dementia patient. It should be noted that there are a number of cases where clinical neuropsychologists and speech-language pathologists are involved in diagnosis and treatment of brain disorders and, although our focus in this section of the chapter will be on patients suffering from dementia, we would be remiss if we did not at least mention some of the other disorders in adulthood where both disciplines provide an important clinical service. Patients with head injury, cerebral vascular disease and stroke, multiple sclerosis, Huntington's chorea, Parkinson's disease, and such neuromuscular disorders as myasthenia gravis and amyotrophic lateral sclerosis, are potential candidates for assessment and rehabilitation by both speech-language pathologists and clinical neuropsychologists.

Diagnosis of Dementing Illnesses

Clinical neuropsychologists play an important role in the diagnosis of dementing illness. Often the neurobehavioral data are the first signs of dementia. The method for achieving a differential diagnosis among dementia, normal changes associated with advancing age, and depression is addressed best by the clinical neuropsychological evaluation (Kaszniak, 1987b; Poon, 1986). Indeed, the diagnosis of dementing illness using the criteria of the *Diagnostic and Statistical Manual of Mental Disorders III–Revised* (*DSM III-R*) (American Psychiatric Association, 1987) requires neurobehavioral data of the kind that are best achieved by a neuropsychological assessment. The range of behavioral deficits necessary for achieving a diagnosis of dementia according to the *DSM III-R* includes impaired abstract reasoning; impaired judgment; and evidence of aphasia, apraxia, and agnosia. These diagnostic signs are very much related to the domains assessed in the neuropsychological evaluation described earlier. It is important to ascertain whether the speech and language deficits are associated with dementia or an aphasic disorder. The role of the speech-language pathologist in the care of the demented patient is that of making diagnoses, monitoring communication deficits, and counseling patients and families (Bayles & Kaszniak, 1987). Collaboration between clinical neuropsychologists and speech-language pathologists is critical. While neuropsychological assessment and speech-language assessment overlap, a neuropsychological battery will include tests of attention, visual perception, motor skills, learning and memory, and abstraction and conceptualization, as well as speech and language tests of anomia, dysarthria, phonology, lexicon, syntax, and semantic knowledge; the speech-language assessment battery will include tests of orientation, auditory discrimination, auditory comprehension, reading comprehension, naming, writing, speech, and expressive language (including some of the areas listed for the neuropsychological battery). It should be obvious that there may be considerable overlap and redundancy in what is evaluated in each assessment. The purpose of assessment, however, differs. Clinical neuropsychologists are primarily interested in cognition and a variety of higher adaptive abilities, whereas speech-language pathologists are concerned primarily with communication and cognition as they affect communication. It is essential that the two disciplines work out a priori what each is going to do in assessment in order to eliminate unwarranted duplication or redundancy.

The role of the speech-language pathologist in assessment and treatment of the dementia patient depends upon a variety of circumstances. The speech-language pathologist is primarily responsible for the comprehensive assessment of the demented patient's communication skills, including comprehension, expressive language, speech, oral function, reading, and writing. Based on what we know about the patient suffering from Alzheimer's disease, for example, the patient may be a candidate for an assessment and may or may not be a candidate for speech-language intervention. At the same time, the families of patients suffering from Alzheimer's disease with manifest communication impairment often are candidates for speech-language counseling in order to learn ways of facilitating communication and to adjust their communicative expectations.

Differential Diagnosis of Dementia and Aphasia

Au, Albert, and Obler (1988) have suggested that the study of language disturbances resulting from brain damage is very much needed. These authors propose that a careful analysis of the speech and language profiles of various forms of dementing illness shows differential patterns of strengths and weaknesses that may aid in discovering how certain brain regions are affected across different illnesses as well as through the course of an illness. Furthermore, they suggest that language deficits that occur in dementia should be viewed as variations of aphasia to enhance the study of aphasia and dementia. Such an examination of speech and language functions may help in the development of more sophisticated brain-based theories of language.

In order to achieve accurate differential diagnosis of dementia patients and aphasic patients, Bayles and Kaszniak (1987) describe some basic assumptions and principles relative to clinical neuropsychology and speech-language pathology. First, contrary to the suggestions of Au et al. (1988), they point out that some speech-language pathologists are "uncomfortable" about calling the communication deficits of dementia patients "aphasia." Second, they suggest that in arriving at an accurate diagnosis, consideration must be given to both the causes and severity of the dementia or aphasia. As with all communication disorders, the best method for optimizing communication with dementia patients should be specified, and these data should be shared with caregivers. The *Arizona Battery for Communication Disorders of Dementia*

(Bayles & Kaszniak, 1987) is designed to differentially diagnose dementia and aphasia patients. Bayles and Kaszniak (1987) extensively discuss assessment of the dementia patient, as well as the responsibilities of clinical neuropsychologists and speech-language pathologists in the care of patients suffering from dementia. In brief, they suggest that sensory perception, receptive language, expressive language, and orientation and memory should be assessed. These authors also provide information for differentiating dementing disorders from aphasic disorders.

Differential Diagnosis of Dementia and Depression

A significant function in which the clinical neuropsychologist is involved is differential diagnosis of dementia and depression (see Caine, 1986; Hart, Kwentus, Wade, & Hamer, 1987; Heaton & Crowley, 1981; Wells, 1979; Wells & Duncan, 1980). Bayles and Kaszniak (1987) suggested from their review of the literature that some neuropsychological procedures can maximize the strength of a clinical diagnosis of dementia versus depression by using instruments like the *Mattis Dementia Rating Scale* (Mattis, 1976, 1988) and the *Comprehensive Assessment and Referral Evaluation* (*CARE*) (Gurland et al., 1977–1978). Gurland, Golden, and Challop (1982) have reported very highly accurate rates on the cognitive impairment and depression scales of the *CARE*. A recent report by McCue, Goldstein, and Shelly (1989) provides some empirical support for the utility of a short form of the *Luria Nebraska Neuropsychological Battery* (*LNNB*) (Golden, Hammeke, & Purisch, 1980) in making a differential diagnosis between Alzheimer's disease and major depression. Similarly, Hart, Kwentus, Wade, and Hamer (1987) have provided data in support of an incidental memory task for the Digit Symbol subtest from the *Wechsler Adult Intelligence Scale–Revised* (Wechsler, 1981) for differentiating mild dementia from depression. Although many advances have been made, there is still a need to replicate these findings and to improve tests in order to be able to make ecologically valid statements about how the identified deficits affect everyday living.

Psychometric Issues

Hertzog and Schear (1989) have described some of the issues that must be considered when examining the literature on tests used with elderly patients. They indicated that professionals must be intelligent users of tests and must be knowledgeable about the technical criteria for interpretation of the results. The technical standards for evaluating tests include validity (the test measures what it purports to measure); reliability (the test consistently measures the construct); background on test development and revision; and information about scores, scales, and norms. See the 1985 *Standards for Educational and Psychological Testing*, jointly authored by the American Educational Research Association, the American Psychological Association, and the National Council on Measurement in Education (American Educational Research Association, 1985). A fundamental part of the graduate training of clinical neuropsychologists and speech-language pathologists involves courses on tests and measurement as well as on the use of scores and scales in clinical assessment. The content of these courses is put to use every day in the work of interpreting test results. Moreover, in order to make good judgments in choosing the best tests to use, clinical neuropsychologists and speech-language pathologists must examine the technical and empirical evidence supporting the validity and reliability of the test procedures they employ in practice. Each professional has a responsibility to be current about developments regarding the test procedures employed in his or her field.

In clinical practice, a rule of thumb is that the test procedures that offer clear evidence of validity for their use with elderly populations are the best tests for each discipline to use. Each has a variety of test procedures at its disposal (see Brookshire, 1986; Davis, 1983; Lezak, 1983). However, a problem confronted by both professional groups is that validity studies in support of these tests for use with the elderly are still very limited. Most studies in neuropsychology and speech-language pathology are based on criterion-related validity. Few studies exist that examine construct validity. Furthermore, studies are needed to examine the relationship between test performance and everyday functioning. More validation work addressing these weaknesses is necessary. Clinicians very much need data that they can use with confidence in their clinical practice.

A separate but related concern involves test norms. Normative data for elderly populations are sparse. In neuropsychology, discussion about the need to develop norms based on "normal" aged people has been seriously considered only in the past decade (Benton, Eslinger, & Damasio, 1981; Kaszniak, 1987a, 1987b; Schear, 1984) even though it has been recognized as an important issue for a much longer time (Pauker, 1977; Reitan, 1973; Vega & Parson, 1967).

At present, several reports have appeared that provide the practitioner with cross-sectional normative data on some of the established tests such as the *Halstead-Reitan Neuropsychological Test Battery* (see Fromm-Auch & Yeudall, 1983; Heaton, Grant, & Matthews, 1986; Reitan, 1979; Reitan & Wolfson, 1985; Russell, 1988; Schear, 1984; Yeudall, Reddon, Gill, & Stefanyk, 1987). However, the need to select norms judiciously is very much warranted; many normative reports are restricted to particular patient subtypes, which limits generalizability. For example, many reports include normal, brain-damaged, psychiatric, and neuropsychiatric populations within the sample. It is not possible to use norms that include such a mix of patient subtypes when attempting to measure an individual patient's test performance. The individual may not represent the target patient population norms.

This problem also exists in speech-language pathology. Thorough normative data on aphasia tests are woefully inadequate. Of the major tests of aphasia, only the *CADL* (Holland, 1980) and the *Porch Index of Communicative Ability* (Porch, 1981) report a clear description of the sample for which norms were reported (Skenes & McCauley, 1985). In addition, the 1983 revision of the *Boston Diagnostic Aphasia Examination* (Goodglass & Kaplan, 1983) added appropriate normative data for most subtests and cited exceptions in performance for individuals 60 years old or over. The recently proposed *Arizona Battery for Communication Disorders of Dementia* (Bayles & Kaszniak, 1987) is an important development in assessment of the geriatric demented patient that deserves attention and that is likely to be enhanced by continued validation work.

It is impossible for a standardized test to include all of the specific psychometric characteristics needed for all patients and for all testing purposes (Messick, 1980). Test results must, therefore, be interpreted in light of the purpose for the testing, the test itself, and the test environment, as well as any patient characteristics that may influence assessment. For example, medical history, age, hearing loss, cognition, socioeconomic status, fatigue, and daily environment may influence a patient's performance during a testing session (Skenes & McCauley, 1985). These variables must be considered for each individual patient and for each assessment. Norms do not exist for every patient in every situation. Evaluation for competency to manage personal affairs requires a different approach to assessment and interpretation than does screening for a communication disorder.

A shared goal of the assessment of aphasia, dysarthria, apraxia, and dementia is to obtain a valid and reliable measurement of communication abilities. It is essential for the psychometric characteristics of a test battery to be evaluated by the clinician according to the purpose of the assessment, the tests to be employed, the testing environment, and patient variability, especially in communication skills. In the latter instance, a representative sample of these skills must then be obtained.

Special Considerations in Testing the Geriatric Patient

We contend that both clinical neuropsychology and speech-language pathology rely upon common clinical practices in assessment. The special case of the geriatric patient requires some additional considerations. There are several excellent sources in the literature that elucidate some of the factors that affect testing (see Aiken, 1980; Albert, 1988a; Beasley & Davis, 1981; Crook, 1979; Hertzog & Schear, 1989; Schear, 1984). We will not attempt to describe this literature in detail here but will restrict ourselves only to some of the most salient factors that are important in testing the geriatric patient.

Factors Adversely Affected by Increasing Age

Behavioral Slowing

A general slowing in behavior is by far one of the most fully demonstrated normative changes that occurs as a function of age (Salthouse, 1985). There has been considerable debate over how much and to what extent behavioral slowing affects test performance. While most of the cross-sectional norms of timed or speeded tests adjust for behavioral slowing, there is little evidence that provides explanations for the impact of, for example, motor speed on complex cognitive test performance. Some have suggested that it is necessary to assess the impact of processing speed on complex test performance because the literature suggests that there is a clear relationship between the

two (Hertzog, 1989; Hertzog & Schear, 1989; Horn, Donaldson, & Engstrom, 1981; Schear & Sato, 1989).

Vision

The literature on vision and aging suggests that there are a number of pathologies that can affect visual acuity of the elderly, including cataracts, glaucoma, and senile retinopathy (Kline & Schieber, 1985). The experimental literature suggests that increasing age results in a decrease in focusing power and a reduction in light sensitivity, image formation, color perception, resistance to glare, contrast sensitivity, and visual search and pattern recognition (Fozard, Wolf, Bell, McFarland, & Podolsky, 1977; Kosnik, Winslow, Kline, Rasinski, & Sekuler, 1988). Kosnik et al. (1988), for example, recently conducted a survey of healthy adults to examine the incidence of this type of visual problems and to determine whether older adults report a higher percentage of such problems than younger adults. They concluded that the five dimensions that declined with increasing age were related to speed of visual processing, light sensitivity, near vision, visual search, and dynamic vision. Each of these problems can represent a significant confounding influence for the test results depending upon the nature of the test and the degree of visual loading the test requires. Unfortunately, few studies have examined the effect of vision and visuoperceptual abilities on cognitive test performance in the elderly, although some work has been conducted with adult patients (for examples of this kind of work, see Glosser, Butters, & Kaplan, 1977; Schear & Sato, 1989).

Audition

Another sensory deficit common in the elderly is hearing loss (Brant, Wood, & Fozard, 1986; Corso, 1977, 1981; Olsho, Harkins, & Lenhardt, 1985). High-frequency hearing loss is common among geriatric individuals and can affect performance on verbal tests of cognition and communication (Granick, Kleban, & Weiss, 1976). Some recent work suggests, for example, that simulated high-frequency hearing loss in healthy young adults resulted in decreased performance in speech sound perception (Schear, Skenes, & Larson, 1988). Similarly, Skenes, Schear, and Larson (1989) also reported that young adults produced more errors in a phrase dictation task under conditions of simulated high-frequency hearing loss than under normal listening conditions. One might expect these results to generalize to older adults with high-frequency hearing loss. Recently, Hutchinson (1989) observed that whereas older subjects as a group profited about as much from contextual cues as younger subjects when listening to sentences in background noise, older listeners still were more adversely affected by the background noise than younger listeners. This experimental literature suggests strongly that clinicians must be cautious about the influence of auditory sensory deficits on tests of higher cognitive and speech-language abilities.

Suggestions for Test Examiners

There are a number of practical issues that both clinical neuropsychologists and speech-language pathologists must consider if they are going to obtain valid and clinically useful data. The testing session has been described as a "clinical process" that demands much effort by patient and clinician alike (Heaton & Heaton, 1981). Testing examiners should work hard to establish rapport with the patient and to administer test procedures in a natural and easy manner. In the testing session, this usually means that test instructions must be memorized in order to present the material in a natural manner without placing undue emphasis on the test instructions, as occurs when they are read from a test manual. Establishing eye contact with the patient and observing signs which suggest that the patient does not understand what to do are important examiner traits. In addition, sufficient time to practice on sample items

before beginning the test is necessary for the geriatric patient.

Motivation is an important factor that should be cultivated with any patient but especially with geriatric patients, because their test-taking approach is often cautious, and characteristically they fail to see how the test materials are relevant. The geriatric patient often requires more information about the purpose of the evaluation and about what to expect than is the case with younger adults. The initial period of the pretest interview, where time is devoted to establishing rapport and providing a framework for the evaluation process, is a critical first step in laying a foundation upon which the administration of the test is based (Hertzog & Schear, 1989; Schear, 1984). Thus, an important prerequisite for gaining valid test data in both neuropsychological or speech-language assessment is to obtain optimal cooperation from the patient and to establish the best motivation for approaching the tests. It is worthwhile to design the order of the tests to be administered so that they reduce stress (administering tests in a balanced manner with a good mix of easy and hard tests, rather than placing difficult tests together). In addition, the test examiner should be an astute observer of the examinee in order to recognize signs of fatigue and should be prepared to schedule multiple testing sessions across separate days (Albert, 1988b; Schear, 1984).

Accommodating for sensory deficits in vision and audition are important. Schear (1984) suggests that patients should undergo visual and auditory screening when visual or auditory deficits are suspected. In the case of visual acuity, if the lighting in the testing room is poor (either too bright or too dark) or the test materials are subject to glare (such as laminated materials that reflect light), then older adults are likely to encounter difficulty. A need for larger-print material may require standard test forms to be modified. Albert (1988b) suggests that if there is a window in the testing room, it should be at the patient's back. It makes good sense to be certain that the geriatric patient can hear the examiner by adjusting both the volume and rate with which instructions are presented to the patient (Schear et al., 1988). Testing should be conducted in a private, quiet setting that is free of unnecessary distraction, either visual or auditory.

Many years ago, Aiken (1980) offered some cogent advice and practical suggestions for dealing with the problems of testing the geriatric patient; these suggestions still are very good advice for any test examiner working with the elderly. They include (a) allowing sufficient time for patients to respond to test items; (b) providing time for them to practice on sample items; (c) using short rest breaks to offset fatigue; (d) providing a lot of encouragement; (e) avoiding repeated failure; (f) keeping the environment free of distraction; and (g) making provisions for auditory, visual, and other sensory deficits.

Conclusions

While neuropsychological and speech and language assessment of the geriatric individual involves consideration of factors unique to older people, the principles of assessment are the same as those for patients of any age regardless of any concomitant deficits. One must ask why a given patient is being assessed, what information is to be obtained, how that information will be gathered, how assessment data will be used, and what confounding patient or testing factors are present. Geriatric patients often have more than one problem and management frequently involves a multi-disciplinary approach (Schear, 1984). As Bayles and Kaszniak (1987) suggest, clinical neuropsychologists and speech-language pathologists have responsibilities in diagnosis, monitoring, treatment, and counseling in the care of the dementia patient. The same holds true for other geriatric patient populations. In general, it is often the clinical neuropsychologist who is primarily responsible for assessment and management of cognitively impaired patients,

whereas the speech-language pathologist is responsible for assessment and management of patients with communication deficits. We have described how each discipline is involved in the diagnosis and treatment of geriatric patients. The disciplines are interdependent and interaction between the two should be frequent and of a collaborative nature for optimum patient care (Porch & Haaland, 1984).

The interface between clinical neuropsychology and speech-language pathology is achieved by a mutual respect for what each discipline has to offer its patients. We have attempted to highlight in this chapter a model for building relationships based on an understanding about the developments in education, training, and credentialing in both fields and an exploration of some of the convergences and divergences in the assessment of elderly patients suffering from brain dysfunction. It should be clear from reading this chapter that our presentation is not exhaustive; it allows for considerable flexibility based on the particular circumstances of any assessment situation. The common ground in delivery of quality services to our patients lies in maximizing what we know about a patient's strengths and weaknesses. Each discipline can provide data for the other in both diagnosis and rehabilitation. We share the attitudes espoused earlier by Porch and Haaland (1984) in their work dealing with the aphasic patient and more recently by Bayles and Kaszniak (1987) in their model for an interface between the two disciplines in communication and cognition in normal aging and dementia. At this time, when each discipline is working hard to establish standards for practice, we feel that it is critical to avoid building artificial walls around ourselves and limiting the scope of service to be offered our patients. The statement adopted by the Division of Clinical Neuropsychology and the American Speech-Language-Hearing Association seems to underscore the mutal respect each discipline has for the other (American Psychological Association, 1990; American Speech-Language-Hearing Association, 1990). As Porch and Haaland (1984) pointed out some time ago, to achieve a viable working relationship between the disciplines requires that individual professionals exert effort to establish the liaison that is needed to achieve optimal patient care.

References

Aiken, L. R. (1980). Problems in testing the elderly. *Educational Gerontology, 5,* 119–124.

Albert, M. S. (1981). Geriatric neuropsychology. *Journal of Consulting and Clinical Psychology, 49,* 835–850.

Albert, M. S. (1988a). Assessment of cognitive dysfunction. In M. S. Albert & M. B. Moss (Eds.), *Geriatric neuropsychology* (pp. 57–81). New York: Guilford Press.

Albert, M. S. (1988b). Cognitive function. In M. S. Albert & M. B. Moss (Eds.), *Geriatric neuropsychology* (pp. 33–53). New York: Guilford Press.

Albert, M. S., & Kaplan, E. (1980). Organic implications of neuropsychological deficits in the elderly. In L. W. Poon, J. L. Fozard, D. Arenberg, L. S. Cermak, & L. W. Thompson (Eds.), *New directions in memory and aging: Proceedings of the George A. Talland Memorial Conference* (pp. 403–432). Hillsdale, NJ: Lawrence Erlbaum.

Albert, M. S., & Moss, M. B. (Eds.). (1988). *Geriatric neuropsychology.* New York: Guilford Press.

Alfano, D. P., & Finlayson, M. A. (1987). Clinical neuropsychology in rehabilitation. *The Clinical Neuropsychologist, 1,* 105–123.

American Educational Research Association, American Psychological Association, & National Council on Measurement in Education. (1985). *Standards for educational and psychological testing.* Washington, DC: American Psychological Association.

American Psychiatric Association. (1987). *Diagnostic and statistical manual of mental disorders* (3rd ed., rev.). Washington, DC: American Psychiatric Association.

American Psychological Association. (1981a). Ethical principles of psychologists. *American Psychologist, 36,* 633–638.

American Psychological Association. (1981b). Specialty guidelines for the delivery of services by clinical psychologists. *American Psychologist, 36,* 640–651.

American Psychological Association. (1987). General guidelines for providers of psychological services. *American Psychologist, 42,* 712–723.

American Psychological Association. (1990). *Division 40 Newsletter, 8*(2), 1.

American Speech-Language-Hearing Association. (1989a). Code of ethics of American Speech-Language-Hearing Association. *Asha, 31,* 27–28.

American Speech-Language-Hearing Association. (1989b). Standards for the Certificates of Clinical Competence. *Asha, 31,* 70–71.

American Speech-Language-Hearing Association. (1990). Interdisciplinary approaches to brain damage. *Asha, 32*(Suppl. 2), 3.

Aronson, A. (1987). The clinical Ph.D.: Implications for the survival and liberation of communicative disorders as a health care profession. *Asha, 29*(11), 35–39.

Au, R., Albert, M. L., & Obler, L. K. (1988). The relation of aphasia to dementia. *Aphasiology, 2,* 161–173.

Bayles, K. A., & Kaszniak, A. W. (1987). *Communication and cognition in normal aging and dementia.* Austin, TX: PRO-ED.

Beasley, D., & Davis, G. A. (Eds.). (1981). *Aging: Communication processes and disorders.* New York: Grune & Stratton.

Benton, A. L., Eslinger, P. J., & Damasio, A. R. (1981). Normative observations on neuropsychological test performance in old age. *Journal of Clinical Neuropsychology, 3,* 33–42.

Brant, L., Wood, J., & Fozard, J. (1986, November). *Age changes in hearing thresholds.* Paper presented at the annual meeting of the Gerontological Society of America, Chicago.

Brookshire, R. (1986). *An introduction to aphasia.* Minneapolis: BRK Publishers.

Caine, E. (1986). The neuropsychology of depression: The pseudodementia syndrome. In I. Grant & K. M. Adams (Eds.), *Neuropsychological assessment of neuropsychiatric disorders* (pp. 221–243). New York: Oxford University Press.

Christensen, A.-L. (1984). The Luria method of examination of the brain-impaired patient. In P. E. Logue & J. M. Schear (Eds.), *Clinical neuropsychology: A multidisciplinary approach* (pp. 5–28). Springfield, IL: Charles C Thomas.

Corso, J. F. (1977). Auditory perception and communication. In J. E. Birren & K. W. Schaie (Eds.), *Handbook of the psychology of aging* (pp. 535–553). New York: Van Nostrand Rheinhold.

Corso, J. F. (1981). *Aging sensory system and perception.* New York: Praeger.

Crook, T. H. (1979). Psychometric assessment in the elderly. In A. Raskin & L. F. Jarvik (Eds.), *Psychiatric symptoms and cognitive loss in the elderly: Evaluation and assessment techniques.* Washington, DC: Hemisphere Publishing.

Darby, J. (Ed.). (1985). *Speech and language evaluation in neurology: Adult disorder.* Orlando, FL: Grune & Stratton.

Davis, G. (1983). *A survey of adult aphasia.* Englewood Cliffs, NJ: Prentice-Hall.

Diller, L., & Gordon, W. A. (1981a). Interventions for cognitive deficits in brain injured adults. *Journal of Consulting and Clinical Psychology, 49,* 822–834.

Diller, L., & Gordon, W. A. (1981b). Rehabilitation and clinical neuropsychology. In S. B. Filskov & T. J. Boll (Eds.), *Handbook of clinical neuropsychology* (pp. 702–733). New York: Wiley.

Emerick, L., & Hatten, J. (1979). *Diagnosis and evaluation in speech pathology.* Englewood Cliffs, NJ: Prentice-Hall.

Fozard, J., Wolf, E., Bell, B., McFarland, R. A., & Podolsky, S. (1977). Visual perception and communication. In J. E. Birren & K. W. Schaie (Eds.), *The psychology of aging* (pp. 497–534). New York: Van Nostrand Reinhold.

Fromm-Auch, D., & Yeudall, L. T. (1983). Normative data on the Halstead-Reitan neuropsychological tests. *Journal of Clinical Psychology, 5,* 221–238.

Gallagher, D., Thompson, L. W., & Levy, S. M. (1980). Clinical psychological assessment of older adults. In L. W. Poon (Ed.), *Aging in the 1980s: Psychological issues* (pp. 19–40). Washington, DC: American Psychological Association.

Glosser, G., Butters, N., & Kaplan, E. (1977). Visuoperceptual processes in brain damaged patients on the digit symbol substitution test. *International Journal of Neuroscience, 7,* 59–66.

Golden, C. J., Hammeke, T. A., & Purisch, A. D. (1980). *The Luria-Nebraska Neuropsychological Battery Manual.* Los Angeles: Western Psychological Services.

Goodglass, H., & Kaplan, E. (1972, 1983). *The assessment of aphasia and related disorders.* Philadelphia: Lea & Febiger.

Granick, S., Kleban, M. H., & Weiss, A. D. (1976). Relationship between hearing loss and cognition in normally hearing aged persons. *Journal of Gerontology, 31,* 434–440.

Grant, I., & Adams, K. M. (Eds.). (1986). *Neuropsychological assessment of neuropsychiatric disorders.* New York: Oxford University Press.

Gurland, B., Golden, K., Challop, J. (1982). Unidimensional and multidimensional approaches to the differentiation of depression and dementia in the elderly. In S. Corkin, K. L. Davis, J. H. Growden, E. Usdin, & R. L. Wurtman (Eds.), *Alzheimer's disease: A report of progress* (pp. 119–125). New York: Raven Press.

Gurland, B., Kuriansky, T., Sharpe, L., Simon, R., Stiller, P., & Birkett, P. (1977–1978). The Comprehensive Assessment and Referral Evaluation (CARE): Rationale, development and reliability. *International Journal of Aging and Human Development, 8,* 9–42.

Hart, R. P., Kwentus, J. A., Wade, J. B., & Hamer, R. M. (1987). Digit symbol performance in mild dementia and depression. *Journal of Consulting and Clinical Psychology, 55,* 236–238.

Heaton, R. K., & Crowley, T. J. (1981). Effects of psychiatric disorders and their somatic treatments on neuropsychological test results. In S. B. Filskov & T. J. Boll (Eds.), *Handbook of clinical neuropsychology* (pp. 481–525). New York: Wiley.

Heaton, R. K., Grant, I., & Matthews, C. G. (1986). Differences in neuropsychological test performance associated with age, education and sex. In I. Grant & K. M. Adams (Eds.), *Neuropsychological assessment of neuropsychiatric disorders* (pp. 100–120). New York: Oxford University Press.

Heaton, S. R., & Heaton, R. K. (1981). Testing the impaired patient. In S. B. Filskov & T. J. Boll (Eds.), *Handbook of clinical neuropsychology* (pp. 526–544). New York: Wiley.

Hertzog, C. (1989). Influences of cognitive slowing on age differences in intelligence. *Developmental Psychology, 25,* 636–651.

Hertzog, C., & Schear, J. M. (1989). Psychometric considerations in testing the older person. In T. Hunt & C. J. Lindley (Eds.), *Testing older adults* (pp. 24–50). Austin, TX: PRO-ED.

Holland, A. (1980). *Communicative Abilities in Daily Living.* Austin, TX: PRO-ED.

Horn, J. L., Donaldson, G., & Engstrom, R. (1981). Apprehension, memory, and fluid intelligence decline in adulthood. *Research on Aging, 3,* 33–84.

Hutchinson, K. (1989). Influence of sentence context on speech perception in young and older adults. *Journal of Gerontology, 44,* 36–44.

Incagnoli, T., Goldstein, G., & Golden, C. J. (Eds.). (1986). *Clinical application of neuropsychological test batteries.* New York: Plenum Press.

INS/APA. (1987). Reports of the INS–Division 40 Task Force on Education, Accreditation, and Credentialing in Clinical Neuropsychology. *The Clinical Neuropsychologist, 1* 29–34.

Kaszniak, A. W. (1987a). Neuropsychological assessment of the dementia patient. In K. A. Bayles & A. W. Kaszniak (Eds.), *Communication and cognition in normal aging and dementia* (pp. 299–323). Austin, TX: PRO-ED.

Kaszniak, A. W. (1987b). Neuropsychological consultation to geriatricians: Issues in the assessment of memory complaints. *The Clinical Neuropsychologist, 1,* 35–46.

Kline, D. W., & Schieber, F. (1985). Vision and aging. In J. E. Birren & K. Warner Schaie (Eds.), *Handbook of the psychology of aging* (2nd ed., pp. 296–331). New York: Van Nostrand Reinhold.

Kolb, B., & Wishaw, I. (1985). *Fundamentals of human neuropsychology* (2nd ed.). New York: W. H. Freeman.

Kosnik, W., Winslow, L., Kline, D., Rasinski, K., & Sekuler, R. (1988). Visual changes in daily life throughout adulthood. *Journal of Gerontology: Psychological Sciences, 43,* P63–P70.

Lezak, M. D. (1983). Neuropsychological assessment (2nd ed.). New York: Oxford University Press.

Lezak, M. D. (1984). An individualized approach to neuropsychological assessment. In P. E. Logue & J. M. Schear (Eds.), *Clinical neuropsychology: A multidisciplinary approach* (pp. 29–49). Springfield, IL: Charles C Thomas.

Logue, P. E., & Schear, J. M. (Eds.). (1984). *Clinical neuropsychology: A multidisciplinary approach.* Springfield, IL: Charles C Thomas.

Matarazzo, J. D. (1988). There is only one psychology, no specialties, but many applications. *American Psychologist, 42,* 893–903.

Mattis, S. (1976). Mental status examination for organic mental syndrome in the elderly patient. In L. Bellak & T. B. Karasu (Eds.), *Geriatric psychiatry* (pp. 77–121). New York: Grune & Stratton.

Mattis, S. (1988). *Dementia Rating Scale: Professional manual.* Odessa, FL: Psychological Assessment Resources.

McCue, M., Goldstein, G., & Shelly, C. (1989). The application of a short form of the Luria-Nebraska Neuropsychological Battery to discrimination between dementia and depression in the elderly. *International Journal of Clinical Neuropsychology, 11,* 21–29.

Meier, M. J. (1974). Some challenges for clinical neuropsychology. In R. M. Reitan & L. A. Davison (Eds.), *Clinical neuropsychology: Current status and application* (pp. 289–323). Washington, DC: V. W. Winston.

Meier, M. J. (1981, September). Report of the task force on education, accreditation and credentialing of the International Neuropsychological Society. *The INS Bulletin,* pp. 5–10.

Meier, M. J. (1983). Education and credentialing issues in neuropsychology. In C. J. Golden & P. J. Vicente (Eds.), *Clinical application of neuropsychological test batteries* (pp. 155–192). New York: Plenum Press.

Meier, M. J., Benton, A. L., & Diller, L. (Eds.). (1987). *Neuropsychological rehabilitation.* New York: Guilford Press.

Messick, S. (1980). Test validity and the ethics of assessment. *American Psychologist, 5,* 1012–1027.

Milberg, W. P., Hebben, N., & Kaplan, E. (1986). The Boston process approach to neuropsychological assessment. In I. Grant & K. M. Adams (Eds.), *Neuropsychological assessment of neuropsychiatric disorders* (pp. 65–86). New York: Oxford University Press.

Obler, L., & Albert, M. (Eds.). (1980). *Language and communication in the elderly.* Lexington, MA: Lexington Books.

Olsho, L. W., Harkins, S. W., & Lenhardt, M. L. (1985). Aging of the auditory system. In J. E. Birren & K. W. Schaie (Eds.), *The handbook of the psychology of aging* (2nd ed., pp. 332–377). New York: Van Nostrand Reinhold.

Pauker, J. D. (1977, February). *Adult norms for the Halstead-Reitan Neuropsychological Test Battery: Preliminary data.* Paper presented at the meeting of the International Neuropsychological Society, Santa Fe, NM.

Poon, L. W. (Ed.). (1986). *Handbook of clinical memory assessment in older adults.* Washington, DC: American Psychological Association.

Porch, B. E. (1967, 1981). *The Porch Index of Communicative Ability*. Palo Alto, CA: Consulting Psychologists Press.

Porch, B. E., & Haaland, K. Y. (1984). Neuropsychology and speech pathology: An examination of professional relationships as they apply to aphasia. In P. E. Logue & J. M. Schear (Eds.), *Clinical neuropsychology: A multidisciplinary approach* (pp. 239–270). Springfield, IL: Charles C Thomas.

Reitan, R. M. (1973, August). *Behavioral manifestations of impaired brain functions in aging*. Paper presented at the meeting of the American Psychological Association, Montreal, Canada.

Reitan, R. M. (1979). *Neuropsychology and aging*. Tucson, AZ: Ralph M. Reitan and Associates.

Reitan, R. M., & Wolfson, D. (1985). *The Halstead-Reitan Neuropsychological Test Battery*. Tucson, AZ: Neuropsychology Press.

Russell, E. W. (1988). *Halstead, Rennick & Russell norms*. Unpublished manuscript.

Salthouse, T. A. (1985). *A theory of cognitive aging*. Amsterdam: North-Holland.

Sarno, M. (1969). *The Functional Communication Profile: Manual of directions*. New York: Institute of Rehabilitation Medicine, New York University Medical Center.

Schear, J. M. (1984). Neuropsychological assessment of the elderly in clinical practice. In P. E. Logue & J. M. Schear (Eds.), *Clinical neuropsychology: A multidisciplinary approach* (pp. 199–236). Springfield, IL: Charles C Thomas.

Schear, J. M., & Sato, S. D. (1989). Effects of visual acuity and visual motor speed and dexterity on cognitive test performance. *Archives of Clinical Neuropsychology, 4*, 25–32.

Schear, J. M., Skenes, L. L., & Larson, V. D. (1988). Effect of simulated hearing loss on speech sounds perception. *Journal of Clinical and Experimental Neuropsychology, 10*, 597–602.

Schuell, H. (1965, 1972). *Minnesota Test for Differential Diagnosis of Aphasia*. Minneapolis: University of Minnesota Press.

Skenes, L., & McCauley, R. (1985). Psychometric review of nine aphasia tests. *Journal of Communication Disorders, 18*, 461–474.

Skenes, L. L., Schear, J. M., & Larson, V. D. (1989). Simulated hearing loss and phrase repetition. *The International Journal of Neuroscience, 47*, 287–293.

Spriestersbach, D. (1989). Professional education and communication disorders. *Asha, 31*, 77–78.

Statement of Executive Committee of Division 40 at APA meeting on August 12, 1988. (1989). Definition of a clinical neuropsychologist. *The Clinical Neuropsychologist, 3*, 22.

Vega, A., & Parson, O. A. (1967). Cross-validation of the Halstead-Reitan tests for brain damage. *Journal of Consulting Psychology, 31*, 619–623.

Wechsler, D. (1981). *WAIS-R manual*. New York: Psychological Corporation.

Wells, C. E. (1979). Pseudodementia. *American Journal of Psychiatry, 136*, 895–900.

Wells, C. E., & Duncan, G. W. (1980). *Neurology for psychiatrists*. Philadelphia: F. A. Davis.

Yeudall, L. T., Redden, J. R., Gill, D. M., & Stefanyk, W. O. (1987). Normative data for the Halstead-Reitan neuropsychological tests stratified by age and sex. *Journal of Clinical Psychology, 43*, 346–367.

Social Aspects of Aging and Communication

5

CHAPTER

Ruth E. Dunkle, PhD, and Cary S. Kart, PhD ■

Communication is a complex task involving more than the simple production of words. Virtually every aspect of an individual's social and physical world contributes to the success of communication. Aging affects communication in a variety of ways. Age-related decline in sensitivity, acuity, and functioning of the sensory system can diminish the quantity and quality of interactions that an older person has with other individuals and the environment (Stone, 1987). Also, changes in the social and physical environment act to withdraw or offer opportunities and means for social interaction (Dreher, 1987). Reduced income in retirement; the loss of friends, siblings, or spouse; or a change in residence may disrupt the communicative interactions of an older person.

When a communicative disorder exists in an older client, the clinician can be most helpful by including a social assessment to aid in the diagnosis and treatment plan. Knowledge about an older client's living arrangements, marital and economic status, and health and functional capacities can provide the clinician with insight into the social processes that influence the client's communication behavior. Understanding the process of socialization to old age, the role transitions experienced by older people, the ways they adapt to these transitions, and the coping resources and styles they employ provides valuable information to a clinician attempting to make a social assessment an integral component of the diagnosis and treatment plan for the communication-impaired elderly. These social dimensions of the aging and health status of the elderly that most directly affect communication are the topics of this chapter.

Social and Demographic Characteristics of Aging That Affect Communication

The U.S. Bureau of the Census projects 31.7 million Americans—12.7% of the total population—to be age 65 or over in 1990. By the year 2000, the aged population is expected to have grown to 35 million or about 13% of the U.S. population. Among the elderly, the 85-plus population is the fastest growing age group. Approximately 3.3 million Americans are now in this oldest-old group, representing an almost 50% increase from 2.2 million in 1980. This population is more likely than the young-old to be female and widowed; at greater risk to be living alone or institutionalized; poor; with multiple health problems, including communication disorders; and in need of health and social services.

Living Arrangements and Marital Status

Patterns of marital status and living arrangements among the aged vary by sex and reflect the greater risk of social isolation for older women. According to the 1983 Current Population Survey, 42% of women aged 75 or over lived alone; the comparable figure for men was 19%. Men in this age group are three times more likely than women to be married and living with their spouse (65% vs. 21%). These male/female disparities are caused by higher age-specific death rates for adult men and the tendency for men to marry younger women. Also, the duration of widowhood experienced by older men is, on average, about one half that of older women (7 vs. 14 years); elderly widowed men have remarriage rates that are seven times those of women. These increased remarriage rates for men make them more likely to receive care from a spouse and be compliant with a medical regimen or rehabilitation program.

Economic Status

The importance of economic status in old age cannot be overestimated. The absence of financial resources has considerable impact on a person's capacity to adjust to the health decrements that may accompany aging. Availability of financial resources can help the elder maintain some degree of control over his or her life, including making decisions about social activities in which to participate, travel, diet, and preventive health care.

The median income of U.S. families with a head of household aged 65 years or over in 1986 was $19,832, representing about 68% of the median income of all families in 1986 ($29,458). While this ratio is about the same as that in 1982, it represents about a 9% improvement from 1977, suggesting that elderly families have enjoyed growth rates in income above the national average in this period. Those elderly who live alone have not done quite as well. The median income for unrelated individuals 65 years of age and over was $7,731 in 1986, or about 64% of the income for unrelated individuals of all ages.

It is one thing to describe how much income the elderly have, and quite another to say what they do with their income and whether or not it is adequate for their needs. The most frequently used measure of income adequacy is the poverty index developed by the Social Security Administration, based on the amount of money needed to purchase a minimum adequate diet as determined by the Department of Agriculture. Food budgets and derivative poverty income cutoff points are estimated for families of differing sizes and compositions adjusted for regional differences. In 1986, 12.4% of the aged population were "officially" defined as impoverished compared to 13.6% of the total U.S. population.

Viewing the elderly as better off financially than the general population is misleading when the poverty level of elderly subgroups is examined. For instance, elderly nonwhites are three times more likely to be living in poverty than are elderly whites (31% vs. 10.7%). Many elderly, including those living dependently with relatives, in institutions, or in group quarters, are not reflected in these official poverty statistics. Clearly, the poor and near-poor elderly have substantial economic difficulties that are likely to manifest themselves in inadequate or low-quality housing, neglect of preventive health care, at-risk nutritional status, and the like.

Health Status

Understanding the etiology of health problems in older persons is a complex task. Genetics, environmental issues, personality, and social context all play a part. Health may be defined in terms of an ability to carry out social roles and performance tasks, as well as in biomedical terms (Parsons, 1958, 1965). Age itself can affect the recognition of physical changes such as the presence of pain or an elevated temperature (Pathy, 1967). Illnesses of older people may be further developed than in younger people at the time the symptoms are first recognized. Overattribution of symptoms to the aging process directs the attention of the elderly person (and health care professionals) away from real disease and/or environmental factors that may affect health (Kart, 1981). Such misattributions may have tragic consequences such as misdiagnosis and subsequent misuse of service, or ultimate death. Among persons with communication disorders these problems can include mistaking aphasia for dementia, misdiagnosing stroke, and believing the person is confused when he or she is hearing impaired.

Data from the 1984 National Health Interview Survey (NHIS) Supplement on Aging (SOA) allow us to examine aspects of the health status of older Americans that are linked directly to communication skills: vision and hearing. Because vision and hearing are connected to perception of the environment, it is very likely that problems in vision and hearing affect the ability to relate to others who share a common view of the person's environment. Examination of the SOA sample shows that hearing and/or vision problems exist among the elderly but vary by age, gender, family income, race, and residence (Table 5.1). The oldest-old are about four times as likely to have hearing trouble (25.5% vs. 6.2%) and

almost five times as likely to have vision trouble (21.2% vs. 4.6%) as the young-old. Older males are more likely to have hearing problems, whereas females are more likely to have difficulties with their vision. Affluence (as defined by a family income of $15,000 or more) seems to protect older people from problems with vision more than is the case for problems with hearing. Elderly whites have a greater incidence of hearing problems than do elderly non-whites (10.5% vs. 5.6%); the reverse is true for vision trouble (7.8% vs. 10.9%). Rural elderly report more difficulties with hearing and vision than is the case for those in the central city and the suburbs.

Socialization to Old Age

All societies divide the lifetime into recognized seasons. Typically, periods of life are identified and defined, age criteria are used to channel people into positions, and rights, responsibilities, privileges, and obligations are assigned based on these culturally specific definitions (Hagestad & Neugarten, 1985). Linton (1942) suggested that the minimal number of age groupings in a society must be four—infancy, childhood, adulthood, and old age.

While life may be a stage and all the men and women merely players, the age-appropriate behaviors that allow us to have our exits and entrances are learned through the process of socialization. This learning is lifelong and includes transmission of the skills and knowledge needed to perform roles that will be occupied in middle and later life (Clausen, 1986). Early socialization or learning is insufficient to prepare a person for the different roles of adulthood in a modern industrial society. Adult socialization stresses the demands that institutions and other members of society make on the individual (Brim, 1968).

Social Roles

The concept of social role describes the expectations we have for individuals who

TABLE 5.1
Percentage Reporting Hearing and/or Vision Troubles by Age, Gender,
Family Income, Race, and Residence

Category	Hearing Trouble (%)[a]	Vision Trouble (%)[b]
Age (Years)		
55–64	6.2	4.6
65–74	8.9	7.4
75–84	13.8	11.2
85+	25.5	21.2
Gender		
Male	12.1	7.3
Female	8.6	8.6
Family Income		
Under $15,000	11.2	10.5
$15,000 or more	9.5	5.8
Race		
White	10.5	7.8
Nonwhite	5.6	10.9
Residence		
Central city	9.0	7.6
Suburban	9.4	7.1
Rural	11.4	9.5

Note. Data taken from "Supplement on Aging to the National Health Interview Survey 1984" by the National Center for Health Statistics, 1986, Bethesda, MD: U.S. Government Printing Office.
[a]Deafness in one or both ears. [b]Trouble seeing in one or both eyes.

occupy a given social position or status. Each distinctive social status has a set of role, or behavioral, expectations attached to it. It is this concept of social role that leads us to expect that in U.S. society parents will act responsibly in providing care and shelter for their young children and that grandparents will live independently and apart from their adult children and grandchildren. It is also the concept that helps us understand how the same individual can juggle the different expectations associated with being a spouse, father, professor, community volunteer, friend, and theater patron all in the same day.

Roles are not acted out in a social vacuum. They are defined in social interaction with others. Knowledge of social roles allows us to anticipate the behavior of others and to respond accordingly. The individual acquisition of social roles is a key element in the socialization process.

Is old age a social role? Do we have behavioral expectations for those who achieve old age? Some have suggested that old age is a formal status in our society with attached behavioral expectations. Others, arguing that there is an absence of expectations for the old, characterize them as occupying a "roleless role." Clearly, when people become old, they continue to occupy many of the social roles held during earlier stages of the life course. They continue to be family members, spouses, parents, siblings, and the like, as well as community volunteers, and some continue to be employed. Perhaps a more appropriate question is, "How does age affect the social roles we occupy?"

As Keith (1982) points out, in many societies, when people can no longer work, they are defined as old; in the United States, the situation is reversed—when people are defined as old, they can no longer work.

Thus, in the United States, chronological age is used to mark the border between work and retirement. Age is employed as an eligibility criterion for social roles. At the same time, it makes us ineligible to work but eligible to occupy the status of retiree. Age also influences our ideas about the appropriateness of certain behaviors. Neugarten (1980), for example, has argued that perceptions in the United States about the behaviors that are appropriate at given ages have relaxed somewhat in recent years. From her view, Americans seem less concerned than ever about the age at which one marries or enters the labor market, or goes to school or has children. Still, Karp and Yoels (1982) argue that a relaxation of age norms should not be equated with the absence of age norms. For example, Americans have fairly rigid ideas concerning who may have intimate sexual relationships with whom. Discrepancies in age between sexual partners is frequently a premise for ridicule. Even in this regard, however, Keith (1987) offers evidence that the age norms that develop in age-homogeneous communities can be quite distinctive when compared to those developed in a broader age-heterogeneous context.

Role Transitions

In most societies, there appears to be a timetable for the ordering of life events and role transitions. Summarizing results of studies begun in the 1950s, Neugarten and Hagestad (1976) reported agreement among respondents about the timing of major role transitions such as marriage and retirement. The timing of role transitions is not static, however. Cohort differences and the effects of historical periods contribute to changes in the timing of role transitions.

For instance, the mean age at widowhood has increased more dramatically for men than for women, although the average duration of widowhood by cohort has remained about the same (Table 5.2). It should be remembered that a much smaller proportion of husbands outlive their wives

than is the case for wives who outlive their husbands.

Changes in the timing of role transitions make it more difficult to assess the importance of being "on-time" or "off-time" in taking on new roles or disengaging from old ones. Some authors have suggested that being "off-time" (early or late) in taking on new roles or exiting old ones may create additional stresses. The source of such stresses may be *internal*, emanating from the individual's internalization of age norms, or *external*, from the reactions of peers or friends (Sales, 1978). Blau (1961) found that women who were widowed relatively early and men who retired earlier than their colleagues had greater disruptions in their social relationships than did those women and men for whom the events occurred on time. Unanticipated role displacement also complicates the transition process. Post-retirement adjustment is generally more problematic when the withdrawal from work is unexpected (see, for example, Streib & Schneider, 1971).

The issues of role transitions are complex for the old and have a clear bearing on the quality of life for those people with communication disorders. When elders struggle with chronic health problems as well as with the changing demands of life brought on by retirement, widowhood, or becoming a grandparent, the stress and strain can be great. Unfortunately, these added strains can prevent or delay their seeking treatment, which may in the long run foster greater impairment.

Stress and Adaptations

Much discussion about the social aspects of aging highlights the stresses associated with role transitions and changing behavioral expectations. The age-linked role transitions that are of particular interest to us here are major life transitions: changes in parental roles as children leave home, grandparenthood, retirement, and widowhood, among others. Coping with the stresses of such

TABLE 5.2
Measures of the Marital Life Cycle of Men and Women for Selected Birth Cohorts: 1908–12 to 1938–42

Item (Years)	Males Cohort (Year of Birth) 1908–12	1918–22	1928–32	1938–42	Females Cohort (Year of Birth) 1908–12	1918–22	1928–32	1938–42
Average age at first marriage	26.2	25.0	23.8	23.3	23.3	22.3	21.1	21.2
Average duration of first marriage	28.7	28.9	28.5	26.1	29.5	29.2	29.7	27.4
Outcome of first marriage (%)								
Divorce	25.1	29.3	33.2	39.4	23.8	27.3	31.5	36.7
Widowhood	22.8	21.1	19.6	17.6	53.0	50.3	48.5	45.1
Death	52.0	49.6	47.3	43.0	23.2	21.2	19.9	18.3
Mean age at								
Widowhood	64.5	66.7	67.8	68.4	64.7	65.6	66.0	66.1
Divorce	40.7	39.7	40.1	38.7	37.4	36.5	37.1	36.5
Mean duration of								
Widowhood	6.6	6.7	6.7	6.6	14.4	14.3	14.4	14.3
Divorce	4.4	4.4	4.5	4.2	8.9	8.7	9.7	9.6

Note. From "Demographic and Socioeconomic Aspects of Aging in the United States" by J. Siegel and M. Davidson, 1984, Table 7-8, p. 97), Current Population Reports, Special Studies Series P-23, No. 138, Washington, DC: U.S. Department of Commerce, U.S. Bureau of the Census.

transitions and adapting to them more or less successfully is an important element in the life course generally, as well as in achieving successful aging. There are various ways to defend against and cope with stressors. *Coping* describes the behaviors individuals use to prevent, alleviate, or respond to stressful situations (George, 1980).

Coping strategies generally take one of two forms: behavioral strategies or cognitive/emotional strategies. Behavioral coping strategies include a wide array of actions that individuals can employ to change or alleviate stress. Personal resources, including finances, health, education, and social supports, provide reserves or assistance that individuals may draw upon in a stressful situation. Cognitive/emotional strategies are ways in which individuals may employ social psychological mechanisms to deal with stress. Clausen (1986) points out that although coming to grips with a problem and finding ways of overcoming it tend to have more favorable consequences for the individual, we are beginning to learn that defensive maneuvers such as denial may also be quite useful. Thus, he suggests that denial of some deficits brought on by old age may be less problematic for a person than dwelling on deficits about which nothing can be done.

This has interesting implications for the older person with a communication disorder. If an elder feels that nothing can be done to restore his or her speech following a stroke, that person may not participate in any rehabilitative regimen. It is very important for the speech or language therapist to help the patient understand the improvement that could result from treatment as well as the additional problems that could occur from lack of treatment.

Pearlin and Schooler (1978) have analyzed the coping strategies individuals employ when they face problems in four areas of life: marriage, parenthood, household economics, and occupational goals and activities. Three broad categories of coping responses were identified: (a) responses that modify situations, (b) responses that

are used to reappraise the meaning of problems, and (c) responses that help individuals to manage tension. The researchers found that the coping responses employed were often specific to an area of household economics where changes in values or goals were required. In the areas of marriage or parenthood, direct action responses were seen as more valuable and effective.

Are specific coping skills or responses associated with old age? It is generally believed that throughout adulthood, "individuals develop and refine a repertoire of workable coping strategies that are compatible with their personal dispositions and lifestyles" (George, 1980, p. 34). A number of researchers have put forth specific models of adjustment or adaptation in later life.

Lieberman and Tobin (Lieberman, 1975; Tobin & Lieberman, 1976) have examined adaptation to changes in living arrangements among older, impaired people. They suggest that change in residence causes *subjective* stress experienced as a sense of loss and *objective* stress experienced as a disruption of customary behavior patterns. Their conceptual model begins with an assessment of personal resources and current functioning. Three adaptive outcomes are possible: (a) enhanced competence, in which functioning is improved after a crisis; (b) homeostasis, in which functioning is at the same level before and after a crisis; or (c) adaptive failure, in which functioning is impaired as a result of a crisis. The basic model was applied in four residential relocation studies. Across all studies, 48 to 56% of the subjects experienced adaptive failure. The authors found the degree of environmental change generated by relocation to be the most important predictor of adaptive outcome; the greater the change, the greater the decline in health or in social or psychological functioning among the residents. Perceptions of stress, personal resources, and coping skills seem relatively irrelevant to the adjustment or adaptation process.

Residential relocation is only one event an individual experiences that requires adaptation to change. According to the life events model of adaptation, "the normal state of the individual is one of homeostasis and . . . life events that require change are crises to the extent that they require time and energy to return to a steady state of functioning" (Whitbourne, 1985). From this perspective, stress is a mediator between an event and adaptation to the event; it causes physical and psychological damage in direct proportion to the disruption of the individual's usual life routine. The life events scales have been used to research variations in the impact of events typically experienced by older adults, including having children move out, death of a spouse, and illness. Age, sex, and socioeconomic status, as well as other personal and social resources, have had a mediating role between such life changes and illness (see, for example, Pearlin, 1980).

The *Social Readjustment Rating Scale* (*SRRS*) has become a common tool to measure the stress of life events (Holmes & Rahe, 1967). It is a checklist of 43 events that have been rated with regard to their intensity and the length of time needed to accommodate to them. Scores on the *SRRS* have generally correlated at a low to moderate level with physical illness and major emotional disturbance. Whitbourne (1985) has itemized a series of criticisms of the life events approach, not the least of which has to do with whether the same life events have a different significance to individuals as they move through the life course.

According to Clausen (1986), the nearest approach to a theoretical statement of the importance of adaptation across the life course is given by Vaillant (1977). Vaillant's essential argument is that if we are to master conflict gracefully and to harness instinctual striving creatively, our adaptive styles must mature. The devices we employ to protect ourselves from painful experiences in childhood will not serve us well in adulthood; instead, we must develop mature ways to cope with unacceptable or painful feelings. We still know too little about the cumulative effects of stress and the costs and benefits of particular coping strategies employed across the life course. Stress is a part of life

for all humans, but particularly for those who have lost a functional ability such as communication.

Social Support

People who suffer from communication disorders often need help beyond that which they receive from health professionals. They need support from their family and friends if they are going to live satisfying lives. The quality and quantity of social support, the different forms it takes, and the structure of social support networks have come to be recognized as important factors in the well-being of older people in general and those with communication disorders in particular. The communication disorders that many older people experience are the result of health problems such as cancer and dementing diseases; the aging process, including hearing and vision loss; and, of course, accidents. The diseases, the process of aging, and accidents often bring other limitations that require support. Social support consists of the particular people or community resources to which an individual turns for emotional, economic, or instrumental assistance. These social support systems have been tied to the mental health and life satisfaction of the elderly.

Social support has been defined as "the degree to which a person's basic needs are gratified through interaction with others" (Thoits, 1982, p. 147). Basic needs include affection, esteem or approval, belonging, identity, and security. This definition extends beyond identifying the quantity of social ties and emphasizes support as the actual fulfillment of needs (Ward, 1985). According to Kaplan's framework, social support may take the form of socioemotional or instrumental aid.

There are a variety of classifications for the types of support available and also numerous dimensions of social networks. In general, the range of factors include structural, functional, or interactional features and type or source of relationship. The most common structural characteristics identified in the literature are size, density, and geographic dispersion. Frequently mentioned interactional properties of networks include complexity, intensity, reciprocity, and a number of temporal variables (frequency, duration, and amount). Social support provision within social networks is also commonly identified by the source of support: primary kin (spouse, children, and siblings) and secondary kin (friends, neighbors, and work acquaintances) (Mitchell & Trickett, 1980). Cohen, Teresi, and Holmes (1985) suggest a fourth category of network characteristics relating to the dynamics or changes in network composition.

Recent research has examined the various characteristics of social networks and the dimensions of social support (Kahn & Antonucci, 1981). Typically researchers treat network members as if they were independent of one another (Cantor, 1983; Litwak, 1985). Often individuals are cognizant of what at least some of the other members are doing with or for the focal person. Even if network members do not communicate directly with one another, they may know about each other. What each is doing for or with the focal person may depend on what others are doing. An adequate network may then be defined not by the numbers of people involved or the various services they provide, but rather in terms of the interaction of the people and services. For example, there is evidence that when a family member is involved in service provision to an elderly relative, friends and neighbors go to greater lengths to provide services to that older person. Apparently, it is beneficial for them to know that if they withdraw from providing the service, someone else will take over (O'Bryant, 1985). A network that includes one close relative, then, may be more supportive than one that does not, even though the relative is only minimally involved in providing support.

The relevance of social support for effective therapy cannot be overemphasized. One of the greatest resources for elders residing in the community is the informal support network of family, neighbors, and friends. Although the family of impaired elders in the community and the institution report their willingness to provide some help, only for the community-residing elderly does the family report the ability and willingness to care for the older person as long as necessary (Smyer, 1980). This fact has significant ramifications for therapy. It means that family members are available to provide transportation as well as the emotional support that can be so helpful to a patient engaged in a protracted period of rehabilitation.

Important unexplored issues in the area of social support include understanding the provider of support, not just the recipient. This has been more extensively examined with regard to the burden the caregiver experiences in the process of providing care to a frail elder. The family is a source of support for many older people, especially when their health begins to deteriorate and they need help in performing the activities of daily living. Family members consistently emerge as the major providers of helping services and in fact provide more assistance to the elderly than do formal organizations. Without the care given by the family, more elderly would need to live in institutions rather than in the community (Brody, 1981; Brody, Poulshock, & Masciocchi, 1978; Horowitz, 1982; Lang & Brody, 1983; Stroller, 1983; Treas, 1977).

While the family caregiving role may be shouldered by any number of relatives, the spouse is the major source of assistance for those who are married (Shanas, 1979). This raises the potential problem of both the spouse and elder having communication disorders. Clearly, the health of the caregiver is a crucial ingredient in the treatment strategy employed with communication-impaired elderly individuals. Especially with speech and language problems that require the patient to perform exercises between treatment sessions, the availability of a care provider who is capable of successful communication is very helpful. When a spouse is unavailable, adult children, and particularly the adult daughter, serve as the primary caregiver (Horowitz,

1982; Johnson, 1983; Robinson & Thurnher, 1979). A third choice of caregiver is other relatives or friends and neighbors (Cantor, 1983).

Regardless of the relationships that link caregiver to elder, burden is a frequent outcome of caregiving. The negative consequences of caregiving have been explored by many researchers (Brody et al., 1978; Fitting, Rabins, Lucas, & Eastham, 1986; George & Gwyther, 1986; Noelker & Wallace, 1985; Zarit, Reever, & Peterson, 1980; Zarit, Todd, & Zarit, 1986). Interestingly, care-related burden varies by type of caregiver (Cantor, 1983; Johnson, 1983; Noelker & Wallace, 1985). Adult child caregivers appear more vulnerable than spouse caregivers, and wives are more burdened in the caregiving role than are husbands (Fitting et al., 1986; Zarit et al., 1986).

In the caregiver arena as well as in other areas, the transaction between the provider of support and the recipient of the support remains unexplored (Coyne, Kahn, & Gotlib, 1984). For example, which behaviors elicit supportive or nonsupportive responses from the network? What consequences are experienced by those who provide support? The negative effects may be substantial, and the provider may become emotionally drained (Belle, 1982). In addition, systematic research is needed to determine whether certain classes of behaviors are supportive or nonsupportive (Kessler, McLeod, & Wethington, 1984).

Brickman, Rabinowitz, Karuza, Cohen, and Kidder (1982) found that supporters offering advice or tangible aid may actually convey to the recipients that they are incapable of handling their own problems. In reality, attempts to support victims of crisis are often ineffective (Wortman & Lehman, 1984). The severity of the recipient's problems may determine the amount of support received. For example, cancer patients with the worst prognosis are less likely to receive support than those in better physical health (Peters-Golden, 1982). On the other hand, those who appear to cope well with life crises are less likely to be judged negatively and avoided by others than those who appear to be having difficulty in coping (Coates, Wortman, & Abbey, 1979).

Social Assessment

A review of the literature on social assessment covers a wide range of topics. The critical issue in assessing an older person's social functioning is its entanglement with physical and mental health functioning. The ability to communicate provides the opportunity to be social, and this facility can be an essential ingredient in promoting the well-being of an older person.

There are many measurement issues involved in social assessment. Unfortunately, the tools currently available are too limited and are often composed of simple checklists. Kane and Kane (1981) provide a comprehensive review of instruments to assess social functioning, discussing their advantages and shortcomings. Their concerns about the use of psychometric instruments in assessing social functioning can be divided into three categories: the design of the instruments themselves, the content included or not included, and the procedure for implementing the survey. The problems inherent in measuring social functioning are related to the complexity of the variables involved and the social, cultural, and personal influences. The clinician must not only choose which variables to assess, but must also incorporate valid judgments and interpretations. The lack of defined roles for the elderly and the lack of substantive age norms make the job of data interpretation difficult. Furthermore, the interactional nature of the clinician and client in the assessment process confounds efforts at determining reliability and validity (Greene, 1986). Even if these hurdles are overcome and an accurate assessment occurs, it does not ensure service use. It is difficult to implement instruments, and they do not entirely predict successful outcomes for intervention. All social assessments, however, include some appraisal of the social support and social networks present in an individual's life.

Unfortunately, our understanding of the complex interactions that make up the social world of the elderly is limited. As Hartman (1978, p. 466) writes: "In attempting to describe the complex system of interacting variables, the meaning and the nature of the integration of the variables, the totality of the event and action is lost." She suggests the use of eco-mapping as a tool for assessing an individual's support system, network, resources, and environmental fit.

Originally developed by Hartman for use by child care workers in assessing the needs of families, the eco-map is a visual representation of social interactions (Figure 5.1). By representing the social network in an illustrative multidimensional framework, it is possible to avoid the tendency to reduce and partialize the dynamic nature of the social system. When used with the geriatric population, the eco-map may provide an opportunity for accurate collection and communication of a person's total interactional system.

The eco-map is a simple paper-and-pencil simulation of an individual and all other persons and organizations with whom he or she interacts. Information can be noted regarding the characteristics for each contact person. The circular repre-

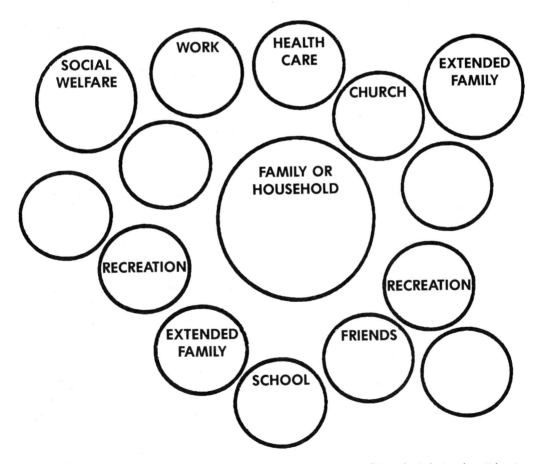

FIGURE 5.1. Eco-map. *Note.* From "Diagrammatic Assessment of Family Relationships" by A. Hartman, 1978, *Social Casework, 59,* pp. 465–477. Copyright 1978 by Family Service America. Reprinted by permission.

sentations of each person or organization in the network are connected by coded lines indicating the nature of the relationship. When it is completed, the eco-map shows not only who is included within the individual's social network, but also the nature of the relationships, the flow of energy within the network, nurturing versus frustrated relationships, the degree of integration within the community, and problem areas where the individual lacks resources.

Not only is the clinician responsible for the accurate assimilation, organization, and interpretation of complex social networks, but he or she must also communicate this information to the service delivery team. The eco-map serves as an effective way of obtaining comprehensive information about an individual's social network and is a dynamic method of representing this information to other members of the service team.

The process of creating an eco-map can contribute to the treatment of the elderly as well. The actual drawing of the eco-map can increase acceptance of self and heighten the emotional importance of the social network for the person (Hartman, 1978). The clinician and the individual work together in drawing the eco-map, making it an interviewing tool and leading to more effective data collection and better rapport.

The eco-map allows the individual and the clinician to identify persons and resources in the social network and to position the elder in his or her environment. Further, the strengths of the relationships as well as their quality are detailed. However, issues of personal coping and subjective well-being are not addressed. This assessment tool and many others are not successfully utilized with all types of clients, who may have varying physical and cognitive abilities. In particular, clients with moderate to severe cognitive impairment cannot describe their lives and their network of support to take advantage of this assessment tool. On the other hand, clients who have communication disorders but who do not have moderate to severe cognitive limitations can relate information

regarding the eco-map through whatever mechanism is used to communicate (e.g., computer or word board).

The review of an individual's eco-map communicates an ecological perspective for discerning treatment approaches. When it is used periodically, the technique allows changes in an individual's life space to be assessed. For the elderly, the diagram will organize a great deal of information; highlight needs, problem areas, and strengths; offer a retrospective index of changes over time; and provide a springboard for mobilizing appropriate services. Unfortunately, although Hartman promotes periodic reassessment, many clinicians view assessment as a one-time occurrence, especially when the client has been placed in a nursing home or becomes severely impaired.

Considering prior life experiences, as well as distinguishing between harmful and helpful social relationships, aids in understanding the quality of the individual's life (Greene, 1986). Whether a person's living alone means isolation or liberation is a question of personal style and values that is rarely investigated in formal assessment surveys (Steinberg & Carter, 1983).

In sum, although an instrument may be helpful in gathering and disseminating data on geriatric populations, there are constraints inherent in interpreting issues of social functioning using psychometric measures.

Social assessment plays an important role in planning services for the elderly. Accurate information about an individual's social functioning and social network contributes greatly to delivery of services that maximize independence, life satisfaction, and quality of life. A social assessment incorporates the evaluation of an individual's social support, social network, social functioning, resources, and integration into his or her environment. The analysis of social support is a complex and difficult task. Formal instruments are used to assess social networks and resources. Practical concerns in using such surveys were noted previously. It is suggested that social assessment should be a continuing process of evaluation, analysis, and reevaluation. Social assessment plays a key role in the comprehensive assessment of the geriatric population.

Conclusions

In conclusion, the social aspects of life as well as their relationship to health status dramatically affect an older person's ability and interest in communicating. Understanding the complex social world and health status of older people facilitates a comprehensive assessment of communication disorders in this population and paves the way for providing successful treatment.

References

Belle, D. (1982). The stress of caring: Women as providers of social support. In L. Goldberger & S. Breznitz (Eds.),*Handbook of stress: Theoretical and clinical aspects* (pp. 496–505). New York: Free Press.

Blau, Z. (1961). Structural constraints on friendships in old age. *American Sociological Review, 26,* 429–439.

Brickman, P., Rabinowitz, B., Karuza, J., Cohen, E., & Kidder, L. (1982). Models of healing and coping. *American Psychologist, 37,* 368–384.

Brim, O. G. (1968). Adult socialization. In J. A. Clausen (Ed.), *Socialization and society* (pp. 182–226). Boston: Little, Brown.

Brody, E. M. (1981). The dependent elderly and women's changing roles. *The Mount Sinai Journal of Medicine, 48,* 511–519.

Brody, S. J., Poulshock, S. W., & Masciocchi, C. F. (1978). The family caring unit: A major consideration in the long-term support system. *The Gerontologist, 18,* 556–561.

Cantor, M. (1983). Strains among caregivers: A study of experience in the United States. *The Gerontologist, 23,* 597–604.

Clausen, J. (1986). *The life course: A sociological perspective.* Englewood Cliffs, NJ: Prentice-Hall.

Coates, D., Wortman, C., & Abbey, A. (1979). Reactions to victims. In I. H. Frieze, D. Bartal, & J. Carroll (Eds.), *New approaches to social*

problems (pp. 21–52). San Francisco: Jossey-Bass.

Cohen, C., Teresi, J., & Holmes, D. (1985). Social networks and adaptation. *The Gerontologist, 25,* 297–304.

Coyne, J. C., Kahn, J., & Gotlib, I. H. (1984). Depression. In T. Jacob (Ed.), *Family interactions and psychopathology.* New York: Plenum Press.

Dreher, B. B. (1987). *Communication skills for working with elders.* New York: Springer.

Fitting, M., Rabins, M., Lucas, M. J., & Eastham, J. (1986). Caregivers for dementia patients: Comparison of husbands and wives. *The Gerontologist, 26,* 248–252.

George, L. K. (1980). *Role transitions in later life.* Monterey, CA: Brooks/Cole.

George, L. K., & Gwyther, L. P. (1986). Caregiver well-being: A multidimensional examination of family caregivers of demented adults. *The Gerontologist, 26,* 253–259.

Greene, R. (1986). *Social work with the aged and their families.* New York: Aldine de Gruyter.

Hagestad, G., & Neugarten, B. (1985). Age and the life course. In R. Binstock & E. Shanas (Eds.), *Handbook of aging and the social sciences* (pp. 35–61). New York: Van Nostrand Reinhold.

Hartman, A. (1978). Diagrammatic assessment of family relationships. *Social Casework, 59,* 465–477.

Holmes, T. H., & Rahe, R. H. (1967). The Social Readjustment Rating Scale. *Journal of Psychosomatic Research, 11,* 213–218.

Horowitz, A. (1982). *Adult children as caregivers to elderly parents: Correlates and consequences.* Unpublished doctoral dissertation, Columbia University, New York, NY.

Johnson, C. L. (1983). Dyadic family relations and social support. *The Gerontologist, 23,* 377–383.

Kahn, R., & Antonucci, T. (1981). Convoys of social support: A life course approach. In S. Keisler, J. Morgan, & V. Oppenheimer (Eds.), *Aging: Social change* (pp. 383–402). New York: Academic Press.

Kane, R. A., & Kane, R. L. (1981). *Assessing the elderly: A practical guide to measurement.* Lexington, MA: Lexington Books.

Karp, D. A., & Yoels, W. C. (1982). *Experiencing the life cycle: A social psychology of aging.* Springfield, IL: Charles C Thomas.

Kart, C. S. (1981). Experiencing symptoms: Attribution and misattribution of illness among the aged. In M. Haug (Ed.), *Elderly patients* and their doctors (pp. 70–78). New York: Springer.

Keith, J. (1982). *Old people as people: Social and cultural influences on aging and old age.* Boston: Little, Brown.

Keith, J. (1987). *Old people, new lives: Community creation in a retirement community.* Chicago: University of Chicago Press.

Kessler, R., McLeod, J., & Wethington, E. (1984). The costs of caring: A perspective in the relationship between sex and psychological distress. In I. G. Sarason & B. R. Sarason (Eds.), *Social support: Theory, research and applications* (pp. 491–506). The Hague: Martinus Nijhof.

Lang, A. M., & Brody, E. M. (1983). Characteristics of middle-aged daughters and help to their elderly mothers. *Journal of Marriage and the Family, 45,* 193–201.

Lieberman, M. A. (1975). Adaptive processes in late life. In N. Datan & L. H. Ginsberg (Eds.), *Life-span developmental psychology: Normative life crises* (pp. 135–160). New York: Academic Press.

Linton, R. (1942). Age and sex categories. *American Sociological Review, 7,* 589–603.

Litwak, E. (1985). *Helping the elderly: The complementary roles of informal networks and formal systems.* New York: Guilford Press.

Mitchell, J., & Trickett, E. (1980). Social networks as mediators of social support. *Community Mental Health Journal, 16,* 27–44.

Neugarten, B. (1980). Acting one's age: New rules for the old. *Psychology Today, 13*(11), 66–74, 77–80.

Neugarten, B., & Hagestad, G. (1976). Age and the life course. In R. H. Binstock & E. Shanas (Eds.), *Handbook of aging and the social sciences* (pp. 35–57). New York: Van Nostrand Reinhold.

Noelker, L. S., & Wallace, R. W. (1985). The organization of family care for impaired elderly. *Journal of Family Issues, 6*(1), 23–44.

O'Bryant, S. (1985). Neighbors' support of older widows who live alone in their homes. *The Gerontologist, 25,* 305–310.

Parsons, T. (1958). Definition of health and illness in the light of American values and social structure. In E. Jaco (Ed.), *Patients, physicians, and illness* (pp. 165–187). New York: Free Press.

Parsons, T. (1965). *Social structure and personality.* New York: Free Press.

Pathy, M. (1967). Clinical presentation of myocardial infarction in the elderly. *British Heart Journal, 29,* 190–199.

Pearlin, L. (1980). Life strains and psychological distress among adults. In N. Smelser & E. Erikson (Eds.), *Themes of work and love in adulthood* (pp. 174–192). Cambridge, MA: Harvard University Press.

Pearlin, L., & Schooler, C. (1978). The structure of coping. *Journal of Health and Social Behavior, 19,* 2–21.

Peters-Golden, M. (1982). Breast cancer: Varied perceptions of social support in the illness experience. *Social Science and Medicine, 16,* 483–491.

Robinson, B., & Thurnher, M. (1979). Taking care of aged parents: A family cycle transition. *The Gerontologist, 19,* 586–593.

Sales, E. (1978). Women's adult development. In I. Freize, J. Parsons, P. Johnson, D. Ruble, & G. Zellman (Eds.), *Women and sex roles: A social psychological perspective* (pp. 157–190). New York: Norton.

Shanas, E. (1979). Social myth as hypothesis: The case of the family relations of old people. *The Gerontologist, 19,* 3–9.

Smyer, M. (1980). The differential usage of services by impaired elderly. *Journal of Gerontology, 35,* 255–259.

Steinberg, R., & Carter, G. (1983). *Case management of the elderly.* Lexington, MA: Lexington Books.

Stone, J. T. (1987). Interventions for psychosocial problems associated with sensory disabilities in old age. In B. Heller, L. Flohr, & L. Zegans (Eds.), *Psychosocial interventions with sensorially disabled persons* (pp. 243–260). New York: Grune & Stratton.

Streib, G., & Schneider, C. (1971). *Retirement in American society: Impact and process.* Ithaca, NY: Cornell University Press.

Stroller, E. P. (1983). Parental caregiving by adult children. *Journal of Marriage and the Family, 45,* 851–857.

Thoits, P. (1982). Conceptual, methodological, and theoretical problems in studying social support as a buffer against life stress. *Journal of Health and Social Behavior, 23,* 145–159.

Tobin, S., & Lieberman, M. (1976). *Last home for the aged.* San Francisco: Jossey-Bass.

Treas, J. (1977). Family support systems for the aged: Some social and demographic considerations. *The Gerontologist, 17,* 486–491.

Vaillant, G. (1977). *Adaptation to life.* Boston: Little, Brown.

Ward, R. (1985). Informal networks and well-being in later life: A research agenda. *The Gerontologist, 25,* 55–61.

Whitbourne, S. K. (1985). The psychological construction of the life span. In J. Birren & K. Schaie (Eds.), *Handbook of the psychology of aging* (pp. 594–618). New York: Van Nostrand Reinhold.

Wortman, C., & Lehman, D. (1984). Reactions to victims of life crises: Support efforts that fail. In I. E. Sarason & B. R. Sarason (Eds.), *Social supports: Theory, research and application* (pp. 463–490). The Hague: Martinus Nijhof.

Zarit, S. H., Reever, K. E., & Peterson, J. B. (1980). Relatives of the impaired elderly: Correlates of feelings of burden. *The Gerontologist, 20,* 649–655.

Zarit, S. H., Todd, P. A., & Zarit, J. M. (1986). Subjective burden of husbands and wives as caregivers: A longitudinal study. *The Gerontologist, 26,* 260–266.

Mental Health and Aging

Richard W. Hubbard, PhD ■

CHAPTER

6

Entire texts and handbooks have been devoted to geropsychology (see, e.g., Birren & Sloane, 1980; Zarit & Tager, 1980), a topic whose diversity and depth of content certainly exceed the dimensions of this chapter. It is also apparent that psychological problems of the elderly overlap with the social and neuropsychological factors discussed at length in other chapters within this text. The focus of this chapter will be on highlighting areas of special importance to professionals in speech and communication disorders by considering emotional well-being in old age, common functional (nonorganic) psychological problems of the elderly, and their implications for clinical practice.

The relatively recent emphasis on multidisciplinary assessment and care of the elderly should result in professionals with backgrounds in speech and communication disorders becoming members of health care teams and increasing their roles in the bio-psychosocial model of health care. The typical older patient represents the strongest case for multidisciplinary approaches; his or her problems are multiple and frequently intertwined, and rehabilitation must reflect this in order to be successful. The acquisition of knowledge and information from our environment and our ability to negotiate for change, reward, and access to our interpersonal worlds are cornerstones of mental health at any age and should make the fields of psychology and communication particularly close allies.

Emotional Well-Being in the Later Years

It has frequently been suggested that as we mature and age we become more like our ''self.'' This notion receives some support

A portion of Hubbard's work was supported by a grant from the Retirement Research Foundation, Chicago, IL.

when we consider the remarkable heterogeneity of the older population on a variety of psychological measures. Tests that measure skills related to learning and memory and those that measure a variety of personality dimensions typically yield wider ranges of scores for older adults than for any other age group (see, e.g., Botwinick, 1984). One interpretation of these results is that normal aging is, in part, a process of self-articulation, which results in each of us becoming more unique as we age. This also makes it difficult to generalize about the older population in research and in clinical practice, where the unique process of self-articulation is critical to accurate assessment and interventions.

Much research has been devoted to a concept referred to as "successful aging" (Rowe & Kahn, 1987). Although there have been a number of complex research and measurement problems associated with this area (Kausler, 1982), the findings are tentative. In fact, the term "successful aging" may be an unfortunate choice, because it can be viewed as implying that aging is something that must be overcome rather than another segment of the life-span. We do not, for example, often hear researchers refer to successful infancy or successful adolescence. Not surprisingly, most of the research results on successful aging point to successful living over earlier stages of the life-span as the best preparation for the later years of life. Thus, those who are still married, in good health, with reasonable income, and with satisfactory family contact seem to do well in old age. Discussing the factors associated with well-being in old age, Botwinick (1984) stresses the importance of the older adult having a confidant, one person with whom he or she has a meaningful, trusting, intimate relationship, as a contributor to successful aging. What is most encouraging about these findings is that each of these factors represents something that is at least partially under our personal control and influence. In other words, what we do in our adult years, the decisions we make, the life-style behaviors we choose, may well have an impact on our life satisfaction and general well-being in old age.

A number of personality theorists and researchers have approached normal aging from a life-span or developmental psychology point of view, in which stages of life are studied in terms of social or psychological tasks or barriers that must be dealt with successfully on the road to emotional well-being. Central to many of these theories as they pertain to the later years of life is an emphasis on the person's capability to *adapt* to the negative changes and losses that confront many elderly on the one hand, and to *attach* to new challenges and sources of intimacy and joy on the other. Thus Erikson (1963) cites choosing ego integrity over despair as a major developmental task for the elderly. Stated briefly, this final stage of life leads the individual either to acceptance and satisfaction with life and correspondingly with mortality, or to an angered disgust and despair characterized by the feeling that time is too short, life too unfinished, or, as Shakespeare's King Richard II puts it: "I wasted time, and now doth time waste me."

Schaie's cognitive development theory (1977) sees the final stage of life as reintegrative. This tendency to simplify life's complexities by organizing and applying cognitive resources on a prioritized basis, with the perceived meaningfulness of the task becoming a critical variable, suggests a movement toward conservation in the later years of life. It is intriguing to consider the possibility that although a well-adjusted older adult may be attached to fewer activities and/or people, the quality of the remaining attachments may in fact be enhanced because there is less competition for attention and commitment. In this framework, disengagement can be viewed as part of a process that results in a reinvestment of resources rather than as an end in and of itself. In other words, the decline and restructuring of activity and emotional investment may be seen as an active coping mechanism rather than a passive retreat.

Havighurst's (1972) developmental tasks for old age place a great deal of emphasis on adjustment and acceptance as they relate to health changes, retirement, death of spouse, and one's own mortality. The awareness and acceptance of one's nearness to death is a theme common to many late-life theories of well-being. While this has an existential sound to it for many young people, it often involves practicalities for older adults such as wills, funeral preparations, and attention to important relationships that may need to be solidified, such as parent–adult child reconciliation.

It would appear that one of the central tasks that must be accomplished in old age is loss transcendence, or finding new ways to meet old needs. Thus the newly widowed may find new roles and relationships to fulfill the need to express nurturance or the need for companionship. The retired may seek new avenues to maintain their sense of productivity. While young people tend to replace losses successfully, many of the losses older adults experience are largely irreplaceable. However, this does not imply that the elderly must accept unfulfilled needs.

Other theorists and researchers have focused on one specific element of psychological development in an attempt to characterize an aspect of the aging process. Neugarten's classic personality study (1973) revealed several personality types that seemed to adjust well to the aging process. Those with integrated personalities tend to be flexible and open to new experiences. These persons may reorganize their lives to maintain a level of activity and attachment that approximates that of their life-style in middle age or they may become focused on fewer activities but remain devoted to investing in others and staying active. Alternatively, they may be disengaged from most activities not because of physical or cognitive limitations but based on what Neugarten calls a self-directed orientation to later life, which results in low activity levels but high self-regard and contentment.

A second personality style that seems to achieve a reasonable level of satisfaction in old age is the armored-defended style. Although individuals with this personality type are characterized as being more anxious and with a greater need to control their impulses and lives, they seem to maintain a high satisfaction with life as long as they are able to hold on to patterns of living they developed in middle age or to fend off impending loss or collapse by constricting their activities.

The other personality styles identified by Neugarten and her colleagues did not fare as well in old age. They tended to exhibit passive-dependent or disintegrated personalities, due in part to physical or mental deterioration but also to the use of passive, accepting coping styles.

Additional perspectives on normal aging are provided by research and theory related to sex role changes in the later years of life where androgyny, the tendency for men to express more feminine characteristics and women to express more masculine ones, may increase (Gutmann, 1977). Finally, health care professionals interested in motivation as it relates to rehabilitation would do well to consider the growing literature on cautiousness in old age as it relates to risk-taking behavior, errors of omission, and the need for certainty in the correctness of a response for older adults (Botwinick, 1966; Okun, Siegler, & George, 1978, Wallach & Kogan, 1961). This growing literature suggests that when older adults are confronted with new tasks, they may require greater certainty prior to responding, more time to respond, and response formats that do not allow them to omit a response but do encourage a best-guess approach.

The Five R's

Birren and Renner (1979) discuss the five R's of emotional well-being in old age based on research and theory in the field. This approach provides a useful framework for considering the overall well-being of the older person. The first R, *review*, represents the importance of older adults having a sense of personal history. The life review process (Butler & Lewis, 1977) is viewed as a natural consequence of aging as the older adult reviews various goals, values, roles, and relationships in his or her life as a way of establishing a sense of meaning for that life and developing an acceptance of mortality.

The second R, *reconciliation,* relates to the fact that in the course of reviewing one's life a form of psychological bookkeeping may evolve in which people tend to ruminate about their own or significant others' failings. Such rumination can lead to guilt, depression, and anger on the part of the older adult, unless it is accompanied by forgiving the self and others for transgressions and letting go of unresolved hurt or anger.

Relevance, the third R, suggests that personal or societal decisions that place the older person in a spectator's role, where he or she is unwilling or unable to participate in family and community functioning, will result in the individual being isolated and out of touch with significant others and events. Relevance as a key to mental well-being endorses *meaningful* activity.

The fourth R, *respect,* addresses some of the emotional needs of this group in terms of their desire for meaningful relationships and for recognition of their worth. Rejected are blind obedience or worship from younger generations, or smothering affection from those who seek to remind them of their supposed dependence.

The fifth R, *release,* emphasizes the need for physical exercise and intimacy as well as the opportunity for a full range of emotional expression.

The five R's provide a helpful conceptual framework for considering normal aging and for gaining perspective on the elderly patient with communication disorders. Clearly, healthy review requires an active listener and the ability to organize, evaluate, and distill large portions of our lives; reconciliation relies on our ability to effectively communicate our meaning to others; relevance requires access to the world around us; respect involves the communication of needs and the development of meaningful relationships; and release is based in part on the ability to express oneself. In evaluating older patients with communication disorders it may be useful to consider which of the five R's are most affected by the problem.

Implications for Practice

It is important for health care professionals to understand normal aging in order to realize that the majority of older adults continue to be satisfied and relatively happy with their lives. A young professional working in a clinical setting will encounter older people with a myriad of psychological, social, and physical health problems and may conclude, incorrectly, that this is what awaits all of us as we age. This kind of misattribution sows the seeds for a type of professional "ageism" that may contribute to professionals leaving the field or developing a significant amount of anxiety about their own aging process.

Our current generation of elderly bring with them some important experiences regarding health care. Such issues are usually referred to as *age-cohort variables.* On one hand, these people grew up at a time when the medical model's view of the patient as a passive recipient of service was predominant, and on the other hand, they have learned to expect great things from health care. The cure of polio, successful treatment for tuberculosis, and the literal revolution in pharmacology all occurred in their lifetimes. As a result they may expect less of themselves and more of health care professionals than current rehabilitation theory, research, and practice allows. Careful and precise explanations of the goals, objectives, and process of therapy in speech and communication disorders is called for.

One clear example of cohort relevance to communication is the non-native language user. Many of our elderly, particularly the old-old, are immigrants who arrived in this country in childhood, adolescence, or adulthood with a principal non-English language already in place. How we assess their skills in old age and whether they may be more fluent in their original language is a matter of some controversy.

However, clinicians need to be aware that researchers do find differences in the abilities of older adults for whom English is not a native language (Bergman, 1980). Obler and Albert (1985) note that researchers consistently find a wider range of scores and diversity of language ability in older populations than in younger groups. Again the heterogeneity of the older population comes into play.

Light (1988) provides a summary of the applications of cognitive psychology to language and aging, in which performance and resource limitations in old age are examined. Of particular importance to clinicians is the relationship between memory and language in old age, which has led some researchers to recommend the use of slow, concrete messages that are shortened to the most relevant and important information (Cohen, 1979). Light (1988) also stresses the intriguing and under-researched area of the style and level of language used in addressing the elderly. In some cases our bias of expecting communication difficulties with the elderly may result in unnecessary and demeaning baby talk; at other times, this approach may in fact be supportive and reassuring (Cohen & Faulkner, 1986; Rubin & Brown, 1975; Ryan, Giles, Bartolucci, & Henwood, 1986).

A similar cohort attitude may be encountered when problems in hearing, vision, or speech are viewed by older adults as a normal part of the aging process. Because today's treatments and prosthetics were unavailable at the turn of the century, it may in fact have been their experience that such losses were normal in a statistical sense (happening to the majority of older persons) and were simply a natural consequence of aging. Taken to an extreme, such attitudes can trigger age denial in an older person and can result in his or her refusing to admit or compensate for losses in auditory or visual acuity even with the use of bifocals or hearing aids. Ventry and Weinstein's (1983) *Hearing Handicap Inventory for the Elderly* represents an important attempt to develop an age-appropriate test for geriatric patients.

Problems in speech and communication not only limit *expression;* they also limit *access* to others. For older adults for whom access is already on the decline because of retirement, death of spouse, or other social exit events, the impact of speech and communication disorders can be particularly devastating. Successful rehabilitation and compensation must focus on enhancing access as well as on expression. The older patient carries a unique and lengthy personal history, which may explain apparently unusual behavior and which may also reveal resources and strengths around which a rehabilitation plan can be developed. When professionals are struggling with an older patient's resistance, noncompliance, or failure to understand a task in rehabilitation, they would do well to consider what they may be doing wrong before asking what is wrong with the older adult. In many cases health care professionals will find that they have made an error of omission, failing to acquire enough personal information or failing to apply a well-grounded model of normal behavior in old age.

The good news in research on the normal aging process is that the older patient will have resources and strengths that can be used in planning treatment. Many areas of skill and ability remain basically intact; the capacity to learn, change, and grow is clearly lifelong in normal populations. What seems necessary and beneficial for today's speech and communication health care professional is to superimpose a sufficient knowledge and skill base in geriatrics, which includes a strong sense of normal aging, on an already well-developed level of training. In general, older adults will be more similar than dissimilar in comparison to younger patients. However, the differences that do exist are usually of significant clinical importance.

Psychological Problems of the Aged

A basic set of guidelines for health care professionals to consider in dealing with the emotionally troubled elderly is given in Figure 6.1. Cohort differences are extremely important not only in mental health but in health care in general. It is not unusual, for example, to encounter overly compliant older adults who never ask questions and always assure the health care professional that they understand everything they have been told, simply because of the authority role they view the professional as filling. As a result, asking an older adult if his or her memory is functioning well may yield very different information from that obtained with a memory-screening test. Older adults may view mental health problems such as depression or anxiety as reflecting on their religious or moral character or that of their family. They may also see mental health treatment as being equivalent to institutionalization. Rather than being irrational, such beliefs are in fact representative of the normative view of mental illness in their adolescence and young adulthood.

It is easy, especially when dealing with individuals who have undergone a serious central nervous system insult such as a stroke, brain disease, or head trauma, to automatically treat any psychological disorders as having as organic etiology. While this may often be the case, it is also possible to encounter psychological problems, especially depression or anxiety, that may be related to the disease but not caused by it. Stroke patients, for example, may be very anxious about doing anything that they feel may cause another stroke; therefore, they severely limit their activities or resist physical therapy, not because of the stroke but because of the fears they associate with it. Similarly, depression may be associated with dementia without being caused by a neurological deficit (Zarit & Tager, 1980).

Having a patient history that includes a review of previous health problems and prior reactions to trauma and crises can be very helpful in predicting the patient's reaction to health and mental health care. In general, one of the best predictors of how individuals will react to their most recent trauma or crisis is the way they have reacted to previous ones. If they withdrew during a previous crisis, they will probably withdraw again; the same can hold true of anger, denial, and other common reactions.

- Be aware of the cohort or general values the older adult may have about mental health/illness.

- In general, more psychologically troubled people become old than do old people suddenly become troubled; look for a history.

- Organic and functional mental illness can coexist.

- Be alert to suicidal statements and indirect self-destructive behavior.

- Drug reviews including over-the-counter, prescription medications and the use of nicotine, caffeine, and alcohol are frequently required in ascertaining the cause of symptoms such as depression or agitation.

- Interview family members to obtain a better history and to evaluate the frequency, intensity, and duration of the problem.

- Try to ascertain the level of depression and/or anxiety present prior to the stroke, surgery, or most recent physical trauma.

- Determine how the individual has dealt with other losses or illnesses.

- Find out how the family has dealt with other losses or illnesses.

FIGURE 6.1. Guidelines for working with older adults experiencing emotional problems.

Knowing whether or not the patient has ever experienced clinical depression, an anxiety disorder, or other psychopathology prior to the current problems is critical in planning treatment. There are vast differences between individuals with lifelong histories of depression or alcohol abuse, for example, and those who are encountering such issues for the first time in old age. Similarly, being able to judge the premorbid level of anxiety or depression in the individual will help to identify the extent of the problems that are directly associated with the current physical disease and resultant loss of function. For example, predicting an acceptable level of recovery in cognitive abilities should include taking the patient's pre-stroke level of functioning into account.

The families of older patients, including not only the spouse but also adult children, can play an important role in the acquisition of knowledge and implementation of a treatment plan for mental health problems. Family members may provide valuable information regarding history that the older adult has forgotten or failed to report because of his or her depression or anxiety. They can also provide information about strategies for motivating and managing the patient that they have found effective. It is important to assess their resources and willingness to act as caregivers in planning for discharge and after-care. If they are already acting as caregivers, they may need to be debriefed regarding their current level of stress, physical health, and the strategies they employ to cope with caregiving as well as their approaches in caring for the patient.

The speech and communication disorders professional will frequently encounter older adults during or subsequent to a major health crisis; therefore, it is important to consider the psychological themes listed in Figure 6.2. The presence of multiple and frequently chronic health problems may be the single most distinguishing factor for the geriatric patient, especially in the age 75+ segment of the population. Approaches to rehabilitation with such individuals should be based in part on a recognition of the patient's belief system and thoughts about illness. For example, it is not unusual for older adults to think catastrophically about relatively minor health problems or functional losses as signifying "the beginning of the end." Loss of autonomy and independence can frequently contribute to a sense of helplessness that is characterized by the belief that all future events are simply up to fate and out of the control of the individual. Obviously, this type of learned helplessness (Guarnera & Williams, 1987; Scheier & Carver, 1985) is counterproductive to motivations for rehabilitation.

The literature on death fears and anxiety in the elderly (Kastenbaum, 1985) indicates that older adults will have more specific and concrete concerns about dying

- Loss of function = loss of autonomy

- Loss of autonomy = institutionalization

- Loss of control: When will the next (stroke, heart attack, seizure, etc.) occur? Can I keep it from happening or is it a randomly occurring event (*it could happen anytime*) over which I have no control (*there is nothing I can do to improve my condition*)?

- How might this disease kill me? Will it be a lingering and painful death?

- Will this disease bankrupt my spouse and me? Will it drain the inheritance I planned to leave my children?

- I know what happens next. My (spouse, mother, friend, etc.) died from this. The treatment you are offering me didn't do her any good!

FIGURE 6.2. Psychological themes in older adults experiencing critical health care problems.

and its practical ramifications than about death itself. In other words, concerns about medical expense, lingering deaths, and their impact on the individual and his or her family are common.

Because the rates of illnesses such as stroke and cardiovascular disease increase with aging, it is not unusual to encounter a patient who has had a spouse, close friend, or family member experience the same disease. Depending on the outcome associated with this prior event, the patient may either be highly motivated or convinced that nothing can be done.

Communication Disorders: Geropsychological Implications

Communication disorders at any point in the life-span may have strong psychological meaning. There are a number of factors that may enhance the devastation for older adults or create unique problems in comparison to younger age groups. First, it is important to note that many older adults have had a lifetime of unfettered communication and are encountering functional limitations and loss for the first time in 70 or 80 years of living. This suggests that their shock and despair may be greater than that of younger counterparts who have not experienced the full range of adult communication.

Second, a communication disorder may be superimposed upon normal or senescent changes in the older adult's vision and hearing, thus limiting his or her ability to compensate with these senses and potentially enlarging the degree of impact the disorder may have. This theme of conditions interacting with each other and creating a set of problems that are broader and potentially more devastating than those found in younger people is common in geriatrics.

The isolation imposed by communication deficits represents another example of the multiple and interacting problems that confront the elderly. Many older adults are already victimized by social isolation as a result of poverty; death of spouse, siblings, and friends; or loss of social roles through retirement and changes in family structure. The addition of communication disorders, even relatively limited ones, may constitute an additional force that essentially seals off the remaining opportunities the individual has for social contact.

Third, rehabilitation relies on the patient as a motivated learner; as a result, therapists need to be aware of some general principles in adult learning and motivation that should influence their approaches with geriatric patient populations. Figure 6.3 summarizes some of these features. Essentially, there is a need to spend more time socializing older adults to therapy—that is, explaining what their role is as well as that of the health care professionals and in very concrete terms describing how each task will improve their function. Ultimately the tasks should be linked to their contribution to the values of independence and staying at home, which the elderly prize. It is also important to apply basic learning techniques such as self-pacing and the use of meaningful tasks in the treatment (see Botwinick, 1984, for an excellent review of learning and the elderly). Older patients may be more sensitive to environmental distractions such as background noise, uncomfortable seating, and other conversations, which are common in institutional settings. It is also important to note that today's older Americans have on average an eighth-grade education, but their years of schooling can range from literally none to postcollege training. Adapting to their educational level is a critical therapeutic modality.

Finally, one of the important psychological functions of communication is that it enables the individual to exert some control over his or her personal environment. A realistic sense of control over what will happen to us and how we can influence our present and future conditions is an essential quality of mental health, as opposed to the feelings of helplessness and hopelessness that are typically a part of depression.

- Older learners tend to respond well to concrete specific explanations, instructions, and tasks.

- Older adults tend to respond well to nonevaluative relaxed instruction that suggests that they are not being tested or compared to others.

- Older adults may be easily distracted by background noise or music, uncomfortable chairs, irrelevant designs and borders on written information, and inadequate or glaring lighting.

- The current generation of elderly place a high value on autonomy and independence; any tasks that they associate with increases in this sphere will be highly valued.

- Self-paced as opposed to timed tasks may tend to enhance older adults' performance.

- The general principles of small linked goals with measurable results work well with aged patients.

- The majority of older adults continue to report that they wish to remain in their own homes as long as possible; interventions associated with this goal will be highly valued.

- Older adults attend and respond well to self-help and support groups.

- Older adults tend to be more motivated when they understand the purpose of the task they are performing.

FIGURE 6.3. The geriatric patient as a motivated learner.

Declines or losses in the older patient's ability to communicate may signify a loss of control, increase in dependence, and continuation of a gradual erosion of power that may have included retirement (loss of power in the workplace), family changes (loss of control over children), and other physical illnesses (loss of control over joints, bladder, etc.). One response to this dilemma on the part of some patients will be an increased effort to manipulate and control their rehabilitation program and the professionals and family members involved in it. Often this can take the form of refusing to participate, sending double messages about the treatment (appearing enthusiastic but never complying with requests), and blaming professionals and family members in an attempt to manipulate through guilt feelings.

Stress and the Elderly

Old age is frequently viewed as a time of increased stress. The increase is not a simple matter of amount; it often includes an increase in the diversity of types of stressors, including physical illness, economic problems, social alienation, and psychological problems. The influence of stress reactions on physical health has been well documented (Siegler & Costa, 1985). One practical implication for work with geriatric populations is their greater likelihood of becoming fatigued as a result of a general decrease in stamina combined with the presence of a significant stress level. This will require briefer periods of rehabilitation training with more rest periods than those used for younger adults. Factors that seem to influence older adults' ability to adapt to stress include their functional reserve for withstanding physical changes, the availability of appropriate coping behaviors, the degree to which the stressful event was expected (e.g., death of a spouse vs. death of a child), and their perception of the stress as controllable or uncontrollable (Kahana & Kahana, 1979; Kasl & Berkman, 1981; Rodin, 1980).

Clearly the effects of environmental or intrapersonal stress are mediated by a variety of factors. Assessment of the amount of stress an individual is under may be too simplistic unless it is accompanied by an analysis of the types of stress and the current level of adaptation and coping that exist. In addition to being stressful events themselves, communication disorders may severely disrupt coping abilities directed at other stressors as well. This restriction of adaptive responses can further increase the burden of additional stressors, initiating a downward spiral of functioning.

Positive events such as grandparenthood or remarriage, especially those with aspects of change in life-style and behavior, can also be stressful. As an example, improvement in health through rehabilitation may restore the older adult to higher levels of functioning and corresponding unwanted increases in responsibility; this may explain the paradoxical resistance to rehabilitation on the part of some patients.

Implications for Practice

Recognizing the impact of speech and communication disorders as stressors and as restraints in adaptation can help the health care professional to conceptualize the relationship between stress, depression, and poor performance in rehabilitation. In all likelihood, patients are experiencing environmental and intrapersonal stress when they are confronted with rehabilitation, which may be viewed as yet another overwhelming stimulus demanding change.

Just as different patients will report varied levels of pain associated with the identical injury, *perceived* levels of stress on the part of patients experiencing the same stressors will vary. It is important to ascertain individual self-perceptions of the levels of stress they are experiencing rather than to impose a professional bias. For instance, the value of activities associated with a functional loss will vary across individuals; hearing loss for a musician or avid music listener may be perceived as being far more stress-

ful than for a voracious reader. A close assessment of premorbid activities will reveal the degree of potential impact the functional limitation may have. A common example of this process among the elderly is the loss of the ability to operate an automobile, which many elderly view as resulting in a great deal of forced dependence; others may only see it as a nuisance that can be compensated for through public transportation and family assistance.

Depression and the Elderly

Although findings related to rates of depression in the older population vary in terms of how depression is defined and diagnosed, there is some agreement that along with organic brain syndromes, where the increase in later years is well documented, depression is one of the most common psychological problems of the elderly (La Rue, Dessonville, & Jarvik, 1985). Before considering depression and its relationship to speech and communication disorders, two notes of caution should be made. First, although a significant number of older adults do become depressed in old age, it is more likely that health care professionals will encounter depressed individuals who have become old. In other words, many persons who have experienced depression periodically throughout their lives encounter additional stressors and losses in old age that may contribute to or trigger an additional episode of depression, whereas a smaller though significant number of patients may be experiencing clinical depression for the first time.

A second caution that must be issued to health professionals concerns the influence of negative personal feelings about aging that may influence their diagnostic skills. If the health care professional views old age as a sad and depressing time of life, he or she may begin to assume that most older people are depressed, interpret any symptom as being part of a depression, or assume that some degree of depression is a natural consequence of aging and does not really warrant treatment. All of these biased perceptions will lead to inaccurate diagnosis and inadequate treatment.

Diagnosis is one of the most important treatment issues related to depression in the elderly. The symptoms of depression are markedly similar to those of dementia and may require a fairly sophisticated differential diagnostic approach, especially since both problems may be present. A great deal of research has been devoted to this area (see, for example, Breslau & Haug, 1983). Of particular import for professionals in the field of speech and communication disorders are the findings indicating that depressed elderly, in contrast to those who are demented, evidence more fluctuation in and rapid onset of cognitive problems, show little fluctuation in mood, and emphasize rather than deny their physical disabilities. Emery (1988) emphasizes the role of language in the diagnosis of pseudodementia. The demented patient typically shows greater loss of complex language skills; therefore Emery encourages the use of word fluency, responsive speech, and sentence completion measures in diagnosis.

Symptoms of depression in the elderly are not vastly different from those of younger adults. Sleep and appetite may increase or decrease. There is a general loss of interest in pleasurable activities such as sexual activity, socializing, and work or hobbies. Emotionally the individual has a pervasive blue mood characterized by feelings of intense sadness, hopelessness, and helplessness. Cognitively the patients view themselves, their present conditions, and the outlook for the future in very negative and pessimistic terms. Behaviorally the clinician will notice a slowing of speech and motor movement; a decline in daily activities; and, especially in the elderly, an increase in somatic complaints such as vague aches and pains. One problem for the clinician lies in the fact that somatic complaints and to some degree a loss of interest in certain activities and changes in sleep patterns have been documented in the nondepressed elderly population as well.

There are several models of depression in old age of which clinicians should be made aware. The *guilt model* suggests that in the course of reviewing their lives and attaching meaningfulness to them and to their mortality some older adults will begin to ruminate about the failures, tragedies, and pain they have experienced and will begin to blame themselves, becoming progressively guilt-ridden in the process. In dynamic terms this process may lead to "anger turned inward"; cognitively, older adults may begin to think of their life and themselves as meaningless and failures and may feel that the problems they encounter in old age are either things they "deserve" or barriers to happiness that cannot be overcome. This model emphasizes the importance of emotional support in therapeutic approaches to the elderly in addition to approaches that enhance self-esteem. Cognitive approaches (Beck, Rush, Shaw, & Emery, 1979) applied to this model involve challenging distorted depressive thinking and emphasizing the use of positive self-statements.

The *loss model* views depression as a response to the irreplaceable losses that many older adults encounter such as death of spouse, mandatory retirement, or reduction of independence due to chronic illness. Such losses are irreplaceable in that it is unlikely that jobs formerly held by spouses (especially husbands) and in some cases previous levels of function can be fully replaced. This is in marked contrast to the attitude of younger adults, who tend to operate on a *loss replacement model*. For the depressed elderly, mourning over losses tends to develop into an abnormal grief reaction characterized by depression, withdrawal, and isolation. The psychosocially oriented model emphasizes the importance of sustaining existing relationships and roles while enhancing the older adult's resources and opportunities for developing new ones.

A more behavioral orientation to depression in the later years could be called the *loss of structure* or *opportunity for reinforcement model*. Essentially this model views the depressed elderly as experiencing a decline in opportunities for pleasant and reinforcing events. This depletion is often caused by a loss of structure in areas where reinforcement was formerly readily available, such as work, child care, and marriage, and also by shrinkage of the individual's significant relationships as a result of the death of family and friends. Individuals may begin to feel that their current and future opportunities for happiness in their daily lives are out of their control. Treatment within this model involves close monitoring of mood, as well as very specific behavioral analysis of events that are reinforcing to the individual and barriers that must be overcome in accessing these events.

Regardless of the model employed, health care professionals should be aware of the emotional, behavioral, cognitive, and physical aspects of depression as it exhibits itself in elderly populations. Rates of depression accompanying physical illness are very high in the elderly and pose an obvious threat to rehabilitation.

The most tragic consequence of untreated depression in older adults is revealed by national statistics, which indicate that the elderly, particularly older white males, complete more suicides than any other age group. Although adolescents have higher rates of attempts, older adults are more likely to complete the act (McIntosh, Hubbard, & Santos, 1981; Osgood, 1985). This alarming trend in completion is caused by a number of factors: The older suicidal person is more physically vulnerable; elderly attempters show a preference for violent methods such as guns and hanging; there is an increased likelihood that the older adult will be living alone and will not be found as quickly or easily after the attempt; and, finally, suicidal older adults may be more intent on and committed to the suicidal act than their younger counterparts.

These trends, when combined with high rates of depression in the elderly population, suggest that all health care professionals in geriatrics need to be sensitive to this problem. Depression alone or combined with alcohol abuse in an elderly person who has also experienced a recent loss (e.g., death of spouse or reduced levels of function due to illness) will place this individual in a potentially high-risk category for suicide. The clinician's concern should be further heightened if a prior attempt is identified for either the individual or his or her family. In addition to direct statements expressing the wish to die, suicidal elderly may express their feelings in more subtle and indirect ways, such as refusing to engage in rehabilitation activities because it "doesn't really matter," saying grateful good-byes to staff and family as though they won't be seen again, or overemphasizing the importance of updating a will and making sure that funeral arrangements are in order. Older patients may also engage in indirect self-destructive behavior such as refusing to eat, take medication, have additional surgery, or comply with a rehabilitation program (McIntosh & Hubbard, 1988). Such death-enhancing actions are potentially devastating to the patient and may in some cases be erroneously labeled as rational acts when in reality they are decisions arrived at without full consideration of the facts and alternatives and within the context of a depressed state.

Implications for Practice

Any loss including those in the sphere of speech and communication functioning will frequently be grieved for by the patient. This is an entirely normal and understandable part of the rehabilitation process. However, when sadness and grief begin to permeate the life-style and choices of the patient, and when symptoms appear in physical, emotional, and cognitive domains, health care professionals should be alert to the possibility of clinical depression and, in particular, the possibility of suicide attempts.

In terms of rehabilitation, it is important to remember that depressed elderly may view new tasks as "just another thing I can't do" or as useless based on their view of their current illness as being "the beginning of the end." Small measurable goals that can produce easily documented improvement, no matter how subtle, should be considered in an attempt to introduce a sense of personal control and likelihood of success into the rehabilitation process. Placing an emphasis on the patient as a collaborator rather than only as a recipient of therapy may also help to combat the negative feelings and withdrawal common to the depressive syndrome.

Correlations between levels of depression and physical illness in the elderly are strong (Jarvik & Perl, 1981) and can be further complicated by side effects from medication and by catastrophic thinking on the part of the older patient and his or her family members. Depression has behavioral, cognitive, and emotional components. Patients who report feeling better but are not thinking or behaving in a less depressed manner will still need treatment.

Anxiety in the Elderly

Older adults who have experienced some degree of physical illness may be hypervigilant about bodily symptoms and functions as their anxiety about real or imagined health crises rises. Such body monitoring can lead to consistent complaints from the elderly that activities related to their rehabilitation may in fact bring on new problems ("If I try too hard I might give myself a heart attack") or exaggerate existing conditions ("I don't want to do anything that might raise my blood pressure any higher. That's what caused my last stroke"). Such concerns may be reinforced by spouse and family members as well.

In other cases it has been noted that some older adults tend to somaticize their emotional problems, leading to an increase in physical complaints during periods of emotional stress. However, high rates of hypochondriasis in the elderly have not been found (Costa & McCrae, 1980). In these situations, providing the patients with emotional support and opportunities to discuss family and personal problems works better than attempts to prove to them that no medical basis for the complaint exists.

It is extremely important to note, however, that underreporting of symptoms is the most typical pattern among the elderly (Kart, 1981). This can have serious medical consequences and is often not considered by health care professionals who falsely believe that most older adults are hypochondriachal. Underreporting of symptoms may be due in part to a belief that the problems are the result of aging and are therefore untreatable.

Implications for Practice

Although rates of anxiety and related disorders do not appear to increase in old age, clinicians in health care and rehabilitation settings will encounter such reactions in elderly patients, particularly when they are in unfamiliar settings such as hospitals. The numerous and subtle physical changes that accompany aging suggest that reported symptoms should be taken seriously even when no physical etiology can be discovered.

Conclusions

The psychological aspects of aging play a central role in diagnosis, treatment planning, and outcome in speech and communication disorder therapy. It is equally important for health care professionals to be aware of the potential psychological impact of working in geriatrics, where they may face issues related to their own as well as their parents' aging and death.

Processing of interpersonal information is critical to emotional well-being at any age. Deficits in input or output reduce the likelihood that both emotional and physical needs will be met. Older adults may be particularly vulnerable to such negative events because they occur in combination with other social, physical, and psychological changes. Communicative ability may decline while opportunities for exchange shrink rather than expand. These problems occur at a time when, more than at any other stage of life, the individual has a rich personal history to share and a strong need to arrive at a sense of meaningfulness by exchanging life stories with significant others.

The psychological aspects of geriatric rehabilitation include careful adherence to principles of learning in later life including personal, physical, and environmental factors. Cohort and motivational issues will also play a role in how the patient approaches and responds to therapy. Similarities outnumber the differences encountered in comparing older and younger patients. However, the differences that do exist are critical to quality care. Above all, it is important for the speech and communication disorders professional and all geriatric health care professionals to remain aware of the fact that older adults can and do learn, change, and improve during the course of treatment.

References

Beck, A., Rush, J., Shaw, B., & Emery, G. (1979). *Cognitive therapy of depression.* New York: Guilford Press.

Bergman, M. (1980). *Aging and the perception of speech.* Baltimore, MD: University Park Press.

Birren, J. E., & Renner, V. J. (1979). *A brief history of mental health and aging.* Washington, DC: National Institute of Mental Health.

Birren, J. E., & Sloane, R. B. (1980). *Handbook of mental health and aging.* Englewood Cliffs, NJ: Prentice-Hall.

Botwinick, J. (1966). Cautiousness in advanced age. *Journal of Gerontology, 21,* 347–353.

Botwinick, J. (1984). *Aging and behavior.* New York: Springer.

Breslau, L. D., & Haug, M. R. (Eds.). (1983). *Depression and aging: Causes, care and consequences.* New York: Springer.

Butler, R. N., & Lewis, M. (1977). *Aging and mental health.* St. Louis, MO: Mosby.

Cohen, G. (1979). Language comprehension in old age. *Cognitive Psychology, 11,* 412–429.

Cohen, G., & Faulkner, D. (1986). Does "Elderspeak" work? The effect of intonation and stress on comprehension and recall of spoken discourse in old age. *Language & Communication, 6,* 91–98.

Costa, P. T., Jr., & McCrae, R. R. (1980). Somatic complaints in males as a function of age and neuroticism: A longitudinal analysis. *Journal of Behavioral Medicine, 3,* 245–257.

Emery, V. O. (1988). Pseudodementia: A theoretical and empirical discussion. In R. W. Hubbard & J. Kowal (Eds.), *Western Reserve Geriatric Education Center Interdisciplinary Monograph Series, 4.* Cleveland, OH.

Erikson, E. (1963). *Childhood and society* (2nd ed.). New York: Norton.

Guarnera, S., & Williams, R. L. (1987). Optimism and locus of control for health and affiliation among elderly adults. *Journal of Gerontology, 42,* 594–595.

Gutmann, D. (1977). The cross-cultural perspective: Notes toward a comparative psychology of aging. In J. E. Birren & K. W. Schaie (Eds.), *Handbook of the psychology of aging* (pp. 302–326). New York: Van Nostrand Reinhold.

Havighurst, F. J. (1972). *Developmental tasks and education* (3rd ed.). New York: McKay.

Jarvik, L. F., & Perl, M. (1981). Overview of physiologic dysfunction and the production of psychiatric problems in the elderly. In A. Levenson & R. C. W. Hall (Eds.), *Psychiatric management of physical disease in the elderly* (pp. 1–15). New York: Raven Press.

Kahana, E., & Kahana, B. (1979). *Person-environment fit revisited: Some new directions for gerontological research and intervention.* Revised version of *A congruence model of person-environment fit.* Paper presented at meeting of Gerontological Society of America, Washington, DC.

Kart, C. (1981). Experiencing symptoms: Attribution and misattribution of illness among the aged. In M. R. Haug (Ed.), *Elderly patients and their doctors* (pp. 70–87). New York: Springer.

Kasl, S. V., & Berkman, L. F. (1981). Some psychosocial influences on the health status of the elderly: The perspective of social epidemiology. In J. L. McGaugh & S. B. Keisler (Eds.), *Aging: Biology and behavior* (pp. 345–377). New York: Academic Press.

Kausler, D. H. (1982). *Experimental psychology and human aging.* New York: Wiley.

La Rue, A., Dessonville, C., & Jarvik, L. F. (1985). Aging and mental disorders. In J. E. Birren & K. W. Schaie (Eds.), *Handbook of the psychology of aging* (2nd ed., pp. 664–702). New York: Van Nostrand Reinhold.

Light, L. L. (1988). Language and aging: Competence versus performance. In J. E. Birren & V. L. Bengtson (Eds.), *Emergent theories of aging* (pp. 177–213). New York: Springer.

McIntosh, J. L., & Hubbard, R. W. (1988). Indirect self-destructive behavior among the elderly: A review with case examples. *Journal of Gerontological Social Work, 13,* 37–48.

McIntosh, J. L., Hubbard, R. W., & Santos, J. F. (1981). Suicide among the elderly: A review of issues with case studies. *Journal of Gerontological Social Work, 1,* 63–74.

Neugarten, B. L. (1973). Personality change in late life: A developmental perspective. In C. Eisdorfer & M. P. Lawton (Eds.), *The psychology of adult development and aging* (pp. 311–338). Washington, DC: American Psychological Association.

Obler, L. K., & Albert, M. L. (1985). Language skills across adulthood. In J. E. Birren & K. W. Schaie (Eds.), *Handbook of the psychology of aging* (2nd ed., pp. 463–471). New York: Van Nostrand Reinhold.

Okun, M. A., Siegler, I. C., & George, L. K. (1978). Cautiousness and verbal learning in adulthood. *Journal of Gerontology, 33,* 94–97.

Osgood, N. J. (1985). *Suicide in the elderly.* Rockville, MD: Aspen.

Rodin, J. (1980). Managing the stress of aging: The role of control and coping. In S. Levine & H. Ursin (Eds.), *Coping and health* (pp. 171–202). New York: Plenum Press.

Rowe, J. W., & Kahn, R. L. (1987). Human aging: Usual and successful. *Science, 237,* 143–149.

Rubin, K. H., & Brown, I. D. R. (1975). A life-span look at person perception and its relationship to communicative interaction. *Journal of Gerontology, 30,* 461–468.

Ryan, E. B., Giles, E., Bartolucci, G., & Henwood, K. (1986). Psycholinguistic and social psychological components of communication by and with the elderly. *Language & Communication, 6,* 1–24.

Schaie, K. W. (1977). Toward a stage theory of adult cognitive development. *Aging and Human Development, 8,* 129–138.

Scheier, M., & Carver, C. (1985). Optimism, coping and health: Assessment and implications of generalized outcome expectancies. *Health Psychology, 4,* 219–247.

Siegler, I. C., & Costa, P. T., Jr. (1985). Health behavior relationships. In J. E. Birren & K. W. Schaie (Eds.), *Handbook of the psychology of aging* (2nd ed., pp. 144–162). New York: Van Nostrand Reinhold.

Ventry, I. M., & Weinstein, B. E. (1983). Identification of elderly people with hearing problems. *Asha, 25,* 37–42.

Wallach, M. A., & Kogan, N. (1961). Aspects of judgment and decision making: Interrelationships and changes with age. *Behavioral Sciences, 6,* 23–36.

Zarit, S. H., & Tager, R. M. (1980). *Aging and mental disorders—Psychological approaches to assessment and treatment.* New York: Free Press.

Older People's Uses of the Environment in Communication

CHAPTER 7

M. Powell Lawton, PhD ■

The study of communication in the personal and social lives of older people has tended to be narrow, having been focused on the direct, technical aspects of the sensory, cognitive, and motor mechanisms involved in communication. This chapter continues a theme begun earlier (Lawton, 1985b) of exploring the sector of communication that involves the environment as a mode of achieving personal and social goals for older people. Throughout the chapter an attempt will be made to depict the older person as both encoder and decoder; that is, environment is seen as a medium through which older people send messages to the world as well as one whose signals shape older people's behavior. A dialectic between need for autonomy and need for support constitutes the central feature of the goal-directed transactions of older people with their environment.

The chapter will begin by defining some relevant constructs from gerontology and environmental psychology. The central position of health in the autonomy-support

dialectic will be noted. The bulk of the chapter will discuss both the core arenas of environment as communication—personal space, territoriality, and personal possessions—and the relevance of this topic to the places where older people live. The chapter will conclude with a brief discussion of how clinical practice might benefit from some of these person-environment considerations.

Environment as Communication: Theoretical Background

The Environment

A substantial claim may be made on theoretical grounds that person and environment as a transactional system cannot be

113

separated (Altman & Rogoff, 1987). Nonetheless, for operational, research purposes they must be measured separately. Thus, for this chapter, environment is defined as all that lies outside the skin of the person—that is, it is "objective" in the sense of being observable, measurable, or countable by people. The environment may be physical, personal (significant others), suprapersonal (the characteristics of aggregates of people in physical proximity to the person), or social-institutional (e.g., the law, social norms, and culture). One important transactional aspect is the "subjective" environment, the person's internally processed representation of the objective environment, whether it is processed through sensory, cognitive, or affective means. A metric for environment may be viewed as "press" (Murray, 1938), or the strength with which an aspect of the environment demands a response from the person.

The Person

In their original statement of an ecological model of aging, Lawton and Nahemow (1973) focused on "personal competence" as the aspect of the person that was most relevant to the behavior of older people. Competence was seen as the person's ability to function in the biological, sensorimotor, and cognitive areas, as evaluated by social-normative standards. Thus, like environment, competence is theoretically observable and measurable.

The outcome of a person-environment interaction was seen as either (a) behavior in a limited number of arenas, again evaluated in terms of social norms, or (b) subjective well-being, requiring the person's evaluation in terms of mental distress or positive affect.

In later elaborations (Lawton, 1980a, 1985a, 1989), a need to account for the more active side of person-environment transactions was acknowledged. Environment also affords resources and the person also has needs (this view was elaborated by Carp, 1984) or "desires" (Reich & Zautra, 1983).

Thus a reactive, or passive, transaction involves an environmental press evoking a response from a person of a given level of competence. A proactive transaction involves a person with a need searching the environment for a resource congruent with his or her needs and competences.

Environmental Communication

The focus of this chapter is on one type of communication, spatial behavior. It specifically excludes linguistics and other aspects of verbal communication that have no spatial component and touches only lightly on kinesics, or communication through the medium of the body alone.

Hall's (1966) definition of proxemics, "the interrelated observations and theories of man's use of space as a specialized elaboration of culture" (p. 1) is broad enough to cover most of the phenomena studied in environmental psychology. A definition of the explicitly communicating aspects of spatial behavior has not come to light. Therefore, let us use the term *proxemic communication* to denote the uses of space, objects, and distances between people as media for encoding and decoding information.

A seminal treatment of proxemic communication was a neglected contribution of Alton DeLong (1972), in which he presented a view of person-environment relationships in terms of structural linguistics. DeLong argued first that environment is a code with three essential aspects: etics, emics, and tactics. *Etics* make up the environment as it exists objectively, where every feature is unique and there is no redundancy; therefore, the environment in these terms alone is so complex as to be without meaning. *Emics* involves groupings of etic aspects of the environment and the imposition of structure by the syntax of the perceiver. It is easy to recognize the definitions of objective and subjective environment in its etic and emic aspects, respectively. Further reduction in complexity of the environmental code is attained by restrictions placed on the ordering and groupings of emics, called *tactics* by DeLong. Thus the structure of communication (though not its content) may be understood in terms of these three basic principles that apply to the environment as well as to other media of communication. Translated into more familiar environmental concepts, etics represents the external aspects of the environment that constitute the raw material for processing by the person; this processing is accomplished by internal biological and socially learned principles of groupings imposed by the perceiver (emics) as well as by differential meanings as a function of the broader context in which the person-environment transaction occurs (tactics).

This linguistic view of environment is not meant to subsume all of its functions, such as the physical provision of shelter; freedom from intrusion; and the instrumental functions of objects, structures, or spaces.

Edward Hall (1966) observed that in American culture space is apt to occupy the same position in covert and overt behavior as sex; it is always there but is talked about much less often. The ways in which environment serves the communication process are likely to be even more covert than the functional processes that relate person and environment. It is thus the intention of the bulk of this chapter to call attention to some of the ways in which environment is involved in the communication processes of older people.

Is Age Relevant to the Coding Functions of Environment?

A milestone in gerontological research was achieved when empirical research, theory, and methodological development culminated in the general acceptance of the idea that many of the negative changes that had been found to be correlated with chronological age were at least partly explainable on the basis of either cohort effects or historical effects (Schaie, 1965). That is, people born at the same calendar time undergo a series of common experiences whose cumulative effects over a lifetime may make them more similar to one another than to people born at other times who have undergone different experiences. Similarly, the time of history in which data are gathered may exert influences on all people at that time, influences that differ across different years of testing. Thus both differences caused by cohort experiences and those resulting from the events of a given time in history may be mistakenly ascribed to age, since they are difficult to separate statistically. The major conclusion from this stream of research was that the extent and timing of cognitive decline associated with chronological age had been greatly overestimated in the past (Eisdorfer & Lawton, 1973). The same ambiguity is possible in every other sphere, for example, in the estimation of psychological well-being, where historical events and cohort-related styles of responding may have profound effects on measured well-being (Costa et al., 1987; Felton & Shaver, 1984).

The same question must be kept in mind as the communicating functions of the environment are discussed. At this point it is fair to say that *no* conclusive evidence is at hand to support the conclusion that age alone changes environmental coding behavior. One should hasten to add that there has been no satisfactory attempt to test this hypothesis. Therefore, it should be understood at the outset that most of the assertions to be made about age in relation to environmental communication are in fact hypotheses; investigation of these relationships among age, cohort, and period effects is vital in accounting for any correlations with chronological age.

Age and Environmental Familiarity

Another source of ambiguity must be acknowledged, which is the difference between an age effect based on the passage of time and an age effect based on accumulated experience. Biological aging viewed in "wear and tear" terms is a generally decremental view of the life-span, where changes in psychological and social functions are viewed as secondary to the winding down of the biological clock. By contrast, however, living longer also brings with it increasing experience in interacting with one's environment. The nature of this interaction may be positive or negative. For example, social stereotyping, ageism, and involuntary retirement would generally be thought of as negative experiences. On the other hand, job experience, practice in the performance of instrumental tasks, and mature judgment may contribute to the accumulation of positive experience. Gerontologists have often based developmental theories on such positive experiential accumulation. Baltes, Dittmann-Kohli, & Dixon (1984) formulated a theory of "selective optimization with compensation," which suggests that people increasingly focus their attention on developing and maintaining expertise in areas most salient to their life goals while relinquishing skills in other areas, compensating for the lost skills in "satisficing" ways (that is, ways that fall short of the ideal but that the person judges to be good enough) (Simon, 1970). Carstensen (1987) has stated a "selectivity" theory of social relationships in adult life, which asserts that people become increasingly skilled in maintaining or enhancing relationships whose outcome is likely to maximize positive affect. Therefore, they are more likely to prefer old relationships to new ones, since the older ones are tried and true, predictable in their more positive nature.

In the area of environmental communication, familiarity is thus posited to play a central role, not because age brings with it an inability to process the unfamiliar, but because familiar aspects of the environment afford several desirable outcomes:

1. Familiarity implies that the meaning of that aspect of the environment has been overlearned. Thus, continued improvement in the cognitive skills for coding the environment enhances adaptive capacity.

2. Familiarity has been shown under some conditions to increase liking (Zajonc, 1980). DeLong (1972) has argued more generally that emotion is a central aspect of the communication process. Affect is thus inseparable from the cognitive aspects of a familiar aspect of the environment.

3. The behavioral implications of an environmental code also are practiced, are overlearned, and become an essential aspect of the person's adaptive capacity.

Thus, cognitive, affective, and behavioral outcomes at least have the ability to be modified by increments of experience in dealing with environmental code. The implications of familiarity for the environmental aspects of cognition, affect, and psychological outcomes will be considered in greater detail.

Cognitive Familiarity

A basic tenet of Piagetian theory (Piaget & Inhelder, 1970) consists of the dialectic processes of assimilation and accommodation. *Assimilation* represents an adaptational process whereby an environmental stimulus is accorded meaning by being fitted into a schema already existent in the person, established on the basis of prior developmental and learning processes. Emics thus involves comprehension of the environment by matching and classifying what is presented; fitting the environment to one's own schemata; and, in fact, altering the environment if its lack of fit is unacceptable. *Accommodation*, on the other hand, is necessary when an etic aspect of the environment cannot be transformed into an existing cognitive template for comprehension but instead forces the person to "accommodate" by altering an existing schema or forming a new one (see the section on Affective Familiarity later in this chapter).

Schematization is obviously an ongoing process, being maintained by the flow of familiar stimuli and augmented by newly formed schemata, which then become familiar. Selective optimization, or selectivity theory, describes what is observed to happen, that is, the maintenance and strengthening of some cognitive templates and the loss of others; in both Baltes's and Carstensen's perspectives, this is an actively managed process. Despite these ''proactivity'' hypotheses (discussed at greater length in Lawton, 1980a, 1985a), there clearly is also schematic attrition of a more passive type, the result of both biological decline and social depression.

Thus, in examining older people's use of the environment for communicative purposes, it is necessary to look separately at how the older person decodes and encodes. In a rough way, decoding is the more reactive stance and encoding the more proactive. While there are many linguistic reasons for studying the disjunction between decoding and encoding, for the present purpose the distinction will be used to pursue the dialectic between the older person as reactor and proactor.

The Older Person as Decoder

To some extent every aspect of the objective environment may function as a potential signal. For the present purpose the discussion will be limited to the decoding tasks that involve other people and their spatial relationship to the older perceiver (proxemics) and to the physical environment as symbol (micro-, meso-, and megaenvironment).

In keeping with the ecological model, the competence of the perceiver is a first matter of concern. Extensive documentation exists regarding sensory changes associated with aging, most of which are decremental and which are often prevalent in older people who are not otherwise impaired either mentally or physically. Comprehensive and updated reviews of this evidence may be found in Fozard (1990). Do poor vision,

hearing, or chemical senses alter the way the environment communicates? Perhaps the most compelling evidence of such an effect is qualitative research on ''the empathic model,'' an attempt to create the sensory competence of an average 75-year-old by applying sensory dampers (coated eyeglass lenses, earplugs, and so on) to younger people (Pastalan, 1979). The experiences reported by subjects going about their day's activities in this manner include severe loss of orientation, anxiety, and dependence on others.

Proxemics

In terms of the communicative functions of proxemics and environmental symbols, there has been relatively little research about the effects of sensory loss. DeLong (1970) reported an extensive qualitative study of the ecology of a treatment area for older people with Alzheimer's disease and other dementing illnesses. The sensory capacity of the specific individuals studied was not measured, however, and the conclusions regarding the relationship between aging and proxemic behavior thus assume sensory limitations without being able to link an individual's sensory loss to his or her proxemic behavior. With this problem acknowledged, a number of creative hypotheses emerged from DeLong's study.

A great deal of the content of environmental psychology has dealt with the messages communicated by others in their spatial positioning with respect to a target person. Many studies began by using Hall's (1966) concept of interpersonal distances and the types of interaction considered appropriate for each:

- Public distance: beyond 12 ft, requiring better than normal sensory amplitudes

- Social distance: from 4 to 12 ft, for ordinary formal social interaction

- Personal distance: the distance from 1.5 to 4 ft, considered appropriate for friendly, relaxed conversation

• Intimate distance: the range where intimate transactions occur, from actual touch to 1.5 ft

DeLong suggested that reductions in visual, auditory, thermal, and olfactory acuity compressed the physical ranges appropriate to these types of social interchange. That is, if the older person cannot see or hear the interaction partner well at a distance of 4 ft, he or she will tend to close the distance. Conversely, where the usual social interaction distances are maintained by the other, the older person will decode the message as one of greater distancing than the other may intend. Or, if the other is forced by a need to perform some hands-on task to reduce interpersonal distance, a message of discomfort or rejection in the other may be conveyed to the older person. DeLong used this paradigm to illustrate sources of tension between staff and residents. For example, direct-care staff of a nursing home, when forced to minister to the resident at an intimate physical distance, may signal their discomfort by arching their head back, looking away from the resident, or conversing with staff rather than the resident.

Quantitative tests of the existence of age- or health-correlated changes in proxemic decoding have been nonexistent. If the focus is broadened to include the uses of space generally, including crowding, the picture does not become appreciably clearer. Aiello (1987) reviewed six age-comparative studies of either actual or preferred interaction distance and found them to vary so widely regarding older people's preferences as to allow no conclusion as to whether age occasioned the need for more or less space.

Suffice it to say that considerable methodological improvement is required, including the use of ecologically valid techniques. The bulk of research on spatial preference has used synthetic methods for representing comfortable interaction distance, such as observing the distance between figures placed on mats, or asking questions like ''How close does this person get to you before you become uncomfortable?''

Thus we end in a still speculative mode. It is reasonable to think that sensory decrements might shrink personal space. An equally tenable hypothesis is that declining sensory functions might reduce the *salience* of interpersonal distance, rather than its metric units. Is it possible that people simply begin to notice such distances less? Reduction of sensory discrimination ability and eventual reduction of cognitive processing capacity might simply erode social decoding ability. A final possibility is a constancy phenomenon, whereby the overlearning that constitutes familiarity enables people to maintain appropriate proxemic behavior in spite of having to use cues of reduced intensity.

Kinesics

Although kinesics cannot be treated adequately in this presentation, it is important to recognize that body signals constitute a significant aspect of Hall's (1966) and DeLong's (1970) conception of proxemics. Included in Hall's proxemic code, for example, are dimensions of posture, body angle, voice loudness, visual contact, touch, thermal contact, and olfactory contact, in addition to distance. In fact, each of these kinesic dimensions has an implied spatial aspect, since each either is a function of distance or changes the distance between people.

Touch in particular has been speculated on by many, especially as an interaction technique in treating older people (Barnet, 1972; deWever, 1977). DeLong (1970) argued that decreased interaction distances forced many older people to reduce the distance to zero, in the absence of sensory or cognitive skills that would allow them to read messages of warmth or acceptance at the usual distances. There is little or no empirical evidence regarding the therapeutic function of touch, yet touching is widely recommended as a signal of acceptance. At the very least, older people are likely to vary in their preferences regarding touch. It would therefore be desirable to subject the use of touch to research evaluation before making any sweeping recommendations that older people should be touched while interacting with them. However, the one research-based study of touch did demonstrate that touching during moderately demented patients' eating increased nutritional intake (Eaton, Mitchell-Bonair, & Friedmann, 1986). Thus it is at least a reasonable hypothesis that a decline in visual, auditory, or cognitive competence may elevate the relatively global touch sense to a more prominent position in the communication hierarchy, because other forms of impairment do not obstruct this type of communication.

Symbolic Codes

The symbolic function of the physical environment is universal, of course. It is unlikely that age alone affects such symbolic communication appreciably. Again, however, what is familiar is likely to convey a clearer message. Thus objects with religious, ethnic, or historical resonances may convey particular meaning to older people. "Nostalgia" is composed partly of feeling ease of communication, and therefore cognitive efficacy, conveyed by a well-known facet of the environment.

Novel aspects of the environment are no doubt more difficult to decode as competence decreases. The symbolic element may thus begin to override the utilitarian message of an object, space, or structure. Becker (1977) has written of the "housing message" conveyed by the exterior of a domicile as perceived by both the occupant and the community at large. A residence radically different from what one has been accustomed to—for example, a multiunit high-rise structure—may communicate strangeness or impersonality. Of course, learning does take place. In fact, a longitudinal study of older people moving into new planned housing demonstrated that their anxious expectation of moving into a

high-rise structure was replaced by a generally positive evaluation of high-rise living a year later (Lawton, 1980b).

The sense of strangeness conveyed by innovative design is often accompanied by a fear that one might fail to master the use of the new object. It is very likely that teaching and practice are necessary to replace such negative symbolic meaning with a sense of efficacy. Thus the automatic banking machine, videotape player, or microwave oven may gain their functional convenience only after the negatively toned symbolic code associated with their novelty has disappeared.

Prosthetic design constitutes a special category of concern in this respect. Many assistive devices have been designed with no particular thought having been given to how they look. Thus their difference from what is usual may be perceived as "deviant" or may connote sickness and therefore discourage their use. Sensitization to such a possibility is needed to guide designers toward creating more acceptable objects for handicapped people.

The Older Person as Encoder

The ability to read the environment as presented is basic to adaptation. This aspect of environment furnishes the subject matter for the major preoccupation of behavioral design, the attempt to construct environments in such a way as to evoke desired behavior or emotions in the user or, in the case of the present chapter, how environments communicate *to* the older person. The way a person shapes the environment to conform to his or her needs, or proactivity, is a topic worthy of greater interest. Creating messages through the medium of the objective environment represents an exercise of autonomy in that the meaning placed by the older person into code has the potential of influencing the behavior of others.

Proxemic behavior is usually interactional, since interpersonal distance may be altered by either party. Curiously absent from proxemic research with older people is any attempt to distinguish between proactivity and reactivity in establishing interaction distance. Although a number of observers have noted clinically that some institutionalized older people offer their hands or touch visitors as they go by, no quantitative study exists to compare such behavior by age. The one relevant publication that was located was a naturalistic study of the proxemic behaviors of pedestrians in five countries (Berkowitz, 1971). Among the findings was the information that people judged to be 50 and over did not differ in frequency of observed touching behavior from adults under 50. Again, however, the study did not record who initiated the behavior.

Territorial behavior is one of the most studied topics in environmental psychology (see review by Brown, 1987). Establishing a territory in public space appears to be one of the most proactive behaviors in institutions, where privacy is a scarce commodity and opportunities to exercise autonomy are few (DeLong, 1970; Lipman, 1968). Despite the high salience of such behavior, territorial marking (i.e., denotation of space ownership in one's absence by an object, possession, or other indicator) by older people in institutions does not seem to have been studied. Older institutional residents apparently decode territorial markers adequately. Nelson and Paluck (1980) demonstrated that a simple tape line dividing a double room in a nursing home resulted in an increase in subjective well-being, presumably because it enhanced the sense of ownership and control.

Establishing a space as one's own is a way of attaining some control over that limited aspect of the environment. Adorning more permanent spaces or structures is another way of communicating to the world the aspects of oneself one wishes to have known. The housing message given by a dwelling in whose look one has had no part may be moderated by the occupant's proactive behavior. For example, Carp (1966) noted that occupants of the first public housing environment for older people, Vic-

toria Plaza in San Antonio, took great pains to have something unique on their door, in their window, or sometimes actually on the walkway of the deck that served as a single-loaded corridor (that is, apartments arrayed on only one side of the hall) for the high-rise building. Patterson (1978) found that older occupants of a high-crime neighborhood who personalized the exteriors of their homes responded to a neighborhood survey in a way that indicated less fear of crime than older occupants who had not made such territorial markings.

Possessions have been the topic of some researchers' attention. Furby (1978) emphasized the control over a limited aspect of the environment afforded by a totally owned object. Like an extension of the body, a possession is one's own to do with what one wishes. Rubinstein (1987) studied 88 older persons' significant objects and found that possessions improved identity and life meaning. There appears to be substantial variation in the meaning of cherished objects as a function of socioeconomic status (Redfoot & Back, 1988). Empirical research has demonstrated that nursing home residents whose rooms were more personalized also showed more positive psychological and social characteristics (Kamptner, 1989; Redondo, Demick, Collazo, Inoue, & Wapner, 1986; Sherman & Newman, 1977–1978).

In addition to these findings regarding the meaning of possessions, it would seem that the communicative aspect of belongings also must be recognized. People engage in a lifelong process of encoding their environment through their possessions with messages regarding the type of person they are. The messages have two objects: other people and the self. Another dialectic is enacted in doing this, the dialectic between communality and individuality (Altman, 1975). By owning and displaying objects that are cultural symbols, people signal their sense of belonging to the wider structures of society, whether they reflect their ethical values, religious affiliations, or socioeconomic status. To varying degrees people also announce to others what is uniquely important to them, such as hobbies, collections, or "good taste."

What is an environmental message to oneself? Such a message is one manifestation of personal identity, about which so much has been written (e.g., Whitbourne, 1987). Virtually all of the meanings discerned by Rubinstein (1987) may be seen as proactive uses of the environment to affirm who one is through one's possessions: relationships with others, past history, symbols of the self and one's accomplishments, defenses against loss, objects to care for, or "mature sensuousness." Knowing who one is clearly is enhanced by daily exposure to and practice with these environmental representations of the complex schemata of the self.

Again, all that has been said thus far about possessions may be true of adults of any age. What is unique about old age is the fact that belongings, for many, slowly evolve into a schema representative of their entire life-span. The temporal self may thus be displayed, reinforcing a sense of continuity with the past. To varying extents, such collections may become selectively representative more of the past than of the present. If "modern" artifacts seem foreign, a sense of security may evolve from the way belongings convey the sense of who one has been (Cumming & Henry, 1961). Such reasoning leads inevitably toward the affective aspects of the environment.

Affective Familiarity

DeLong (1972) suggested that emotion is an intrinsic aspect of communication. When the environment provides a novel stimulus for which a personal schema is not available, thus preventing assimilation of its meaning, the stream of behavior is interrupted. The interruption *is* emotion, DeLong argues. To this reasonable thought it may be added that matching an environmental stimulus to an internal schema also has an affective aspect, whether it is a posi-

tive evaluation of the familiarity of the stimulus or a negative response to the meaning previously accorded the stimulus.

Recent theory (Scherer, 1984) has called into question whether cognition and affect are really divisible and whether the question of temporal priority is as salient as has been suggested (Lazarus, 1982; Zajonc, 1980). It should simply be noted that the proxemic and symbolic functions of the environment discussed here are capable of including affective as well as cognitive content. For example, close physical proximity has been shown to increase autonomic activation and presumably emotional arousal (McBride, King, & James, 1965), but once again, we know little about whether aging affects such a tendency. Another example may be found in the functions of possessions, especially those related to personal identity (Rubinstein, 1987).

Still another example of the affective aspect of environmental messages helps us to comprehend further the already much-researched phenomenon of age grading in social relationships. One facet of the objective environment proposed in the ecological view of aging (Lawton, 1970) was the "suprapersonal environment," consisting of the modal characteristics of other people who are in physical proximity to the person. Age is one of the most salient of all such suprapersonal environmental characteristics. Research on age mixing (age integration vs. age segregation) has generally identified a number of favorable social and psychological outcomes associated with older people having large numbers of age peers in their immediate environment (Lawton, Moss, & Moles, 1984; Rosow, 1967; Teaff, Lawton, Nahemow, & Carlson, 1978). Shared values, common historical experiences, and age-appropriate social norms are among the mechanisms responsible for the higher levels of social interaction of older people in age-dense as compared to age-sparse environments. The basic underlying integrative process, however, is the confluence of communicative functions that begins with the visual image of people one's own age (etics) and extends through an immense array of verbal, proxemic, and kinesic messages of familiarity (emics). DeLong (1974) builds a case in favor of a learned parallel between intracultural sharing of environmental codes and central nervous system functioning that ensures positive affective experience in interchanges involving one's own group: "What coding accomplishes . . . is that it renders the behavior of members of a group *familiar* and *predictable.* Members of a group, through the mechanisms of socialization, insure themselves that they will know what to *expect* in the behavior of others. They may not know *what* others will communicate, but they know that if others are to behave meaningfully their behavior must conform to a variety of expectations" (p. 104).

Thus, although most older people do not actually reside in age-segregated residences, there is neurological, cognitive, and affective affinity among age peers by virtue of the shared meanings of communication at all levels.

The encoding role of the older person in relation to achieving a preferred suprapersonal environment may be seen first in the active choice by about 8% of the 65-and-older population of planned, age-segregated housing (Lawton, 1990). An even larger, though less exactly estimatable, proportion migrates to areas of the country that are "retirement destinations" both geographically and socially, in terms of age density (Biggar, 1980). In parallel with the general demographic age trends of the United States, increasing numbers of older people attend senior centers and participate in other age-conscious group activities. Finally, wherever they may live, older people demonstrate a measurable tendency to overchoose friends of their own age (Fischer, 1982; Rosow, 1967). Although this is not usually interpreted in terms of coding behavior, the individual choices of these people are actively creating, or encoding, the suprapersonal environments that in turn are decoded by others as age-dense environments. Thus the collective individ-

ual encoding behaviors of these people result in a powerful environmental code.

The autonomy-security dialectic is also well illustrated in the individual's response to age homogeneity. On one hand, age homogeneity conveys the message of safety and security. In fact Lawton et al. (1984) showed that those who preferred age-segregated living tended to be less healthy and of more disadvantaged status than those who preferred age-heterogeneous environments. On the other hand, once they attain such security, these people seem to experience a liberating effect that encourages more socialization and participation in activities (Rosow, 1967; Teaff et al., 1978).

To conclude this section, "familiarity" as it is frequently used to explain some preferences by older people, is seen to be a multifaceted, dynamic process that describes cognitive, affective, and behavioral outcomes associated with encoding and decoding. Although this analysis does not suggest that novelty and learning of new codes are undesirable just because a person is chronologically old, the assertion that length of exposure and practice in communication enhance learning and positive emotion does seem reasonable.

Using the Environment in Clinical Practice

By combining proxemic and kinesic perspectives, personal interactions may be modified in many ways. Intrinsic to some types of communication therapy is a close interaction distance between therapist and patient. Such distances are usually determined by the professional; for example, the worker may move closer so that a visually or aurally handicapped person can obtain some of the cues from the worker's facial expression or voice quality that risk being filtered out by the disability. Some workers are very uncomfortable in this situation without being aware of the origin of their discomfort. Direct use of proxemic principles during the training of staff, together with role playing in adapting to foreshortened interaction distances, will help to alleviate the worker's anxiety. Well-documented defensive reactions of unaware staff may include looking beyond the subject, arching the body away from the subject, or signaling tension in the facial muscles.

Ambiguities regarding the effects of touching older clients have already been noted. It may be that communication professionals are in the best position to be able to judge how different patients may prefer to be treated in terms of touch; they are trained to observe facial and body movements and may thus gain good ideas about whether a specific individual warms to a hand on the shoulder. It seems at least worth the experimental effort to see whether such a therapist could become the team specialist in "proxemic therapy," that is, a judge of how patients might respond and the person to whom staff might turn in discussing how to use touch.

Familiarity as a positive value might be introduced as a part of professional practice. For example, some types of eyeglasses or hearing aids are more familiar than others. The worker should at least be sensitive to making such choices available. On the other side, the low acceptability of novel environmental features must be recognized. Prosthetic and assistive devices and technologically advanced equipment often have this negative effect on older people. A deliberate attempt to provide multiple exposures to such novelty, or to allow new objects to be viewed before requiring them to be manipulated or allowing them to touch the person, may pay off with some clients.

Furnishings in an office or waiting room can be made to communicate familiarity and warmth. If the locus for therapy is the person's home, there are many opportunities for the worker to observe a need for environmental changes and to work with the client to effect them. It is especially appropriate for the impaired person to exercise proactivity in rearranging furniture or possessions. Resistance is usual when an outsider simply comes in and tells the person how the room can be brightened, how he or she can read better, and so on. A joint effort is much more likely to succeed. A good starting point might be the worker's asking the client to conduct a tour of the home, during which the client is encouraged to tell the professional what he or she does in each place. In conversational form, the older person can be encouraged to talk about what is good and bad in each space, can describe what is important about the space and furnishings, and perhaps can be enlisted in further efforts to redesign the interior. Although redesign for safety and improvement of function make up the usual focus of such conversations, it is sometimes possible for the person to verbalize the symbolic and aesthetic aspects of such concerns. This direction for the communication professional should be looked on as experimental for the time being. There would seem to be a great need to add such professionals to the multidisciplinary home adaptation team that more usually includes a designer, an environmental psychologist, an occupational therapist, and a social worker.

Conclusions

The way environment functions in communication for older people appears to be similar to the way it functions for people in general. What may change relationships between the person and the environment are factors like health (especially sensory changes), which impede decoding, and age cohort, which has a strong effect on the learning, decoding, and encoding of environmental meaning. Despite the reasonableness of these assertions, relatively little empirical research has been performed that would definitively test cross-sectional age differences, to say nothing of the virtually absent longitudinal research.

This chapter asserts that environment is a neglected agent in the autonomy-security dialectic that characterizes older people's goal-seeking behavior. Decoding behavior, particularly the cognitive ability to glean information from environmental signals, has been the focus of more attention than encoding behavior. Encoding is suggested as the point where autonomy is typically exercised (proactive behavior). Older people show considerable ability to construct physical environments that provide meaning to others and to themselves. Meaning provided to the self by the self-constructed environment is one aspect of identity.

The new large body of research on the paradigmatic environmental psychology issues of proxemics, territoriality, crowding, and other spatial transactions constitutes a sufficient base from which age-comparative research can flow. A mandatory aspect of such a long-term research program is to extend it into the longitudinal and sequential research designs that have informed so well our conception of cognitive aging.

References

Aiello, J. (1987). Human spatial behavior. In D. Stokols & I. Altman (Eds.), *Handbook of environmental psychology* (pp. 389–504). New York: Wiley.

Altman, I. (1975). *The environment and social behavior.* Monterey, CA: Brooks/Cole.

Altman, I., & Rogoff, B. (1987). World views in psychology: Trait, interactional, organismic, and transactional perspectives. In D. Stokols & I. Altman (Eds.), *Handbook of environmental psychology* (Vol. 1, pp. 7–40). New York: Wiley.

Baltes, P. B., Dittmann-Kohli, F., & Dixon, R. A. (1984). New perspectives on the development of intelligence in adulthood. In P. B. Baltes & O. G. Brim (Eds.), *Life-span development and behavior* (Vol. 6, pp. 33–76). New York: Academic Press.

Barnet, K. (1972). A theoretical construct of the concepts of touch as they relate to nursing. *Nursing Research, 21,* 102–110.

Becker, F. D. (1977). *Housing messages.* Stroudsburg, PA: Dowden, Hutchinson, & Ross.

Berkowitz, W. R. (1971). A cross-national comparison of some social patterns of urban pedestrians. *Journal of Cross-Cultural Psychology, 2,* 129–144.

Biggar, J. C. (1980). Reassessing elderly sunbelt migration. *Research on Aging, 2,* 177–190.

Brown, B. B. (1987). Territoriality. In D. Stokols & I. Altman (Eds.), *Handbook of environmental psychology* (pp. 505–532). New York: Wiley.

Carp, F. M. (1966). *A future for the aged.* Austin, TX: University of Texas Press.

Carp, F. (1984). A complementary/congruence model of well-being or mental health for the community elderly. In I. Altman, M. P. Lawton, & J. Wohlwill (Eds.), *Human behavior and the environment: The elderly and the physical environment.* New York: Plenum Press.

Carstensen, L. L. (1987). Age-related changes in social activity. In L. L. Carstensen & B. A. Edelstein (Eds.), *Handbook of clinical gerontology* (pp. 222–237). New York: Pergamon Press.

Costa, P. T., Jr., Zonderman, A. B., McCrae, R. R., Cornoni-Huntley, J., Locke, B. Z., & Barbano, H. E. (1987). Longitudinal analyses of psychological well-being in a national sample: Stability of mean levels. *Journal of Gerontology, 42,* 50–55.

Cumming, E., & Henry, W. (1961). *Growing old.* New York: Basic Books.

DeLong, A. J. (1970). The microspatial structure of the older person. In L. A. Pastalan & D. H. Carson (Eds.), *Spatial behavior of older people* (pp. 68–87). Ann Arbor: University of Michigan Institute of Gerontology.

DeLong, A. J. (1972). The communication process: A generic model for man-environment relations. *Man-Environment Systems, 2,* 263–313.

DeLong, A. J. (1974). Environments for the elderly. *Journal of Communication, 24,* 101–112.

deWever, M. K. (1977). Nursing home patients' perception of nurses' affective touching. *Journal of Psychology, 96,* 163–171.

Eaton, M., Mitchell-Bonair, I. L., & Friedmann, E. (1986). The effect of touch on nutritional intake of chronic organic brain syndrome patients. *Journal of Gerontology, 41,* 611–616.

Eisdorfer, C., & Lawton, M. P. (Eds.). (1973). *The psychology of adult development and aging.*

Washington, DC: American Psychological Association.

Felton, B. J., & Shaver, P. (1984). Cohort variation in adults' reported feelings. In C. Z. Malatesta & C. E. Izard (Eds.), *Emotion in adult development* (pp. 103–124). Beverly Hills, CA: Sage.

Fischer, C. S. (1982). *To dwell among friends: Personal networks in town and city.* Chicago: University of Chicago Press.

Fozard, J. L. (1990). Vision and hearing in aging. In J. E. Birren & K. W. Schaie (Eds.), *Handbook of the psychology of aging* (3rd ed., pp. 150–170). New York: Academic Press.

Furby, L. (1978). Possessions: Toward a theory of their meaning and function throughout the life cycle. In P. B. Baltes (Ed.), *Lifespan development and behavior* (Vol. 1). New York: Academic Press.

Hall, E. T. (1966). *The hidden dimension.* Garden City, NY: Doubleday.

Kamptner, N. L. (1989). Personal possessions and their meanings in old age. In S. Spacapan & S. Oskamp (Eds.), *The social psychology of aging* (pp. 165–196). Beverly Hills, CA: Sage.

Lawton, M. P. (1970). Ecology and aging. In L. A. Pastalan & D. H. Carson (Eds.), *Spatial behavior of older people* (pp. 40–67). Ann Arbor: University of Michigan Institute of Gerontology.

Lawton, M. P. (1980a). Environmental change: The older person as initiator and responder. In N. Datan & N. Lohmann (Eds.), *Transitions of aging* (pp. 171–193). New York: Academic Press.

Lawton, M. P. (1980b). *Social and medical services in housing for the elderly.* Washington, DC: U. S. Government Printing Office.

Lawton, M. P. (1985a). The elderly in context: Perspectives from environmental psychology and gerontology. *Environment and Behavior, 17,* 501–519.

Lawton, M. P. (1985b). Environment as communication. In H. Ulatowska (Ed.), *The aging brain* (pp. 7–19). Austin, TX: PRO-ED.

Lawton, M. P. (1989). Environmental proactivity and affect in older people. In S. Spacapan & S. Oskamp (Eds.), *Social psychology of aging* (pp. 135–164). Beverly Hills, CA: Sage.

Lawton, M. P. (1990). Knowledge resources and gaps in housing for the aged. In D. Tillson (Ed.), *Aging in place* (pp. 287–309). Glenview, IL: Scott, Foresman.

Lawton, M. P., Moss, M. S., & Moles, E. (1984). The suprapersonal neighborhood context of older people. *Environment and Behavior, 16,* 84–109.

Lawton, M. P., & Nahemow, L. (1973). Ecology and the aging process. In C. Eisdorfer & M. P. Lawton (Eds.), *Psychology of adult development and aging* (pp. 619–674). Washington, DC: American Psychological Association.

Lazarus, R. S. (1982). Thoughts on the relations between emotion and cognition. *American Psychologist, 37,* 1019–1024.

Lipman, A. (1968). A socio-architectural view of life in three homes for old people. *Gerontologia Clinica, 10,* 88–101.

McBride, G., King, M. G., & James, J. W. (1965). Social proximity effects of galvanic skin responses in adult humans. *Journal of Psychology, 61,* 153–157.

Murray, H. A. (1938). *Explorations in personality.* New York: Oxford University Press.

Nelson, M. N., & Paluck, R. J. (1980). Territorial markings, self concept, and the mental status of the institutionalized elderly. *The Gerontologist, 20,* 96–98.

Pastalan, L. A. (1979). Sensory changes and environmental behavior. In T. O. Byerts, S. C. Howell, & L. A. Pastalan (Eds.), *The environmental context of aging* (pp. 118–126). New York: Garland.

Patterson, A. H. (1978). Territorial behavior and fear of crime in the elderly. *Environmental Psychology and Nonverbal Behavior, 2,* 131–144.

Piaget, J., & Inhelder, B. (1970). *The psychology of the child.* New York: Basic Books.

Redfoot, D. L., & Back, K. W. (1988). The perceptual presence of the life course. *International Journal of Aging and Human Development, 27,* 155–170.

Redondo, J. P., Demick, J., Collazo, J. A., Inoue, W., & Wapner, S. (1986, August). *Role of cherished possessions in adaptation to the nursing home.* Paper presented at the annual meeting of the American Psychological Association, Washington, DC.

Reich, J., & Zautra, A. (1983). Demands and desires in daily life: Some influences on well-being. *American Journal of Community Psychology, 11,* 41–58.

Rosow, I. (1967). *Social integration of the aged.* New York: Free Press.

Rubinstein, R. L. (1987). The significance of personal objects to older people. *Journal of Aging Studies, 1,* 225–238.

Schaie, K. W. (1965). A general model for the study of developmental problems. *Psychological Bulletin, 64,* 92–107.

Scherer, K. R. (1984). On the nature and function of emotion: A component process approach. In K. R. Scherer & P. Ekman (Eds.), *Approaches to emotion* (pp. 293–317). Hillsdale, NJ: Lawrence Erlbaum.

Sherman, E., & Newman, E. S. (1977–1978). The meaning of cherished personal possessions for the elderly. *International Journal of Aging and Human Development, 8,* 181–192.

Simon, H. A. (1970). Style in design. In J. Archea & C. Eastman (Eds.), *EDRA 2: Proceedings of the second Environmental Design Research Association Conference.* Stroudsburg, PA: Dowden, Hutchinson, & Ross.

Teaff, J. D., Lawton, M. P., Nahemow, L., & Carlson, D. (1978). Impact of age integration on the wellbeing of elderly tenants in public housing. *Journal of Gerontology, 33,* 126–133.

Whitbourne, S. K. (1987). Personality development in adulthood and old age. In K. W. Schaie (Ed.), *Annual review of gerontology and geriatrics* (Vol. 7, pp. 181–216). New York: Springer.

Zajonc, R. B. (1980). Feeling and thinking: Preferences need no inferences. *American Psychologist, 35,* 151–175.

Caregiver Stress and Communication Management in Alzheimer's Disease

CHAPTER

Lynn W. Clark, PhD ■

A lzheimer's

Pronounce it Alzheimer's
Color it grey
Diagnose it only at death

Do brain scans
To show shrinkage.
Diffuse atrophy.

See neurons all tangled,
Plaques intertwined,
Absence of acetylcholene.

Call it dementia, madness
A disease
That kills not one, but two.[1]

Caregiving of the person with Alzheimer's disease has become one of the largest personal and professional issues of the 1980s and beyond. With a greater percentage of the population living to an old age and developing chronic impairments such as Alzheimer's disease, more families will have to provide care, and with it face varying degrees of burden and stress on their personal health and their social and economic resources. The progressive decline of cognitive, behavioral, and eventually physical functioning that characterizes Alzheimer's disease diminishes the quality of life not only for persons with the disease but for their families as well.

The sheer numbers of caregivers of persons with Alzheimer's disease mandates that health professionals provide effective caregiver intervention to reduce the impact caregiving has on the physical and emotional health of the caregiver. Only recently have health care professionals begun to explore the sources of caregiver stress and to implement intervention programs designed to reduce the caregiver's stress (Gallagher, Lovett, & Zeiss, 1989; Zarit & Anthony, 1986).

[1]From B. Morgan, 1984, *Generations,* 4(Winter), p. 55. Copyright 1984 by WGS, ASA. Reprinted by permission of Generations, 833 Market St., Suite 516, San Francisco, CA 94103.

The professional role of the speech-language pathologist in working with the caregivers of persons with Alzheimer's disease remains ill defined. In the future, in order for speech-language pathologists to work effectively with these caregivers, they must have a clear understanding of who the caregivers are and what their burdens are, including those associated with the communication changes of Alzheimer's disease. Thus, the first objective of this chapter is to review the complex interactions that exist between the clinical symptoms of the Alzheimer's patient; the caregiver's characteristics and social roles; the social support, financial resources, and health care services available within the caregiving environment; and the caregiver's emotional and physical reactions to providing care. Within this review, assessment tools for measuring the caregiver's burden and well-being will be highlighted.

The second objective of this chapter is to illustrate, through a review of the literature, why the communication changes associated with Alzheimer's disease may act as a critical source of caregiver stress, requiring intervention. The last section of the chapter provides the speech-language pathologist with a communication stress management approach for the caregiver.

Who Are the Caregivers?

Families and Caregiving

Caregivers of individuals with Alzheimer's disease have been a neglected and invisible group. Contrary to lingering myths, families do not abandon their older relatives to institutions. Of the 1.5 million Americans afflicted with Alzheimer's disease, one-half million are cared for at home (Katzman, 1976). Further, 80 to 90% of the home care of persons with Alzheimer's disease is directly performed by families, with a significant portion of caregivers spending at least 40 hours a week in the direct personal care of their relatives (Brody, 1985).

Changes in Family Roles

Given the heterogeneity among family caregivers, no single pattern of response to caregiving exists. The role that the person with Alzheimer's disease played in family relations prior to the diagnosis of the disease changes after diagnosis (Chenoweth & Spencer, 1976). Besides overtly maintaining instrumental family tasks (e.g., housekeeping, transportation, or financial management), the person may have covertly maintained the cohesiveness and emotional needs of family members (Zarit, Orr, & Zarit, 1985). Power and dominance in family relationships change; as the disease progresses, the caregiver must gradually take over many role behaviors and tasks that were formerly performed by the person with Alzheimer's disease. This can be particularly difficult when a spouse must begin to take over unfamiliar gender-specific roles or when an adult child must take over former parental roles (Circirelli, 1986).

The Effect of Cultural-Ethnic Backgrounds

Research on adult caregiving in general has demonstrated that the emotional stress of the family caregiver is minimized in minority families (e.g., blacks, Hispanics, Pacific Islanders, and Asians) as compared to non-minority families (Cantor, 1979; Mindel & Wright, 1980; Weeks & Cuellar, 1981). To date, only one study of minority black caregivers of persons with Alzheimer's disease has been conducted (Morycz, 1985). Collectively, results of studies suggest that minority caregivers report less emotional stress because they traditionally have had to assume a caregiver role throughout their entire life cycle as part of their culture's system.

Gender and Caregiving

It is no surprise that 85% or more of caregivers are female spouses and daughters, followed by male spouses, many who themselves are elderly. In some instances, sisters, daughters-in-law, nieces, and friends also act as caregivers through a paid surrogate. Given increased geographic mobility, decreases in family size, increase in participation of middle-aged women in the work force, and increasing divorce rates, who the caregivers are in the future will inevitably change.

A number of researchers have shown that differences exist in the type and degree of stress experienced by male and female caregivers (Boutselis & Zarit, 1984; Brody, 1985; Rabins, Mace, & Lucas, 1982; Zarit, 1982). Even when female spouses with Alzheimer's disease are more severely impaired than male spouses, male spouse caregivers remain less physically burdened and emotionally distressed than female spouse caregivers (George & Gwyther, 1984; Gwyther & George, 1986; Zarit, 1982). Although male spouse caregivers are distressed over not being able to interact with their female spouse as they once did, they adopt a more instrumental approach to everyday caregiving. As the disease progresses, male spouse caregivers increase their level of tolerance toward the changes caused by the disease, psychologically accept their caregiving limitations, and seek daily assistance from family members and paid household assistance (Zarit, Todd, & Zarit, 1986). On the other hand, female spouse caregivers are reluctant to seek help and fail to use support services even when they are available, because they traditionally view caregiving as a woman's role and more specially as a female spouse's responsibility (Morycz, 1985). For the female spouse caregiver, emotional and physical stress results from social isolation, the physical burden of daily caregiving, and the changing of their husband's role from one of independence to dependency.

Age and Relationship of the Caregiver

The life stage or age of the caregiver, and the relationship of the caregiver to the person with Alzheimer's disease, interact together as a predictor of stress. As one would expect, the better the prior relationship between the caregiver and the person with Alzheimer's disease, the less the caregiver burden (Fitting, Rabins, & Lucas, 1984; Fitting, Rabins, Lucas, & Eastham, 1986). However, the closer the family member, such as a spouse or adult child, is to the person with Alzheimer's disease, the greater the stress is for the caregiver (Cantor, 1983).

Intergenerational caregivers are more likely to suffer from role conflicts, whereas intragenerational caregivers suffer role entrenchment and isolation (Brody, 1985; Jarrett, 1985; Rabins, 1984). Spouses are emotionally distressed over the changes they observe in their impaired spouse. Further, their impaired spouse reminds them of their own mortality. Adult children, particularly middle-aged females, experience emotional stress because of the competing demands and additional role responsibilities placed on them (Brody, 1985). Although adult children feel a moral obligation to care for their parent, they find the caregiving responsibility an additional burden because they often are married and are still caring for their own children (Jarrett, 1985).

Caregiver Burden and Stress

Definitions

Alzheimer's disease has been identified as one of the most socially disruptive ailments because of the severe burdens it may place on families (Brody, 1981). Although the mean number of hours spent providing care may be similar for caregivers of other physically and mentally disabled persons, caregivers of persons with Alzheimer's disease report more stress and negative feelings (Given, Collins, & Given, 1988).

The term "caregiver burden" is used to describe the physical, psychological, emotional, social, and financial problems that are experienced by family members caring for persons with Alzheimer's disease (George & Gwyther, 1986). Burdens result from several factors: the tasks of caregiving, the way in which these tasks impose on other role obligations, and the manner in which the caregiver views both the patient and the legitimacy of the caregiving obligations. Given et al. (1988) conceptualize caregiving reactions as psychological responses or "stresses" that influence the caregiving relationship, as well as in terms of the impact that caregiving has on the actual physical and emotional health of the caregiver. The nature and severity of caregiver reactions appear to be related to the interaction between the prior and present characteristics of both the caregiver and the person with Alzheimer's disease. The caregiving environment further impinges upon this interaction (Poulshock & Deimling, 1984; Zarit, Reever, & Bach-Peterson, 1986).

The Burdens of Caregiving

Not all caregivers of persons with Alzheimer's disease find the same problems burdensome. Where some caregivers are bothered by the small behavioral and social changes of their relatives, others tolerate and effectively manage the major changes associated with the disease such as incontinence and agitation (Zarit et al., 1985). Further, some families who have been followed over time report that what bothered them in the past no longer bothers them (Jenkins, Parham, & Jenkins, 1985). Social support for the caregiver (Zarit & Zarit, 1983), the utilization of home health and community services for persons with Alzheimer's disease (Poulshock & Deimling, 1984), and the caregiver's perceived level of satisfaction with the help received for the relative with Alzheimer's disease (Gilhooly, 1984; Hirschfield, 1983) directly correlate with caregiver morale and mental health.

Nature, Severity, and Duration of the Disease Symptoms

Although George and Gwyther (1986) found no relationship between the duration of the disease and the caregiver's level of burden, Gilhooly (1984) correlated the duration of the caregiving experience with the caregiver's mental health. As opposed to what one would have anticipated, the longer the caregiving period, the better the caregiver's morale. Over time, by effectively using coping strategies, caregivers learned to adjust better to the disease's symptoms.

While Zarit (1982) found no correlation between the severity of the cognitive and behavioral symptoms associated with Alzheimer's disease, more recent investigations have shown that these symptoms do in fact negatively affect the caregiver (Colerick & George, 1986; Deimling & Bass, 1986; Poulshock & Deimling, 1984). The major disease symptoms reported were aggressive and dangerous behavior, low level of social functioning, mental confusion, catastrophic reactions, paranoia, and accusations.

The burden felt by the caregiver depends upon the amount and type of daily assistance and supervision required of the caregiver by the person with Alzheimer's disease. Collectively, several studies describe assistance in the following areas: feeding and eating, incontinence, wandering, inability to care for grooming needs, immobility, and abnormal sleep patterns (Chenoweth & Spencer, 1976; Isaacs, Livingstone, & Neville, 1972; Rabins et al., 1982; Sanford, 1975).

Financial Burdens

Families do not report the financial burden as being as troublesome as the daily caring for their relative (Cantor, 1980; Ory et al., 1985). However, in situations where family caregivers are employed, they may stop working to care for their relative, suffering the financial loss of their salary. If they continue working, they must bear the brunt of the additional financial costs for day care, home custodial care, or even institutionalization for their relative. There are a host of related legal issues such as guardianship and property ownership with which they must deal (Pratt, Schmall, & Wright, 1987). Over time, financial resources may be virtually drained so that the caregivers are left, in many instances, with no money to care even for themselves.

Measures of Burden

Various instruments have been specifically designed to measure the degree of burden that caregiving has on the caregiver of the person with Alzheimer's disease. Illustrative of these measures are the *Burden Interview*, the *Caregiver Strain Index* (Robinson, 1983; Zarit et al., 1985), the *Caregiver Social Impact Scale* (Poulshock & Deimling, 1984), and the *Caregiving Hassles Scale* (*CHS*) (Kinney & Stephens, 1989). With these instruments, the caregiver is asked to indicate on a point scale which caregiving situations and patient behaviors occur most frequently and how burdensome the caregiver perceives them to be. Both the *Burden Interview* and the *Caregiver Strain Index* (a) focus explicitly on the caregiving situation (e.g., asking questions on how caregiving influences the respondent's life), (b) tap the many dimensions in which burden can be experienced (e.g., physical and emotional health, social activities), and (c) yield total scores indicating the overall burden level.

The *CHS* differs from the two aforementioned measures in that it focuses solely on how the minor irritants of the daily caregiving experience burden the caregiver. It provides not only a total burden score but also subscale burden scores (e.g., activities of daily living, independent activities of daily living, cognitive status, behavior of the person with Alzheimer's, and social network of the caregiver). The *Caregiver Social Impact Scale* assesses the degree of interference that results in the caregiver's daily social life because of the caregiving role (e.g., negative personal reactions of caregiving such as anger and resentment, and restriction in social activity).

The Stresses of Caregiving

While some relationship exists between the nature and severity of the symptoms associated with Alzheimer's disease and caregiver stress, the care needs of the person with Alzheimer's disease do not tell the whole story. It is the subjective perception of burden by the caregiver, rather than the objective care needs of the person with Alzheimer's disease, that creates stress for the caregiver (Montgomery, 1985; Quayhagen & Quayhagen, 1988).

Lack of Family and Community Support

Social support can take many forms for the caregiver, both direct and indirect. Family and friends provide informal support. Respite support for the caregiver can be derived from homemaking services and respite and day care for the person with Alzheimer's disease. Professional support for the caregiver comes through psycho-educational counseling; the community can provide support group programs. Without adequate family and community support, the caregiver becomes socially isolated (Chenoweth & Spencer, 1976; Lazarus, Stafford, Cooper, Cohler, & Dysken, 1981; Morris, Morris, & Britton, 1989; Poulshock & Deimling, 1984; Zarit, 1983).

A Funeral That Never Ends

Long before the disease proves fatal, a psychological death occurs in the family. Cath (1978) describes the experience of caretakers as they cope with the declining process of a loved one:

> . . . witnessing the death of a beloved ego is even more intolerable than the experience of physical death. Senility (Alzheimer's disease) represents a progressive and agonizingly slow death of the human side of existence, for its ultimate residue is no longer recognizable as a person. (p. 28)

Having to live daily with the loss of personality of their relative with Alzheimer's disease can be a stress as great as or even greater than the actual physical death of the person. This psychological death, which often causes caregivers to describe their relatives as the "walking dead," has a profound impact on the caregiver (Kapust, 1982). Although relatives of the person with Alzheimer's disease grieve for the loss of the person they once knew, their mourning is incomplete (Pollack, 1984). It has been suggested that caregivers go through a normal and predictable process of grieving, with behavioral stages similar to those described by Kubler-Ross (1969). Gallagher, Lovett, and Zeiss (1989) suggest that caregiving of persons with Alzheimer's disease can be viewed on a psychological level as an anticipatory mourning process. Healthy resolution of the normal mourning process includes a sense of psychological closure and acceptance (Vaillant, 1982). For caregivers of persons with Alzheimer's disease, this closure is not possible; the caregiver has emotionally lost the person he or she once knew, yet the person still physically lives (Kapust, 1982). Lezak (1978) summarizes this dilemma:

> The spouse can not mourn decently. Although he lost his mate as surely and permanently as if by death, since the familiar body remains, society neither recognizes the spouse's grief nor provides the support and comfort that surrounds those bereaved by death. (p. 595)

Cohen, Kennedy, and Eisdorfer (1984) suggest several phases of change as Alzheimer's disease progresses, with corresponding family caregiver adaptive mechanisms. They postulate that before diagnosis of the disease, recognition, concern, and even fear of the unknown are typical of both patient and caregiver. Once the diagnosis is confirmed, denial occurs, followed by anger, guilt, and sadness. In the terminal stages of the disease, a degree of "maturation" occurs, followed by a separation of self in which the caregivers accept their relative as a greatly changed person who will never again be the particular person they loved as a parent or spouse.

Lack of Adequate Information for the Caregiver

Barnes, Raskind, Scott, and Murphy (1981) identified the lack of information and the misperceptions that families have regarding the nature and course of Alzheimer's disease as a major source of stress for the families, particularly in the early stages of the disease. Further, families report feelings of total hopelessness when the actual diagnosis is given and they are told that "nothing can be done." On the other hand, those families who receive complete information regarding Alzheimer's disease tend to have more realistic expectations about what their relative is capable of, successfully use coping strategies to deal with their relative's symptoms, and report lower levels of stress (Zarit et al., 1985).

Stress from Institutionalization

Contrary to public belief, families do not readily abandon their older Alzheimer's relatives when they become institutionalized. Nursing home placement does not relieve the stresses felt by families but rather changes the type of stresses they experience. Just seeing their relative in an institution is in itself stressful. Families take on the burden of visiting their relative in the institution, interacting with staff, and maintaining strong supervision over the quality of care and the well-being of their relative (Brody, 1983; Zarit & Zarit, 1983). For some, the high cost of care is devastating.

The Physical and Emotional Impact of Caring

A number of physical and emotional conditions have been reported by caregivers of persons with Alzheimer's disease (Colerick & George, 1986; Eisdorfer & Cohen, 1981; Fitting et al., 1986; Hirschfield, 1983). Depression, the use of psychotropic drugs, alcohol abuse, and chronic fatigue are major conditions reported by caregivers (Cohen & Eisdorfer, 1988; Coppel, Burton, Becker, & Fiore, 1985; Deimling & Bass, 1986; Eisdorfer, Kennedy, Wisnieski, & Cohen,

1983; George & Gwyther, 1984; Goldman & Luchins, 1984; Zarit, 1982). Both Chenoweth and Spencer (1976) and Sluss-Radbaugh, Lorenz, Wells, and Hooper (1983) report that 18 to 20% of their caregivers experienced decreases in their general physical health. Health conditions included heart attacks, high blood pressure, tension headaches, obesity, nervous breakdowns, ulcers, and complete physical exhaustion.

Measures of Well-Being

Unlike the subjective instruments that measure the caregiver's burden, standardized instruments are used to measure the degree to which caregiving leads to decrements in various areas of well-being for the caregiver. As opposed to the "burden" measures, well-being measures can also be administered to other types of groups (e.g., single parents). In this way, it can be determined whether caregivers of persons with Alzheimer's disease are any worse off than other groups of caregivers. Further, well-being measures can separately assess specific areas, such as mental as compared to physical health. To date, "burden" measures yield only a total severity level of burden.

Illustrative of well-being measures, George and Gwyther (1986) used four separate measures to assess the well-being of caregivers of persons with Alzheimer's disease: (a) physical health (e.g., number of physician visits in 6 months), (b) mental health (e.g., psychotropic drug usage, psychiatric symptom checklist), (c) social participation (e.g., frequency of family visits and phone contacts), and (d) financial resources (e.g., household income). Recently the *Brief Symptom Inventory* (Derogatis & Spencer, 1982) has been used to assess the well-being of caregivers of persons with Alzheimer's disease (Anthony-Bergstone, Zarit, & Gatz, 1988; Zarit, Anthony, & Boutselis, 1987). This scale, which was originally developed for use with psychiatric patients, can separately assess the frequency of specific symptomatic distress (e.g., depression, anxiety, and hostility) that caregivers experience.

Communication Problems and the Caregivers

Evidence of Communicative Stress

No published studies have been conducted by speech-language pathologists to determine whether, how much, and when the communication changes associated with Alzheimer's disease emotionally affect the caregiver. Findings of five studies completed by other health care professionals seem to suggest that the communication changes do indeed have an emotional impact (Hirschfield, 1983; Kinney & Stephens, 1989; Levine, Dastoor, & Gendron, 1983; Rabins, 1982; Zarit, 1982). Researchers grouped the communication problems with other patient problems and behaviors to derive a total measure of burden. Thus, with the exception of Rabins's study (1982), it is impossible to determine from the results of these studies the exact nature of the communication problems and their impact on the caregiver. Further, many of the assessment tools consisted of predetermined lists of patients' symptoms. Therefore, the communication problems listed may not have included those problems that create the most communicative stress for the caregiver.

In Levine et al.'s study (1983), 7 out of his 10 caregivers reported communication problems in general as a major source of caregiver stress. Further, only 3 of the 7 caregivers in this study felt that they knew how to effectively cope on their own with the communication problems. Zarit (1982) developed a checklist of memory and behavior problems to assess the frequency of patient behaviors and caregivers' emotional reactions to such behaviors. Three of the 29 patient behaviors listed dealt with communication difficulties (e.g., being constantly talkative, talking little or not at all, asking repetitive questions). Caregivers listed their reactions to these communication behaviors at higher stress levels (particularly the latter item) than other patient behaviors. In assessing whether cognitive problems associated with Alzheimer's disease caused caregiver stress, Hirschfield (1983) included questions dealing with communication problems. Although Hirschfield found that cognitive problems generally created more stress than many of the other patient behaviors listed, it could not be determined whether communication was a primary contributor to this stress, since only a total cognitive score was calculated. Kinney and Stephens's *Caregiving Hassles Scale* (1989) included five "hassle" items that could be directly associated with communication (e.g., not making sense) and another three items that could be indirectly inferred as being associated with communication (e.g., talking about seeing things that aren't "real"). Again, the actual impact of these communication changes could not be ascertained from the results of the study since all items were grouped together to derive subscale and total scale scores.

Unlike those investigators who provided caregivers with a predetermined list of behaviors for assessing burden, Rabins et al. (1982) asked caregivers to list the problems that created the greatest sources of stress. Out of the 20 most significant behaviors reported, caregivers rated a general communication impairment as the sixth major source of stress. Catastrophic reactions were listed by caregivers as the second most stressful symptom. If one defines a catastrophic reaction as being an emotional reaction precipitated by a task failure, then possibly the communication failures associated with Alzheimer's disease, such as not being understood or not understanding others, could have been the source of some of the catastrophic reactions reported by caregivers. While not directly assessing burden, eight other studies cite the general communication problems associated with Alzheimer's disease as being a reported source of stress for the caregiver (Aronson, Levin, & Lipkowitz, 1984; D. Cohen, 1983; Colerick & George, 1986; Hayter, 1982; Pratt, Schmall, Wright, & Cleland, 1985; Reifler & Wu, 1982; Scott, Roberto, & Hutton, 1986; Steuer & Clark, 1982).

Need for Intervention

Many of the stressful communication difficulties caregivers experience may merely result from a failure to adequately understand the nature and progression of the communication problems associated with Alzheimer's disease. Typically families receive little, if any, information about the nature and progression of their relative's communication impairments when the diagnosis is initially made, or even later as the disease progresses. Even on those rare instances where caregivers may be provided with such information, they may not retain or accept the information, because they are already in a state of shock over their relative's diagnosis. Thus, they may (a) develop misconceptions about the communication changes, (b) fail to develop appropriate coping strategies for dealing with their relative's communicative behaviors, (c) develop unrealistic expectations about their relative as a communicator, (d) develop false hope that their relative's communication abilities are improving, and (e) develop a sense of loss for the communication interactions they once had with the person with the disease.

The following examples illustrate the need of the speech-language pathologist to educate caregivers and their families. By the very simple fact of not understanding their relative's communication strengths and weaknesses, families may develop too high or low expectations of what their relative is capable of doing as a communicator. Too high an expectation by the caregiver may lead to catastrophic reactions by the person with Alzheimer's disease. Further, the caregiver's style of interaction may be the ignition to set off such reactions. For example, during the visit of a grandson to his grandparents, the child's grandmother said to her spouse, ''Why don't you explain to Timmy how you make a sailor's knot?'' The grandfather started to explain, but in his frustration at trying to find the exact words, he forgot where he had left off in his explanation. Because his grandson had always looked up to him, he felt embarrassed over his inadequacies in explaining to his grandson about the knot. As a result, he lost his temper and yelled at his wife, ''You just wanted to make me look like a fool in front of my own grandson!''

On the other hand, caregivers may think that their relative is totally helpless and unable to communicate adequately. To illustrate, a person with Alzheimer's disease complained, ''Because I can't make connections quickly to get my thoughts out in normal conversation, every time I go to say something, someone's thought of it first. So now I've become the silent partner, since I don't want any eggs on my face.''

In many instances, caregivers create unnecessary and early communicative dependency situations for their relative, which in turn add a further daily burden to their caring role. The person with Alzheimer's disease fails to receive adequate social communication stimulation because the caregiver fails to involve him or her in activities. The caregiver feels either embarrassed or protective of his or her relative in these situations. Communication stimulation is important to any person, whether cognitively intact or not. If persons with Alzheimer's disease are not allowed to use their residual communicative abilities, these abilities may be prematurely lost.

Often caregivers fail to understand that the neurological damage of the disease is what creates some of their relative's communicative behaviors. Rather, they believe that behaviors such as failing to respond immediately to a question or asking the same question repeatedly are intended to gain attention. When it is explained to the caregiver that the relative may be repeating a question because he or she may not have comprehended the question, may not have remembered the question, may be demonstrating perseverative behavior, or may not

remember what was said, the caregiver may become more tolerant of the person's communicative behavior.

Caregivers often comment that they feel disheartened at not being able to communicatively interact with their relative as they once did. They must understand that they can still interact at some level; however, in order to do so, they must change their own communicative approach as their relative's communication abilities progressively decline. Further, they must learn that what may be an appropriate communication strategy at one stage of the disease may no longer be successful at another stage.

Intervention and Stress Management

The Communication Stress Management Approach

Unfortunately, an unjustified tradition has prevailed that nothing can be done for persons with a nonreversible dementia such as Alzheimer's disease. Although current medical treatment for persons with Alzheimer's disease cannot alleviate the clinical communication symptoms associated with the disease, family members can alter their own and their relative's communication behaviors in ways that make the communication difficulties less burdensome for both persons.

As Zarit et al. (1987) point out, in addition to psychological counseling and social support for the caregiver, an educational stress management approach is also in order if caregiver stress is to be reduced. The purpose of any stress management approach is to improve the caregiver's ability to manage the patient's behavior and to increase the caregiver's own social supports (Glosser & Wexler, 1985; Lovett & Gallagher, 1988; Pinkston & Linsk, 1984; Safford, 1980; Zarit et al., 1985).

The specific implementation of a communication stress management approach involves the use of three treatment strategies and three modalities for providing treatment. The strategies are (a) educating the caregiver, (b) increasing problem-solving abilities, and (c) emotionally supporting the caregiver. The modalities include (a) individual counseling with the primary caregiver, (b) family meetings, and (c) participation in a support group. How these strategies and modalities are used will depend on the characteristics and needs of a particular caregiver and his or her family.

Educating the Caregiver

The provision of appropriate direct communication intervention for the caregiver and family and indirect intervention for the person with Alzheimer's disease calls for knowledge, understanding, and acceptance of the nature and progression of the communication impairment associated with the disease.

The inconsistent nature of the communication changes associated with Alzheimer's disease increases stress for the caregiver by setting up false hopes. Persons with Alzheimer's disease often have sporadic appropriate verbal responses in their unintelligible speech. The change from nonsensical verbal responses to sudden episodes of appropriate speech may confuse caregivers and cause them to believe that their relative is improving. When their relative reverts back to the usual pattern of unintelligible speech, they sway from feelings of hope to those of utter hopelessness and even may wonder whether their relative is "faking it." Caregivers must learn that their relative has no control over these fluctuations.

Caregivers often ask whether there are any medicines to alleviate their relative's communication problems. A successful intervention depends on having caregivers understand two basic principles: first, that there are no "cures" currently available to effectively treat their relative's communication problems, and second, that it is the caregivers who have to make changes in their own communication.

Imparting information also includes helping families to understand and relabel the problem communication behaviors. For example, many families view "asking repeated questions" as an intentional behavior rather than a behavior that may result from the difficulty their relatives have in remembering what they have said.

It is preferable for the speech-language pathologist to educate families about the nature and progression of the communication changes as part of an interdisciplinary team of health professionals. In this way, if stresses other than those of communication arise, the professionals who are more knowledgeable in these areas can answer the caregivers' questions. Further, an interdisciplinary approach places the caregivers' stresses in a holistic perspective rather than fragmenting management for the individual caregiver.

Instead of presenting material to caregivers in a lecture style, the speech-language pathologist should first let them ask questions, in order to avoid overloading them with too much information and to learn what they already know. Some notes of caution: The speech-language pathologist should be direct but positive regarding the progression of the communication changes. For example, the pathologist should state what abilities are maintained at each level rather than listing those that are absent. Unrealistic optimism should not be conveyed to the caregivers or encouraged; this only serves to set up the false hope that there is a "magical" solution. Discussions dealing with their feelings of stress concerning the communication changes should be supported.

Problem Solving

Problem solving is a process through which the caregivers (and families) identify the communication problems that create the most stress for the caregivers and determine to what extent these communication problems may be modified (Morrissey, 1983; Pratt et al., 1985; Zarit et al., 1985). There are three steps to problem solving. The first step is to *identify the communication problems.* By keeping a daily record, the caregiver determines what the communication problems are, and when, where, and how often they occur. This record serves as a baseline against which intervention can be measured. When the antecedents and consequents (e.g., events that trigger or reinforce the communication problem) are analyzed, intervention strategies emerge for the caregivers. The caregivers can also record their emotional reaction to each communication problem, such as feeling upset, stressed, or frustrated. The communication problems that are the most disturbing to the caregivers can then be targeted for intervention. In instances where the caregivers may have some initial difficulty in keeping records, communication behavioral checklists can be developed, similar to those developed by Zarit et al. (1985) and other researchers.

The second step is for the caregiver and speech-language pathologist to *develop effective strategies* for managing the communication behaviors that are the most disturbing to the caregivers. Speech-language pathologists are in error when they decide that they know what is best for the caregivers. They must consider the caregivers' real needs and wishes. With a stress management approach, rather than having the speech-language pathologist give advice on dealing with problems, strategies are derived from active assessment of the problem by the caregivers. The eventual goal is for the caregivers to apply the problem-solving process from one communicative problem to another and not to become dependent on the speech-language pathologist for every solution. Problem solving also leads to cognitive rehearsal, in which the caregivers mentally carry out the steps leading toward solution of the problem. Cognitive rehearsal successfully allows caregivers to anticipate communicative problems that might arise and to provide a strategy that will prevent these problems from occurring. Problem solving also involves generating as many solutions or strategies as possible to the problem in order to explore the advantages

and disadvantages each strategy might provide.

The third step is for the caregivers to *evaluate the effectiveness of a strategy.* If the problem is occurring less frequently than its baseline measure, the strategy may have had a positive effect. If there is no change, an alternative strategy is warranted. It is important for the speech-language pathologist to remember that inappropriate strategies can in some instances lead to increased stress on both caregivers and the relative with Alzheimer's disease.

Supporting the Caregiver

Individual Counseling

Initially, it is recommended that the speech-language pathologist and other health care professionals meet with the caregiver on an individual basis rather than in a group setting. Not all caregivers or their families share identical problems and concerns regarding the communicative behaviors of their relative. Therefore, the educational component of the management program must be individualized as much as possible to meet the specific needs of caregivers.

Family Counseling

Often relatives and friends are willing and able to help but have no idea how to do so, and caregivers are hesitant or embarrassed to ask for help. Once the caregiver receives individual counseling, family meetings may be beneficial to bring the family's level of information about the communication changes up to that of the caregiver's.

Support Groups

Once the caregivers begin the problem-solving process, they may be ready for group sessions in which they can learn about new coping strategies from other group members. Problem solving is often very effective in groups because caregivers may be more willing to accept suggestions from another group member than from a professional. The group also provides a structure in which members can role play various strategies with each other (Hayter, 1982). As Witte (1986) has effectively demonstrated, use of videotapes showing different communication strategies is also helpful to caregivers. The group setting provides a social support system where they can socialize, share information, vent frustrations, and regain self-esteem (Aronson et al., 1984; Bergman, Foster, & Matthews, 1978; Cobb, 1976; P. M. Cohen, 1983; Hayter, 1982). With this type of group, the speech-language pathologist should not assume a full leadership role, but should allow the group to strengthen its own leadership.

Duration of Intervention

Stress management programs are "time-limited," varying from 7 weeks to 6 months, depending on whether individual and family counseling is later followed by a group experience. Sessions should be scheduled during the evening or on weekends so that attendance does not become an additional burden for the caregiver. It may be beneficial for the caregiver if it can be arranged for the relative with Alzheimer's disease to be seen for social communicative group sessions at the same time that the caregiver attends his or her own individual or group sessions (Aronson et al., 1984).

Program Failures

Some caregivers may not respond to a stress management approach to lessen their stress and burdens. For example, if the caregiver's expectations are initially too high, he or she may become disappointed if the intervention does not alleviate the problems. Other caregivers may be too overwhelmed to try new coping strategies. In some cases, their relative's communication impairments may be too severe to be managed by the caregiver without overwhelming hardship. Despite these cautions, a communication stress management approach should assist in reducing the stress that the caregiver experiences.

Conclusions

In the future, the profession of speech-language pathology must begin to conduct research to determine the extent to which the communication changes associated with Alzheimer's disease emotionally affect the caregiver. As described in this chapter, the caregiver experiences stresses that are significant and that come from many sources. Because communication is a vehicle for social interaction, improves independent functioning, and provides a way to vent one's feelings and emotions, it would seem that the communication changes associated with Alzheimer's disease may be one of the primary sources of caregivers' stress. If this is the proven case, then a communication stress management program for the caregiver may be an important professional service for the speech-language pathologist to provide. In providing communication intervention services directly to caregivers and thus indirectly to the person with Alzheimer's disease, speech-language pathologists may help to improve the quality of life for both caregivers and their relative. This mandates future objective documentation of the relative effectiveness of such an approach.

References

Anthony-Bergstone, C., Zarit, S. H., & Gatz, M. (1988). Symptoms of psychological distress among caregivers of dementia patients. *Psychology and Aging, 3,* 245–248.

Aronson, M. K., Levin, G., & Lipkowitz, R. (1984). A community-based family/patient group program for Alzheimer's disease. *The Gerontologist, 24,* 339–342.

Barnes, R. F., Raskind, M. A., Scott, M., & Murphy, C. (1981). Problems of families caring for Alzheimer patients: Use of a support group. *Journal of the American Geriatrics Society, 19,* 80–85.

Bergman, E. M., Foster, A. W., & Matthews, V. (1978). Management of the demented elderly patient in the community. *British Journal of Psychiatry, 132,* 441–449.

Boutselis, M., & Zarit, S. H. (1984). *Burden and distress of dementia caregivers: Effects of gender and relationship.* Paper presented at the meeting of the Gerontological Society of America, San Antonio, TX.

Brody, E. (1981). Long-term care institutions. In N. Miller & G. Cohen (Eds.), *Clinical aspects of Alzheimer's disease and senile dementia* (pp. 103–112). New York: Raven Press.

Brody, E. M. (1983). *Testimony on the effects of Alzheimer's disease on caregiving families.* Paper presented to the Committee on Energy and Commerce, Subcommittee on Health and the Environment, and the Select Committee on Aging, Subcommittee on Long-Term Care, Washington, DC.

Brody, E. M. (1985). Parent care as a normative stress. *The Gerontologist, 25,* 19–29.

Cantor, M. H. (1979). Social and family relationships of black aged women in New York City. *Journal of Minority Aging, 4,* 50–61.

Cantor, M. H. (1980). *Caring for the frail elderly: Impact on family, friends, and neighbors.* Paper presented at the 33rd Annual Scientific Meeting of the Gerontological Society of America, San Diego, CA.

Cantor, M. H. (1983). Strain among caregivers. A study of experience in the United States. *The Gerontologist, 23,* 597–604.

Cath, S. (1978). The geriatric patient and his family. *Journal of Geriatric Psychiatry, 1,* 25–46.

Chenoweth, B., & Spencer, B. (1976). Dementia: The experience of family caregivers. *The Gerontologist, 26,* 267–272.

Circirelli, V. G. (1986). Family relationships and care management of the dementing elderly. In M. L. M. Gilhooly, S. H. Zarit, & J. E. Birren (Eds.), *The dementias: Policy and management* (pp. 93–109). Englewood Cliffs, NJ: Prentice-Hall.

Cobb, S. (1976). Social support as a moderator of life stress. *Psychosomatic Medicine, 38,* 300–314.

Cohen, D. (1983). Management of stress in families caring for relatives with Alzheimer's disease and related disorders. In G. Landsberg (Ed.), *Preventing mental health problems in the elderly: Directions and strategies* (pp. 79–85). Englewood Cliffs, NJ: Hoffman-Laroche.

Cohen, D., & Eisdorfer, C. (1988). Depression in family members caring for a relative with Alzheimer's disease. *Journal of the American Geriatric Society, 36,* 885–889.

Cohen, D., Kennedy, G., & Eisdorfer, C. (1984). Phases of change in the patient with Alzheimer's dementia: A conceptual dimension for defining health care management. *Journal of the American Geriatrics Society, 32,*11–15.

Cohen, P. M. (1983). A group approach for working with families of the elderly. *The Gerontologist, 23,* 248–250.

Colerick, E., & George, L. (1986). Predictors of institutionalization among caregivers of patients with Alzheimer's disease. *Journal of the American Geriatrics Society, 34,* 493–498.

Coppel, D. B., Burton, C., Becker, J., & Fiore, J. (1985). Relationships of cognitions associated with coping reactions to depression in spousal caregivers of Alzheimer's disease patients. *Cognitive Therapy and Research, 9,* 253–266.

Deimling, G., & Bass, D. (1986). Symptoms of mental impairment among elderly adults and their effects on family caregivers. *Journal of Gerontology, 41,* 778–784.

Derogatis, L., & Spencer, P. (1982). *The Brief Symptom Inventory.* Baltimore, MD: Johns Hopkins University School of Medicine, Clinical Psychometric Research Unit.

Eisdorfer, C., & Cohen, D. (1981). Management of the patient and family coping with dementing illness. *Journal of Family Practice, 12,* 831–837.

Eisdorfer, C., Kennedy, G., Wisnieski, W., & Cohen, D. (1983). Depression and attributional style in families coping with the stress of caring for a relative with Alzheimer's disease. *The Gerontologist, 23,* 115–116.

Fitting, M. D., Rabins, P. V., & Lucas, M. J. (1984). *Caregivers for dementia patients: A comparison of men and women.* Paper presented at the 37th Annual Scientific Meeting of the Gerontological Society of America, San Antonio, TX.

Fitting, M. D., Rabins, P. V., Lucas, M. J., & Eastham, J. (1986). Caregivers for dementia patients: A comparison of husbands and wives. *The Gerontologist, 26,* 248–252.

Gallagher, D., Lovett, S., & Zeiss, A. (1989). Interventions with caregivers of frail elderly persons. In M. Ory & K. Bond (Eds.), *Aging and health care: Social science and policy perspectives* (pp. 167–190). New York: Tavistock.

George, L. K., & Gwyther, L. P. (1984). *Family caregivers of Alzheimer's patients: Correlates of burden and the impact of self-help groups.* Paper presented at the Meeting of the Gerontological Society of America, Durham, NC.

George, L. K., & Gwyther, L. P. (1986). Caregiver well-being: A multidimensional examination of family caregivers of demented adults. *The Gerontologist, 26,* 253–259.

Gilhooly, M. L. M. (1984). The impact of caregiving on care-givers: Factors associated with the psychological well-being of people supporting a dementing relative in the community. *British Journal of Medical Psychology, 57,* 35–44.

Given, C. W., Collins, C. E., & Given, B. A. (1988). Sources of stress among families caring for relatives with Alzheimer's disease. *Nursing Clinics of North America, 23,* 69–82.

Glosser, G., & Wexler, D. (1985). Participants' evaluation of educational/support groups for families of patients with Alzheimer's disease and other dementias. *The Gerontologist, 25,* 232–236.

Goldman, L. S., & Luchins, D. J. (1984). Depression in the spouses of demented patients. *American Journal of Psychiatry, 141,* 1467–1468.

Gwyther, L., & George, L. (1986). Caregivers for dementia patients: Complex determinants of well-being and burden. *The Gerontologist, 26,* 245–247.

Hayter, J. (1982). Helping families of patients with Alzheimer's disease. *Journal of Gerontological Nursing, 8,* 81–86.

Hirschfield, M. (1983). Homecare versus institutionalization: Family caregiving and senile brain disease. *International Journal of Nursing Studies, 20,* 23–32.

Isaacs, B., Livingstone, E. M., & Neville, Y. (1972). *Survival of the unfittest: A study of geriatric patients in Glasgow.* London: Routledge & Kegan Paul.

Jarrett, W. H. (1985). Caregiving within kinship systems: Is affection really necessary? *The Gerontologist, 25,* 5–10.

Jenkins, T. S., Parham, I. A., & Jenkins, T. (1985). Alzheimer's disease: Caregivers' perceptions of burden. *Journal of Applied Gerontology, 4,* 40–57.

Kapust, L. R. (1982). Living with dementia: The ongoing funeral. *Social Work Health Care, 7,* 79–91.

Katzman, R. (1976). The prevalence and malignancy of Alzheimer's disease. *Archives of Neurology, 33,* 217–218.

Kinney, J. M., & Stephens, M. A. P. (1989). Caregiving Hassles Scale: Assessing the daily hassles of caring for a family member with dementia. *The Gerontologist, 29,* 328–332.

Kubler-Ross, E. (1969). *On death and dying.* New York: Macmillan.

Lazarus, L. W., Stafford, B., Cooper, K., Cohler, B., & Dysken, M. (1981). A pilot study of an Alzheimer patient's relatives discussion group. *The Gerontologist, 21,* 353–358.

Levine, N. B., Dastoor, D. P., & Gendron, C. E. (1983). Coping with dementia: A pilot study. *Journal of the American Geriatrics Society, 1,* 12–18.

Lezak, M. (1978). Living with the characterologically altered brain injured patient. *Journal of Geriatric Psychiatry, 3,* 101–104.

Lovett, S., & Gallagher, D. (1988). Psychoeducational interventions for family caregivers: Preliminary efficacy data. *Behavior Therapy, 19,* 321–330.

Maddox, G. L. (in press). Mutual health groups for caregivers in the management of senile dementia: A research agenda. In J. Wertheimer (Ed.), *Senile dementia in the next 20 years.* New York: Alan R. Liss.

Mindel, C. H., & Wright, R. (1980). *Intergenerational factors in the utilization of social services by black and white elderly: A causal analysis.* Paper presented at the 33rd Annual Meeting of the Gerontological Society of America, San Diego, CA.

Montgomery, R. J. V. (1985). Caregiving and the experience of subjective and objective burden. *Family Relations, 34*(1), 19–25.

Morris, L. W., Morris, R. G., & Britton, P. G. (1989). Social support networks and formal support as factors influencing the psychological adjustment of spouse caregivers of dementia sufferers. *International Journal of Geriatric Psychiatry, 4,* 47–51.

Morrissey, E. R. (1983). *Depression and happiness among spouses of Alzheimer's disease patients: The impact of coping resources.* Paper presented at the Annual Meeting of the American Sociological Association, Detroit, MI.

Morycz, R. K. (1985). Caregiving strain and the desire to institutionalize family members with Alzheimer's disease: Possible predictors and model development. *Research on Aging, 7,* 329–362.

Ory, M. G., Williams, T. F., Emr, M., Lebowitz, B., Rabins, P., Salloway, J., Sluss-Radbaugh, T., Wolff, E., & Zarit, S. (1985). Families, informal supports, and Alzheimer's disease. *Research in Aging, 7,* 623–644.

Pinkston, E. M., & Linsk, N. L. (1984). Behavioral family intervention with the impaired elderly. *The Gerontologist, 24,* 576–583.

Pollack, R. (1984). Dealing with the emotional turmoil of Alzheimer's disease. In M. Aronson (Ed.), *Understanding Alzheimer's disease* (pp. 163–172). New York: Scribner's.

Poulshock, S. W., & Deimling, G. T. (1984). Families caring for elders in residence: Issues in the measurement of burden. *Journal of Gerontology, 39,* 230–239.

Pratt, C., Schmall, V., & Wright, S. (1987). Ethical concerns of family caregivers to dementia patients. *The Gerontologist, 27,* 632–638.

Pratt, C., Schmall, V., Wright, S., & Cleland, M. (1985). Burden and coping strategies of caregivers to Alzheimer's patients. *Family Relations, 14,* 32–33.

Quayhagen, M., & Quayhagen, M. (1988). Alzheimer's stress: Coping and caregiving role. *The Gerontologist, 28*(3), 396.

Rabins, P. (1982). Management of irreversible dementia. *Psychosomatics, 22,* 591–597.

Rabins, P. V. (1984). Management of dementia in the family context. *Psychosomatics, 25,* 369–375.

Rabins, P. V., Mace, N. L., & Lucas, M. J. (1982). The impact of dementia on the family. *Journal of the American Medical Association, 248,* 333–335.

Reifler, B. V., & Wu, S. (1982). Managing families of the demented elderly. *The Journal of Family Practice, 14,* 1051–1056.

Robinson, B. C. (1983). Validation of a caregiver strain index. *Journal of Gerontology, 38,* 344–348.

Safford, F. (1980). A program for families of mentally impaired elderly. *The Gerontologist, 20,* 656–660.

Sanford, J. R. A. (1975). Tolerance of debility in elderly dependents by supporters at home: Its significance for hospital practice. *British Medical Journal, 23,* 471–473.

Scott, J. P., Roberto, K. A., & Hutton, J. T. (1986). Families of Alzheimer's victims: Family support to the caregivers. *Journal of the American Geriatrics Society, 34,* 348–354.

Sluss-Radbaugh, T., Lorenz, G., Wells, S., & Hooper, F. (1983). *The helping study: Tasks,* *helpers and consequences.* Paper presented at the 11th Annual Meeting of the American Public Health Association, Dallas, TX.

Steuer, J., & Clark, E. (1982). Family support groups within a research project on dementia. *Clinical Gerontologist, 1,* 87–95.

Vaillant, G. E. (1982). Attachment, loss and rediscovery. *Psychiatric Times, 3,* 1–3.

Weeks, J., & Cuellar, J. (1981). The role of family members in the helping networks of older people. *The Gerontologist, 21,* 388–394.

Witte, K. (1986). *Using the past and present to enhance family visits.* Workshop presentation at the Hebrew Home for the Aged at Riverdale, Riverdale, NY.

Zarit, J. M. (1982). *Predictors of burden and distress for caregivers of senile dementia patients.* Unpublished doctoral dissertation, University of Southern California, San Diego.

Zarit, S. H. (1983). *Families, informal supports and Alzheimer's disease.* Position paper submitted to the National Institute on Aging, Washington, DC.

Zarit, S. H., & Anthony, C. R. (1986). Interventions with dementia patients and their families. In M. L. M. Gilhooly, S. H. Zarit, & J. E. Birren (Eds.), *The dementias: Policy and management.* Englewood Cliffs, NJ: Prentice-Hall.

Zarit, S., Anthony, C., & Boutselis, M. (1987). Intervention with caregivers of dementia patients: Comparison of two approaches. *Psychology of Aging, 3,* 225–232.

Zarit, S. H., Orr, N. K., & Zarit, J. M. (1985). *The hidden victims of Alzheimer's disease: Families under stress.* New York: New York University Press.

Zarit, S. H., Reever, K. E., & Bach-Peterson, J. (1986). Relatives of the impaired elderly: Correlates of feelings of burden. *The Gerontologist, 20,* 649–655.

Zarit, S. H., Todd, P. A., & Zarit, J. M. (1986). Subjective burden of husbands and wives as caregivers: A longitudinal study. *The Gerontologist, 26,* 260–266.

Zarit, S. H., & Zarit, J. M. (1983). Families under stress: Interventions for caregivers of senile dementia patients. *Psychotherapy, 19,* 461–471.

Speech Production and Aging

SECTION

Joel C. Kahane, PhD ∎

This section on speech production and aging consists of five chapters, which examine several aspects of the involutional changes that result in alterations of speech and voice. The first three chapters deal with structural and functional changes in the respiratory, laryngeal, and supralaryngeal components of the speech mechanism. They are followed by two chapters that address possible alterations in speech motor control and central programming that may influence production and flow of speech in the elderly.

The first chapter in this section is "Aging and the Respiratory System," by Rochet. The chapter begins with a critical review of the literature dealing with structural changes of the skeleton and viscera of the respiratory system, followed by a discussion of the functional (mechanical) consequences of these alterations. The latter include a description of general ventilatory changes as well as a discussion of alterations in speech breathing and the compensatory changes in respiratory function that result from disease. The chapter concludes with a discussion of problems associated with the assessment and measurement of respiratory function.

The next chapter, "The Aging Larynx and Voice," by Kahane and Beckford, addresses conditions found in the older larynx, including physical changes in structure and clinical conditions that are frequently observed in older persons. The voice quality of the older larynx is discussed in light of the physical changes that may be present in the larynx and contributed to by other body systems. The chapter concludes with a discussion of the significance of research and clinical findings to therapeutic management of the older individual with laryngeal impairment and voice deficits.

The third chapter in this section is "The Aging Oropharyngeal System," by Sonies. The chapter begins with a brief discussion of basic biological considerations in the study of aging, followed by a review of salient age changes in the pharyngeal cavities. A discussion of involutional changes that affect chemosensory and somatosensory functions follows. The chapter concludes with a discussion of how age-related sensorimotor changes affect speech, mastication, and swallowing.

In the fourth chapter, "Speech Motor Control and Aging," Weismer and Liss discuss age-related changes in speech production by attempting to explain how structural changes in the peripheral speech mechanism and nervous system contribute to or influence the quality and level of motor control operation during speech and voice production. They discuss several possible explanations for compromised or adapted motor control that help us to understand the kinematic characteristics of speech production in aging individuals.

The final chapter in this section, "Fluency, Dysfluency, and Aging," by Rosenfield and Nudelman, presents a neurocybernetic model to explain fluency and dysfluency in aging speakers. This model centers around motor instability in the speech motor control mechanism. The authors then go on to discuss how injury to the nervous system, aging, and several neurological diseases present with different manifestations of disruption in speech flow.

Aging and the Respiratory System

Anne Putnam Rochet, PhD ■

". . . the respiratory system is resilient. . . . In the absence of major acute and chronic diseases, the aging lung adequately adapts to aging and permits a full range of activities." (Lebowitz, 1988, p. 263)

Advancing age in the human organism expresses itself in the respiratory system, as in many others. This chapter will review the age-related changes that have been documented to occur among the components of the respiratory system and their implications for functional changes in respiratory capabilities for ventilation and speech. The primary focus will be on the literature documenting changes in the respiratory systems of elders at the healthy end of the physiological continuum (Ramig, 1983). The complicating and compromising effects of poorer health conditions on the aging respiratory system will be mentioned at the end of the chapter.

Respiratory function is a complex phenomenon. There is no easy middle ground, for the writer or the reader, between a superficial and a substantive consideration of its facets. To facilitate the presentation of the information that follows, a brief review of some salient terms and concepts is included here and elsewhere in the chapter. The reader is referred to the work of Hixon (1987a), Morris, Koski, and Johnson (1971), or Wilson (1985) for more detailed information about the respiratory system, pulmonary functions, and their measurements.

The respiratory system has two major components, the *pulmonary system*, consisting of the lungs and lower airways, and the *chest wall*, consisting of the rib cage and the diaphragm-abdomen. A state of dynamic tension normally exists between these components, such that the chest wall's tendency to expand is counteracted by the lungs' tendency to collapse. These interactive forces normally are mediated by a liquid interface between the parietal and visceral pleurae. So long as the integrity of this interface is maintained, the resting volume of the respiratory system represents a compromise

145

between the relaxation forces of the chest wall and the lungs. This resting volume normally is achieved at the end of a quiet, tidal expiration; the volume remaining in the lung at that point constitutes the *functional residual capacity* (FRC). The FRC is just one of a number of terms of reference for subdivisions of the pulmonary system that will recur throughout this chapter. Other subdivisions, or compartments, of the lung volume include the *vital capacity* (VC) or *forced vital capacity* (FVC), *residual volume* (RV), *total lung capacity* (TLC), *tidal volume* (TV, or V_T), *expiratory reserve volume* (ERV), and *inspiratory capacity* (IC). In addition, a number of dynamic ventilatory maneuvers are relevant to this discussion because their values change as the age or respiratory health of the performer increases. These include *maximum voluntary ventilation* (MVV), *forced expiratory flow* (FEF, referenced to some percentage of the FVC already exhaled), and *forced expiratory volume* (FEV, referenced to a certain period of time; for example FEV_1, where $1 = 1$ s). Definitions, terms, and abbreviations for these and many other pulmonary functions, lung volumes, ventilatory maneuvers, and associated blood gas measurements have been suggested by the American College of Chest Physicians/American Thoracic Society and are tabulated by Wilson (1985).

Numerous investigators have studied changes in pulmonary and chest wall mechanics with age. These efforts have focused particularly on the phenomena of elastic recoil and compliance. Such studies have been plagued by problems associated with the natural history of any biological tissue system: disease residuals, environmental factors, genetic heritage, and the physical activity habits of the human subjects whose respiratory systems have been studied. Disease residuals include inhalation injuries and the permanent sequelae of pulmonary infections. For example, a history of pediatric respiratory illness is an important predictor of respiratory disease in an adult (Ferris, 1978). Environmental factors include altitude, nutritional history, and the "slowly acting toxins" of ambient

atmospheric pollutants (Dhar, Shastri, & Lenora, 1976), as well as those associated with occupational and domestic environments, such as industrial fumes and cigarette smoke. Genetic factors include inherited characteristics that may predispose an individual to pulmonary system disorder, such as alpha$_1$-antitrypsin-deficiency heterozygosity. In its severe form, this disorder may be associated with pulmonary emphysema (Knudson, Clark, Kennedy, & Knudson, 1977). Furthermore, evidence is accumulating to suggest that a person's physical activity habits and exposure to endurance training may influence certain characteristics of the aging process in the respiratory system (Belman & Gaesser, 1988; Fleg & Lakatta, 1988; Hagberg, Yerg, & Seals, 1988; Shock et al., 1984).

The methodological tools used to study respiratory behavior in humans include instruments to measure subdivisions of the lung volume, intrapulmonary pressures, dynamic ventilatory tasks, chest wall compliance, and chest wall motion during respiratory maneuvers. Frequently cited methods include spirometry, pneumotachometry, nitrogen or helium dilution methods using single or multiple breaths, static and dynamic chest wall compliance measurements, static measurements of pulmonary pressure at various levels of the lung volume, dynamic records of inspiratory and expiratory flow, respiratory-inductive or whole-body plethysmography, and surface motion magnetometry. See Lebowitz (1988) for a review of methods. Plethysmography and magnetometry (Hixon, 1987b) are particularly useful in the study of speech breathing behaviors because they do not encumber the airway openings or the articulators. It is, however, important to note that descriptive studies have been the source of much of this information, and subject variables known to influence pulmonary function have not always been well controlled or consistent across the accumulated database. Furthermore, the techniques used to obtain information themselves may introduce artifacts or be unreliable within and across subjects

(Gibson, Pride, O'Cain, & Quagliato, 1976; Mittman, Edelman, Norris, & Shock, 1965; Morris et al., 1971; Wilson, 1985). Finally, it should be noted that animals such as horses, rabbits, and rats may be used to study aging in the respiratory system because they exhibit some changes in lung physiology with age that are comparable enough to those exhibited by humans to allow them to serve as adequate models for some aging effects (Brody & Thurlbeck, 1986). These animal models obviously are limited, however, in their usefulness for static and dynamic measurements of respiratory performances that are peculiar to humans, such as speech.

Morphological Changes

Morphological changes associated with advancing age have been documented for the musculoskeletal framework of the respiratory apparatus as well as for the soft tissues of the pulmonary system. In general, the cellular components of the respiratory system follow an aging schedule that is comparable to other somatic systems of the human body. According to Lynne-Davies (1977), such cells reach senescence after about 50 doublings of their population. Functional decline, however, may begin to occur before the capacity for cell division has been exhausted.

The Chest Wall

The chest wall reportedly exhibits a decrease in compliance from infancy to senescence (Islam, 1980; Jones, Overton, Hammerlindl, & Sproule, 1978; Kenney, 1982; Lynne-Davies, 1977; Mittman et al., 1965), although this may be more or less obvious from one individual to the next and may be exaggerated by factors other than those provoked by natural aging. Degenerative changes in chest wall morphology associated with aging include osteoporosis of the vertebral bodies, thinning of the inter-

vertebral discs, and calcification of costal cartilages at the sternal and vertebral interfaces (Lebowitz, 1988; Reddan, 1981; Shephard, 1987). These degenerative changes are thought to encourage kyphoscoliosis of the vertebral column, resulting in an increase in the anteroposterior dimension of the thorax, and also to reduce the overall compliance of the chest wall (Brody & Thurlbeck, 1986; Klocke, 1977; Shephard, 1987). A few decades ago, this kyphotic change was given the unfortunate name of *senile* (or *postural*) emphysema because it resembled changes in the thoracic musculoskeletal form that accompany obstructive pulmonary emphysema. Recently, however, use of the term *senile emphysema* has been discouraged because its implication of pulmonary disease in clinically asymptomatic elderly individuals is misleading (Colebatch, Greaves, & Ng, 1979; Klocke, 1977; Stanescu et al., 1968).

An increase in chest wall stiffness with natural aging implies that more elastic work is required to deform the chest wall of an older person than of a younger person for the same ventilatory behavior (Jones et al., 1978; Kenney, 1982). Buskirk (1985), Lebowitz (1988), and Shephard (1987) speculate that as the rib cage stiffens with aging, the diaphragm assumes more responsibility for inspiratory gestures, and that anything that alters intra-abdominal pressure—such as body position, a large meal, a truss, or a girdle—may compromise the diaphragm's ability to contribute to ventilation. In addition, several authors have reported a flattening of the diaphragm and caudal descent of pulmonary structures with age (Macklin & Macklin, 1942; Shephard, 1987). This change may compromise the efficiency of the diaphragm for quick inspiratory gestures, such as those used during speech (Hixon, Goldman, & Mead, 1987).

The decrease in chest wall compliance with age may be accompanied by a decrease in respiratory muscle strength (Jones et al., 1978; Kenney, 1982; Reddan, 1981). Lebowitz (1988) has summarized changes in the voluntary muscles of the chest wall with age. They are consistent with age-related changes in skeletal muscle elsewhere in the human body and include decreases in the size of motor units (Kenney, 1982), prolonged contraction and relaxation times, and loss of muscle mass (Fleg & Lakatta, 1988; Shephard, 1987). Such changes are realized as reductions in voluntary respiratory muscle forces and maximal respiratory pressures (Black & Hyatt, 1969; Dubois & Alcala, 1964; Kenney, 1982). The fact that the timed ventilatory functions and rates of expiratory flow of elderly persons are reduced compared to those of younger subjects has been attributed, in part, to this reduction in chest wall muscle mass and strength with age. Most researchers in this area agree, however, that reduction in respiratory muscle mass alone cannot account for the changes in pulmonary function and dynamic ventilatory behaviors that accompany aging (Gibson et al., 1976; Jones et al., 1978).

The Pulmonary System

Lungs, Bronchioles, and Associated Tissues

The lungs have been described as undergoing a series of involutional changes with aging (Stanescu et al., 1968). These are associated with a redistribution of pulmonary volumes and alterations in pulmonary functions. Not unexpectedly, however, considerable differences of opinion exist about the nature of such changes. For example, recall that the respiratory surfaces of the lungs include the respiratory (terminal) bronchioles, the alveolar ducts, and the alveolar sacs, the walls of which are pitted with tiny pulmonary alveoli (Zemlin, 1988). Apparently the total number of one's alveoli is related to height (Knudson et al., 1977) and remains constant beyond about the 5th year of life (Kenney, 1982; Radford, 1964). Nevertheless, the available respiratory surface of the lung changes with age. Klocke (1977) reports that it declines beyond age 20

at a rate of about 0.27 m²/yr. This corresponds to a similar prediction by Shephard (1987), who projects a decrease in functional respiratory surface from 75 m² in the young adult to 60 m² in a person 70 years of age. A number of explanations have been offered for the loss of ventilatory surface area, though they are not all compatible, nor are clinical reports of reduction in ventilatory capacity in elders necessarily consistent with the explanations. Many writers attribute the decrease in respiratory surface to an increase in the volume of the alveolar ducts and respiratory bronchioles at the expense of alveolar volume; the alveoli become broadened and shallow (Kenney, 1982; Radford, 1964; Shepard, 1987). This phenomenon, referred to as "ductectasia" (Ryan, Vincent, Mitchell, Filley, & Dart, 1965, as cited in Klocke, 1977), has been noted in lungs older than 40 years (Klocke, 1977), and the frequency of its appearance reportedly increases with age beyond that milestone. In addition, a proliferation of the pores of Kohn in the alveolar tissue, or an increase in their size, has been noted with age, presumably at the expense of respiratory tissue surface (Brody & Thurlbeck, 1986; Radford, 1964). Furthermore, aging alveolar membranes reportedly become thinner (Shephard, 1987) and may even separate from their basement membranes (Reddan, 1981). These alterations have been attributed to changes in the resiliency and tensile properties of tissues at the interface of alveolar ducts and sacs (Klocke, 1977; Radford, 1964; Shephard, 1987). It also has been suggested (Radford, 1964) that there are changes in surface tension forces with age (for example, reduced surfactant production or activity) that affect respiratory function, although research has not yet substantiated this hypothesis (Lebowitz, 1988; Turner, Mead, & Wohl, 1968).

Age changes also have been noted in the vascular tissues of the lungs. Several authors (Heath, 1964; Shephard, 1987) report that the pulmonary venules and arterioles become increasingly less compliant with age. The capillary intima may become fibrotic due to collagen deposition or hyalinization (Lebowitz, 1988; Reddan, 1981; Shephard, 1987). These changes may increase vascular resistance and contribute to an increase in the alveolar-arterial oxygen (PO_2) gradient that is noted with aging (Kenney, 1982; Lebowitz, 1988; Lynne-Davies, 1977; Pierce & Ebert, 1958). Robinson (1964), on the basis of his studies of lungs from elderly men, suggested that changes in this gradient reflected an increasing resistance to diffusion of gas through the capillary walls and pulmonary epithelium. This diffusion disorder may be complicated by uneven alveolar ventilation and reduced respiratory surface area resulting from the aforementioned changes in the pulmonary tissues themselves. Other authors have offered similar interpretations for the pulmonary ventilation-perfusion imbalance that is exaggerated by aging (Brody & Thurlbeck, 1986; Kenney, 1982; Lebowitz, 1988; Pierce & Ebert, 1958).

Lebowitz reports that the mucociliary clearance mechanism of the lower airways is affected by aging, although he suggests that the nature of the effect is not completely understood. Kenney refers to a reduced effectiveness of the "mucus escalator" (1982, p. 47) with age. This has been attributed to a loss of cilia, reduction in the efficiency of ciliary action, or both. In addition, Kenney reports that macrophages at the alveolar level may be less efficient with age, although Lebowitz (1988) denies that anything is known about the effects of age on alveolar macrophage behavior. Reddan (1981) reports that mucous glands may actually proliferate with age, while Lebowitz (1988) contends that there is mucosal atrophy. Obviously much has yet to be learned about age-related changes in the clearing mechanism of the lower airways. The significance of deficits in mucous clearing is that accumulation of inhaled debris and residual mucus in the pulmonary airways may constitute another source of compromise for the ventilatory surfaces of the respiratory bronchioles, alveolar ducts, and alveolar sacs.

Fibrous Connective Tissues: Elastin and Collagen

Perhaps the most intensely investigated aspect of lung morphology associated with aging consists of the changes in the fibrous connective tissues of the pulmonary system that are thought to influence its elastic recoil characteristics. Most studies of respiratory function in aging persons document a decrease in pulmonary elastic recoil (or an increase in static compliance). (See, for example, Bode, Dosman, Martin, Ghezzo, & Macklem, 1976; Colebatch et al., 1979; Knudson et al., 1977; Pierce & Ebert, 1958, 1965; Turner et al., 1968.) Not all investigators agree on the reasons for, or implications of, this reduced pulmonary elasticity. Furthermore, its implications for changes in pulmonary function depend on associated age-related changes in chest wall compliance. Select studies will be reviewed here to exemplify the effects of aging on the structures and functional relationship of the lung and chest wall.

The major connective tissue proteins in the lungs are collagen, elastin, and reticulin. The first two have been studied extensively using histological and biochemical techniques, although the methods themselves are not without criticism and artifact (see Brody & Thurlbeck, 1986; Turner et al., 1968). Some reports suggest that elastin and collagen function in independent networks; that is, resiliency of elastic fibers are responsible for the slope of the pressure-volume curve at low and midlevel lung volumes, while collagenous networks limit pulmonary distension at high lung volumes (Turner et al., 1968; Wilson, 1985). This explanation remains inferential, however.

Collagen is thought to be in highest concentration among the resilient lung fibers. It is not readily distensible but is very responsive to lateral force deformation. In association with elastin, collagen forms the alveolar septa, the capillary support beds of the respiratory parenchyma, and is the major structural protein of the pleurae, the larger pulmonary blood vessels, and the lower airways. The concentration of collagenous protein in these tissues is not thought to change with age (Brody & Thurlbeck, 1986; Kohn, 1964). Aging collagen does exhibit an increase in cross-linking among neighboring fibers, however, forming aggregates that are thought to be less compliant for laterally directed forces (Kenney, 1982; Kohn, 1964). These cross-linkages also have been associated with an overall increase in the resting length of collagenous fibers (Shephard, 1987).

The amount of elastin in the lungs has been reported by some to decrease and by others to increase with age. Wright (1961), for example, reported a reduction in the number and thickness of elastic fibers in aging lung tissues. Although he reported this reduction as progressive, generalized, and uniform, he went on to say that it was more obvious in the region of the alveolar ducts and the alveoli themselves. Pierce and Ebert (1965) studied changes in the amount of elastin and collagen in the respiratory parenchyma (respiratory bronchioles, alveolar ducts, alveoli, and associated capillaries) and in the pleurae of dried human lung tissues. Their data indicated that the ratio of collagen to elastin in the respiratory parenchyma remained stable across their tissue sample age range (9–76 years), but that the ratio decreased in the pulmonary pleurae and septa with age due to an apparent increase in the proportion of elastin in those tissues.

Since the provocative reports of Pierce and Ebert (1965) and Wright (1961), the consensus seems to be that there may be some increase in the proportion of *total* (i.e., bulk) elastin relative to collagen in the lungs with age, although the physiological mechanism, anatomical distribution, and technical verification of this remain to be demonstrated. Researchers continue to pursue explanations for the discrepancy between a quantitative change in pulmonary elastin and a noticeable decrease in the lungs' elastic recoil with age.

Blumenthal, Yu, and Ridley (1964) compared changes in the elastic tissues of some major arteries, including the aorta, pulmonary arteries, and veins, with changes in pulmonary system tissues, including portions of the visceral pleurae, lobular septa, pulmonary airways, vestibules of the alveolar ducts, and walls of the alveoli. They noted that with increasing age, the quantity of elastic tissue increased overall in the lungs more consistently than in the arterial system and hypothesized that repeated mechanical stress constitutes a stimulus for formation of new elastic tissue. Similar processes appear to be operating in the development of pleural adhesions and myocardial scars.

Radford (1964) reported that although an overall increase in the amount of lung elastin may occur with age, a selective decrease occurs in the region of the alveolar ducts and alveoli. He attempts to resolve the discrepancy by noting that ''the elastic effects of tissue fibers may depend more on their location and anatomical arrangement, particularly with adjacent collagen, than on the absolute amount of fibers in the lung'' (p. 154).

Radford goes on to suggest that loss of lung elastic recoil with age is a complex phenomenon related to changes in alveolar dimensions as well as to the integrity of elastic tissue in and around the alveolar walls. If elasticity is reduced because of a loss of fibers locally or a change in the resiliency of existing fibers, the recoil pressure of the alveolar tissue will vary as the dimension of an alveolus varies, according to Laplace's law: Recoil pressure in a spherical segment is directly proportional to tension but inversely proportional to the radius of curvature of the sphere. Therefore, as air distends the alveolus, its radius of curvature will increase and its recoil pressure will decrease.

Turner et al. (1968) reached conclusions similar to Radford's. They infer from other reports that the total mass of resilient fibrous proteins (collagen and elastin) in the lungs does not change with age in adults, and that any change in lung surface forces that accompanies aging is not documented well enough to explain the loss of elastic recoil. Instead, they prefer to conclude that changes in the linkages between collagenous and elastic fibers significantly alter lung function and that the distribution of elastin fibers, rather than the total amount, within the lung parenchyma is the critical determinant.

It is appropriate to conclude this review of research on change in the lungs' resilient character with a cautionary note by Colebatch et al. (1979). They suggest that the change in elasticity in human lungs with age is small relative to the normal variation in elasticity across individuals of the same age, and that before definitive statements can be made about changes in the fibrous structure of the lungs vis-à-vis changes in their elastic recoil properties, a large sample of lung tissues across a large age range must be studied.

Functional (Mechanical) Changes

Knudson and colleagues have written that "the aging effect would seem to be statistically significant and inexorable but yet not very profound" (1977, p. 1059). In this section, the functional and clinical significance of the morphological changes cited previously will be discussed.

Changes in Pulmonary Volumes

The most commonly documented age-related changes in pulmonary volumes and ventilatory functions include (a) a reduction in the absolute VC and in the ratio of the VC to the TLC; (b) an increase in the absolute RV and in the ratio of the RV to the TLC; (c) an increase in the ratio of FRC to VC; (d) reduced MVV (L/min); (e) reduced volumes on timed FEV tasks, including FVC

and FEV_1; and (f) reduced maximum expiratory flows, particularly at low lung volumes. Among these, the most noticeable and statistically robust changes include the decrease in VC, the increase in RV, and the reduction in FEV_1. The relentless reduction in VC begins in the 4th decade and decreases by a mean of 26.4 ml/yr for males and 21.6 ml/yr for females, with a similar rate of decline for both sexes (Klocke, 1977). Thus, Kenney (1982) reckons that between the ages of 20 and 60 years, the aging respiratory system loses about 1 L of VC. The RV has been estimated to increase by a factor of about 40% between 20 and 70 years of age (Lynne-Davies, 1977). Dhar et al. (1976) and Shephard (1987) report the average loss in FEV_1 as 32 ml/yr for men and 25 ml/yr for women, with a related decrement in the FEV_1/FVC ratio.

Elastic Recoil of the Lung

One of the earliest studies of the mechanical properties of the lungs in elders was that of Cohn and Donoso (1963). Their subjects included old (> 60 years) and young (< 40 years) men, of whom some were cigarette smokers. Cohn and Donoso observed numerous differences between these two subject groups, including decreased VC; decreased IC; and increased FRC, RV, and RV/TLC among the elder subjects compared to the younger ones. In addition, the older subject group exhibited reduced maximum inspiratory pressures and increased mean pulmonary airway resistance for a flow of 1 L/s at FRC. Cohn and Donoso also measured dynamic compliance[1] of the lungs under several conditions in which rate and volume of tidal respiration were varied. During normal quiet breathing, the dynamic compliance of the lungs of the elders was significantly higher than that of the young men. When the breathing rate for

---

[1]According to the American College of Chest Physicians/American Thoracic Society, *dynamic compliance* is measured at the mouth at the moment of zero air flow during breathing. The breathing rate should be specified. This differs from the measurement of *static compliance* that is made during conditions of air flow interruptions at specific lung volumes. See Wilson (1985, pp. 125–136) for further explanation.

the usual volume exchange was doubled, dynamic compliance of the elderly subjects' lungs decreased significantly; when tidal volumes were increased while breathing frequency was kept usual or slower, the dynamic compliance of the elderly subjects' lungs increased significantly. Cohn and Donoso attributed changes in dynamic compliance with breathing rate and tidal volume, and the difference in overall dynamic compliance between the old and the young subjects, to alterations in the elastic matrix of the older lung tissues. Furthermore, they proposed that these alterations are unevenly distributed in that the lungs of the elderly are composed of units with nonuniform pressure/volume characteristics. Thus, tidal volume distribution among the alveoli would be expected to vary with breathing rate, tidal volume, and lung volume level. When breathing frequency is rapid, dynamic compliance is measurably decreased because the uneven distribution of air realizes a smaller alveolar volume. When breathing frequency is slow or tidal volumes are large, however, distribution reaches more alveoli and dynamic compliance is measurably increased. A number of researchers in the decades since the publication of Cohn and Donoso's paper have noted that elderly subjects achieve more efficient ventilation when tidal respiration is deep and slow (Shephard, 1987).

Turner et al. (1968) and Knudson et al. (1977) documented that the decrement in pulmonary elastic recoil with age is more noticeable at higher lung volumes, although the rate of recoil decrement in the data of Knudson et al. (1977) was less than that reported a decade earlier by Turner et al. (1968). One explanation for this discrepancy may be that Turner et al.'s subjects included smokers as well as nonsmokers, whereas all those of Knudson et al. were lifetime nonsmokers. Furthermore, according to Knudson et al., when data are corrected for lung size, no sex difference emerges in older subjects' tendency to lose pulmonary elastic recoil properties, despite earlier reports to the contrary (Bode et al., 1976). Knudson et al. also reported that maximum flow did

not show a decrement until 70% of the VC had been expired. Hence, in spite of reduced elastic recoil in older lungs at higher lung volumes, maximum flow rate was preserved.

Colebatch et al. (1979) used a single exponential function to derive an index of pulmonary compliance that represents "true nonlinear elastic behavior of the lungs over a substantial range [upper 50%] and is independent of the size of the lungs" (p. 687). They applied their exponential analysis to a study of elastic recoil in 124 lifetime nonsmoking men and women, 17–82 years of age. They report an increase in the index of lung compliance with age, regardless of gender, and attribute this change to an increase in the resting length of the alveoli and a reduction in the number of elastic fibers in the region of the alveoli and alveolar ducts, or some change in their resilient nature.

Chest Wall and Pulmonary Compliance

Many writers have reported that the chest wall becomes less compliant and the pulmonary system more compliant with age. Mittman et al. (1965) investigated the relationship among pulmonary compliance, chest wall compliance, and age in 42 men (24–78 years of age) who were free of signs of cardiopulmonary or neurogenic disease. Pulmonary compliance differences were not significant between the young and old subjects at FRC. At higher lung volumes (that is, close to 75% TLC), however, pulmonary compliance decreased more in the young subjects than in the old. Mittman et al. acknowledge that elderly subjects' failure to exhibit as large a decrement in pulmonary compliance between FRC and 75% TLC as young subjects could be attributed to a decrement in lung elastic recoil with age. They also argue, however, that this finding could be attributable to a decrease in chest wall compliance in the elderly. This implies that TLC should be limited in the older subjects, and they report a nonsignificant trend to that effect. This is controversial, because TLC is thought to remain relatively stable across the natural history of the respiratory system with age. Their data for chest wall compliance exhibited a significant decrease with age, and the authors attribute age-associated decrements in VC and increases in RV to this acquired chest wall stiffness. Their report includes some useful comments about the difficulties inherent in the measurement of chest wall compliance. Its assessment, regardless of the exact technique used, requires subjects to relax the chest wall musculature completely at various lung volumes. Subjects at any age may have difficulty accomplishing this. Hence, chest wall compliance data may be unreliable across repeated measures, particularly for static compliance maneuvers, and may be contaminated by a voluntary neuromuscular component.

Turner et al. (1968) combined their data on the relationship between lung elasticity and age with those of Mittman et al. (1965) for pulmonary and chest wall compliances to produce ''ideal'' clinical examples of the combined effects of changes in both phenomena with age. In a 20-year-old, the lungs are less compliant than the chest wall within the range of spontaneous breathing. By 60 years of age, the reverse is true. The chest wall's increase in stiffness is slightly greater than the lung's decrease in stiffness, however, so the 60-year-old's total respiratory system is less compliant overall than that of the 20-year-old. Hence, Turner et al. propose that the older subject would have to do 20% more elastic work at a given level of ventilation than the 20-year-old, but would expend 70% of the total elastic work on moving the chest wall, whereas this job for the 20-year-old would ''cost'' only 40% of the total elastic work. Figure 9.1 is taken from Turner et al. Panels A and B illustrate changes in the static recoil volume-pressure relationship of the lung and chest wall for ''ideal'' 20- and 60-year-old subjects. Composite data are displayed in part C of the figure.

Turner et al. (1968) point out that the increase in lung compliance at high lung volumes normally is counteracted rather comparably by a decrease in chest wall compliance. This explains the apparent stability of TLC across the aging process, the arguments of Mittman et al. (1965) notwithstanding. At lower lung volumes, however, the altered mechanics of the lungs and chest wall favor the recoil tendency of the wall. Thus, the resting lung volume of the respiratory system, or FRC, increases from about 50% TLC in a 20-year-old person to about 60% TLC in a 70-year-old person (Kenney, 1982; Lynne-Davies, 1977; Turner et al., 1968).

Lower Airways

Airway behavior related to mechanical changes in the aging pulmonary system is an important research area because the airways reportedly are less stable with age. Interpretations of this instability differ depending on the nature of the respiratory task, the lung volume at which airway behavior was measured, and whether the dependent measurement is airway compliance, conductance, or resistance. Furthermore, it is not clear whether altered airway stability, when it can be reliably measured, is a function of changes in the walls of the airways themselves, changes in parenchymal forces normally influencing their patency, or some combination thereof that varies with the lung volume at which the measurements are made. With respect to the larger airways, Lebowitz (1988) reports reduced compliance of the trachea. Some reports claim that the dimensions of the larger airways are unaltered (e.g., Shephard, 1987), whereas others report an increase in large airway diameters and therefore larger physiological ''dead space.'' Lebowitz (1988) reports that with increasing age, there is a reduction in bronchiole diameter and an increase in alveolar duct volume, which result from localized changes in elastic recoil.

The most valuable information on age-related changes in airway aeromechanical behaviors comes from studies of expiratory

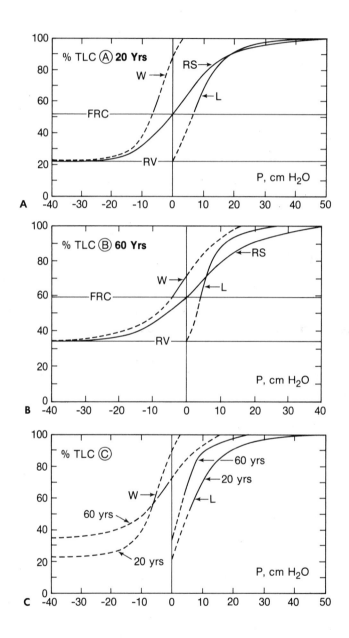

FIGURE 9.1. Rahn diagrams of static volume-pressure relationships of lungs (L), chest wall (W), and total respiratory system (RS) for "ideal" 20- and 60-year-old subjects, based on the present data (Turner, Mead, & Wohl, 1968) plus that of Mittman, Edelman, Norris, and Shock (1965). The diagrams are given separately (A & B) and in combination (C) for direct comparison. *Note.* From "Elasticity of Human Lungs in Relation to Age" by J. M. Turner, J. Mead, and M. E. Wohl, 1968, *Journal of Applied Physiology, 25,* pp. 664–671. Copyright 1968 by The American Physiological Society. Reprinted by permission.

flow limitations and closing volume (i.e., that point in the lung volume when small airways cease to ventilate and are presumed closed). Appreciation of the research devoted to this complex topic warrants some background information.

Dynamics of Conductance and Resistance

In the human lung, several physical gradients related to transpulmonary pressures and airway conductance/resistance are known to affect closing volume and dynamic compliance. That is, transpulmonary pressure decreases from apex to base, airway diameter becomes progressively smaller from apex to base, and airway resistance becomes progressively higher from apex to base and as the flow rate increases. The tiny distal airways of the lung have no skeletal structure and must depend, to some extent, on elastic recoil for their patency. These so-called "dependent" regions tend to be lower in the lung because of the aforementioned apical-to-basal gradients. As a person goes low in the lung volume during an expiratory maneuver, airway collapse occurs first in these dependent regions. The loss of elastic recoil with aging makes these dependent airways more susceptible to collapse. Therefore, it is easier for an older person to reach a point in the flow/volume performance curve when an increase in expiratory effort is not associated with an increase in expiratory flow. As one ages, this point "creeps" higher in the lung volume. In young humans, the closing volume as a percentage of the VC is well below FRC and should not influence normal ventilation. In older subjects, however, closing volume may be above FRC (depending on the rate of breathing, and therefore the rate of flow) and may alter the distribution of ventilation in the tidal breathing range (Kenney, 1982; Pierce & Ebert, 1958; Stanescu et al., 1968). In addition, lung emptying is less efficient: FVC, MVV, peak expiratory flow rates, and FEV_1 all are reduced, while RV is increased (Jones et al., 1978; Lebowitz, 1988).

Begin, Renzetti, Bigler, and Watanabe (1975) described changes in the dynamic compliance of the lungs with respect to closing volume. They studied 66 lifetime nonsmoking men and women, ages 20–82, who were asymptomatic for respiratory disease and otherwise healthy. (For those who may be interested, they also studied a smaller group of smokers who were younger, overall, than the nonsmoking group). They report that closing volume was dependent on the expiratory flow rate and increased with age. These results for single-breath measurements for closing volume correlated strongly with those for dynamic compliance at two breathing rates, normal (0.5 L/s) and fast (1.5 L/s). That is, dynamic compliance exhibited a decrease with a breathing rate increase that was significant for subjects in the 5th decade and beyond. This has implications for the elderly with respect to tidal ventilation. Begin et al. use an example of a 68-year-old person in whom closing volume would occur in the tidal volume range at an expiratory flow of 0.5 L/s, a rate comparable to peak flow at a common frequency of 15 breaths per minute (BPM). At higher breathing frequencies, which logically are associated with higher flow rates, it is likely that closing volume would increase. Begin et al. suggest that the interplay between airway compliance and resistance during breathing becomes more nonuniform with age and may effect asynchronous behavior with respect to airway closing and opening in the tidal volume range.

The implications for this observation may be relevant not only to ventilation but also to breathing for speech. The frequency dependence of compliance when closing volumes are above FRC may have implications for the depth of prespeech inspiration, as well as for prolonged speech tasks or those loaded with sound segments associated with high expiratory flows (e.g., obstruent consonants). This is discussed further below, when the speech breathing data of Hoit and Hixon (1987) for young and old persons are considered.

The work of Knudson et al. (1977) also has shed light on the extent of elastic recoil changes in the lung and lower airways with age. Their discussion (pp. 1060–1061) provides insight into the interdependence of elastic forces within the lung parenchyma and pulmonary airways and the influence of these forces on airway caliber and airway resistance as intrapulmonary pressure changes during expiration throughout the lung volume. Knudson et al. note that recoil of the lung parenchyma provides external support for the intrapulmonary airways. Hence, if the parenchyma alone lost elastic recoil with age, airway caliber might be compromised by high flow rates at high lung volumes. In the results of Knudson et al., however, maximum expiratory flow rates were not limited in their elderly subjects at high lung volumes, even though elastic recoil was reduced at high lung volumes for the elders. Maximum expiratory flow was only limited after 70% of the VC had been expired. Knudson et al. propose that the loss of elastic recoil with age must affect both intrapulmonary airways and parenchymal tissues. They suggest that the maximum flow limitations experienced by the elderly only at low lung volumes were a function of the location of the so-called "equal pressure point" (EPP), at which intrapulmonary and transpulmonary pressures are equal. In young lungs, the EPP tends to move upstream toward the alveoli as the lung empties during a maximum expiratory maneuver. With increasing compliance of the intrapulmonary airways, however, the EPP remains in more central airways as the lung empties. This effectively produces a longer airway upstream of the EPP that will exhibit higher resistance to expiratory flow. In addition, the less compliant airways downstream of the EPP would be more vulnerable to dynamic compression and collapse, limiting further upstream migration of the EPP. Both these factors would be consistent with maximum flow limitations exhibited by elderly subjects at low lung volumes. Gibson et al. (1976) also speak to this phenomenon.

Lynne-Davies (1977) interprets these data relative to decreased ventilation/perfusion efficiency with age. Higher closing volumes result in decreased efficiency of ventilation in dependent lung regions. This alteration in the distribution of ventilation is not necessarily compensated for, or offset by, changes in pulmonary blood perfusion patterns, however. This discrepancy explains part of the decrease in arterial oxygen tension (PaO_2) seen with age. She notes that most of the studies of expiratory flow limitations and closing volumes have been done on subjects in the seated body position and argues that a further reduction in efficient ventilation/perfusion may be expected when elders assume a recumbent position and experience its associated decrease in FRC. In this position, higher closing volumes (relative to FRC) and reduced PaO_2 together may induce a hypoxemia that could contribute to the nocturnal confusion exhibited by some elders.

Aging and Speech Breathing

The comprehensive report of Hoit and Hixon (1987) is the first in the literature to assess the effects of aging on breathing for speech per se. These researchers used surface motion magnetometry and the principles of respiratory kinematics (Hixon, Goldman, & Mead, 1987) to study aspects of general respiratory function and speech breathing behaviors in 30 healthy men representing young (25 ± 3 years), middle-aged (50 ± 3 years), and old (75 ± 3 years) English-speaking, white Americans. Hoit and Hixon compared static measurements of a number of subdivisions of the lung volume among the three subject groups, including TLC, VC, IC, FRC, ERV, and RV. They found that absolute values of RV were significantly smaller in the youngest subjects than in either of the older groups. Furthermore, when subjects' lung volume divisions were normalized to a percentage of TLC, the youngest subjects exhibited a mean RV/TLC that was significantly smaller, and a mean VC/TLC that was significantly larger, than those of the oldest subjects. Dynamic observations of tidal volumes, tidal breathing rates, minute volumes, and relative volume contributions of the rib cage to tidal volume exchange revealed no significant differences among the subject groups, however. In addition, the authors noted no differences among the subjects of this study, nor between them and subjects of previous kinematic studies, with respect to the background configuration of the chest wall at the resting tidal end-expiratory level, or with respect to the continuum of chest wall configurations displayed by subjects during tidal inspiration that reflect rib cage and abdominal contributions to tidal volume intake. Certainly the trends in the Hoit and Hixon data for static respiratory functions are consistent with the literature on changes in pulmonary function with age. For example, VC was reduced and RV was increased with aging, a finding that recapitulates other reports of the last 2 decades, regardless of subject health or history. Hoit and Hixon attribute such changes in RV and VC with age to mechanical factors, namely, reduced elastic recoil in the lung parenchyma and lower airways, and reduction in lower airway conductance resulting from higher small airway closing volumes with age. In addition, their data show trends toward an increase in absolute and normalized values for FRC, a decrease in absolute and normalized values for IC, and a reduction in ERV with age, although these trends did not reach statistical significance. Hoit and Hixon also noted a stability of TLC across the age range observed. They interpreted the implications of the age-related differences they noted in general respiratory functions for speech breathing as follows:

> . . . it is probably the age-related reduction in VC that carries the greatest impact. For any act requiring volitional expenditure of air, such as speech production, the volume of air available to perform the act is, by definition, the vital capacity. Therefore, it fol-

lows that older individuals must operate within a more limited range of volumes for speech production. (1987, p. 362)

The Hoit and Hixon (1987) experimental protocol for speech breathing assessment included data collection for repeated measures of extemporaneous speech and for reading aloud. The material for reading was a paragraph constructed to provide opportunities for a large number of expiratory breath groups of variable syllable numbers and is included in an appendix to their report. Among the data for extemporaneous speaking, significant differences were noted between the youngest and oldest subjects for lung volume excursions and syllables produced per breath group, as well as for the percentage of the VC exchanged per syllable. Specifically, the oldest subjects produced fewer syllables per breath group but expended a larger percentage of the VC per syllable and therefore exhibited larger lung volume excursions per breath group than the youngest subjects. In association with this observation, it was noted that the oldest subjects tended to initiate speech at higher lung and rib cage volumes than the youngest subjects. Among the data for reading aloud, the only difference observed was the percentage of the VC expended per syllable.

Hoit and Hixon (1987) attribute the age-related differences in speech breathing behaviors to several possible interactive phenomena: (a) changes in the elders' linguistic output (viz., fewer syllables per breath group); (b) reduced efficiency of laryngeal and/or upper airway valving (viz., larger lung volume excursions and a larger percentage of VC/syllable expenditures); and (c) anticipatory adjustments in the breathing apparatus (e.g., higher lung volume initiation levels to accommodate larger lung volume excursions associated with reduced laryngeal or upper airway valving efficiency). The higher lung volume initiation levels also may relate to the increase in closing volume with aging, noted earlier in the chapter. If closing volume is above FRC, elders may initiate speech at a higher lung volume to avoid closing volume limitations. Unfortunately, no data for speaking rate across subject groups are included in the Hoit and Hixon (1987) report, so it is not known if this factor may have affected the group differences they noted in the number of syllables per breath group and lung volumes exchanged on the speaking tasks. This would seem to be a relevant issue in light of earlier reports such as those of Ramig (1983) and Smith, Wasowicz, and Preston (1987), which indicate that speaking and reading rates may slow with aging.

In summary, Hoit and Hixon (1987) were able to describe differences in speech breathing functions that distinguished elderly subjects from younger ones. On the basis of their data, the clinician might expect an elderly talker to initiate speech at higher lung and rib cage volumes, expend larger lung and rib cage volumes, produce fewer syllables per breath group, and expend a greater average lung volume per syllable than a young talker. Furthermore, these differences might be more readily distinguished if the speech on which these variables were measured was extemporaneous rather than read aloud, so that subjects would be free to make whatever linguistic and respiratory adjustments were necessary to compensate for any respiratory, laryngeal, or articulatory limitations acquired with age. It is also of interest to note that the most significant differences seen by Hoit and Hixon (1987) were between the youngest and oldest subjects, with an occasional significant difference between the youngest and middle-aged groups. The 50- and 75-year-old groups were not significantly different on any of the general respiratory or speech breathing variables studied. This is consistent with observations in the literature that age-related changes in pulmonary function, at least, begin to become measurable after about 40 years of age. Little is known as yet, however, about the linearity of the progression of age-related decline in respiratory function beyond that point, or about the ways in which various influential factors of environmental and personal health and life-style contribute to that decline. Part of this ignorance is a limitation in the ability of cross-sectional research designs to elucidate these trends (Birren & Renner, 1977; Lebowitz, 1988; Shock, 1985).

Aging Respiratory Function Complicated by Disease

Most of the information reviewed so far in this chapter relates to aging and respiratory changes in healthy persons. A few comments are warranted about disease phenomena that tend to occur with age and that may complement or exaggerate natural senescent changes in respiratory system function. Among diseases of the lung that may occur with aging, there are two major classes (Lebowitz, 1988): *airway obstructive diseases* and *restrictive lung diseases*. Airway obstructive diseases are more common; they are most prevalent in the 7th and 8th decades. They include the chronic obstructive pulmonary or lung diseases (COPD or COLD): emphysema and chronic bronchitis (and, in some listings, bronchiectasis). Asthma and bronchiolitis obliterans also are included in this category. The less common restrictive lung diseases, such as pneumoconioses, usually occur in elders as a result of some occupational exposure. Pulmonary function testing using spirometry or pneumotachometry may be helpful in distinguishing between the obstructive and restrictive disorders when they are combined with an aging affect.

The onset and expression of airway obstructive diseases in elders may be gradual and insidious or variably acute; clear-cut diagnoses are influenced by the patient's gender, smoking history, and allergic sensitivities. Cigarette smoking is the variable most often associated with the presence and development of COPD (Ferris, 1978) and appears to accelerate the physiological changes associated with aging (Lebowitz, 1988). Age-related changes in immunologic integrity are reflected in reports that the prevalence of asthma increases with age, as does the incidence of malignancies. The reader is referred to reviews by Dhar et al. (1976), Lynne-Davies (1977), Wilson (1985), and Lebowitz (1988) for more details about the effects of pulmonary disease on respiratory function in elders. Among these, the Lebowitz (1988) summary is particularly enlightening with respect to the appearance and strength of these trends in cross-sectional versus longitudinal studies, as they reflect cohort and survival effects, and as they are skewed by smoking and respiratory diseases. He also notes philosophically that the signs of aging in the respiratory system are, inevitably, a function of its job description in life:

> The lungs are the primary defense against external toxic agents, are the primary depository for many toxic particles and fibers, and are important for eliminating various metabolic byproducts and wastes. Whatever enters the lung, and from there enters the circulation, may well affect the lungs in the process. (1988, p. 269)

Pitfalls in the Assessment of Respiratory Function

It is important to comment briefly on the factors that are important to the assessment and measurement of respiratory functions, in general, and the study of those functions in elderly persons, in particular. In clinical practice, a person's performance on tests of pulmonary functions, timed forced ventilatory tasks, and compliance maneuvers forms the basis for considerable inference about the status of that person's respiratory health. Therefore, it is important (a) to obtain accurate information about the respiratory health and history of the person under scrutiny, (b) to ensure that the testing methods used follow standardized procedures so that the data obtained are valid reflections of the function under test, and (c) to verify the reliability of the data obtained and the measurements made from them.

With respect to the standardization of epidemiological record keeping and procedures, a useful reference is the Epidemiology Standardization Project (Ferris, 1978), sponsored by the American Thoracic Society and supported by the Division of Lung Diseases, National Heart, Lung and Blood Institute (of the National Institutes of Health). The published project includes two standard questionnaires on respiratory health history and status (one for children and one for adults), recommended standardized procedures for tests of pulmonary function, and recommended procedures for chest radiographs obtained by epidemiological programs studying nonoccupational lung diseases. Of particular interest to readers of this text are the adult questionnaire and the procedures for testing pulmonary function. The questionnaire is designed for interviewer administration to, or self-completion by, persons aged 13 years and older. It includes questions about respiratory health; occupational, smoking, and family histories; and demographic-environmental factors. The use of this and complementary screening instruments pertinent to a specific study (see, for example, Hoit & Hixon, 1987) would ensure that an adequate picture of a subject's respiratory history and current status was obtained. This information, in turn, influences the choice of relevant clinical tests, accurate interpretation of test results, and comparisons of results with the appropriate cohort group. The standards for pulmonary function testing provided by the Epidemiology Standardization Project also constitute a valuable resource. Throughout this chapter, allusions have been made to the reliability problems inherent in respiratory function testing. It is gratifying but rare to see comments about subject variability and performance reliability in published studies of pulmonary function and compliance testing. Yet many of these tasks are tedious, require considerable rehearsal, and deserve repeated measurement during the actual data collection (see caveats in Kent, Kent, & Rosenbek, 1987; Morris et al., 1971; Wilson, 1985). Thus, whether one is obtaining such data or just reading reports based on their collection and measurement, standardization of the procedures used and the reliability of the data obtained affect the validity of the results.

A study that attempted to consider all these factors—subject heterogeneity, procedural standardization, and performance reliability—is that of Morris et al. (1971). It is a source of prediction formulas for a number of routine clinical pulmonary function tasks, and a sobering reflection of the vagaries of measuring respiratory behaviors. Morris et al. reported data from a particularly well-controlled cross-sectional study of 988 subjects who followed a life-style that prohibited smoking and resided in an area of low elevation that was free of urban air pollutants. The population included men and women, aged 20 to 84 years; their performances presumably reflect the biological effects of aging independent of atmospheric pollution, respiratory disease, or cigarette smoking. These researchers assessed pulmonary volumes and forced expiratory flows using methods of spirometry that are frequently used in clinical practice. Not unexpectedly, they found that performance on these measures correlated positively with height and *negatively with age*. Their report includes prediction formulas based on height and age for the expiratory flows and volumes studied, although they suggest that their sample of elders was too limited for statistically valid prediction equations at that end of the age continuum. They candidly include cautionary notes about the limitations of any predictors in light of the large standard errors of estimate associated with their data, the size and homogeneity of their subject group notwithstanding. They conclude: "The wide range of normal values seriously impairs the usefulness of spirometry in reliably detecting impairment of ventilatory function in asymptomatic individuals" (Morris et al., 1971, abstract. See also Comroe, 1974; Shephard, 1987).

Another study that sheds light on variability in respiratory function, particularly among elderly individuals, is that of Tobin,

Mador, Guenther, Lodato, and Sackner (1988). They report a series of experiments in which they used respiratory inductive plethsmography to study the breath-to-breath and day-to-day variability of resting breathing patterns in healthy subjects. One of their experiments observed the effects of age on breathing pattern variability by comparing data from young (aged 21–50) and old (aged 60–81) subjects for measures of respiratory timing, volume, and respiratory drive. The elderly subjects distinguished themselves by exhibiting greater breath-to-breath variability than the young subjects on most of the measures taken; the strength of this difference was particularly robust for breath-by-breath ventilation, inspiratory time, and the ratio of inspiratory time to total breathing cycle time. Tobin et al. interpret this observation in light of research by Peterson, Pack, Silage, and Fishman (1981), whose elderly subjects exhibited abnormal ventilatory responses to conditions of hypercapnia (increased CO_2) and hypoxia (decreased O_2), and to the work of Tack, Altose, and Cherniack (1981), who documented a decreased perceptual sensitivity to respiratory loads in elderly subjects. There are insufficient data at this time, however, to conclude that the increased variability noted in the resting breathing patterns of elderly subjects represents an abnormality in respiratory control rather than simply an increase in the intra- and intersubject variability noted in other studies of elders (see, for example, Weismer, 1984).

It is useful and frequently necessary to consider the problematic issues of respiratory function assessment in light of related and larger issues associated with the study of aging humans. The reader is referred to Shock's critical treatise on longitudinal studies of aging (1985) for insight into, and a historical perspective on, a number of pertinent research models. As a prototypic example, he reviews in detail the *Baltimore Longitudinal Study of Aging* (Shock et al., 1984), a valuable resource of information about changes in respiratory function with age in the context of many other variables.

Conclusions

A number of changes in the respiratory system occur naturally with age. Those changes that are major and well documented include a decrease in the VC and an increase in the RV, while the TLC remains relatively stable across the years. In addition, the FRC, which reflects the resting level of the respiratory system, increases, as does the closing volume of the peripheral airways during forced expiratory maneuvers. Furthermore, forced expiratory volumes, including the FVC and FEV_1, and associated flow rates, exhibit a natural reduction with aging. These changes appear to be related to decreased elastic recoil of the lung parenchyma and pulmonary airways, decreased chest wall compliance, reduced stability in the distal airways subject to dynamic compliance, and decreased respiratory muscle mass and strength. Finally, such mechanical alterations, combined with morphological changes in the respiratory tissues themselves, affect the respiratory system's efficiency for gas exchange, thereby exaggerating a ventilation-perfusion imbalance that increases with age. No decrements in speech intelligibility or communication effectiveness have been associated with these changes in the respiratory system in the absence of complicating factors such as neurological or neuromuscular disorders. Some reports have even suggested that prolonged endurance training into senescence may forestall some of this decline. These natural changes in respiratory system function may be complicated, exaggerated, or accelerated, however, by acute and chronic respiratory diseases, neurological and neuromuscular diseases that influence chest wall muscle strength, smoking, occupational exposures to damaging inhalants, and, to some extent, environmental exposures to airborne pollutants. In the final analysis, Lebowitz (1988) writes,

> In the absence of cigarette smoking, major occupational exposures, and disease, there is a reduction of both volume excursions and instantaneous expiratory flow rates (at different parts of the flow-volume curve) with age. The typical reduction does not reach the level of clinical disease, even in the elderly, for even the lower segment of the distribution in the asymptomatic nonsmoking population. (p. 263)

Furthermore, Colebatch et al. (1979) note that while age-related decreases in elastic recoil and diffusing capacity and changes in some portions of the pulmonary subdivisions do share a qualitative similarity with changes induced by pulmonary emphysema, it would take an average healthy subject about 140 years to attain a pulmonary compliance value comparable to that of an emphysematous subject, and perhaps 220 years for the healthy subject's static recoil pressure at 90% of the TLC to decline to that of a person with clinically obvious pulmonary emphysema. They conclude that "the average lung can provide useful function for a period well beyond the present human life span, and that the process which we recognize as aging in the lungs does not determine longevity" (1979, p. 691).

References

Begin, R., Renzetti, A. D., Jr., Bigler, A. H., & Watanabe, S. (1975). Flow and age dependence of airway closure and dynamic compliance. *Journal of Applied Physiology, 38,* 199–207.

Belman, M. J., & Gaesser, G. A. (1988). Ventilatory muscle training in the elderly. *Journal of Applied Physiology, 64,* 899–905.

Birren, J. E., & Renner, V. J. (1977). Research on the psychology of aging: Principles and experimentation. In J. E. Birren & K. W. Schaie (Eds.), *Handbook of the psychology of aging* (pp. 3–41). New York: Van Nostrand Reinhold.

Black, L. F., & Hyatt, R. E. (1969). Maximal respiratory pressures: Normal values and relationship to age and sex. *American Review of Respiratory Disease, 99,* 696–702.

Blumenthal, H. T., Yu, S. Y., & Ridley, A. M. (1964). Comparison of aging changes in elastic tissue of the lungs and arteries. In L. Cander & J. H. Moyer (Eds.), *Aging of the lung* (pp. 21–40). New York: Grune & Stratton.

Bode, F. R., Dosman, J., Martin, R. R., Ghezzo, H., & Macklem, P. T. (1976). Age and sex differences in lung elasticity, and in closing capacity in nonsmokers. *Journal of Applied Physiology, 41*, 129–135.

Brody, J. S., & Thurlbeck, W. M. (1986). Development, growth and aging of the lung. In P. T. Macklem & J. Mead (Eds.), *Handbook of physiology, section 3: The respiratory system, Vol. 3, Part I—Mechanics of breathing* (pp. 355–386). Bethesda, MD: American Physiological Society.

Buskirk, E. R. (1985). Health maintenance and longevity: Exercise. In C. E. Finch & E. L. Schneider (Eds.), *Handbook of the biology of aging* (2nd ed., pp. 894–924). New York: Van Nostrand Reinhold.

Cohn, J. E., & Donoso, H. D. (1963). Mechanical properties of lung in normal men over 60 years old. *Journal of Clinical Investigation, 42*, 1406–1410.

Colebatch, H. J. H., Greaves, I. A., & Ng, C. K. Y. (1979). Exponential analysis of elastic recoil and aging in healthy males and females. *Journal of Applied Physiology: Respiratory, Environmental and Exercise Physiology, 47*, 683–691.

Comroe, J. H. (1974). *Physiology of respiration* (2nd ed.). Chicago: Year Book Medical Publishers.

Dhar, S., Shastri, S. R., & Lenora, R. A. K. (1976). Aging and the respiratory system. *Medical Clinics of North America, 60*, 1121–1139.

Dubois, A. B., & Alcala, R. (1964). Airway resistance and mechanics of breathing in normal subjects 75–90 years of age. In L. Cander & J. H. Moyer (Eds.), *Aging of the lung* (pp. 156–162). New York: Grune & Stratton.

Ferris, B. G. (1978). Epidemiology Standardization Project. *American Review of Respiratory Disease, 118* (Suppl.), 1–53.

Fleg, J. L., & Lakatta, E. G. (1988). Role of muscle loss in the age-associated reduction in $VO_{2\ max}$. *Journal of Applied Physiology, 65*, 1147–1151.

Gibson, G. J., Pride, N. B., O'Cain, C., & Quagliato, R. (1976). Sex and age differences in pulmonary mechanics in normal nonsmoking subjects. *Journal of Applied Physiology, 41*, 20–25.

Hagberg, J. M., Yerg II, J. E., & Seals, D. R. (1988). Pulmonary function in young and older athletes and untrained men. *Journal of Applied Physiology, 65*, 101–105.

Heath, D. (1964). Structural changes in the pulmonary vasculature associated with aging. In L. Cander & J. H. Moyer (Eds.), *Aging of the lung* (pp. 70–76). New York: Grune & Stratton.

Hixon, T. J. (1987a). Respiratory function in speech. In T. J. Hixon et al. (Eds.), *Respiratory function in speech and song* (pp. 1–54). San Diego, CA: College Hill Press.

Hixon, T. J. (1987b). Some new techniques for measuring the biomechanical events of speech production: One laboratory's experiences. In T. J. Hixon et al. (Eds.), *Respiratory function in speech and song* (pp. 55–91). San Diego, CA: College Hill Press.

Hixon, T. J., Goldman, M. D., & Mead, J. (1987). Kinematics of the chest wall during speech production: Volume displacements of the rib cage, abdomen and lung. In T. J. Hixon et al. (Eds.), *Respiratory function in speech and song* (pp. 93–133). San Diego, CA: College Hill Press.

Hoit, J. D., & Hixon, T. J. (1987). Age and speech breathing. *Journal of Speech and Hearing Research, 30*, 351–366.

Islam, M. S. (1980). Mechanism of controlling residual volume and emptying rate of the lung in young and healthy elderly subjects. *Respiration, 40*, 1–8.

Jones, R. L., Overton, T. R., Hammerlindl, D. M., & Sproule, B. J. (1978). Effects of age on regional residual volume. *Journal of Applied Physiology: Respiratory, Environmental and Exercise Physiology, 44*, 195–199.

Kenney, R. A. (1982). *Physiology of aging: A synopsis*. Chicago: Year Book Medical Publishers.

Kent, R. D., Kent, J. F., & Rosenbek, J. C. (1987). Maximum performance tests of speech production. *Journal of speech and hearing disorders, 52*, 367–387.

Klocke, R. A. (1977). Influence of aging on the lung. In C. Finch & L. Hayflick (Eds.), *Handbook of the biology of aging* (pp. 432–444). New York: Van Nostrand Reinhold.

Knudson, R. J., Clark, D. F., Kennedy, T. C., & Knudson, D. E. (1977). Effect of aging alone on mechanical properties of the normal adult human lung. *Journal of Applied Physiology: Respiratory, Environmental and Exercise Physiology, 43*, 1054–1062.

Kohn, R. R. (1964). Changes in connective tissue. In L. Cander & J. H. Moyer (Eds.), *Aging of the lung* (pp. 13–20). New York: Grune & Stratton.

Lebowitz, M. D. (1988). Respiratory changes of aging. In B. Kent & R. N. Butler (Eds.), *Human aging research* (pp. 263–276). New York: Raven Press.

Lynne-Davies, P. (1977). Influence of age on the respiratory system. *Geriatrics, 32,* 57–62.

Macklin, C. C., & Macklin, M. T. (1942). Respiratory system. In E. V. Cowdry (Ed.), *Problems of ageing* (2nd ed., pp. 185–253). Baltimore, MD: Williams & Wilkins.

Mittman, C., Edelman, N. H., Norris, A. H., & Shock, N. W. (1965). Relationship between chest wall and pulmonary compliance and age. *Journal of Applied Physiology, 20,* 1211–1216.

Morris, J. F., Koski, A., & Johnson, L. C. (1971). Spirometric standards for healthy nonsmoking adults. *American Review of Respiratory Disease, 103,* 57–67.

Peterson, D. D., Pack, A. I., Silage, D. A., & Fishman, A. P. (1981). Effects of aging on ventilatory and occlusion pressure responses to hypoxia and hypercapnia. *American Review of Respiratory Diseases, 124,* 387–391.

Pierce, J. A., & Ebert, R. V. (1958). The elastic properties of the lungs in the aged. *Journal of Laboratory and Clinical Medicine, 51,* 63–71.

Pierce, J. A., & Ebert, R. V. (1965). Fibrous network of the lung and its change with age. *Thorax, 20,* 469–476.

Radford, E. P., Jr. (1964). Static mechanical properties of lungs in relation to age. In L. Cander & J. H. Moyer (Eds.), *Aging of the lung* (pp. 152–155). New York: Grune & Stratton.

Ramig, L. A. (1983). Effects of physiological aging on speaking and reading rates. *Journal of Communication Disorders, 16,* 217–226.

Reddan, W. G. (1981). Respiratory system and aging. In E. L. Smith & R. C. Serfass (Eds.), *Exercise and aging: The scientific basis* (pp. 89–107). Hillside, NJ: Enslow.

Robinson, S. (1964). Physical fitness in relation to age. In L. Cander & J. H. Moyer (Eds.), *Aging of the lung* (pp. 287–301). New York: Grune & Stratton.

Shephard, R. J. (1987). *Physical activity and aging* (2nd ed.). Rockville, MD: Aspen.

Shock, N. W. (1985). Longitudinal studies of aging in humans. In C. E. Finch & E. L. Schneider (Eds.), *Handbook of the biology of aging* (2nd ed., pp. 721–743). New York: Van Nostrand Reinhold.

Shock, N. W., Gruelich, R. C., Andres, R. A., Arenberg, D., Costa, P. T., Jr., Lakatta, E. G., & Tobin, J. D. (1984). *Normal human aging: The Baltimore Longitudinal Study of Aging* (NIH Publication No. 84-2450, pp. 45–57). Washington, DC: U.S. Government Printing Office.

Smith, B., Wasowicz, J., & Preston, J. (1987). Temporal characteristics of speech of normal elderly adults. *Journal of Speech & Hearing Research 30,* 522–529.

Stanescu, S., Dutu, St., Jienescu, Z., Hartia, L., Nicolescu, N., & Sacerdoteanu, F. (1968). Investigations into changes of pulmonary function in the aged. *Respiration, 25,* 232–242.

Tack, M., Altose, M. D., & Cherniack, N. S. (1981). Effect of aging on respiratory sensations produced by elastic loads. *Journal of Applied Physiology, 50,* 844–850.

Tobin, M. J., Mador, M. J., Guenther, S. M., Lodato, R. F., & Sackner, M. A. (1988). Variability of resting respiratory drive and timing in healthy subjects. *Journal of Applied Physiology, 65,* 309–317.

Turner, J. M., Mead, J., & Wohl, M. E. (1968). Elasticity of human lungs in relation to age. *Journal of Applied Physiology, 25,* 664–671.

Weismer, G. (1984). Articulatory characteristics of parkinsonian dysarthria: Segmental and phrase-level timing, spirantization, and glottal-supraglottal coordination. In M. R. McNeil, J. C. Rosenbek, & A. E. Aronson (Eds.), *The dysarthrias: Physiology, acoustics, perception, management.* San Diego, CA: College Hill Press.

Wilson, A. F. (1985). *Pulmonary function testing indications and interpretations.* Orlando, FL: Grune & Stratton.

Wright, R. R. (1961). Elastic tissue of normal and emphysematous lungs: A tridimensional histologic study. *American Journal of Pathology, 39,* 355–367.

Zemlin, W. R. (1988). *Speech and hearing science.* Englewood Cliffs, NJ: Prentice-Hall.

The Aging Larynx and Voice

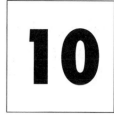

CHAPTER

Joel C. Kahane, PhD, and Neal S. Beckford, MD ■

One of the markers of old age is a change in the voice, frequently characterized as a loss of robustness, or as possessing a tremulous, frail, or thin quality. Although these perceptions abound, their origins are not well understood. Simply stated, little is known about the biology of the aging larynx. Although aging is not a pathological process, involutional changes may not only alter the biomechanical properties and capacities of the tissues of the larynx, resulting in voice changes, but may also predispose them to certain medical and pathological conditions that require medical attention. These conditions may overtly cause the older person to experience dysphonia or, at the very least, contribute to some level of mechanical instability in an otherwise finely tuned sound generator.

It is clearly acknowledged that vocal function and voice disorders should not and cannot be viewed as residing exclusively in the larynx. The contributions of the respiratory and supralaryngeal structures of the vocal tract must be considered as integral contributors to the final voice product; as such, they are addressed separately in this volume. However, it would appear to be valuable to examine the voice science and laryngologic changes that are associated with aging in order to provide a more complete description of the geriatric larynx. This chapter attempts to address this by

1. Describing the aging larynx in terms of its physical changes and accompanying alterations and perceptions as a sound generator

2. Identifying laryngologic problems that are frequently encountered or that are particular to older individuals and explaining their potential contributions to voice deviations

3. Discussing treatment and management strategies for older dysphonic speakers

Structural and Functional Changes in the Aging Larynx

The larynx changes throughout the lifespan; however, relatively little information is available about the details of the structural changes (Kahane, 1983a) associated with vocal aging. Visual descriptions of the older larynx as it is revealed through laryngologic observations are summarized in Table 10.1. It should be noted that even with relatively simple observational techniques, skilled observers have been able to identify characteristic changes in the epithelium, the lamina propria, and the degree of approximation of the vocal folds during voicing. Among these observations, bilateral bowing of the vocal fold is probably the most characteristic feature of the involution of the larynx. These observations raise an impressive list of questions about the nature, quality, gender specification, and onset of physical changes occurring in the larynx with advancing age. The following discussion[1] attempts to identify the significant physical changes in the larynx that occur with age and the resultant vocal changes that characterize the aging voice.

Hately, Evison, & Samuel, 1965; Keen & Wainwright, 1958; Roncollo, 1949) of hyaline cartilages in the larynx. The epiglottis, the only elastic cartilage, does not become ossified or calcified. Ossification has been observed in both sexes and occurs earlier in the male than in the female, where it is less extensive. In the male, these intrinsic changes in the cartilages have been observed to begin as early as the 3rd decade and to continue throughout adulthood.

Significant age-related changes have also been found in the cricoarytenoid joint (CAJ) (Kahane, 1988; Kahane & Hammons, 1987; Kahn & Kahane, 1986). Age changes in the cricothyroid joint have not yet been written about. Changes in the CAJ include thinning of the articular surfaces, breakdown in and disorganization of the collagen fibers in the cartilage matrix, and surface irregularities. Kahane and Hammons (1987) have also noted age-related changes in the synovial membrane of the CAJ. Taken together, these structural changes in the CAJ may influence the extent of approximation of the vocal folds and the smoothness with which vocal fold adjustments may be made during voicing. Segre (1971) indicated that aging causes loosening of the joint capsule of the CAJ but presented no empirical data to support this contention.

Structural Changes

The Laryngeal Cartilages

The cartilaginous skeleton of the larynx undergoes changes from birth through adulthood into old age (Kahane, 1983a). The principal changes are calcification (Ardran, 1965; Malinowski, 1967) and/or ossification (Chamberlain & Young, 1935;

The Intrinsic Laryngeal Muscles

Limited information is available on age changes in the intrinsic muscles of the larynx. The consensus among investigators is that laryngeal muscles undergo atrophy and that some degeneration occurs with advancing age (Bach, Lederer, & Dinolt, 1941; Carnevalle-Ricci, 1937; Ferreri, 1959; Hommerich, 1972). Several investigators attribute these changes to disturbances in vascular supply to the muscle (Ferreri, 1959;

---

[1]This discussion was presented at the Research Symposium on Communication Sciences and Disorders and Aging in September 1988 in Washington, DC. It appears as part of chapter 9 of ''Age Related Changes in the Peripheral Speech Mechanism: Structural and Physiological Changes'' by J. C. Kahane, 1990, *Proceedings of the Research Symposium on Communication Sciences and Disorders and Aging*, ASHA Reports, No. 19, Rockville, MD: American Speech-Language-Hearing Association.

TABLE 10.1

Summary of Laryngoscopic Observations of Aging Human Vocal Folds

Author	Epithelium	Bowing/Gap	Lamina Propria	Edema	Atrophy	Other
Behrendt & Strauch (1965)	Keratosis		Increase in collagenous and elastic fibers			Fatty degeneration of vocal folds
Segre (1971)	Yellow discoloration	Present	Decrease in elasticity			Vestibular fold atrophy
Honjo & Isshiki (1980)	Darkening of mucosa	Present 67% Male 58% Female	Sulcus vocalis	Present 56% Male 74% Female	Present 67% Male 26% Female	

Hommerich, 1972; Leutert, 1964). Bach et al. (1941), however, suggest that under-nourishment of the laryngeal musculature arises from disturbances in the vasomotor fibers of the sympathetic nerves supplying these vessels.

The Neurovascular Supply

Little is known about the effects of aging on the innervation of the larynx. Recent work by Malmgren and Ringwood (1988) on aging of the recurrent laryngeal nerve (RLN) of the rat provides interesting information about the machanisms that may be at work. They found that in old RLN there is an increase in the number of completely degenerated fibers, evidence of the regeneration of small numbers of neurons and significant increases in the size of the endoneurial extracellular space. These disturbances suggest that regulatory mechanisms in the nerve involving ionic and oxidative processes may be disrupted in the older nerves.

Changes in blood supply to the laryngeal nerves have been reported to occur with increasing age (Ferreri, 1959; Hommerich, 1972; Leutert, 1964). These changes consisted of thickening of the capillary walls and reduction in the diameter of the vessels. Leutert noted them as early as the 5th decade.

The Glands

Laryngeal glands, mainly from the vestibular folds, lubricate and protect the mucosal surfaces of the vocal folds. Not much is known about the involution of these glands. Hommerich (1972) and Ruckes and Hohmann (1963) reported that mucous glands in the larynx degenerate or atrophy after age 70. Bak-Pedersen and Nielsen (1986) did not find significant changes based on sex or age. Recently, Gracco and Kahane (1989) examined changes in the male vestibular glands and found that they involute with increasing age. Serous and mucous acini were found to atrophy or degenerate and to become replaced by adipose and connective tissue. The resultant changes are believed to affect the amount and quality of the secretions, which in turn may cause the epithelial surface of the vocal folds to become dried or less hydrated. This may contribute to a clinical condition seen in geriatrics called *laryngeal sicca* (atrophic laryngitis). Diminished glandular secretions may make epithelial surfaces less well protected against abrasive forces produced during effort closure and vocalization and against aerodynamic forces developed during vocalization. In addition, these epithelial changes may adversely affect the surface topography of the leading edges of the vocal folds, causing them to vibrate irregularly.

Vocal Folds

The Epithelium

Disagreement exists about age changes in the epithelium of the vocal folds. Some reports (Eggston & Wolff, 1947; Hommerich, 1972) note that laryngeal epithelia increase in thickness with age, while others (Hirano, Kurita, & Nakashima, 1983; Noell, 1962; Ryan, McDonald, & Devine, 1956) indicate no significant changes. Segre (1971) noted that after middle age, the laryngeal mucosa becomes thin and yellowing in appearance. Of interest are Noell's observations that with increasing age, the laryngeal epithelium becomes less firmly attached to the underlying lamina propria. This could introduce a decrease in structural support to the cover of the vocal fold, which may increase perturbation during phonation (Wilcox & Horii, 1980).

The Lamina Propria

The three layers of subepithelial connective tissues of the vocal folds—the lamina propria—have been shown to be essential to vocal fold function during voice production (Hirano, 1974). These layers are composed of collagenous and elastic fibers that are arranged in different arrays and that have different mechanical properties. Age-related changes have been noted in the lamina propria (Hirano et al., 1983; Kahane, 1982, 1983b, 1987; Kahane, Stadlan, & Bell, 1979). Mueller, Sweeney, and Barbeau (1985) studied morphological characteristics of aged male postmortem laryngeal specimens. Twenty-five old larynges (mean age 81 years) and 10 young specimens (mean age 44.7 years) were studied. Mueller and associates reported several involutional changes, which included bowing, atrophy, and cordal sulcus of the vocal folds. They reported that 75% of the older group exhibited an arrowhead configuration of the rima glottidis which was not found in the younger group. Lederer and Hollender (1951) refer to variations in cadaveric forms of the rima glottidis attributed to Fein (no citation given). Two arrowhead configurations were among the 10 configurations presented. Thus, the arrowhead configuration of the rima glottidis, described by Mueller et al. (1984) as reflecting involutional change, may simply represent one form of postmortem fixation of the vocal folds. There may, however, be some predilection to that configuration and further research may provide an explanation for it.

In general, changes in the lamina propria are greater in the male than in the female. The connective tissues in the different layers of the lamina propria involute differently. Connective tissues in the superficial layer thicken and then become edematous (Hirano et al., 1983). They represent the greatest changes in the cover of the vocal folds. The intermediate layer of the lamina propria becomes thinner after age 40 (Hirano et al., 1983). This is occasioned by a decrease in the density of the fibers and deterioration in their contour. Kahane et al. (1979) and Kahane (1983b) reported that after age 50, elastic and collagenous fiber bundles began to lose their well-defined weave. Collagenous fibers showed a greater tendency toward separation and waviness, whereas elastic fibers frequently showed fragmentation and breakdown.

Significant changes have been found in the deep layer of the lamina propria in the male, whereas little change appears to take place in the female (Hirano et al., 1983; Kahane, 1982, 1983b). After age 50, in the male, appreciable changes occur in collagenous fibers, which are the principal fiber component in this layer (Hirano et al., 1983; Kahane, 1983b). These consist of a breakdown in fiber organization (fibrotic, according to Hirano et al., 1983) and increased density of collagenous fibers. The latter may result from the clumping together or spreading apart of usually tightly bound fibers.

It is likely that changes in the lamina propria contribute to bowing of the vocal folds and irregularities in the medial (vibratory) surfaces of the vocal folds. These structural alterations provide an opportunity for the development of aperiodicity, irregularities in vocal fold vibration, and incomplete approximation of the vocal folds.

The Vocalis Muscle

Vocalis fibers of the thyroarytenoid muscle (the so-called ''vocalis muscle'') have been shown to be the most functionally significant component of the muscle during voice production. Because of their mechanical and functional properties, the vocalis fibers of the thyroarytenoid muscle are referred to as the body of the vocal folds (Hirano, 1974). Specific age-related changes have been reported in the thyroarytenoid muscle (Ferreri, 1959; Hommerich, 1972; Kersing, 1984; Leutert, 1964; Sato & Tauchi, 1982). These include atrophy, degeneration, decrease in fiber diameter (Ferreri, 1959; Hommerich, 1972; Leutert, 1964; Sato & Tauchi, 1982), and breakdown in fibrous support of the muscle (Hommerich, 1972; Kahane, 1982; Leutert, 1964; Segre, 1971). Histochemical studies of aging vocal fold musculature (Kersing, 1984; Sato & Tauchi, 1982) have shown that type 1 and type 2 fibers decrease significantly in the vocal fold in addition to other intrinsic and metabolic changes in the thyroarytenoid muscle. Sato and Tauchi (1982) reported that these changes were greatest after age 80. Another factor contributing to involution of laryngeal muscles may be alterations in the blood supply to them (Ferreri, 1959; Hommerich, 1972; Leutert, 1964).

Functional Changes

The myriad changes in the connective tissues, muscles, and articular surfaces of joints in the larynx appear to contribute to several alterations in vocal performance (Kahane, 1987). Weismer and Fromm (1983) have shown how the effects of aging of the larynx manifest themselves in the segmental and nonsegmental characteristics of speech. The following discussion summarizes data on changes in the level and stability of fundamental frequency, vocal range, and glottal efficiency.

Perception of Pitch and Measurement of Fundamental Frequency

Of all vocal parameters, pitch has been studied most extensively. Ptacek, Sander, Maloney, and Jackson (1966) found that trained listeners perceived that older male speakers had lower pitch than younger counterparts. Seven out of 10 judges deemed pitch level to be an important vocal characteristic for differentiating the age of the speaker. This finding was not supported by data from Hollien and Shipp (1972), who provide convincing evidence that after the 5th decade of life, fundamental frequency increases in males.

Age-related changes in fundamental frequency in the female are not as well defined as in the male. Some investigators have reported little noticeable change (McGlone & Hollien, 1963) while others (Endres, Bambach, & Flosser, 1971; Honjo & Isshiki, 1980; Saxman & Burk, 1967) have shown that there is a slight lowering of fundamental frequency with increasing age. More recent work has shown that elderly speakers exhibit a decrease in fundamental

frequency stability (Linville & Fisher, 1985a, 1985b; Stoicheff, 1981; Wilcox & Horii, 1980) compared to younger counterparts. Linville (1987a) has recently reported that in women, decreased frequency stability becomes a significant factor only after middle age.

More discrete analyses of cycle-to-cycle variation in fundamental frequency (jitter) have been interpreted as an expression of control or mechanical stability of the vocal folds. Increased pitch variability has been observed in males and was seen to accompany increased age (Mysak, 1959; Mysak & Hanley, 1958). Whereas a slight decrease in pitch variability has been reported in older female voices (McGlone & Hollien, 1963), Wilcox and Horii (1980), using computer extraction techniques, reported increases in both sexes of mean perturbation values.

Ramig and Ringle (1983) point out that chronological age may not be the key determinant of cycle-to-cycle variation in fundamental frequency. They found that the physical condition of the older speaker (biological age or condition) was most important and was most closely associated with increased jitter values. Amplitude variation (shimmer), however, was not significantly increased in persons with poor physical conditions, suggesting that other mechanisms may be operating.

Pitch control and pitch range have been shown to depreciate with increasing age. Endres et al. (1971) conducted a 20-year longitudinal study on several female subjects and found that these speakers lose their ability to vary fundamental frequency. Linville and Fisher (1985a, 1985b) and Linville (1988) reported corroborating data. In addition, older speakers also exhibited more restricted pitch range than younger counterparts (Endres et al., 1971; Linville, 1987b; Ptacek et al., 1966).

Measures of laryngeal control such as voice onset time have shown that there is no significant difference in voice onset times (VOT) for single-word tasks between young and old male and female adults (Sweeting & Baken, 1982). No significant differences in VOT were found between younger and older female subjects (Morris & Brown, 1987; Neiman, Klich, & Shuey, 1983).

There have been a few reports about voice quality changes that accompany aging. Hoarseness has been perceived as an identifying characteristic of older male voices (Hartman & Danhauer, 1976; Ptacek et al., 1966). Honjo and Isshiki (1980) have shown that hoarseness characterized the voices of 20 Japanese women with a mean age of 75 or older, but was not perceived in comparably aged older male voices. It appears that hoarseness may be associated with geriatric voice quality but may not be a characteristic feature of it.

Deficiencies in laryngeal valving in older males, reported by Melcon, Hoit, and Hixon (1988), may also contribute to voice difficulties and reduced glottal efficiency. These investigators found that in older men, reduced glottal resistance and increased respiratory effort associated with adjustment in the length of the breath group was used during speech. This reduction in laryngeal valving may affect phonation time and loudness and may be a partial factor in the observations of several investigators who have characterized vocal performance in older males as ''hypofunctional'' (Benjamin, 1980), tense (Ryan & Burk, 1974), and reduced in phonation time (Ptacek et al., 1966). Kruel (1972) reported that this reduction in phonation time amounted to as much as 26% for sustained vowel productions.

Pathological Changes

The aforementioned structural and vocal changes in the aging larynx represent only part of the total picture of laryngeal senescence. One must not forget, however, that the aging larynx is susceptible to various disease processes that are wholly separate from normal involutional changes. A comprehensive assessment of the entire vocal tract is necessary to assure that voice change is part of the natural involution and not due to some underlying disease process.

The following is a discussion of the laryngologic considerations of examination of the older individual and is a review of some of the most commonly observed laryngeal pathologies found in the geriatric population.

The Medical History

Characterization of the specific vocal complaint should be undertaken first, because this can often delineate the nature and severity of the problem and direct further questioning. The patient should be encouraged to relate what it is about his or her voice quality that is disturbing. Changes in loudness, pitch, vocal texture, or strength all point to differing pathologies in the vocal tract. Symptom onset, duration, frequency, and progression should be assessed temporally if possible. Specific precipitating and relieving factors are also helpful in assessing the full scope of the problem. A vocal history is essential in order to characterize the voice use pattern of the individual.

A good general medical history complements the vocal assessment and often helps explain the cause of the patient's initial complaint. The patient should be questioned as to the presence of chronic medical problems such as heart disease, arthritis, and diabetes. Of particular importance are conditions that directly affect the vocal folds, such as reflux esophagitis, sinusitis, and allergic problems. Previous surgeries involving the vocal tract, chest, and any point along the course of the recurrent laryngeal nerve should be noted. A history of malignancy—especially in the larynx, lung, thyroid, or brain—is important and should be investigated thoroughly as to the extent of disease and the treatment received. Cataloging the geriatric patient's medications is essential. These individuals often are dependent on a multitude of drugs that may cause problems either individually or collectively. A brief psychosocial evaluation can also be helpful in uncovering deep-seated problems that contribute to a strong functional component of the patient's difficulties.

The Physical Examination

Examination of the upper aerodigestive tract is the next step in the comprehensive assessment of the vocal tract. Of paramount importance is the visualization of all structures involved in voice production that are available for inspection. This includes the oral cavity, the oropharynx (including the velum and tongue base), the nasopharynx, and the hypopharynx/larynx area. All structures should be viewed in a dynamic as well as static mode. The salient observations that should be included in a physical examination of the upper aerodigestive tract are summarized in Table 10.2.

TABLE 10.2
Structures and Clinical Determinations Made in Examination of the Upper Aerodigestive Tract (UADT)

Section of UADT	Structures Examined	Clinical Determinations
Oral cavity	Lips Tongue Hard palate Cheek Teeth/gingiva	Mucosal integrity (texture, color) Mass lesions Tongue mobility Status of dentition/occlusion
	TMJ[a]	Mandibular excursion Joint crepitus Tenderness to palpation Related musculoskeletal tenderness
Nasopharynx	Posterior wall Lateral wall Torus tubarius	Mass lesions Mucosal irregularities Velopharyngeal port abnormalities
Oropharynx	Tonsils Soft palate Posterior pharynx	Mass lesions Mucosal integrity Palate movement Sensory changes Symmetry
Hypopharynx	Pyriform sinus Postcricoid area Lateral pharynx	Mass lesions Mucosal irregularities Pooling of secretions
Larynx: Supraglottis	Epiglottis Aryepiglottic folds Vestibular folds Ventricle	Mass lesions Mucosal irregularities Deviation/displacement
Glottis	Vocal folds	Color Contour Mobility Mass lesions Mucosal integrity
Subglottis		Mass lesion restricting subglottic airway

[a]Note that the temperomandibular joint is not a part of the UADT but contributes to oral cavity functioning.

Careful and detailed evaluation of the larynx is essential for accurate diagnosis of dysphonia. Traditionally, laryngeal examination has been performed with the indirect technique, using a small mirror to reflect the image of the larynx to the examiner's eye. This time-honored method is still very acceptable and allows the examiner to obtain a clear and often unobstructed view of laryngeal structures. Many clinicians today, however, are using fiberoptic technology to obtain a better view of the larynx. This technique affords the clinician better visibility, dynamic as well as static imaging, and the ability to record findings with still and/or video photography. Greater patient comfort is usually afforded by the use of this newer technique.

For examination purposes, the larynx is divided into supraglottal, glottal, and subglottal regions. The contiguous hypopharynx must be carefully examined. Supraglottic examination requires inspection of both the lingual and laryngeal surfaces of the epiglottis, aryepiglottic folds, vestibular folds, and laryngeal ventricle. Any irregularities in morphology or color should be noted. Excess muscular tension in the supraglottis may be exacerbated by medialization of the vestibular folds, posterior displacement of the petiole of the epiglottis, or advancement of the arytenoid/corniculate cartilage complex. These dynamics should be described in detail. The pyriform sinuses, postcricoid area, and lateral walls should be inspected separately as part of examining the hypopharynx.

The vestibular folds and the ventricle of Morgagni must be thoroughly examined to rule out tumors and benign lesions such as cysts. In addition, excessive supraglottal tension in hyperfunctional dysphonia may be accompanied by medialization of the vestibular folds. This may, on occasion, result in their participation in vocalization, resulting in a condition called *dysphonia plicae ventricularis*.

In the glottal region, the vocal folds must be examined carefully, giving particular attention to their morphology, color, and function. In particular, the contour of the vocal fold edges, the amount of vocal fold bowing, the size of the glottic chink, and the presence of any topographical abnormalities should be assessed. Any departure from normal should be well described in the medical record, preferably with a drawing or photograph. Stroboscopic laryngoscopy is helpful in assessing fine details of the vocal fold mucosal structure and function by detailing the amplitude of vibration, amount of vocal wave, and regularity of vibration.

The subglottal area should be inspected to ensure that no lesions are present and that no diminution of the airway exists such as that caused by edema or inflammation.

Examination of the vocal tract should conclude with careful palpation of the neck to rule out any cervical adenopathy, thyromegaly, or other abnormalities.

Disorders of the Geriatric Larynx

Among the common complaints expressed by older speakers is that their voice is weak, hoarse, gravelly, or breathy. They will frequently say, ''My voice doesn't sound like me.'' This poses a great challenge to the laryngologist and the voice pathologist, because it is necessary to distinguish an individual's perception and expectation of vocal inefficiency from the realities of normal intrinsic change as well as from a number of medical conditions that may cause dysphonia. It is not uncommon to have normal involutional changes in the larynx exacerbated by some form of pathology. Thus, it appears valuable to review some of the more common problems seen in the practice of laryngology that may contribute directly to the vocal complaints of older persons.

Psychogenic Etiologies of Dysphonia in Elderly Speakers

Functional dysphonia in the elderly speaker may result from several sources. These behaviors may be the source of dysphonia or may exacerbate a physically weakened laryngeal mechanism. Cooper (1970) notes that among the important contributors to functional dysphonia in the aged are body fatigue resulting in poor respiratory support during speech; an inappropriate vocal image; and such emotional states as grief, despair, and resignation. Cooper believes that at the center of these problems is the use of inappropriate pitch levels and poor tone focus. In attempts to deal with an inefficient voice, older speakers frequently develop muscular tension in the upper thoracic, neck, and suprahyoid areas that contributes to an effortful, throaty, weak voice that is both inefficient and displeasing to the speaker.

Compensatory Strategies Used by Older Speakers

Morrison, Rammage, and Nichol (1989) have identified several results of unsuccessful compensatory strategies used by older speakers to improve the quality of their voice. These strategies appear to differ between male and female speakers. In the male, there are attempts to drop fundamental frequency and the development of a gravelly, breathy voice characterized by vocal fry. This results in appreciable vocal fatigue. In the female, compensatory attempts include raising pitch by using a squeeze/strain voice to compensate for a hypofunctioning glottal valve; the use of effortful voice; and, in severe cases, the possible development of ventricular fold phonation.

Organic Etiologies of Dysphonia in the Elderly

Mass Lesions

Lesions of the vocal folds cause dysphonia via a number of mechanisms. Mass loading disrupts normal orderly vocal fold vibration; changes are then transmitted throughout the remainder of the vocal tract. Depending on mass size, lesions can prevent glottic closure to varying degrees. Clinical presentation with breathiness, stridor, or frank airway obstruction is common. Although they are not restricted to older individuals, many lesions are more common in the elderly. The dysphonia caused by mass lesions is most important in that misdiagnosis or even delayed diagnosis can have life-threatening sequelae. One of the most common of these changes is polypoid degeneration of the vocal fold.

Polypoid Degeneration

Noxious upper airway stimuli such as cigarette smoking, alcohol abuse, and constant exposure to particulate material can lead to the development of a pattern of progressive vocal fold mucosal degeneration. The development of laryngeal polyps is the end-stage result of these changes. Polypoid degeneration appears most commonly in both sexes after middle age; however, in the United States and Europe, most patients are women (Bennett, Bishop, & Lumpkin, 1987; Fritzell & Hertegard, 1986; Lumpkin, Bishop, & Bennett, 1987; Yates & Dedo, 1984). Although the etiology of polypoid degeneration, also called Reinke's edema or polypoid corditis, is not completely understood, most otolaryngologists agree that it results from long-term cigarette smoking and is frequently accompanied by vocal abuse or misuse. Polypoid degeneration is characterized by chronic diffused edema that extends the full length of one or both vocal folds. The pathology is located in the superficial layer of the lamina propria. The precise mechanism for this condition is not known; however, a widely held explanation is Kleinsasser's (1982), who indicates that the polyposis results from chronic irritation and trauma of the vocal fold mucosa, which alters the permiability of the capillary walls and allows extravasation of blood and fluids into Reinke's space. This disturbs the mechanical properties of the cover of the vocal folds, increasing its mass and compliance.

Polypoid degeneration progresses from the development of small nodular structures on the vibrating edges of the vocal folds to uniform epithelial changes and finally irreversible mucosal polypoid transformation. Severe cases demonstrate either excessive true vocal fold swelling, gross polypoid degeneration, or irregular diffuse fibrotic thickening. Vocal symptoms attributable to polypoid degeneration (Bennett et al., 1987; Lumpkin et al., 1987) include significant reduction in fundamental frequency and phonational range, with the upper end of the range being most affected.

Although several surgical approaches may be used to treat polypoid degeneration, no one procedure appears to bring about the best result (Bennett et al., 1987). Treatment requires microlaryngoscopy with careful removal of abnormal tissue. Surgery is often performed in two stages to avoid creation of a fibrous anterior glottic web. Vocal folds with changes of chronic fibrosis do not always benefit from removal to the epithelial cover; however, laryngoscopy is essential to rule out malignant transformation. Bennett and associates point out that surgery improves the voice by bringing about increases in fundamental frequency (30–60 Hz), significantly decreasing hoarseness and increasing patients' satisfaction with their own voice. They add, however, that postoperative fundamental frequency did not reach normal levels for nonspeaking females aged 40–70 years; instead, it closely resembled the mean fundamental frequency (167 Hz) of women who smoked but did not have polypoid degeneration. Thus, polypoid degeneration in general, but particularly in older individuals, is quite a debilitating condition, and the resulting dysphonia is not likely to be fully reversed. Elimination of smoking is essential and vocal rehabilitation appears to be limited to developing good vocal hygiene and minimizing the development of vocal hyperfunction (Bouchayer & Cornut, 1987).

Intubation Granuloma

Given that geriatric patients often have had surgical procedures that require a general anesthetic, intubation granulomas are uncommon but not rare causes of voice change. More common in females because of the smaller diameter of the glottis, these lesions stem from irritation of the posterior glottis during placement of the endotracheal tube or from static pressure from that tube on the vocal processes. Ulceration develops in the vocal process area, with variable amounts of exposed cartilage at the base. A combination of trauma from repeated vocal process adduction and infection stimulate the formation of granulation tissue. The amount of reactive granulation formed determines whether a contact ulcer, intubation polyp, or granuloma develops. Patients usually present with dysphagia and gross dysphonia. Some pedunculated lesions will react in a ball-valve fashion, flipping up above the glottis during exhalation and causing disruption of airflow above the glottis and a muffled type of dysphonia. When the lesion is below the glottis, phonation can be near normal. Treatment requires simple endoscopic removal. Some clinicians believe that injection of cortisone into the base of the lesion will prevent recurrence (Paperella & Shumrick, 1980; Snow, Harano, & Balogh, 1966).

Leukoplakia or Keratosis

Literally translated as "white plaque," these lesions present as whitish raised irregularities of vocal tract mucosa. Most common in the oral cavity, they are often found in the glottic larynx. All nonkeratinizing squamous epithelial surfaces in the larynx are susceptible to the development of these lesions. This excludes the laryngeal ventricle and subglottis, which are lined by pseudostratified ciliated columnar epithelium. Although they often carry a premalignant connotation, the great majority of these lesions are benign. Microscopically, they run the gamut from an increase in the number of cells in particular layers of mucous membranes to marked cytoarchitectural abnormalities to frank carcinoma. It must be emphasized that this is a clinical diagnosis, not a histological one. Benign lesions that demonstrate abnormal cellular changes can become malignant over time even after treatment. Their clinical significance then lies in the fact that these mucosal irregularities are associated with the later development of malignancy or can mask the presence of a carcinoma, even though they are not malignant in and of themselves.

Laryngeal keratosis is usually found in men over 50 years of age with a history of smoking and/or significant vocal abuse. As the number of women who smoke increases, the incidence in this population is growing. Lesions can present as a small, flat focus on one aspect of the vocal fold mucosa or as raised lesions that virtually cover the entire mucosal surface of the vocal folds. Clinically these patients will present with varying degrees of dysphonia, often related to the degree of vocal fold mass effect. As leukoplakia doesn't often have a large third dimension, airway distress is not a common clinical finding. Treatment requires direct laryngoscopy with biopsy to determine the histological nature of the lesion. Microsurgical techniques are used to remove all the disease possible with care taken to preserve the vocal fold architecture. Improvement in dysphonia usually results with minimal morbidity for the patient. If no evidence of malignancy is found, the patient is encouraged to stop smoking and refrain from vocally abusive behavior. A thorough speech assessment with therapy, if necessary, is warranted. Medical follow-up should be carried out on a regular basis to rule out recurrence of disease (Batsakis, 1979).

Malignant Lesions

Maisel (1986) notes that nearly half the cancers of the head and neck are of the larynx, with peak incidence between the ages of 50 and 70. The commonest and earliest symptom of laryngeal carcinoma is hoarseness. Over 90% of malignant vocal fold lesions are squamous cell carcinoma. English (1976) notes that 50% of laryngeal tumors occur on the vocal fold; of these,

75% originate in the anterior half of the fold. Nonetheless, tumors can occur in any area of the larynx and can have symptoms related to their respective locations. Laryngeal carcinomas are divided into three types: supraglottic, glottic, and subglottic. Symptoms depend on the location and size (stage) of the tumor growth. Lesions of the supraglottic larynx (epiglottis, aryepiglottic folds, and false vocal folds) may present with a muffled vocal quality, dysphagia, and odynophagia. Referred pain to the ear and weight loss are not uncommon. As abundant lymphatic vessels course through the supraglottis, these patients are prone to develop cervical metastases presenting as neck masses. Lesions of the glottic larynx are not predisposed to lymphatic spread and tend to stay localized. Patients with pure glottic lesions present with a gravelly voice. Subglottic lesions often present with stridor and airway obstruction. Bulky lesions of the glottis and/or supraglottis also can present with airway distress. Tumors can travel along the mucosa to involve adjacent areas or invade deep into the soft tissue and spread submucosally. Paraglottic spread of disease often results in vocal fold paralysis, thus contributing to dysphonia and glottic compromise (Batsakis, 1979).

Patients with squamous cell carcinomas that are restricted to the vocal folds almost invariably have a history of cigarette smoking. Those with supraglottic tumors often have histories of considerable alcohol consumption. Lesions are more common in males than females, although as the number of women smokers increases, the number developing malignant lesions is increasing as well. Squamous cell carcinoma has a variety of appearances that run the gamut from an exophytic, cauliflower-like tumor to an erythematous, ulcerative crater. Abnormal redness or erythroplasia of the laryngeal mucosa is positive in 50% of cases. The diagnosis is made by biopsy using direct laryngoscopy (Templer, 1987). Small lesions are equally well treated with surgery or radiation therapy. Larger tumors, especially those that cause vocal fold fixation, are best treated with surgery with or without postoperative irradiation. Supraglottic tumors necessitate some type of neck dissection or neck irradiation to counter lymphatic spread of disease. Survival depends on the size of the lesion on presentation, its location, and the presence or absence of neck metastases.

Systemic Problems

Rheumatoid Arthritis

Rheumatoid arthritis can develop anytime during life; however, 70% of the cases occur between the 3rd and 7th decades (Thorne, 1977). In the early decades, females are more affected than males (3:1), although there is increased frequency in males in the later decades. Rheumatoid arthritis may involve the larynx in up to 20% of all patients (Koopmann, 1986) and typically affects the CAJ. It is an inflammatory disease of the joints, usually involving the synovial membrane, which may cause destruction (erosion) of the articular surfaces and fibrosis of connective tissues in the joint capsule; the joint may become ankylosed. Laryngeal arthritis (Montgomery & Lofgren, 1963) most often results from generalized rheumatoid arthritis, but may also result from acute infection of the larynx or hypopharynx and trauma. Hoarseness is the most common symptom. Frequently, notable throat pain on swallowing and speech also are present. The disease usually presents itself by restricting movements of the CAJ and forming granulomatous lesions, rheumatoid nodules, in the vocal fold mucosa. Restricted movement of the CAJ may reduce vocal fold movement or may fix the vocal fold at some position lateral to midline. Thus in the early stages of the disease, patients may present with symptoms similar to those of vocal fold paralysis. Physical examination shows edema and mild erythema of the arytenoid/corniculate cartilage complex. As the disease progresses, edema subsides and joint dysfunction becomes apparent. In rare instances, rheumatoid nodules form on the vibrating surfaces of the vocal folds, produc-

ing perceived vocal changes similar to those of other mass loading lesions. Treatment is primarily symptomatic, with salicylates and nonsteroidal anti-inflammatory agents. Corticosteriods are given in severe cases. Bilateral CAJ fixation causing airway obstruction is treated surgically by arytenoidectomy or arytenoidopexy. These procedures improve airway competency but produce a weakened breathy voice (Montgomery, 1963).

Hypothyroidism

Voice changes have long been associated with hypothyroidism. An early sign of this condition is a slowly progressive deepening of the voice and a slight huskiness that may make the voice sound dull. This change is less conspicuous in men than in women. Vocal fold movements are normal, but the vocal folds demonstrate increases in bulk. Although the pathophysiology is unclear, animal studies imply that this process involves the deposition of mucopolysaccharide substances into the submucosa of the vocal fold (Ritter, 1964). Heinemann (1969) studied 49 cases of dysphonia resulting from hypothyroidism and noted that if the condition and voice are permitted to deteriorate substantially, there will be an irreversible change in the voice despite the administration of thyroxin. Vocal improvement can be achieved by removal of abnormal tissue; however, return to normal vocal status is very uncommon. Surgery should not be performed without some plan to correct the underlying thyroid deficiency.

Laryngitis Sicca

The aging larynx loses moisture secondary to involution of seromucinous glands (Gracco & Kahane, 1989). These glands produce the thin, watery secretions that lubricate the vibrating surfaces of the vocal folds. Loss of this fluid results in decreased pliability of the vocal fold mucosa and an inability of the vocal folds to vibrate in a vocally efficient manner. Efforts at compensating for this glottic compromise are often evidenced by the development of glottic and supraglottic constriction. Treatment is directed at decreasing the factors that contribute to vocal fold desiccation. Increasing hydration is a prime mode of treatment with patients in whom additional fluid intake is not otherwise medically contraindicated. Mucolytic drugs like guiafenesin (Humibid®) decrease the viscosity of the thicker laryngeal secretions and tend to decrease the effects of gland involution. Compromise in normal nasal airflow will force dry, unhumidified air to be taken in through the mouth and presented to the larynx. Over time, this can cause significant drying of laryngeal mucosa. Careful assessment of the nasal airflow will sometimes reveal a nasoseptal deformity or some other cause of nasal obstruction. Correction will often improve laryngeal symptoms. Finally, increases in ambient moisture can be achieved by reducing the amount of forced, dry air heating that the patient is exposed to and encouraging the use of either a central or stand-alone room humidifier.

Reflux Laryngitis

Vocal fold irritation and subsequent dysphonia can be caused by chronic exposure to gastric acid. This reflux of fluid is common in overweight, elderly individuals who have lost the competence of the lower esophageal sphincter. This esophageal incompetence is exacerbated by conditions that increase the amount of gastric acid produced, such as stress, smoking, and alcohol consumption. Assuming a recumbent position defeats the forces of gravity that prevent the retrograde passage of fluid into the esophagus and allows the larynx to be bathed in this irritating fluid. Patients often complain of a bitter taste or halitosis in the morning. A feeling of a lump in the throat and frank pain are not uncommon and are often accompanied by an upset stomach. Physical examination often shows erythematous arytenoids and vocal processes along with chronic irritation on the true vocal folds. Contact ulcerations on the vocal processes are not uncommon. Intrinsic and extrinsic laryngeal muscular hyperfunction may be evident in an effort to compensate for vocal tract dysfunction.

The diagnosis is confirmed by contrast radiographic studies and/or esophagoscopy. Examination of the stomach is important to rule out the presence of ulceration or malignancy. Treatment is directed at decreasing the amount or the acidity of the gastric acid. This can be accomplished by ingesting a substance that neutralizes the acid (Maalox®, Mylanta®, Carafate®, etc.) or using medication that decreases the amount of gastric acid produced (Cimetidine®, Ranitidine®). Sleeping with four to six bricks under the head of the bed enables gravity to keep the gastric contents in the stomach and avoid reflux. Life-style modification including avoidance of late and spicy meals, caffeine, alcohol, and tobacco is recommended. Weight loss can also assist in decreasing symptoms.

Neurogenic Problems

Vocal Fold Paralysis

Symptoms of breathiness, dysphonia, and sometimes aspiration suggest the presence of vocal fold paralysis. Although certainly not limited to the geriatric population, it is nonetheless a fairly common cause of dysphonia in this age group. The diagnosis is easily made, because the lack of vocal fold movement is fairly obvious. Investigation should include a review of all pathological processes that may affect the recurrent laryngeal nerve along its course from the brainstem to its endpoint in the larynx. Iatrogenic injury after thyroidectomy is still the most common cause. Surgery need not be recent to account for symptoms. Patients often develop successful postoperative compensation for vocal fold paralysis and may not realize that function has been compromised until much later. Clinical symptoms may only appear when other effects of laryngeal senescence are present. In addition to the symptoms mentioned here, patients can also present with decreased exercise tolerance and shortened phonation times. Barring a history of thyroid surgery, other neck or chest surgery, or intracranial disease, the clinician's index of suspicion should be high for malignancy. Advanced lung tumors will often damage the nerve in the mediastinum, causing paralysis. Thyroid carcinomas invade the nerve in the tracheoesophageal groove. Rarer lesions, such as glomus tumors, sarcomas, and neuromas, can be found in the posterior fossa, skull base, and neck. Lesions of the larynx usually immobilize the vocal fold by invasion of the paraglottic musculature. Large mass lesions of the vocal folds may give the impression of paralysis by physically restricting vocal fold movement. The true status of the restricted fold is discovered only after the fold is surgically debulked.

After indirect laryngectomy, diagnostic imaging studies are imperative. Chest X rays to rule out mediastinal disease are obtained first. Computerized tomography (CT) of the chest will often detect disease that is not apparent on chest X ray. Additional CT studies from the clivus to the clavicle are helpful in detecting occult disease in these areas. Thyroid scans can be helpful in detecting subclinical thyroid malignancies. If no obvious causes are detected, the paralysis is often attributed to some type of viral infection or considered idiopathic.

After treatment of the underlying cause is complete, the paralysis itself can be addressed. Treatment involves some means of moving the paralyzed fold medially into a more physiologically favorable position. This can easily be accomplished by injecting the vocal fold with an inert material such as Teflon®. Isshiki, Okamura, and Ishikawa (1975) have popularized a procedure whereby the vocal fold is medialized by surgically inserting Silastic® or some other substance between the lateral thyroid cartilage and its inner perichondrium. Both techniques are highly successful in experienced hands. The use of neuromuscular pedicle grafts for reinnervation of laryngeal musculature has been described. Its efficacy, however, has not been demonstrated by a majority of clinicians and subsequently has not received universal endorsement (Rontal & Rontal, 1977; Titche, 1976).

There are several focal and progressive neurogenic disorders affecting the geriatric population that can have associated dysphonias. Cerebrovascular accidents and many dysarthrias acquired later in life have laryngeal disabling effects. Since these are not usually typically found in the otherwise normal aging person, the interested reader is directed to discussions in Darley, Aronson, and Brown (1975) and Aronson (1985) for more detailed discussions of central and peripheral neuropathies affecting speech and voice production. An excellent review of central neurological dysfunction involving the larynx is found in Ward, Hanson, and Berci (1981).

The following discussion summarizes several neurological conditions and disorders occuring in older adulthood that present with dysphonia and that the laryngologist and voice pathologist are likely to be involved in treating.

Parkinson's Disease

Parkinson's disease is a significant neurological disease of the extrapyramidal tract that has a peak incidence between the ages of 55 and 80. Several forms of the disorder exist, inducing postencephalic, arteriosclerotic, and idiopathic disorders. Ward et al. (1981) note that on visual examination of the larynx, quivering involuntary movements of the interarytenoid muscles and ventricular folds may be well established. This tremor produces a quivering voice quality. There is a full range of vocal fold movement (adductory and abductory) in these patients. Ward et al. note that patients with the idiopathic form of hypokinetic Parkinsonism have weak breathy voices as a result of air loss, which causes phrasing to be limited. Visualization of the larynx reveals a normal range of motion of the vocal folds with an inability to tense the vocal folds, which sometimes exhibit marked bowing. These Parkinson patients have difficulty changing pitch and have voices that do not present with a significant tremor. The disorder is a progressive motor disease whose major symptoms are resting tremor, rigidity, and akinesia. A related form, called senile Parkinsonism, is thought to result from atherosclerosis. The patient presents with dysarthria and dysphonia accompanied by respiratory (speech breathing) deficits. The voice becomes monotonous and is weak and soft. Respiration is rapid and shallow and speech output is staccato, occurring in bursts through phrases, rather than full sentences. These patients frequently exhibit swallowing deficits (dysphagia) that result from hypokinesia of the oral and pharyngeal musculature.

Shy-Drager Syndrome

Shy-Drager syndrome is sometimes confused with Parkinsonism because of similar symptoms caused by lesions in the substantia nigra of the extrapyramidal system. Ward et al. (1981) note that patients with Shy-Drager syndrome typically present with progressive abductor paresis, which may ultimately result in complete abductor paralysis. They report that the typical course of the laryngeal abnormality is a progressive loss of voluntary and respiratory abductor function and loss of voicing control. Ludlow and Bassich (1983) studied the speech of Parkinson and Shy-Drager patients. They found that the Shy-Drager patients were more impaired on all acoustic and perceptual measures of voice than their Parkinson counterparts. These measures included breathiness, loudness stress, and rate of speech. Both groups of patients were equally impaired on ratings of monopitch and uncontrolled loudness.

Meige's Syndrome

Meige's syndrome, according to Klawans and Tanner (1984), is the most common dystonic disorder of old age. Onset of this syndrome is after age 60 and is characterized by oromandibular dystonia and blepharospasm. The hypopharyngeal muscles are frequently involved, resulting in pharyngeal-stage dysphagia. Aphonia and other vocal disturbances may be caused by impaired laryngeal muscles. Golpher, Nutt, Rau, and Collman (1983) found that 5 out of 10 patients studied presented with laryngospasm. Their dysphonia shared characteristics with spasmodic dysphonia such as strained/strangled voice and voice stoppages during phonation.

Organic (Essential) Voice Tremor

Organic voice tremor is observed in the voices of some older individuals. This condition may accompany tremor in other parts of the body, such as the upper limbs, head, face, and neck musculature. As such, this tremorous condition must be differentiated from those of Parkinsonism or cerebellar disease. The onset of organic voice tremor may be gradual or rapid (Brown & Simonson, 1963); it is characterized as a quavering intonation that generally occurs at a frequency of 5–6 Hz. In severe cases, there may be rhythmic voice arrests that are caused by sudden vocal fold adduction. Laryngoscopically, the vocal folds appear normal in structure. Vocal tremor may be masked in contextual speech but may become more manifest during sustained or prolonged phonation. The tremors increase in severity with increase fatigue and emotional stress. This condition should be differentially diagnosed from spasmodic dysphonia, with which it may be mistaken. Dynamic fiberoptic imaging may be beneficial in describing the character of the tremor over time.

Spasmodic Dysphonia

A profoundly debilitating voice disorder affecting middle-aged and older adults is spasmodic dysphonia. This is a particularly troublesome disorder to diagnose and treat because of its early presentation and the problems usually associated with its onset. In addition, spasmodic dysphonia may be brought on by psychogenic factors and must be distinguished from more systemic neurological disorders such as organic voice tremor and from several forms of dystonia, including Meige's syndrome, spasmodic torticollis, and mixed dystonia tremor. The interested reader is directed to an excellent summary of this disorder by Aronson

(1985). A brief summary of spasmodic dysphonia follows to highlight its characteristics and distinguish it from among other neuromotor disrupting conditions in the older larynx.

Spasmodic dysphonia is a condition with onset in middle age (40–50 years), although it also has a significant presence among 50- to 60-year-olds. It affects males and females in the ratio of 1:1 to 1:2, depending on the study consulted. Aronson (1985) notes that this voice is characterized as having strained, strangled, effortful, staccato phonation. These voice qualities vary from individual to individual and may range in severity from mild to severe, although most patients present with severe vocal impairment. The onset is usually gradual, presenting initially as a nonspecific hoarseness with fluctuation of symptoms and intervening periods of normal voice. This is followed by progressively longer periods of dysphonia, which ultimately reach a plateau. Upper respiratory infections (Izdebski, Dedo, & Boles, 1984) or severe emotional upset—such as death of a relative or work, marital, or social stress—are often associated with the development of spasmodic dysphonia. Once the initial symptoms present, improvement rarely occurs. Stabilization of symptoms usually occurs between 9 and 24 months after the onset, although fluctuations in severity are exacerbated by stress or physical labor.

Abductor and adductor types of spasmodic dysphonia have been identified, with the adductor variety being by far the most common. Abductor spasmodic dysphonia, first described by Aronson (1973), is a distinctive form of spasmodic dysphonia in which a normal or hoarse voice is suddenly interrupted by brief periods of breathy or whispered voice. In contrast, adductor spasmodic dysphonia is characterized by hyperadduction of the vocal folds, often accompanied by supraglottal and vocal tract hyperfunction. The etiologies and onset for both types are similar; however, unlike adductor spasms, which occur throughout all forms and contexts of phonation, abductor spasms occur most frequently on unvoiced consonants, to a lesser degree during voiced consonants, and least on vowels.

The most common laryngoscopic observations of the vocal folds in spasmodic dysphonia (Finitzo & Freeman, 1989) are the presence of rapid, twitch-like movements, which are sometimes accompanied by or solely represented by forceful spasm-like jerking of the vocal folds and arytenoid cartilages. These spasms are frequently superimposed on by regularly occurring twitches (6–8 Hz). McCall, Skolnick, and Brewer (1971) also observed abnormal movements in vocal tract structures during quiet respiration that became exacerbated during phonation.

Prognosis is poor for patients with spasmodic dysphonia, although some surgical therapies (Dedo, 1976) have had variable success. Recent use of Botulinum toxin injection into the vocal folds (Blitzer, Brin, Fahn, & Lovelace, 1988) has produced significant reductions in symptoms and voice; however, to date, these results last for only short intervals of time (3–6 months) and reinjection is needed. The long-term effectiveness is not known at this time.

Management Strategies for the Older Dysphonic Speaker

Older persons experiencing voice problems frequently do not seek help or may not be referred by their physicians, who may not recognize the existence of their voice problems. In addition, the aging person frequently has other medical problems that cause fatigue, breathing problems, depression, anxiety, and cognitive deficits.

Thus, plannng the treatment of the older dysphonic patient requires a thorough knowledge of the patient *as a person*. This includes information about the patient's physical condition and health care, the family and emotional support system, the home living circumstances, the nature and extent of the patient's social activities, and a realistic appraisal of his or her vocal needs.

Nonmedical treatments may consist of the following:

1. Helping to develop strategies for daily communication

2. Improving breath support

3. Reducing vocal hyperfunction and developing appropriate habitual pitch levels

4. Improving loudness and projection

5. Reducing vocal fatigue

6. Providing counseling to encourage compliance with therapy, providing information about communication deficits, or simply offering a sympathetic ear

Medical treatment is sometimes necessary to help the patient with vocal deficits. Frequently this consists of appropriate referral to a medical specialist such as a pulmonologist, gastroenterologist, neurologist, or psychiatrist. The otolaryngologist may provide significant relief to patients with dysphonia who experience acute or chronic sinusitis. Drainage from this condition can cause irritation to the vocal folds, resulting in hoarseness, chronic throat clearing, and discomfort during voicing. In addition, this condition and other upper respiratory tract infections may lead to middle ear conditions that can affect proper monitoring of the voice and the use of appropriate levels of vocal loudness. Pharyngeal discomfort and dental or temporomandibular joint dysfunction may contribute to unsuitable compensations that may cause supralaryngeal muscle tension, leading to strain on phonation. Management of esophageal reflux can result in significant improvement from the discomfort and hoarse-inefficient voice frequently associated with reflux laryngitis.

Surgical intervention to improve glottal competency of the aging is rarely employed or indicated; however, however, two procedures may be of value. These are collagen injections and thyroplasty. Injection of bovine collagen into the vocal fold may be useful in medializing the vocal fold to correct glottal gaps, correcting irregularities in the margins of the vocal folds, and adding bulk to them if they become atrophied. An alternative to this procedure, thyroplasty, involves placing small pieces of inert materials between the thyroid cartilage proper and its inner perichondrium, thereby moving the adjacent vocal fold medially. This has the advantage of being reversible if relief of the bowing is not satisfactory. The anticipated benefit of this procedure is increased vocal efficiency resulting from enhanced vocal fold stability, improved mucosal wave dynamics, and reduction in air loss.

Treating the aging person with a voice disorder is a clinical challenge. Diagnosis and treatment are frequently complicated by other physiological deficits and often are accompanied by emotional and psychological factors. The key to successful management is accurate appraisal, realistic goal setting, and, most importantly, a patient and understanding attitude.

References

Ardran, G. (1965). Calcification of the epiglottis. *British Journal of Radiology, 38,* 592–595.

Aronson, A. E. (1973). *Psychogenic voice disorders.* Philadelphia: Saunders.

Aronson, A. E. (1985). *Clinical voice disorders* (2nd ed.). New York: Thieme.

Bach, A., Lederer, F., & Dinolt, R. (1941). Senile changes in the laryngeal musculature. *Archives of Otolaryngology, 34,* 47–56.

Bak-Pedersen, K., & Nielsen, K. (1986). Subepithelial mucous glands in the adult human larynx. *Acta Otolaryngologica, 102,* 341–352.

Batsakis, J. G. (1979). *Tumors of the head and neck—Clinical and pathological considerations.* Baltimore, MD: Williams & Wilkins.

Behrendt, W., & Strauch, G. (1965). Die Feinstruck des menschlichen Stimmbandes abhängig vom Lebensalter. *Archiv Ohren Nasen Keklkofheilkd, 184,* 510–520.

Benjamin, B. (1980). *Acoustic, aerodynamic and perceptual characteristics of geriatric speech.* Unpublished doctoral dissertation, Pennsylvania State University, University Park, PA.

Bennett, S., Bishop, S. G., & Lumpkin, S. M. M. (1987). Phonatory characteristics associated with bilateral diffuse polypoid degeneration. *Laryngoscope, 97,* 446–450.

Blitzer, A., Brin, M. F., Fahn, S., & Lovelace, R. E. (1988). Localized injections of Botulinum toxin for the treatment of vocal laryngeal dysphonia (spastic dysphonia). *Laryngoscope, 98,* 193–197.

Bouchayer, M., & Cornut, G. (1987). Microsurgery for benign lesions of the vocal folds. *Ear, Nose, and Throat Journal, 67*(6), 446–466.

Brown, J. R., & Simonson, J. (1963). Organic voice tremor. *Neurology* (Minneapolis), *13,* 520–525.

Carnevalle-Ricci, R. (1937). Osservazioni isopatologiche sulla laringe nella senescenza. *Archivo Italiana di Otologia, Rhinologia e Laringologia, 49,* 1.

Chamberlain, W., & Young, B. (1935). Ossification (so-called ''calcification'') of normal laryngeal cartilages mistaken for foreign bodies. *American Journal of Roentgenology, 33,* 441–450.

Cooper, M. (1970). Voice problems of the geriatric patient. *Geriatrics, 25*(1), 107–110.

Darley, F., Aronson, A., & Brown, J. (1975). *Motor speech disorders.* Philadelphia: Saunders.

Dedo, H. H. (1976). Recurrent laryngeal nerve section for spastic dysphonia. *Annals of Otology, Rhinology and Laryngology, 85,* 451–459.

Eggston, A., & Wolff, D. (1947). *Histopathology of the ear, nose and throat.* Baltimore, MD: Williams & Wilkins.

Endres, W., Bambach, W., & Flosser, G. (1971). Voice spectrographs as a function of age, voice disguise, and vocal imitation. *Journal of the Acoustical Society of America, 49,* 1842–1848.

English, G. M. (1976). Malignant neoplasms of the larynx. In G. M. English (Ed.), *Otolaryngology: A textbook* (ch. 48). New York: Harper & Row.

Ferreri, G. (1959). Senescence of the larynx. Italian General review of *Oto-Rhino-Laryngology, 1,* 640–709.

Finitzo, T., & Freeman, F. (1989). Spasmodic dysphonia, whether and where: Results of seven years of research. *Journal of Speech and Hearing Research, 32,* 541–555.

Fritzell, B., & Hertegard, S. (1986). A retrospective study of treatment for vocal fold edema: A preliminary report. In J. A. Kirchner (Ed.), *Vocal fold histopathology: A symposium* (pp. 57–64). San Diego, CA: College Hill Press.

Golpher, L. C., Nutt, J. G., Rau, M. T., & Collman, R. O. (1983). Focal cranial dystonia. *Journal of Speech and Hearing Disorders, 48,* 128–134.

Gracco, C., & Kahane, J. (1989). Age related changes in the vestibular folds of the human larynx: A histomorphometric study. *Journal of Voice, 3*(3), 204–212.

Hartman, D. E., & Danhauer, J. L. (1976). Perceptual features of speech for males in four perceived age decades. *Journal of the Acoustical Society of America, 59,* 713–715.

Hately, B., Evison, G., & Samuel, E. (1965). The pattern of ossification in the laryngeal cartilages: A radiological study. *British Journal of Radiology, 38,* 585–591.

Heinemann, M. (1969). Myxoedem und Stimme. *Folia Phoniatrica, 21,* 55–62.

Hirano, M. (1974). Morphological structure of the vocal cord as a vibrator and its variations. *Folia Phoniatrica, 26,* 89–94.

Hirano, M., Kurita, S., & Nakashima, T. (1983). Growth, development, and aging of human vocal folds. In D. M. Bless & J. H. Abbs (Eds.), *Vocal fold physiology: Contemporary research and clinical issues.* San Diego, CA: College Hill Press.

Hollien, H., & Shipp, T. (1972). Speaking fundamental frequency and chronological age in males. *Journal of Speech and Hearing Research, 15,* 155–159.

Hommerich, K. (1972). Der alternde Larynx: Morphologische Aspekte. *Hals Nasen Ohrenaerzte, 20,* 115–120.

Honjo, I., & Isshiki, N. (1980). Laryngoscopic and voice characteristics of aged persons. *Archives of Otolaryngology, 106,* 149–150.

Isshiki, N., Okamura, H., & Ishikawa, T. (1975). Thyroplasty type I (lateral compression) for dysphonia due to vocal fold paralysis or atrophy. *Acta Otolaryngologica, 80,* 465–473.

Izdebski, K., Dedo, H. H., & Boles, L. (1984). Spastic dysphonia: A profile of 200 cases. *American Journal of Otolaryngology, 5,* 12–20.

Kahane, J. C. (1982). Age related changes in the elastic fibers of the adult male vocal ligament. In V. Lawrence (Ed.), *Transcripts of the Eleventh Symposium: Care of the professional voice.* New York: Voice Foundation.

Kahane, J. C. (1983a). Postnatal development and aging of the human larynx. *Seminars in Speech and Language, 4,* 189–203.

Kahane, J. C. (1983b). A survey of age related changes in the connective tissues of the adult human larynx. In D. M. Bless & J. H. Abbs (Eds.), *Vocal physiology* (pp. 44–49). San Diego, CA: College Hill Press.

Kahane, J. C. (1987). Connective tissue changes in the larynx and their effects on voice. *Journal of Voice, 1,* 27–30.

Kahane, J. C. (1988). Age related changes in the human cricoarytenoid joint. In O. Fugimura (Ed.), *Vocal physiology: Voice production, mechanisms and functions.* New York: Raven Press.

Kahane, J. C., & Hammons, J. (1987). Developmental changes in the articular cartilage of the human cricoarytenoid joint. In T. Baer, C. Sasaki, & K. Harris (Eds.), *Laryngeal function in phonation and respiration.* San Diego, CA: College Hill Press.

Kahane, J. C., Stadlan, E. M., & Bell, J. S. (1979). *A histological study of the aging human larynx.* Scientific exhibit, Annual Meeting of The American Speech-Language-Hearing Association, Atlanta.

Kahn, A. R., & Kahane, J. C. (1986). India ink pinprick assessment of age-related changes in the cricoarytenoid joint (CAJ) articular surfaces. *Journal of Speech and Hearing Research, 29,* 536–543.

Kaplan, H. (1971). The oral cavity in geriatrics. *Geriatrics, 26,* 96–102.

Keen, J., & Wainwright, J. (1958). Ossification of the thyroid, cricoid, and arytenoid cartilages. *South African Journal of Laboratory and Clinical Medicine, 4,* 83–108.

Kersing, W. (1984). Vocal musculature, aging and development aspects. In J. Kirchner (Ed.), *Vocal fold histopathology* (pp. 11–16). San Diego, CA: College Hill Press.

Klawans, P. J., & Tanner, C. M. (1984). Movement disorders in the elderly. In M. L. Albert (Ed.), *Clinical neurology of aging.* New York: Grune & Stratton.

Kleinsasser, O. (1982). Pathogenesis of vocal cord polyps. *Annals of Otology, Rhinology and Laryngology, 91,* 378–381.

Koopmann, C. F. (1986). Geriatric otolaryngology. In A. Katz (Ed.), *Manual of otolaryngology—Head and neck therapeutics* (ch. 12, pp. 431–445). Philadelphia: Lea & Febiger.

Kruel, E. J. (1972). Neuromuscular control examination (NMC) for Parkinsonism: Vowel prolongations and diadochokinetic and reading rates. *Journal of Speech and Hearing, 15,* 72–83.

Lederer, F. L., & Hollender, A. R. (1951). *Textbook of the ear, nose and throat* (3rd ed., p. 523). Philadelphia: F. A. Davis.

Leutert, G. (1964). Über die histologische Biomorphose der menschlichen Stimmlippen. *Morphologisches Jahrfach, 106,* 11–72.

Linville, S. E. (1987a). Acoustic-perceptual studies of aging voice in women. *Journal of Voice, 1,* 44–48.

Linville, S. E. (1987b). Maximum phonational frequency range capabilities of women's voices with advancing age. *Folia Phoniatrica, 39,* 297–301.

Linville, S. E. (1988). Intraspeaker variability in fundamental frequency stability: An age related phenomenon? *Journal of the Acoustical Society, 83*(2), 741–745.

Linville, S. E., & Fisher, H. (1985a). Acoustic characteristics of perceived versus actual vocal age in controlled phonation by adult females. *Journal of the Acoustical Society of America, 78*(1), 40–48.

Linville, S. E., & Fisher, H. B. (1985b). Acoustic characteristics of women's voices with advanced age. *Journal of Gerontology, 3,* 324–330.

Ludlow, C. L., & Bassich, C. J. (1983). The results of acoustic and perceptual assessment of two types of dysarthria. In W. R. Berry (Ed.), *Clinical dysarthria* (pp. 121–151). Austin, TX: PRO-ED.

Lumpkin, S. M. M., Bishop, S. G., & Bennett, S. (1987). Comparison of surgical techniques in the treatment of polypoid degeneration. *Annals of Otology, Rhinology and Laryngology, 96,* 254–257.

Maisel, R. H. (1986). Carcinoma of the larynx and laryngopharynx. In D. G. McQuarrie, G. L. Adams, A. R. Shans, & G. A. Browne (Eds.), *Head and neck cancer: Clinical reasons and management principles.* Chicago: Year Book Medical Publishers.

Malinowski, A. (1967). The shape, dimensions and process of calcification of the cartilaginous framework in relation to age and sex in the Polish population. *Warzawa Folia Morphologica, 26,* 118–128.

Malmgren, L., & Ringwood, M. (1988). Aging of the recurrent laryngeal nerve: An ultrastructural morphometric study. In O. Fujimura (Ed.), *Vocal physiology: Voice production, mechanisms and function* (Vol. 2). New York: Raven Press.

McCall, G., Skolnick, L., & Brewer, D. (1971). A preliminary report of some atypical movement patterns in the tongue, palate, nasopharynx and larynx of patients with spasmodic dysphonia. *Journal of Speech and Hearing Disorders, 36,* 466–470.

McGlone, R., & Hollien, H. (1963). Vocal pitch characteristics of aged women. *Journal of Speech and Hearing Research, 6,* 164–170.

Melcon, M. C., Hoit, J. D., & Hixon, T. (1988). *Age and laryngeal airway resistance during vowel production.* Unpublished manuscript.

Montgomery, W. (1963). Cricoarytenoid arthritis. *Laryngoscope, 73,* 801–836.

Montgomery, W. W., & Lofgren, R. H. (1963). Usual and unusual causes of laryngeal arthritis. *Archives of Otolaryngology, 77,* 29–33.

Morris, R. J., & Brown, W. S. (1987). Age-related measures among adult women. *Journal of Voice, 1,* 38–43.

Morrison, M. D., Rammage, L. A., & Nichol, H. (1989). Evaluation and management of the voice disorders in the elderly. In J. Goldstein, H. J. Kashima, & C. F. Koopmann (Eds.), *Geriatric otolaryngology.* Toronto: B. C. Decker.

Mueller, P. B., Sweeney, R. J., & Barbeau, L. J. (1985). Acoustic and morphologic study of the senescent voice. *Ear Nose Throat Journal, 63,* 71–75.

Mysak, E. D. (1959). Pitch duration characteristics of older males. *Journal of Speech and Hearing Research, 2,* 46–54.

Mysak, E. D., & Hanley, T. P. (1958). Aging process in speech: Pitch and duration characteristics. *Journal of Gerontology, 13,* 309–313.

Neiman, G. S., Klich, R. J., & Shuey, E. M. (1983). Voice onset time in young and 70-year-old women. *Journal of Speech and Hearing Research, 26,* 118–123.

Noell, G. (1962). On the problem of age related changes of the laryngeal mucosa. *Archiv fuer klinische und experimentelle Ohren-Nasen-und-Kehlkopfheilkunde, 179,* 361–365.

Paperella, M., & Shumrick, D. (1980). *Otolaryngology* (p. 2452). Philadelphia: Saunders.

Ptacek, P., Sander, E., Maloney, W., & Jackson, C. (1966). Phonatory and related changes with advanced age. *Journal of Speech and Hearing Research, 9,* 353–360.

Ramig, L. A., & Ringle, R. L. (1983). Effects of physiological aging on selected acoustic characteristics of voice. *Journal of Speech and Hearing Research, 26,* 22–30.

Ritter, F. N. (1964). The effect of hypothyroidism on the larynx of the rat. *Annals of Otology, Rhinology and Laryngology, 73*(3), 404–416.

Roncollo, P. (1949). Researches about ossification and conformation of the thyroid cartilage in men. *Acta Otolaryngologica, 103,* 169–171.

Rontal, E., & Rontal, E. M. (1977). Lesions of the vagus nerve—Diagnosis, treatment and rehabilitation. *Laryngoscope, 87,* 72.

Ruckes, J., & Hohmann, M. (1963). On the topography and presence of squamous fatty tissue in the human superior vocal cord in relation to age, weight and disease. *Anatomischer Anzeiger, 112,* 405–425.

Ryan, R., McDonald, J., & Devine, K. (1956). Changes in laryngeal epithelium: Relation to age, sex and certain other factors. *Mayo Clinic Proceedings, 31,* 47–52.

Ryan, W., & Burk, K. (1974). Perceptual and acoustic correlates of aging in the speech of males. *Journal of Communication Disorders, 7,* 181–192.

Sato, T., & Tauchi, H. (1982). Age changes in human vocal fold muscles. *Mechanisms of Aging Development, 18,* 67–74.

Saxman, J., & Burk, K. (1967). Speaking fundamental frequency characteristics of middle aged females. *Folia Phoniatrica, 19,* 167–172.

Segre, R. (1971). Senescence of the voice. *Eye, Ear, Nose & Throat Journal, 50,* 62–68.

Snow, J., Harano, J., & Balogh, K. (1966). Post-intubation granuloma of the larynx. *Anesthesia and Analgesia, 45,* 425–429.

Stoicheff, M. L. (1981). Speaking fundamental characteristics of nonsmoking adults. *Journal of Speech and Hearing Research, 24,* 437–441.

Sweeting, P., & Baken, R. (1982). Voice onset time in a normal-aged population. *Journal of Speech and Hearing Research, 25,* 129–134.

Templer, J. (1987). Clinical evaluation of the larynx. In S. Thawley, W. R. Panie, J. G. Batsakis, & R. B. Lindberg (Eds.), *Comprehensive management of head and neck tumors.* Philadelphia: Saunders.

Thorne, G. W. (1977). *Harrison's principles of internal medicine* (p. 2051). New York: McGraw-Hill.

Titche, L. (1976). Causes of recurrent laryngeal nerve paralysis. *Archives of Otolaryngology, 102*(5), 259–261.

Ward, P. H., Hanson, D. G., & Berci, G. (1981). Observations on central neurologic etiology for laryngeal dysfunction. *Annals of Otology, Rhinology and Laryngology, 90,* 430–441.

Weismer, G., & Fromm, D. (1983). Acoustic analysis of geriatric utterance: Segmental and nonsegmental characteristics that relate to laryngeal function. In D. M. Bless & J. H. Abbs (Eds.), *Vocal fold physiology: Contemporary research and clinical issues* (pp. 317–332). San Diego, CA: College Hill Press.

Wilcox, K., & Horii, Y. (1980). Age and changes in vocal jitter. *Journal of Gerontology, 35,* 194–198.

Yates, A., & Dedo, H. (1984). Carbon dioxide enucleation of polypoid vocal cords. *Laryngoscope, 94,* 731–735.

The Aging Oropharyngeal System

Barbara C. Sonies, PhD ∎

A discussion of the salient parameters of aging and their effects on the oropharynx and its primary functions (speech, swallowing, and taste) must also take account of our general knowledge of the aging process. Two seemingly discrepant theories of aging emerge. The first is that aging is an irreversible process that somehow reflects, in some predictable stepwise fashion, changes in a number of biomarkers of the process of aging. These biomarkers are determined from analysis of a variety of biochemical, cellular, genetic, and physiological events (Wilson, 1988). These events may serve to cause change in metabolic, immunologic, and neurological functions in various ways so that the life-span is either maximized at its termination, extended in mean value, or changed in regard to the aging of a single system (Baker & Sprott, 1988). It is acknowledged in this view that chronological age is, by itself, an invalid predictor of functional age (Baker & Sprott, 1988). The second, currently less accepted, view of aging is based upon the idea that

age is a disease with implicit changes or decrements of a pathological nature, so that as one ages the expectation of disease increases. These views could be simplified into a *developmental* or nonpathological view versus a *decremental* or pathological view of aging. To date there are no truly valid biomarkers of age within the human species that can account for some of the more readily observable changes such as skin wrinkles, gray hair, slowing of motor reaction time, and reduced muscle mass (Baker & Sprott, 1988; Masoro, 1988). Curiously, within the human species, some individuals in their 70s are more like their younger counterparts in their 50s, while some 50-year-olds are more like those in their 7th decade. It is certain that no single explanation (environmental, cellular, nutritional, genetic, or psychological) can suffice to explain these variations. In spite of this lack of clarity in determining a salient underlying hypothesis of age-related change, we can still delineate a variety of changes that appear to be most commonly associated with longevity in humans. Some of these changes have an effect on the morphological (cellular, tissues), chemosensory (taste, smell, salivation), somatosensory (temperature, touch), and sensorimotor (speech, mastication, swallowing) functions of the oropharynx. Each of these functions and their relationship to age will be discussed in turn.

Overview

For the purposes of this chapter, the *oropharyngeal system* will be anatomically described as beginning at the alveolar ridge and extending to the pharyngoesophageal segment. It includes the mucosal lining of the entire oral cavity and the pharynx; the sensory end-organs embedded in the mucosal linings; the velum; the larynx; the tonsils, fauces, palate, and tongue; the taste receptors; and the salivary glands, as well as the bones (mandible, maxilla, and hyoid), cartilages (epiglottis, thyroid, cricoid, arytenoid), teeth, and cervical vertebrae (see Figure 11.1).

The oral and pharyngeal cavities are essentially open and air-filled and can be closed for short periods of time by a series of valves. Valving can be created by the opposition of the various soft tissues and/or bony structures (lips, tongue/teeth, tongue/palate, velum/pharynx, tongue base/pharynx, epiglottis/laryngeal aditus). The lowermost pharyngeal valve remains closed except when it relaxes to permit a bolus to

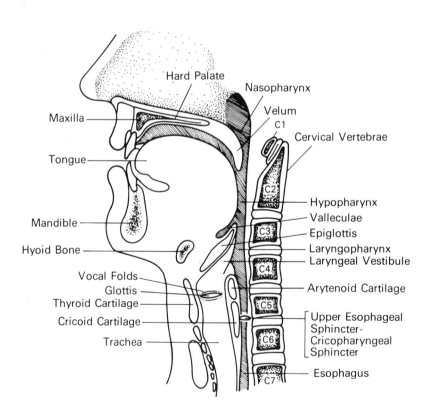

FIGURE 11.1.   Oropharyngeal structures.

enter the esophagus. There are several purposes for these valving actions. One is to change the turbulence or flow of air through this air-filled tube and create resonatory and phonatory patterns that are distinguished as articulated speech. Another purpose for valving in the oropharynx is to move food materials (liquid and solid) from the mouth through the pharynx into the esophagus. This is accomplished by a series of muscular contractions, often called *peristalsis*, that move food through the tubelike oropharynx. Peristaltic activity is generated by air pressure and by lingual force.

Morphological Considerations

Cellular Changes: General Principles

Functional changes that begin at the level of the cell are numerous and relate to the many and varied components of human physiology, from biochemistry to behavior. Thus, given the unequivocal fact that aging begins at the level of the cell (and is undeniable, even in normals), we have begun an exploration of aging starting at the microcosm (the cell). The composition of a normal cell evolves and changes with time. Normal cells duplicate in a fixed pattern and some eventually die or mutate. Some cells can change permeability or rates of metabolism. Although the rate of cell reproduction varies, there does not appear to be such a phenomenon as cell immortality in human organs; cells have a set number of reproductions or doublings before they die. Accordingly, an inverse relationship exists between age and the number of doublings possible (Hayflick, 1987, 1989). Although all human cells have a limited ability to reproduce, Hayflick (1989) states that certain ''decrements in physiologic function . . . appear before cells lose their capacity to replicate'' (p. 13), which are the true causes of aging

at the cellular level. These variations occurring at the cellular level may increase the susceptibility of the cell to pathological intrusions.

The Oral Mucosa

Although the oral mucosa may thicken or thin out, become drier, and change slightly in appearance, there appears to be no conclusive evidence that these changes can be attributed solely to the normal aging process (Baum, 1984a; Ofstehage & Magilvy, 1986). The effects of the oral environment, including the traumas of long years of mastication, poorly fitting or ill-maintained prostheses, smoking, and a host of medications, have, however, been found to produce the changes seen in the oral mucosa (Baum, 1984b; Breustedt, 1983). Some of the mucosal changes typically seen as one ages include ulcerations, increased varicosities, malignancies, and susceptibility to diseases and infections of the oral mucosa.

The mucosal lining of the oral cavity can be classified into several broad categories: (a) slightly keratinized and freely movable, as in the labial and buccal mucosa and mouth floor; (b) well keratinized and adhering to bone, as in the lining that covers the gingiva and palate; (c) specialized, as in the tongue dorsum; (d) masticatory; and (e) lining mucosa (Baum, 1984b; Breustedt, 1983). Some investigators have determined that with advancing age, cellular changes occur that cause all of these types of oral mucosa to be less able to function in various metabolic, sensory, and neuromotor tasks (Breustedt, 1983). The elderly may be more apt to have denture-induced mucosal changes and be less aware of thermal, chemical, and pressure stimuli in the oral cavity than younger persons. Common opinion is that if major changes appear in the oral mucosa they are the result of drugs, diseases, or pathological conditions and not the aging process. This seems to be supported by observations that in healthy older persons with excellent oral hygiene who do not smoke, few changes in the oral mucosa are evidenced.

Bony Structures

Bone changes both in structure and in its mechanical properties with age. Women incur greater degrees of bone loss than men. It is not uncommon to find losses in women that may equal a reduction of bone volume of up to 8% per decade (Norton, 1988). These losses are most likely due to an imbalance between resorption and replacement of bone at the cellular level. As the bone loss increases, the number of osteoclasts increases and the mineralization rate decreases, changing the quality of the bone matrix (Norton, 1988).

According to Lyles (1989), osteoporosis, the decrease in bone mineral and matrix associated with normal nondisease aging, is the most common metabolic bone change in the elderly. Osteoporosis is most frequent in women who have reached menopause and causes fracturing of the bones, even after minimal trauma. Although the entire bony skeleton can be affected by changes in bone composition, the changes seen with age most often affect the hip, distal forearm, vertebrae, and long weight-bearing leg bones. Norton (1988) reported that the structure of all the facial bones changes with age as the bone matrix becomes air-filled (pneumatized), causing the sinus cavities to increase, The alveolar bone of older persons exhibits decreased trabeculation (or support) because of either tooth loss or osteoporotic change (Greenwell & Bissada, 1989). There is no clear evidence that suggests that the hyoid bone will become osteoporotic. Evidence in case reports exists to suggest that arthritis may affect the cervical vertebrae and the temporomandibular joint as well as the articular surfaces between the laryngeal cartilages and thus may affect vocal fold function (de Bont, Liem, & Boering, 1985). (Because age and voice will not be discussed in this chapter, the reader should see chapter 10 for this information.) The appearance of osteo-phytes, bony outgrowths, in the cervical region (C3–C5) are more common in the elderly. Since osteophytes protrude anteriorly, they impinge into the pharynx. This causes pain and obstructs the flow of a bolus during swallowing. In general, these bony changes have been noted to have only minimal effects on the physiology of the oropharynx.

Muscular Structures

The major muscles of the oropharyngeal system can be grouped as *labial* (orbicularis oris, platysma), *facial/masticatory* (masseter, temporalis, pterygoid, buccinator), *floor of the mouth* (geniohyoid, mylohyoid), *palatal* (levator veli palatini, tensor veli palatini, musculus uvulae, palatoglossus, palatopharyngeus), *lingual* (genioglossus, hyoglossus, styloglossus, superior and inferior longitudinal, transverse, vertical), and *pharyngeal* (superior, middle and inferior constrictors, stylopharyngeus, salpingopharyngeus, palatopharyngeus). The *cricopharyngeus* muscle, which is part of the inferior constrictor, is attached to the cricoid cartilage and acts as a sphincter between the pharynx and esophagus during swallowing (Williams, Warwick, Dyson, & Bannister, 1989). The extrinsic laryngeal muscles elevate and protectively posture the larynx during swallowing. Action of the aryepiglotticus and thyroepiglotticus muscles may also influence closure of the entrance into the larynx (the vestibule) during swallowing.

It is acknowledged that the mass or bulk of most muscles diminishes in old age. These changes, in addition to skin wrinkling, are a major but expected component of later development. Reductions in muscle mass have been linked to reduced strength and lessened ability to learn new motor behaviors in the elderly.

Muscle atrophy, characterized by a decrease in the number of muscle fibers, is typical in individuals above age 60. Studies have found that there is a progressive decline in the number of functional motor units after the 5th decade, which appears to be the contributing factor in the wasting and weakness of aging muscles (Campbell, McComas, & Petito, 1973). Other investigators have found that a decline in muscle strength appeared before morphological changes were measurable. This finding suggests that both genetic (endogenous) and environmental (exogenous) factors can be involved in the aging of the muscular system (Larsson, 1978). Larsson postulated that these muscle changes related to differences in the amounts of ribonucleic acid and deoxyribonucleic acid in aging cells as well as changes in cellular protein metabolism. Other changes in muscles that have been related to age include extended contraction time and reduced muscle tension (Campbell et al., 1973; Larsson, 1978).

Several studies serve to confirm that similar types of change occur in the muscles of the oropharynx. Using electromyography (EMG) of the orbicularis oris superior and inferior muscles of the lips and face in healthy women aged 70 to 75 years, young adults, and children, one group of investigators found that their oldest group demonstrated the greatest amount of variability in EMG recordings (Rastatter, McGuire, Bushong, & Loposky, 1987). They concluded that the variability was due to a loss of general muscle function of the facial area caused by the facial muscle atrophy evidenced in the elderly. In another study the masseter and medial pterygoid muscles were shown to be reduced by a range of 35–47% in both area and density on cross-sectional computerized axial tomography studies (Newton, Abel, Robertson, & Yemm, 1987). Increases in lipid pigment (lipofuscin) accumulation were found in aging lip and tongue muscles (Dayan, Abrahami, Buchner, Gorsky, & Chimovitz, 1988). Similarly, changes in muscle fiber type and reduced density of muscle fibers were found in the muscles of the pharyngeal constrictors and the esophagus (Leese & Hopwood, 1986) and atrophic changes have been described in the bilabial tissues (Fanous, 1987).

These changes in muscle fiber density, muscular tension, muscle strength, and muscular contraction can affect the functions of the oropharynx. Decreased muscle function can slow mastication, impede oral bolus preparation, weaken lingual motion, and slow bolus motility through the pharynx. We will describe the effects of age on these functions in later sections.

Chemosensory Functions

Salivary Function

Saliva is essential in maintaining the physiology and anatomy of the oral cavity, the mucous membranes, and the teeth. A distinction is made between the *major* salivary glands lying distant to the oral mucosa (parotids, submandibular, sublingual) and the *minor* glands embedded in mucosa or submucosa (Williams et al., 1989). Saliva serves to aid speech and swallowing by providing several functions that are important for the tissues within the oral cavity. These functions, as described by Baum (1986, 1989), include lubrication of the oropharyngeal mucosa, remineralization of the teeth, antibacterial and antifungal control, dissolving of food, presenting taste stimuli to the taste buds, and food bolus formation and translocation. Diminished salivary flow has numerous consequences on normal oral physiology. For example, reduced lubrication of the oropharyngeal mucosa causes dryness, friability, and altered oral sensation. Caries increase and tooth loss can be rampant if the remineralization ability is altered or if antimicrobial function is diminished (Baum, 1989). Tooth decay and xerostomia affect food bolus preparation, formation, and transportation, causing oral phase dysphagia. Studies of salivary gland hypofunction have revealed significant durational changes in oropharyngeal swallowing (Caruso, Sonies, Fox, & Atkinson, 1989; Hughes et al., 1987). Interestingly, Baum (1989) states that little is currently known about the normal range of salivary flow. He says that basal salivary flow rates can vary by a factor of 100, whereas stimulated parotid flow rates may vary by a factor of 10–20. Important to the study of the effects of reduced saliva is the investigation of concomitant oral motor function and patients' subjective complaints about whether they perceive oral dryness or have difficulty swallowing. Studies using ultrasound to noninvasively image the oropharyngeal swallow revealed durational differences between stimulated and unstimulated swallows in normal aging adults that are directly related to the amount of oral lubrication, but not to age itself (Hughes et al., 1987; Sonies, Parent, Morrish, & Baum, 1988; Sonies, Ship, & Baum, 1989).

Numerous reports can be found suggesting that a common component of aging is reduction in salivary flow (Bertram, 1967; Meyer, Golden, Steiner, & Necheles, 1937), but more recent studies using better collection techniques do not confirm this earlier supposition (Baum, 1986, 1989; Ganguly, Stablein, Lockey, Shamblin, & Vargas, 1986). While no age-related decrements in salivary flow rate can be found in collections taken from stimulated or unstimulated parotid glands, evidence currently suggests that this may not be the case for submandibular gland flow rates (Pedersen, Schubert, Izutsu, Mersai, & Truelove, 1985). Accordingly, when historical studies are performed that look at the structural and cellular composition of salivary glands, changes are found in aged subjects (DeWilde, Baak, van Houwellingen, Kater, & Slootweg, 1986; Ganguly et al., 1986; Pedersen et al., 1985; Scott, Flower, & Burns, 1987). These changes may shed some light on why the elderly have oral infections, oral lesions, and loose teeth more often than their younger counterparts. However, frank diminution of salivary flow is rarely found in healthy persons and is thus suggestive of systemic pathology (Sjogren's syndrome) or use of pharmacological agents.

Smell

The sense of smell has been found to decline and change with age in all of the studies conducted to assess perception of odorants. Disagreement exists as to whether the losses in smell are homogeneous across all odorants (Cain & Stevens, 1989) or heterogeneous and specific to particular odorants (Stevens & Cain, 1986a; Wysocki & Gilbert, 1989). Since detection of odors can be measured using several tasks (threshold determination, magnitude estimation, similarity judgments, and identification tasks), results of studies vary according to the type of task used (Cowart, 1989; Wysocki & Gilbert, 1989). It is widely accepted that declines in smell occur in the late 50s or early 60s, causing the elderly to be impaired in their ability to detect certain noxious odors, including leaking gas and smoke (Leopold et al., 1989). Evidence suggests that the mucous membranes lining the nasopharynx atrophy and therefore become less able to serve as a barrier to nasal congestion and infection. Although loss of nerve fibers in the olfactory bulb and tract occur with age, evidence suggests that the olfactory system can regenerate its epithelial cells (Leopold et al., 1989, Wysocki & Gilbert, 1989). The work of Cowart (1989), using both basic threshold measures and detection of odorants above threshold levels, continues to suggest age-related decrements; it is of interest that these decrements were found to correlate with educational level as well as with age. The question of the contribution of the oral cavity in detection of odors was examined in elderly subjects by a study requiring judgments of magnitude of odors with nostrils occluded and unoccluded (Stevens & Cain, 1986b). The elderly subjects' ability to detect smells was equally impaired whether input was nasal and oral or oral alone, thus suggesting a possible reason why the elderly often complain of food being bland or distorted in taste.

Taste

Taste buds can be found within the epithelial lining of the tongue, soft palate, faucial arches, posterior epiglottis, and posterior wall of the oropharynx. They are most frequent on the tongue tip and dorsum and relatively rare in the midportion of the tongue, soft palate, epiglottis, and pharynx (Williams et al., 1989). Several types of taste buds have been described and are found on papillae of several types: *Fungiform* papillae are found primarily near the anterior portion of the tongue; *foliate* papillae lie behind them and also laterally on the tongue margins; *filiform* papillae are found at the tongue tip and in rows at the tongue dorsum parallel to the *circumvallate* papillae, which are large and few in number (8–12) and only appear on the tongue dorsum in a V-shaped row (Miller, 1989; Williams et al., 1989). Several qualities of taste can be measured: salty, (NaCl), sweet (sucrose), bitter (quinine hydrochloride), and sour (citric acid). A loss of taste is termed *ageusia* and diminution is called *dysgeusia*. Studies investigating the morphological changes in taste buds with age are conflicting. Some investigators find anatomical differences in fungiform papillae (Satoh & Seluk, 1988) whereas others find none that are correlated with age alone (Kullaa-Mikkonen, Koponen, & Seilonen, 1987; Miller, 1988; Mistretta, 1989).

The issues of age-related losses in taste are not as clearly related to advanced aging as is smell. Most investigators find that although taste changes occur, they are generally more specific to the tastant than uniform across all substances. According to Bartoshuk (1989) the thresholds for taste detection increase with age. However, it is not necessarily true that there are any differences in taste ability in elderly persons at levels above threshold intensity. Chauhan and Hawrysh (1988), looking at suprathreshold detection of ''sour'' in young and old healthy subjects, found significant differences in this one tastant, where the elderly subjects perceived stronger stimuli

as less intense. Another study of suprathreshold detection of all four tastes using magnitude matching (sound intensity and taste intensity were matched) did not reveal significant age decrements (Bartoshuk, Rifkin, Marks, & Bars, 1986). Thus, studies of taste must be critically examined as to the choice of the response method used as well as the tastant used. Weiffenbach and colleagues (Weiffenbach, Cowart, & Baum, 1986; Weiffenbach, Tylenda, & Baum, in press) suggest that one way to correct for inherent statistical biases in interpreting results based upon averaging across individuals and the slope of the average linear trend is to use an analysis of variance on the individual estimates or on the slopes of the individual linear regression functions (Weiffenbach et al., 1986, p. 461). Using this method, the investigators agreed that there were some measurable aspects of taste that diminished with age but stated that subjective taste decrements could occur in the absence of true sensory changes.

Murphy (1985) found that older subjects performed more poorly than younger subjects when identifying blended foods using both taste and smell. She suggested that these declines related to the combined contributions of olfactory/trigeminal, gustatory, and cognitive factors. It must be noted, however, that significant decrements in the ability to taste in elderly populations are generally found only in those individuals who either are suffering from systemic conditions or neurological, nutritional, or cognitive disorders or are taking various medications (Miller 1989; Spitzer, 1988).

These reductions or losses in acuity of taste, smell, and temperature may cause some elderly persons to have severe reductions in appetite and become anorectic (Morley & Silver, 1988; Schiffman & Warwick, 1988). Schiffman and Warwick have reasoned that anorexia and the concomitant reduction of oral sensory input not only may lead to malnutrition, but may reduce the turnover rate of receptors on the tongue and nasal lining, which in turn further reduces taste and smell. These researchers suggest that "flavor enhancement," or amplification of flavor and smell in table food for persons aged 70–79, increased food preference by as much as 75%. Flavor additives might then be an excellent and natural way to increase appetite and foster nutrition in the undernourished elderly.

Somatosensory Functions

The oral cavity and oropharynx, along with the other body structures, has sensory receptors for a range of stimuli, including thermal (hot/cold) and tactile-vibratory (touch/pressure/texture/shape), which provide information about the material that is ingested. These sensory functions are necessary to monitor mastication and swallowing and to protect against ingestion of noxious substances. Oral sensory mechanisms also serve to provide input regarding the location of the articulators during monitoring of speech production.

Studies of somatosensory perception of stimuli presented to the hands and feet of elderly subjects showed that general sensitivity to a variety of stimuli was reduced in the oldest group for all stimuli, except for thermal (cold) sensitivity (Kenshalo, 1986). Fucci, Petrosino, Harris, & Randolph-Tyler (1987) examined suprathreshold lingual vibrotactile sensation magnitudes in four age groups (ages 5 to 64) using cross-modal matching (sound plus vibrotactile stimuli). Their results indicated that the upper power functions became steeper in the older group, which they related to reduced neural density in the peripheral receptors of the tongue and auditory system in the elderly. Weiffenbach et al. (in press) conducted a study of oral sensory changes in aging. They also used cross-modal matching judgments of intensity of four types of oral stimuli (taste intensity, thermal intensity of water, viscosity of water, and intensity of local pressure on the tongue dorsum). They did not find age-specific decrements in intensity judgments for taste, temperature, or viscosity; both older and younger sub-

jects were able to make correct intensity judgments of these qualities. Only one of the measurements, lingual pressure, was sensitive to age. Older subjects made consistently smaller distance judgments to characterize their perception of lingual pressure (in agreement with the work of Fucci and colleagues, 1987). Since the ability to detect localized lingual pressure declines with age, it could follow that some effect might be found in the major functions of the tongue during speech or swallowing. This finding could also cause the elderly to produce extra lingual gestures to initiate a swallow, as suggested by the work of Sonies et al. (1988).

Pain is less well understood in aging, but evidence exists suggesting that complaints of oral pain increase in the elderly. However, increased pain may be related to increases in periodontal disease, neuralgias, and oral infection.

Sensorimotor Functions

Motor Functions

There is an extensive body of literature describing the changes that occur in general motor performance as one ages (Walshe, 1987). Primary among these motor changes is widespread slowing of performance in fine and gross motor tasks; slowed reaction times; and changes in muscular strength, tone, and endurance (Welford, 1984, 1988). Welford (1984) reasons that these changes, especially the ones that slow behavior, are caused by some central nervous system (CNS) mechanism whereby the brain is less able to distinguish between an actual electrical signal and the random activity generated within the CNS itself. He stated that this difficulty in distinguishing between a signal and noise in the system tends to predispose the elderly to adopt "higher criteria" for responding and to spend more time monitoring their actions (p. 73). Mortimer (1988) has determined that this central mechanism is most likely located in the dopaminergic system (the caudate nucleus and the putamen), which shows age-related reductions in synthesis of dopamine in biochemical studies. Mortimer compared the speeded movement behaviors of normal aging adults and adults with Parkinson's disease and found that normals did show declines in motor speed. However, their patterns were unlike those of the Parkinson's patients, who had greater degrees of slowed movement along with rigidity and tremors not seen in the normals. This chapter will not focus on the oropharyngeal effects of neuromotor disorder seen in neurological patients (e.g., Parkinson's, stroke, pseudobulbar palsy, Alzheimer's, Huntington's); rather, our focus is on normal age-related changes. The reader is referred to other works that discuss the dysarthrias, apraxias, and other symptoms of oromotor dysfunction that may appear in advanced age (Albert, 1984; Berry, 1983; Johns, 1978; McNeil, Rosenbek, & Aronson, 1984; Rosenbek, McNeil, & Aronson, 1984; Sonies, 1987).

Speech

Speech articulation does not change with age unless CNS or peripheral nervous system (PNS) pathology exists. This highly redundant motor system seems impervious to either exogenous or endogenous influences during the lifetime. If changes exist in the motor patterns that underly speech production in the elderly, they are imperceptible to the listener. A study of tongue movement in the elderly by Sonies, Baum, and Shawker (1984) using ultrasound imaging revealed that tongue position and displacement patterns differed for young and old subjects on the production of various selected phonemes but that these differences did not alter speech intelligibility, nor were they detected by sophisticated clinicians. Because of the ability of the tongue to produce various combinations of motion, numerous adjustments of the lingual surface can produce similar phonemes (Stone, 1990).

Mastication

Mastication depends upon the integrity and the alignment of the maxilla, mandible, and teeth. In order to chew food to a swallow-ready consistency, correct occlusal relationships must exist so that proper biting force can be exerted. The presence of correct dental alignment is needed during speech to produce stops, affricates, fricatives, and sibilants. A full set of teeth is more cosmetic than essential; several missing teeth have little effect on food preparation or speech. Adjustments in biting surfaces, changes in lingua-dental contact, and use of remaining teeth to bite can compensate for most partial tooth loss.

The teeth may dramatically change in appearance from the forces of wear, dental restoration, exposure to pollutants, smoke, and food. The teeth often appear shorter, darker, discolored, and worn from continual abrasion. This is especially true in the anterior arch. Wear on the molars may create a collapsed bite, closed-mouth appearance, wrinkled skin, and deepened nasolabial folds (Reiter & Weintraub, 1984). Advancing age may change the perception of temperature by the teeth. A study by Kollmann and Mijatovic (1985) used electrically controlled thermodes to stimulate the front teeth for cold and hot/warm temperatures. Differences were found in the amount of time taken to identify a cold stimulus and in the magnitude of perception of cold for the older subject group. This change in thermal perception can be attributed to changes in the dental hard tissues, tooth pulp, innervation, and vascularization (Norton, 1988).

Perhaps a major problem in aging, especially after age 70, is that of periodontal disease and subsequent tooth loss (Papapanou, Wennstrom, & Grondahl, 1988). The periodontum is composed of gingiva, the periodontal ligament, cementum, and alveolar bone. Greenwell and Bissada (1989) report that with age, cellular changes occur to all of the periodontal tissues. The gingiva thin and become keratinized. Connective tissue decreases in cellularity and the alveolar bone matrix is diminished. However, inflammation of the gingiva and bone loss have recently been linked to buildup of dental plaque, which is not solely a phenomenon of normal aging (Greenwell & Bissada, 1989).

On a positive note, it appears that the majority of these age-related changes do not have to occur and can indeed be prevented by good oral hygiene. Since the introduction of fluorine into drinking water, the rate of caries has declined significantly. More elderly persons are retaining their natural teeth and senior citizens in the next several decades are less likely to have periodontal disease because of flossing, special plaque-destroying solutions, and new tooth-brushing systems (Baum, 1984a; Greenwell & Bissada, 1989).

Swallowing

Unlike speech, which is relatively impervious to the effects of age, swallowing, even in healthy adults, shows some decrements with time. Many of these decrements do not seriously impede the swallowing process, but they may alter food selection. Many elderly people prefer soft, bland, warm foods rather than hard, hot or cold, or spicy foods. In normals, slight alterations in pharyngeal swallowing can be detected. These changes can be viewed with instrumental or diagnostic procedures that can uncover subtle deficits. Many of these changes are subclinical and do not constitute disorder. It is, however, widely acknowledged that the incidence of frank swallowing problems in the elderly can be attributed, in the main, to various neurological, neuromotor, or systemic conditions, and *not* as part of normal aging.

We will discuss the oropharyngeal swallowing of normal aging individuals before we discuss pathological conditions. The oropharyngeal swallow will only be briefly summarized; it has been aptly described anatomically and physiologically by numerous investigators (Blitzer, 1989; Buchholz, Bosma, & Donner, 1985; Kennedy & Kent, 1985; Larson, 1985; Logemann, 1983; Morrell, 1984; Sonies et al., 1988).

In brief, the oropharyngeal swallow can be viewed as consisting of several phases: oral preparation, oral, pharyngeal, and esophageal. These are not discrete phases but are continuous and overlap with one another. Solid food is first prepared to a swallow-ready consistency by mastication, salivary lubrication, and lingual motions. The masticated bolus is located centrally in a groove in the tongue and transported posteriorly. Liquids, needing no preparation, are rapidly transported from the front to the back of the mouth, and then into the pharynx by gravity. The initiation of the oropharyngeal swallow occurs when the bolus reaches the faucial pillars, velum, and posterior pharynx, causing a reflex to occur that starts the bolus on its passage through the pharynx. As the bolus is moved backward over the tongue, the velum elevates to meet the posterior pharyngeal wall and impedes nasal regurgitation. The hyoid bone elevates anteriorly and superiorly under the mandible, thus elevating the larynx, lowering the epiglottis, and assisting in closing off the laryngeal sphincters to prevent tracheal penetration or aspiration. Pressure changes in the oropharynx are created by the motions of the tongue and propel the bolus into the pharynx, where gravity and muscle contractions propel the bolus to the esophagus. The cricopharyngeal muscle relaxes when the head of the bolus reaches the pharyngoesophageal (PE) segment. When the PE segment relaxes, the bolus enters the esophagus. The duration of the combined oral and pharyngeal phases is approximately 2–3 s. Swallowing consists of both voluntary and involuntary neural control components. The voluntary components terminate as the bolus enters the upper pharynx and laryngopharynx. The remainder of the swallow is primarily involuntary. Coughing is a protective mechanism to expel material that has entered the laryngeal vestibule.

The chemosensory (taste and smell) and somatosensory (temperature, touch) functions are essential in the preparatory phase of swallowing. The sensorimotor functions (lingual motion, peristalsis, muscle contractions, and valving of the nasopharynx and laryngopharynx) are needed in bolus passage.

Some changes have been noted in the speed and efficiency of swallowing in older persons. Videofluoroscopic studies performed on normal elderly persons have demonstrated that small amounts of barium may remain in the valleculae (pair of depressions at the junction of the base of the tongue and the epiglottis) and that peristaltic action may become slowed. A pilot study by Tracy et al. (1988) evaluated the effects of age and increasing bolus size on swallowing. They observed that elderly subjects had delayed pharyngeal reflexes, longer laryngeal closure times, and prolonged PE segment openings. They also observed that their elderly subjects held the bolus farther back in the oral cavity, often near the valleculae, which shortened the time needed to transport the bolus through the pharynx. They did not observe changes in pharyngeal peristalsis with age but did find that increasing the size of the bolus to 20 ml was the major variable in producing the observed changes.

Sonies and colleagues (Sonies, Stone, & Shawker, 1984; Sonies et al., 1988) studied the effects of normal aging on the oropharyngeal swallow using ultrasound imaging to measure motion of the tongue and hyoid bone from initial rest to final resting position, thus demarcating the entire oropharyngeal swallow. Significant differences were found in swallow duration in both studies between younger and older subjects. In the 1988 study, a larger population was studied and comparisons were made between unstimulated (dry) and stimulated (wet) 10-cc bolus swallows. Dry swallows were longer than wet swallows across all age groups. Elderly males and females did not exhibit the same durational patterns. Women ages 55–74 showed a significant increase in swallow duration when compared to either of the other age groups and to the males on both wet and dry swallows.

The most striking age-related finding in this study was that all elderly subjects (age 55+) presented with multiple gestures of the hyoid (Sonies et al., 1988). These extraneous gestures were seen primarily in the initial phase of the swallow and were associated with extra effort and tongue motions. We believe that these findings are not indicative of oropharyngeal pathology but reflect decreases in generalized motor performance that contribute to delays in the initiation of motor activity by suprahyoid and/or tongue muscles. We also believe that these delays in motor performance are ''probably attributable to subtle changes in the neurologic substrates needed for any muscular series of events'' (Sonies et al., 1988, p. 7) typical in the elderly.

Except for reductions in contractile force (peristaltic activity) of the esophagus and increases in gastroesophageal reflux, the esophageal phase of swallowing remains basically stable throughout life (Eastwood, 1984; Thomson & Keelan, 1986). Since many elderly people exhibit muscular weakness and changes in muscle mass, reduced esophageal motility is common in the elderly (Pelemans & Vantrappen, 1985). There are a host of symptoms of esophageal disease that are usually found in persons over age 50 and that are caused primarily by neuromuscular disease or structural abnormalities (Eastwood, 1984; Pelemans & Vantrappen, 1985). For example, the upper esophageal sphincter (the PE sphincter, also called the *cricopharyngeal sphincter*) becomes hypotonic with age; thus sphincter relaxation and bolus passage from pharynx to esophagus may be slowed (Pelemans & Vantrappen, 1985). A common esophageal abnormality in elderly persons, pharyngoesophageal diverticulae (Zenker's), is more common in persons over age 65 because there are several weak areas in the pharyngeal wall musculature where the muscles attach. These areas have been described by Pelemans and Vantrappen (1985) as the triangle of Killian and the triangle of Laimer, which are above and below the attachment of the cricopharyngeal muscle. It is in these two locations, but more prevalent in the lower region, that diverticulae appear in the elderly.

A variety of CNS disorders are more common in older persons (Figure 11.2). These disorders are likely to cause oropharyngeal dysphagia because they can impair the neuromuscular, sensorimotor, and chemosensory control systems needed to swallow (Elliott, 1988). Following is a partial list of these CNS disorders: Parkinson's disease, cerebrovascular accident, Huntington's chorea, brainstem strokes, Shy-Drager syndrome, Steele-Richardson's syndrome, Meige syndrome, amyotrophic lateral sclerosis, multiple sclerosis, lingual-facial-buccal dyskinesia, pseudobulbar palsy, and cortical tumors (see Sonies, 1987, for a description of these diseases and their symptoms). In addition to neurological conditions, the following immunologic conditions can cause dysphagia: Sjogren's syndrome, polymyositis, and arthritis. The incidence of head and neck cancers and iatrogenic deficits from chemotherapy, radiation therapy, and toxic medications also increases in the elderly, thus providing another set of causes for dysphagia.

Blitzer (1989) has noted that the elderly are also more susceptible to aspiration because of muscle weakness and an increased incidence of neuromuscular dysfunction. The aspiration may be secondary and occur after the swallow from residue in the valleculae and pyriform sinus, or it may be caused by incomplete laryngeal adduction or paralysis of the true and false vocal cords. Reduced sensation in the oral cavity caused by CNS and PNS lesions can impede triggering of the protective cough and the swallow relex, thereby causing aspiration.

The actual incidence of swallowing disorders in the elderly ranges from 25 to 50% and has been shown to be substantial in nursing home residents (Siebens, Trupe, Siebens, et al., 1986) and in institutions (Groher & Bukatman, 1986). With increased longevity in the population, these percentages may increase in the next decade in elderly nonhealthy persons who are unable to live in their own residence.

*Neurogenic	
Vascular	— Stroke
Degenerative	— Movement disorders
	upper motor neuron
	lower motor neuron
Traumatic	— Acquired injury
	Postoperative
Systemic	— Poliomyelitis
Metabolic	— Diabetes
	Wilson's disease
	Thyroid
Infectious	— Meningitis, diphtheria
Neoplastic	— Tumors
Toxic	— Chemical burns
	Noxious substances
Autoimmune	— Polymyositis
	Dermatomyositis
	Lupus
	Arthritis
	Guillain-Barre
	AIDS
Neurodevelopmental	— Cerebral palsy
	Arnold-Chiari
Congenital	— Structural, genetic
	Cleft palate
Neuropathies	— Cranial nerve
*Psychiatric	— Globus hystericus
	Anorexia
	Bulimia
*Dementias	— Alzheimer's
	Psychosis
*Obstructive	— Non-CNS tumors
	Bony growths
	Cervical displacement
	Esophageal rings and webs
	Diverticula
*Acute Inflammations	— Temporary
*Postsurgical	— Laryngectomy
	Oral surgery
*Iatrogenic	— Toxins
	Therapies
	Treatments
	Pharmacological
*Salivary	— Xerostomia
	Postradiation
*Pain	— Odynophagia
	Ulcerations, tumors
	Infections, lesions
	Gastric reflux

FIGURE 11.2. Etiologies of dysphagia.

Conclusions

We have reviewed the range of age-related changes in the oropharynx starting from basic morphological changes and progressing to chemosensory, somatosensory, and sensorimotor processes. It is the basic contention from reviewing this vast body of knowledge that, even though changes occur at the cellular and structural levels with age, the basic functions of the oropharynx remain intact. Age alone does produce modifications in general rate of response, reductions in sensory threshold sensitivity, and muscular coordination. However, any significant diminution in oropharyngeal function is caused by some type of pathology, exposure to the environment, or medication. Thus, the developmental view of aging is supported.

In determining whether the studies reviewed in this chapter are truly representative of the developmental changes that occur across the life-span in the population of normal, healthy, aging persons, several unavoidable facts must be acknowledged. In conducting studies on any population, unavoidable sources of error may occur in either subject selection, design, or instrumentation. First, as one example, it is well known that cohort comparisons may influence results, and in the elderly, longitudinal and cross-sectional designs yield different information (Sonies & Caruso, 1990). Past life-style, nutrition, medications, chronic health problems, environmental exposure, and the presence of decrements in auditory and/or visual acuity create possible sources of error in making across-subject comparisons in older persons. Second, there is another set of within-subject, age-related sources of error that, again, cannot be controlled in those who are over age 65. Among these are the following: delayed motor response; diminished reflexes; obesity; skin laxity, which can reduce the skin contact needed for placement of devices; postural changes, which may affect head control and positioning; a tendency toward fatigue; difficulty in maintaining postures for long time periods; partial (or complete) edentulousness; and poorly fitting dental appliances. Third, within-subject sources of error can be coupled with added sources of error that are generated by alterations in electrophysiology, histological changes in muscle composition, reduced conductivity of muscles, and

changed bone matrices in the elderly. Fourth, some studies of elderly self-selected volunteers represent an extreme of the population in that these people are often the super-healthy, the better educated, and the most perfect specimens of the aged, who are almost too fit for realistic comparisons. On the other hand, some of the elderly who are studied are at the opposite extreme and are institutionalized with chronic diseases and conditions; they do not represent the average elderly individual either. It is possible, then, that certain design flaws and biases make our current data unrepresentative of the majority of the elderly.

As we have previously discussed, a major function of the oropharyngeal system is to prepare and transport food from the mouth to the stomach, supporting the nutritional needs of all humans. An issue of continuing consideration for the elderly is how to increase the life-span and maintain better health and quality of life. A provocative suggestion to accomplish this goal, *dietary restriction* (DR), has been derived from work with animal models. DR, or undernutrition, has retarded aging and extended the life-span in every species so far tested (Weindreich & Walford, 1988). In this practice, caloric restriction, rather than the reduction of specific types of nutrients, increases the life-span. It has been postulated that DR slows down the cell turnover rate and thus could decrease the rate of aging while also reducing the production of free radicals by restricting caloric intake (Weindreich & Walford, 1988). Although no studies currently exist in humans, researchers have argued for this theory in humans because of observations regarding the Japanese people of Okinawa, who have a diet that is lower in calories (sugars and cereals) and much higher in fish and green and yellow vegetables than their mainland counterparts. These people are smaller, live longer, and have less vascular disease and fewer malignancies. It is suggested that by reducing smoking and reducing caloric intake in humans to 1,500 to 1,800 Cal a day, body weight would be reduced and longevity increased. Reduced caloric intake might also reduce the demands on the digestive system; less sugar intake could improve gums, teeth, and oral mucosa; and reduced fats might maintain blood supply to the oral tissues and muscles and a better generalized status of the aging oropharynx. It is possible to speculate that in a generally healthy elder individual, the 1990s and beyond may not bring substantial change to either the morphological, chemosensory, or sensorimotor activities of the oropharynx and that if changes are exhibited, they can be linked more conclusively to various pathological conditions than to normal life-span developmental changes.

References

Albert, M. R. (Ed.). (1984). *Clinical neurology of aging*. New York: Oxford University Press.

Baker, G. T., & Sprott, R. L. (1988). Biomarkers of aging. *Experimental Gerontology, 23,* 233–240.

Bartoshuk, L. M. (1989). Taste: Robust across the age span? In C. Murphy, W. S. Cain, & D. M. Hegsted (Eds.), *Nutrition and the chemical senses in aging: Recent advances and current research needs* (pp. 65–75). New York: Annals of the New York Academy of Sciences.

Bartoshuk, L. M., Rifkin, B., Marks, L. E., & Bars, P. (1986). Taste and aging. *Journal of Gerontology, 41,* 51–57.

Baum, B. J. (1984a). The dentistry-gerontology connection. *Journal of the American Dental Association, 109,* 899–900.

Baum, B. J. (1984b). Normal and abnormal oral status in aging. *Annual Review of Gerontology and Geriatrics, 4,* 87–105.

Baum, B. J. (1986). Salivary gland function during aging. *Gerodontics, 2,* 61–64.

Baum, B. J. (1989). Salivary gland function secretion during aging. *Journal of the American Geriatric Society, 37,* 453–458.

Berry, W. (Ed.). (1983). *Clinical dysarthria*. Austin, TX: PRO-ED.

Bertram, U. (1967). Xerostomia. *Acta Odontologica Scandanavia, 25*(Suppl. 49).

Blitzer, A. (1989). Swallowing disorders and aspiration in the elderly. In J. Goldstein, H. Kashima, & C. Koopmann (Eds.), *Geriatric*

otorhinolaryngology (pp. 124–133). Toronto: B. C. Decker.

Breustedt, A. (1983). Age-induced changes in the oral mucosa and their therapeutic consequences. *International Dental Journal, 33*(3), 272–280.

Buchholz, D. W., Bosma, J. F., & Donner, M. W. (1985). Adaptation, compensation, and decompensation of the pharyngeal swallow. *Gastrointestinal Radiology, 10,* 235–239.

Cain, W. S., & Stevens, J. C. (1989). Uniformity of olfactory loss in aging. In C. Murphy, W. S. Cain, & D. M. Hegsted (Eds.), *Nutrition and the chemical senses in aging: Recent advances and current research needs* (pp. 29–338). New York: Annals of the New York Academy of Sciences.

Campbell, M. J., McComas, A. J., & Petito, F. (1973). Physiological changes in aging muscles. *Journal of Neurosurgery and Psychiatry, 36,* 174–182.

Caruso, A. J., Sonies, B. C., Fox, P. C., & Atkinson, J. (1989). Objective measures of swallowing in patients with primary Sjogren's syndrome. *Dysphagia, 4*(2), 101–105.

Chauhan, J., & Hawrysh, Z. J. (1988). Suprathreshold sour taste intensity and pleasantness perception with age. *Physiology and Behavior, 43,* 601–607.

Cowart, B. J. (1989). Relationship between taste and smell across the adult life span. In C. Murphy, W. S. Cain, & D. M. Hegsted (Eds.), *Nutrition and the chemical senses in aging: Recent advances and current research needs* (pp. 39–55). New York: Annals of the New York Academy of Sciences.

Dayan, D., Abrahami, I., Buchner, A., Gorsky, M., & Chimovitz, N. (1988). Lipid pigment (lipofuscin) in human perioral muscles with aging. *Experimental Gerontology, 23,* 97–102.

de Bont, L. G. M., Liem, R. S. B., & Boering, G. (1985). Ultrastructure of the articular cartilage of the mandibular condyle: Aging and generation. *Oral Surgery, Oral Medicine, Oral Pathology, 60,* 631–641.

DeWilde, P. C. M., Baak, J. P. A., van Houwellingen, J. C., Kater, L., & Slootweg, P. J. (1986). Morphometric study of histological changes in sublabial salivary glands due to aging process. *Journal of Clinical Pathology, 39,* 406–417.

Eastwood, G. L. (1984). G. I. problems in the elderly. *Geriatrics, 39*(5), 59–60, 64, 69–70.

Elliott, J. L. (1988). Swallowing disorders in the elderly: A guide to diagnosis and treatment. *Geriatrics, 43,* 1, 95–100, 104, 113.

Fanous, N. (1987). Aging lips—Esthetic analysis and correction. *Facial Plastic Surgery, 4,* 179–183.

Fucci, D., Petrosino, L., Harris, D., & Randolph-Tyler, E. (1987). Effects of aging on responses to suprathreshold lingual vibrotactile stimulation. *Perceptual and Motor Skills, 64,* 683–694.

Ganguly, R., Stablein, J., Lockey, R. F., Shamblin, P., & Vargas, L. (1986). Defective antimicrobial function of oral secretion in the elderly. *The Journal of Infectious Diseases, 153,* 163–164.

Greenwell, H., & Bissada, N. F. (1989). Factors influencing periodontal therapy for the geriatric patient. *Dental Clinics of North America, 33*(1), 91–100.

Groher, M. E., & Bukatman, R. (1986). The prevalence of swallowing disorders in two teaching hospitals. *Dysphagia, 1,* 3–6.

Hayflick, L. (1987). The cell biology and theoretical basis of human aging. In L. L. Carstensen & B. L. Edelstein (Eds.), *Handbook of clinical gerontology* (pp. 3–17). New York: Pergamon Press.

Hayflick, L. (1989). Cell biology of human aging. In J. Goldstein, H. Kashima, & C. Koopmann, Jr. (Eds.), *Geriatric otorhinolaryngology* (pp. 8–18). Toronto: B. C. Decker.

Hughes, C. V., Baum, B. J., Fox, P. C., Marmary, Y., Yeh, C., & Sonies, B. C. (1987). Oral-pharyngeal dysphagia: A common sequela of salivary gland dysfunction. *Dysphagia, 1,* 173–177.

Johns, D. F. (Ed.). (1978). *Clinical management of neurogenic communicative disorders.* Austin, TX: PRO-ED.

Kennedy III, J. G., & Kent, R. D. (1985). Anatomy and physiology of deglutition and related functions. In W. H. Perkins & J. L. Northern (Eds.), *Seminars in speech and language* (pp. 257–273). New York: Thieme.

Kenshalo, D. R., Sr. (1986). Somesthetic sensitivity in young and elderly humans. *Journal of Gerontology, 41,* 732–742.

Kollmann, W., & Mijatovic, E. (1985). Age-dependent changes in thermoperception in human anterior teeth. *Archives of Oral Biology, 30*(10), 711–715.

Kullaa-Mikkonen, A., Koponen, A., & Seilonen, A. (1987). Quantitative study of human fungiform papillae and taste buds: Variation with aging and in different morphological forms of the tongue. *Gerodontics, 3,* 131–135.

Larson, C. (1985). Neuro-physiology of speech and swallowing. In W. H. Perkins & J. L. Northern (Eds.), *Seminars in speech and language* (pp. 275–291). New York: Thieme.

Larsson, L. (1978). Morphological and functional characteristics of the aging skeletal muscle in man. A cross-sectional study. *Acta Physiologica Scandanavia, 457*(Suppl.), 1–36.

Leese, G., & Hopwood, D. (1986). Muscle fibre typing in the human pharyngeal constrictors and oesophagus: The effect of aging. *Acta Anatomica, 127,* 77–80.

Leopold, D. A., Bartoshuk, L., Doty, R. L., Jafek, B., Smith, D. V., & Snow, J. B. (1989). Aging of the upper airway and the senses of taste and smell. *Otolaryngology—Head and Neck Surgery, 100*(4), 287–289.

Logemann, J. (1983). *Evaluation and treatment of swallowing disorders.* Austin, TX: PRO-ED.

Lyles, K. W. (1989). Osteoporosis. In W. N. Kelly (Ed.), *Internal medicine* (Vol. 2, pp. 2601–2607). Philadelphia: Lippincott.

Masoro, E. J. (1988). Physiological system markers of aging. *Experimental Gerontology, 23,* 391–394.

McNeil, M. R., Rosenbek, J. C., & Aronson, A. E. (Eds.). (1984). *The dysarthrias: Physiology, acoustics, perception, management.* San Diego, CA: College Hill Press.

Meyer, J., Golden, J. S., Steiner, N., & Necheles, H. (1937). The ptyalin content of human saliva in old age. *American Journal of Physiology, 119,* 600–602.

Miller, J. I., Jr. (1988). Human taste bud density across adult age groups. *Journal of Gerontology: Biological Sciences, 43,* B26–B30.

Miller, J. I., Jr. (1989). Variation in human taste bud density as a function of age. In C. Murphy, W. S. Cain, & D. M. Hegsted (Eds.), *Nutrition and the chemical senses in aging: Recent advances and current research needs* (pp. 307–319). New York: Annals of the New York Academy of Sciences.

Mistretta, C. M. (1989). Anatomy and neurophysiology of the taste system in aged animals. In C. Murphy, W. S. Cain, & D. M. Hegsted (Eds.), *Nutrition and the chemical senses in aging: Recent advances and current research needs* (pp. 277–290). New York: Annals of the New York Academy of Sciences.

Morley, J. E., & Silver, A. J. (1988). [Review of *Anorexia in the Elderly*]. *Neurobiology of Aging, 9,* 9–16.

Morrell, R. M. (1984). The neurology of swallowing. In M. E. Groher (Ed.), *Dysphagia: Diagnosis and management* (pp. 3–35). Stoneham, MA: Butterworth.

Mortimer, J. A. (1988). Human motor behavior and aging. *Annals of the New York Academy of Sciences, 515,* 54–66.

Murphy, C. (1985). Cognitive and chemosensory influences on age-related changes in the ability to identify blended foods. *Journal of Gerontology, 40,* 47–52.

Newton, J. P., Abel, R. W., Robertson, E. M., & Yemm, R. (1987). Changes in human masseter and medial pterygoid muscles with age: A study by computed tomography. *Gerodontics, 3,* 151–154.

Norton, L. A. (1988). The effects of aging cellular mechanisms on tooth movement. *Dental Clinics of North America, 32*(3), 437–446.

Ofstehage, J. C., & Magilvy, K. (1986). Oral health and aging. *Geriatric Nursing, 7*(5), 238–241.

Papapanou, P. N., Wennstrom, J. L., & Grondahl, K. (1988). Periodontal status in relation to age and tooth type. A cross-sectional radiographic study. *Journal of Clinical Periodontology, 15,* 469–478.

Pedersen, W., Schubert, M., Izutsu, K., Mersai, T., & Truelove, E. (1985). Age-dependent decreases in human submandibular gland flow rates as measured under resting and post-stimulation conditions. *Journal of Dental Research, 64*(5), 822–825.

Pelemans, W., & Vantrappen, G. (1985). Oesophageal disease in the elderly. *Clinical Gastroenterology, 14*(4), 635–656.

Rastatter, M. P., McGuire, A., Bushong, L., & Loposky, M. (1987). Speech-motor equivalence in aging subjects. *Perceptual and Motor Skills, 64,* 635–638.

Reiter, D., & Weintraub, G. S. (1984). Cosmetic considerations of dental arch form and function in managing the aging face. *Ear, Nose and Throat Journal, 63*(9), 432–439.

Rosenbek, J. C., McNeil, M. R., & Aronson, A. E. (Eds). (1984). *Apraxia of speech, physiology, acoustics, linguistics: Management*. San Diego, CA: College Hill Press.

Satoh, Y., & Seluk, W. L. (1988). Taste threshold, anatomical form of fungiform papillae and aging in humans. *Journal of Nihon University School of Dentistry, 30,* 22–29.

Schiffman, S. S., & Warwick, Z. S. (1988). Flavor enhancement of foods for the elderly can reverse anorexia. *Neurobiology of Aging, 9,* 24–26.

Scott, J., Flower, E. A., & Burns, J. (1987). A quantitative study of histological changes in the human parotid gland occurring with adult age. *Journal of Oral Pathology, 16,* 505–510.

Siebens, H., Trupe, E., Siebens, A., et al. (1986). Correlates and consequences of eating dependency in institutionalized elderly. *Journal of the American Geriatric Society, 24,* 192–198.

Sonies, B. C. (1987). Oral motor problems. In H. G. Mueller & V. C. Geoffrey (Eds.), *Communication disorders in aging: Assessment and management* (pp. 185–213). Washington, DC: Gallaudet University Press.

Sonies, B. C., Baum, B. J., & Shawker, T. H. (1984). Tongue motion in the elderly: Initial *in situ* observation. *Journal of Gerontology, 39*(3), 279–283.

Sonies, B. C., & Caruso, A. J. (1990). The aging process and its potential impact on measures of oral sensorimotor function. *ASHA Reports, 19,* 114–125.

Sonies, B. C., Parent, L. J., Morrish, K., & Baum, B. J. (1988). Durational aspects of the oral-pharyngeal phase of swallow in normal adults. *Dysphagia, 3,* 1–10.

Sonies, B. C., Ship, J. A., & Baum, B. J. (1989). Relationship between saliva production and oropharyngeal swallow in healthy, different-aged adults. *Dysphagia, 4*(2), 85–89.

Sonies, B. C., Stone, M., & Shawker, T. (1984). Speech and swallowing in the elderly. *Gerodontology, 3*(2), 115–123.

Spitzer, M. E. (1988). Taste acuity in institutionalized and noninstitutionalized elderly men. *Journal of Gerontology: Psychological Sciences, 43,* P71–P74.

Stevens, J. C., & Cain, W. S. (1986a). Aging and the perception of nasal irritation. *Physiology and Behavior, 37,* 323–328.

Stevens, J. C., & Cain, W. S. (1986b). Smelling via the mouth: Effect of aging. *Perception and Psychophysics, 40*(3), 142–146.

Stone, M. (1990). A three-dimensional model of tongue movement based on ultrasound and X-ray microbeam data. *Journal of the Acoustical Society of America, 87*(5), 2207–2217.

Thomson, A. B. R., & Keelan, A. (1986). The aging gut. *Canadian Journal of Physiology and Pharmacology, 64*(1), 30–38.

Tracy, J. F., Logeman, J. A., Kahrilas, P. J., Jacob, P., Kobasa, M., & Krugler, C. (1988). *Preliminary observation on the effects of age on oropharyngeal deglutition.* Paper presented at American Speech-Language-Hearing Association National Conference, Boston.

Walshe, J. M. (1987). Neurologic examination of the elderly patient. Signs of normal aging. *Postgraduate Medicine, 81*(4), 375–378.

Weiffenbach, J. M., Cowart, B. J., & Baum, B. J. (1986). Taste intensity perception in aging. *Journal of Gerontology, 41,* 460–468.

Weiffenbach, J. M., Tylenda, C., & Baum, B. J. (in press). Oral sensory changes in aging. *Journal of Gerontology.*

Weindreich, R., & Walford, R. L. (1988). *The retardation of aging and disease by dietary restriction.* Springfield, IL: Charles C Thomas.

Welford, A. T. (1984). Between bodily changes and performance: Some possible reasons for slowing with age. *Experimental Aging Research, 10*(2), 73–88.

Welford, A. T. (1988). Reaction time, speed of performance, and age. *Annals of the New York Academy of Sciences, 515,* 1–17.

Williams, P. L., Warwick, R., Dyson, M., & Bannister, L. H. (1989). *Gray's anatomy.* London: Churchill Livingstone.

Wilson, D. L. (1988). Aging hypothesis, aging markers and the concept of biological age. *Experimental Gerontology, 23,* 435–438.

Wysocki, C. J., & Gilbert, A. N. (1989). National Geographic smell survey: Effects of age are heterogenous. In C. Murphy, W. S. Cain, & D. M. Hegsted (Eds.), *Nutrition and the chemical senses in aging: Recent advances and current research needs* (pp. 12–28). New York: Annals of the New York Academy of Sciences.

Speech Motor Control and Aging

CHAPTER

Gary Weismer, PhD, and Julie M. Liss, PhD ■

This chapter deals with speech motor control in aged individuals. When we use the term "speech motor control," we refer to a larger domain of inquiry than might be assumed by some contemporary researchers. For example, the edited text *Speech Motor Control* (Grillner, Lindblom, Lubker, & Persson, 1982) contains a number of papers that discuss the electromyographic and kinematic characteristics of speech production behavior. This is the kind of work that many speech scientists would take to be the proper domain of "speech motor control research." Presumably, the assumption that other types of speech production analyses (e.g., acoustic) cannot reveal much about motor control processes derives from the intense effort among neurophysiologists to identify the precise neural mechanisms underlying movement. There is a good deal of thought, however, that systems should not be con-ceptualized as having a level or levels of analysis that are more important than other levels for an ultimate understanding of a phenomenon or process (Bunge, 1977). All levels of a process—like communication—are regarded as equally important to the understanding of that process, and the goal of reducing the phenomena of one level to those of another level is viewed as counterproductive. This antireductionist, scientific program has been summarized succinctly by Gardner (1985, p. 286): ". . . one cannot have an adequate theory about anything the brain does unless one also has an adequate theory about that activity itself."

For the purposes of this chapter, the domain of speech motor control is taken to include, or be affected by, (a) anatomical factors—that is, possible remodeling of speech mechanism structures, both central and peripheral, as a function of aging; (b) peripheral physiological factors—that is, the

The writing of this chapter was supported in part by NIH Awards Nos. 18797 and 22345.

muscular contraction patterns that are reflected in the force, movement, and aerodynamic characteristics of respiratory, laryngeal, and supralaryngeal function for speech; and (c) cognitive factors—that is, computational changes (Cerella, 1985) that are assumed to reflect the various changes in the central nervous system that are a consequence of aging. Obviously these three factors are not mutually exclusive, but our discussion will at times necessitate an artificial separation of their potential effects on speech motor control. In summary, we regard speech motor control as a process that is affected by a broad array of factors that bear on the production of spoken language.

This chapter is divided into sections dealing with age-related anatomical and physiological changes that occur in the respiratory, laryngeal, supraglottal, and nervous systems. Within each of these sections, the available data will be reviewed, and some attempt will be made to develop reasonable predictions regarding the effects of these changes on the speech of the aged. Where possible, these predictions will be compared to the available data, but as will become clear, there is not an abundance of data on speech production characteristics in aging individuals. One of the main purposes of this chapter is to provide a research map for future studies of speech motor control in the aged.

General Anatomical Changes with Aging

Many of the anatomical changes to be discussed in this section are not specific to the speech mechanism, but are characteristic of the aging animal. In general, striated muscle fibers atrophy and lose elasticity and contractile power because of decrements in sensorimotor innervation and increased density of connective tissue. The working surfaces of joints become eroded with age, leading to increased friction with movement and a consequent reduction in range of motion. Nonmuscular tissue, including cartilage, tendons, membranes, and specialized tissue (such as alveolar structures) tend to become stiffer. As will be discussed in the following sections of this chapter, these changes are characteristic of structures at all levels of the speech mechanism. Because these structural changes are treated in detail in other chapters of this volume, the strategy here will be only to identify the *relevant* structural changes that occur with age and to address in greater depth the functional consequences for speech motor control.

Speech Breathing

Table 12.1 contains a brief synopsis of the anatomical changes associated with aging in the respiratory system and their functional implications. The first column of the table lists relevant structural changes, the second column the associated functional implications, and the third column the expected influences on speech breathing.

Anatomically, the aging respiratory system is characterized by decreased elasticity of lung tissue, an increase of the connective tissue of muscle, ossification of cartilaginous structures, and degeneration of nerve fibers and sensory receptors (see Knudson, 1989, for a review). The known functional effects of these changes on general respiratory function are that overall alveolar relaxation pressures are *higher* at corresponding lung volumes when compared to young adults,[1] muscle strength is diminished, and ventilatory frequency is much more variable. In addition, it is likely that diminished sensorimotor integrity of the respiratory system

---

[1]We have found no published studies that provide a direct comparison of alveolar relaxation pressures in older and younger subjects. It may be inferred from studies of aging effects on chest wall and pulmonary compliance (e.g., Mittman, Edelman, Morris, & Shock, 1965) that, at corresponding lung volumes, older subjects have higher alveolar relaxation pressures than younger subjects.

TABLE 12.1
Synopsis of Age-Related Anatomical Changes in the Respiratory System, the Functional Changes Associated with These Changes, and the Implications for Speech Breathing

Anatomical Changes	Functional Changes	Implications for Speech
Increased stiffness of respiratory structures	Increased relaxation pressure at corresponding lung volumes	Adjustments in starting lung volumes for speech
Muscular weakness Atrophy and increased fibrotic content of muscle	Diminished pressure-generating capability at a given lung volume	Reduced stress contrasts; less extreme "posturing" of chest wall for speech production
Degeneration of nerve fibers and sensory receptors	Loss of appreciation of absolute lung volumes, lung volume changes, and precision of motor commands	Less efficient and more variable lung volume usage for utterance
Less efficient gas exchange	Higher breathing frequency	Short phrases

would lead to decreased appreciation for respiratory positions and volumes.

Given these changes, one might predict the following changes in speech breathing with aging. First, it might be expected that starting lung volumes for utterances would be lower than those observed in young adults because of the greater stiffness of the aged system. It has been found that younger speakers typically initiate their utterances at roughly 60% of vital capacity, a lung volume at which alveolar relaxation pressures closely approximate the subglottal pressure requirements of speech (Hixon, Goldman, & Mead, 1973; Weismer, 1985). If older speakers were to inspire for utterance initiation to comparable lung volumes, they would not only have to work harder to reach that point, but the alveolar relaxation pressure at that lung volume might be somewhat in excess of the desired subglottal pressure for speech. The small amount of data that exist on starting lung volumes for utterance in older subjects indicates, however, that geriatric men actually initiate their utterances at *higher* lung volumes than young adults (Hoit & Hixon, 1987).

Hoit and Hixon (1987) explain this finding in terms of compensation for a leaky laryngeal valve, which they infer from larger volumes per syllable expired by the

older men during utterance (see also Benjamin, 1986). It is possible, however, that both the higher starting lung volumes and greater volume per syllable might be explained by greater phonatory intensities (i.e., higher subglottal pressures) among old as compared to young speakers. Because Hoit and Hixon (1987) did not report data on phonatory intensity or subglottal pressure, the effect of this variable on their data is unknown.

Another explanation for the counterintuitive finding of higher starting lung volumes for older speakers is that the decreased elasticity of lung tissue in older speakers potentially decreases the sensitivity of lung stretch receptors, making sensory feedback for lung volume less efficient; speakers then seek out higher starting lung volumes for utterances to augment the sensory feedback using stretch receptors in the chest wall (e.g., muscle spindles). The notion that speakers may adjust their starting lung volumes for speech to enhance sensory feedback from respiratory stretch receptors has been posited previously by Hixon (1982) to explain the low starting lung volumes exhibited by deaf individuals. One way to test the hypothesis of decreased appreciation of lung volumes for speech breathing would be to test subjects' abilities to match starting lung volumes across trials or to replicate lung volume excursions across trials for various types of utterance. The prediction would be that older adults would be less proficient (less accurate and more variable) in these tasks when compared to younger adults. To our knowledge, such studies have not been performed.

Although the relevant data are not available, there are other characteristics of speech breathing in the aged that might be expected from the anatomical and physiological changes just described. Phrase length, for example, is often measured either by the number of syllables produced per breath group or by the duration of the breath group. It should be obvious that neither of these measures can be related to lung volume usage for speech in a simple way. A small number of syllables per breath group could be produced over a small or large range of lung volumes, depending on the speaking rate, and the duration of a breath group may be affected by the efficiency of downstream valving at the larynx and upper articulators. In addition, changes in respiratory sensation with age may affect lung volume usage for utterances. That is, faulty or diminished sensory feedback could influence the breath group component of linguistic planning, use of afferent information to guide respiratory motor behavior, or both. For example, one prediction would be that the amount of lung volume displaced for utterances would be more variable for older than for younger speakers.

Hoit and Hixon (1987) have reported that elderly speakers use greater lung volume ranges for utterances and produce fewer syllables per breath group, when compared to young adult speakers. They attribute these differences to the elderly speakers' need to compensate for a less efficient laryngeal valve. If the reported age differences in lung volume usage remained after older and younger speakers were matched on laryngeal resistance (Smitheran & Hixon, 1981), speaking rate, and speech output level, this compensation hypothesis would not be supported. The speaking rate issue is important, because it is known that

older subjects speak more slowly than younger subjects (Smith, Wasowicz, & Preston, 1987), and the Hoit and Hixon data could be explained on the basis of age-related differences in speaking rate, which are not reported in their study. There is controversy in the literature regarding the phonatory intensities of older speakers (Hollien, 1987), which emphasizes the need to control this variable in speech breathing experiments.

In physiological terms, linguistic stress is classically associated with an increase in subglottal pressure and vibratory rate of the vocal folds (Lehiste, 1970). One might expect that a stiffer respiratory system associated with advanced age would reduce the elderly speaker's ability to raise the subglottal pressure above the "background" pressure and thus create a perceptual impression of reduced stress contrasts or monotony. However, perceptual studies of age identification from speech samples (e.g., Hartman, 1979; Hartman & Danhauer, 1976; Ryan & Burke, 1974) have not identified lack of stress contrasts or monotony as a significant feature of aged speech, and Benjamin (1986) has actually reported that elderly speakers use larger fundamental frequency (F0) swings in speech compared to younger speakers. This suggests that the age-related changes in the respiratory system are not sufficiently great to affect prosodic integrity, or that speakers compensate for the changes in an effective way.

If decreased muscle strength in the respiratory system has an effect on speech breathing, it may be seen in the chest wall configurations adopted for speech production by aged individuals. Hixon et al. (1973) have shown that normal, young adult speakers use a substantial amount of abdominal muscle activity to "posture" the chest wall for speech production. It may be that the older speaker does not use such extensive contraction of the abdominal muscles during speech (see Figure 12.1). Because Hixon, Mead, and Goldman (1976) have argued that the abdominal contraction seen in younger individuals serves to place

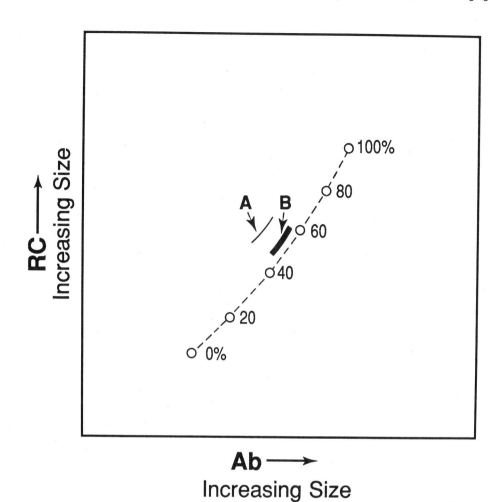

FIGURE 12.1. Schematic example of how weakened muscles of the respiratory system might affect chest wall configuration for speech production. A *motion-motion* diagram (Hixon, Goldman, & Mead, 1973) is shown, in which abdominal size is shown on the abscissa and rib cage size on the ordinate. The dotted line connecting open circles is the *relaxation configuration* of the chest wall throughout the vital capacity range; 20% increments of vital capacity are indicated along this function. This function shows the simultaneous rib cage–abdomen sizes when all muscles are relaxed. The line labeled "A" shows the successive chest wall configurations (i.e., simultaneous rib cage–abdomen size) for a hypothetical utterance produced by a young adult. Note that this trace is substantially to the *left* of the relaxation line, indicating a large amount of abdominal muscle contraction (smaller abdominal size) as a "posturing" of the chest wall for speech. The trace labeled "B" shows a hypothetical utterance for a geriatric speaker. Note that this utterance is closer to the relaxation configuration, indicating less forceful contractions of the abdominal musculature. A general prediction that follows from weaker respiratory muscles in older, as compared to younger, speakers is that utterances produced by older speakers will tend to fall closer to the relaxation configuration than utterances produced by younger speakers.

the diaphragm in an optimal position for inter-utterance, inspiratory refills, we might expect the older speaker to produce shallower and slower inspiratory refills. Unfortunately, observations of chest wall configuration and inter-utterance inspiratory behavior have not been reported for older individuals.

Laryngeal Function

Table 12.2 contains a synopsis of age-related laryngeal changes and their functional implications. Excellent reviews of the effects of aging on the human larynx have been written by Kahane (1981, 1987; Kahane & Beckford, chapter 10 of this volume). These changes include increases in the stiffness of laryngeal structures as a result of ossification of cartilages, decreased elasticity of connective tissue in muscle, and erosion of joint surfaces and basement membrane (see also Kahn & Kahane, 1986). There is also a decrease in the number of mucous glands, leading to an increased viscosity of the vocal folds (see Gracco, 1988). We would also presume, based on general patterns of nerve degeneration with aging, degeneration of nerve fibers subserving afferent and efferent functions of the larynx. The functional implications of these changes are a decreased mobility of the overall laryngeal framework, decreased efficiency of muscle contraction, reduced range of motion at laryngeal joints, increased viscosity of vocal fold tissue, and diminished sensorimotor integrity.[2]

These changes may explain some well-known alterations in phonatory function that are associated with aging. Examples of these alterations include changes in habitual F0 (Hollien & Shipp, 1972; McGlone & Hollien, 1963); changes in voice quality, usually characterized by increased noise in the glottal spectrum (perceptually, increased breathiness—see Ramig, 1986); modification of the articulatory function of the larynx (Weismer & Fromm, 1983); and loss of stability in laryngeal function, as evidenced by increased jitter, shimmer, and F0 variability in the aged population (Linville, 1988; Ramig, Scherer, & Titze, 1986; Wilcox &

Horii, 1980). In addition, it might be expected that the dynamic range for fundamental frequency and phonatory intensity would be reduced with age, but relevant data are lacking.

Because phonation requires complex coordination among muscles, joints, and mucosal surfaces, it is difficult to determine precisely which age-related anatomical changes correspond to phonatory changes. It is likely, however, that increased stiffness of laryngeal structures could account for all the phonatory changes described above. The increased viscosity of the vocal folds would have an effect on their vibratory pattern, and hence on the glottal spectrum and voice quality. The degeneration of the nervous supply of the larynx may contribute, at least in part, to all the changes described above, with perhaps most specific effects on the articulatory function of the larynx.

For the purposes of this chapter, the articulatory function of the larynx will be taken to include the production of sentence-level F0 contours, the marking of syntactic boundaries by laryngealization, and the devoicing of voiceless obstruents (the laryngeal devoicing gesture). Intuitively, one might expect increased stiffness of the laryngeal structures to result in a relative flattening of F0 contours in aged persons. One relevant study, however, suggests that older subjects produce *larger* swings in sentence-level F0 when compared to young adult speakers (Benjamin, 1981, 1986). It is possible, however, that in the production of "laboratory utterances" this difference represents a social cohort effect (Birren & Cunningham, 1985) whereby older persons value expression in formal speaking situations more than young adults. One possible way to corroborate Benjamin's findings under more natural circumstances would be

---

[2]It must be noted that aging effects on the larynx are quite different for men and women. Specifically, males seem to lose elasticity and mass of the vocal fold because of increased connective tissue in muscle and ossification of cartilage, whereas postmenopausal women seem to gain vocal fold mass, primarily as a result of edema (Honjo & Isshiki, 1980). These facts may explain why the F0 of males rises with age and the F0 of women decreases or stays roughly constant with age (Hollien, 1987; Hollien & Shipp, 1972; McGlone & Hollien, 1963). Morrison and Gore-Hickman (1986) have also argued that the general deterioration of the larynx with age is worse in males than in females. The implication of these considerations is that theories of the effects of aging on laryngeal control for speech will have to be sex-specific.

TABLE 12.2
Synopsis of Age-Related Anatomical and Functional Changes in the Larynx and Their Implications for Speech Production

Anatomical Changes	Functional Changes	Implications for Speech
Ossification of cartilages	Decreased mobility of laryngeal framework	Reduced ability to change pitch; decreased dynamic ranges
Increased stiffness of muscle tissue, due to thinning and increased connective tissue	Decreased efficiency of muscle contraction; loss of vibratory mass	Higher F0 (men); reduced adductory force for vocal fold closure; reduced abductory force for laryngeal devoicing gesture (LDG)
Increased edema	Increase of vibratory mass	Lower F0 (women)
Erosion of joint surfaces	Reduced range of motion at joints	Shortened LDG; reduced maximum range for F0
Decrease in number of mucous glands	Increased viscosity of vocal fold tissue	Increased jitter and shimmer; thus "noisy" glottal spectra
Degeneration of nerves and sensory receptors	Less efficient sensorimotor function	Increased jitter, plus variability of F0

to examine F0 swings in the casual speech of older and younger subjects. Morgan and Rastatter (1986) investigated the variability of F0 of women who were producing spontaneous speech (a description of the Cookie Thief picture on the *Boston Diagnostic Aphasia Examination*), and found that the older women had *less* F0 fluctuation than the younger women, apparently contradicting Benjamin's finding. Additional work in this area is required to understand better the effect of age on F0 and intensity variability in aged speakers.

Laryngealization, a variant of the glottal stop (Priestly, 1976; Umeda, 1982), is often used to mark the onset of a syntactic phrase that is initiated by a vowel (Umeda, 1982). It is possible that the compression of laryngeal structures required to produce the laryngeal configuration for laryngealization would be compromised by the increased stiffness (see Kahane, 1987, p. 28) and decreased integrity of the laryngeal nervous supply in aged speakers. An acoustic study of the occurrence of laryngealization in

casual speech could also provide insight into this issue.

The laryngeal devoicing gesture is a relatively slow opening and closing gesture of the vocal folds that occurs during the production of voiceless obstruents (Weismer, 1980). The gesture is produced by an interplay between the posterior cricoarytenoid muscle, which initiates the separation of the folds, and the interarytenoids, which are active during the closure phase of the gesture (Hirose, 1976). There is evidence that the degree of movement at the cricoarytenoid joint is diminished in elderly speakers, and perhaps especially in elderly males. The reduction of movement is probably the result of several factors, including decreased efficiency of the posterior cricoarytenoid muscles and reduced range of motion at the cricoarytenoid joints. One consequence of reduced range of motion at the cricoarytenoid joint for speech motor control is that the laryngeal devoicing gesture will be shorter in older, as compared to younger, speakers. Several different types of acoustic data support this prediction. Weismer and Fromm (1983) found that the *voiceless interval*—the acoustic measurement that is an index of the duration of the laryngeal devoicing gesture—was significantly shorter in older, as compared to younger, speakers. These data are consistent with other reports (Liss, Weismer, & Rosenbek, 1990; Smith et al., 1987; Sweeting & Baken, 1982) suggesting that older speakers have shorter voice-onset times (VOTs) than younger speakers. Most of these acoustic studies have been done using male speakers, but at least one comparison of older and younger female speakers (Neiman, Klich, & Shuey, 1983) did not find an age-related VOT difference, raising the possibility that the age effect described above is sex-specific. This issue may have some theoretical importance because of the notion in the literature that the male larynx ages more rapidly than the female larynx (Kahane, 1987; and see Footnote 2).

The investigation of changes of the articulatory function of the larynx with age may also be important for the understanding of neurogenic disorders such as Parkinson's disease. Weismer (1984) found that the voiceless interval duration and the VOT in Parkinson's disease were substantially shorter than they were in elderly men (aged 65–82 years). This was interpreted as reflecting the exaggeration of aging effects of the larynx that may accompany Parkinson's disease. This notion was addressed by Liss et al. (1990), who studied selected acoustic characteristics of very old males (aged 87–93 years) who were free of neurogenic disease and found that the VOTs were more like those of Weismer's (1984) Parkinson's patients than they were like those of his younger geriatric speakers. This suggests that at least some of the pathological changes associated with Parkinson's disease occur to some degree with advanced age. The implication is that the study of speech characteristics in Parkinson's dysarthria may provide insights into the changes in speech motor control that occur with aging.

Supraglottal Function

Table 12.3 provides a synopsis of supraglottal changes with age and their functional effects. Unfortunately, there has been little anatomical work in this area. One way to conceptualize these effects is in terms of (a) changes in the articulators (where articulators are defined as moving structures) and (b) changes in the oropharyngeal environment. A general summary statement concerning the nonbony supraglottal articulators (including the pharynx, velum, tongue, and lips) is that the muscles tend to become atrophied and fibrotic with age, and the associated oral mucosa of some of these structures becomes keratinized (Baum, 1981; Cohen & Gitman, 1959; Massler, 1971). The jaw, the only bony articulator, undergoes remodeling with age. This remodeling is characterized by bone growth, in the form of a lengthening of the body of the mandible (Israel, 1971), and bone resorption, most notably associated with tooth loss in the alveolar region (Langer, 1976). Movement of the jaw is potentially affected by degenerative changes in the relevant muscles (such as the pterygoids, masseter, and temporalis) and in the way these muscles act upon a degenerating temporomandibular joint (Blackwood, 1969; Moffett, Johnson, McCabe, & Askew, 1964).

Changes in the oral environment with age include loss of elasticity of the oral mucosa, general drying of oropharyngeal tissues resulting from diminished function of the salivary glands (Baum, 1981; Massler, 1971), and the possibility of a general increase in vocal tract size (Israel, 1971). In addition, loss of teeth in old age changes the dimensions and boundaries of the working space in the oral cavity. Another possible source of modification of the dimensions and boundaries of the vocal tract would be the atrophy of sublingual, buccal, velar, and pharyngeal musculature.

It can be inferred from certain functional data that the neural supply of the orofacial region also deteriorates with age. There is

TABLE 12.3
Synopsis of Age-Related Anatomical and Functional Changes in Supraglottal Structures and Their Implications for Speech Production

Anatomical Changes	Functional Changes	Implications for Speech
Atrophy and fibrosis of muscle	Reduced range, speed, and accuracy of structural movement	Reduced phonetic working space; slowness of articulatory movements
Keratinization of oral mucosa; drying of oral tissue	Increased viscosity between mucosal surfaces	Increased phases of articulatory contacts
Remodeling of jaw; degeneration of temporomandibular joint	Potential changes in muscle-load relations; reduced range and ease of motion	Reorganization of coordinative function of articulators
Modification of vocal tract dimensions, including tooth loss	Rescaling of structural movements	
Degeneration of nerves and sensory receptors	Diminished appreciation for and efficiency of structural position, movement, and contact	Variability in force of articulatory contacts; loss of precision in articulatory contacts; changing patterns of interarticulatory coordination

a documented decrease with age of touch, pressure, and vibratory sensitivity (see Baum & Bodner, 1983; Curtis & Fucci, 1983; and Kahane, 1981, for reviews), indicating a decrease in the integrity of peripheral and/or central sensory function for orofacial structures. Although there is a limited amount of actual histological work on the status of orofacial sensory nerves throughout the life-span, the functional data reviewed above as well as age-related neural degeneration evidenced in other portions of the body (e.g., Ronge, 1943, cited in Kahane, 1981) suggest this kind of degeneration in orofacial structures. Information regarding neuromotor deficits with aging is equally sparse. As Kahane (1981) notes in his review, there may be some neuronal loss in cranial nerve nuclei that subserve motor functions in orofacial musculature, resulting in muscle weakness. Although some investigators have attempted to separate orofacial sensory mechanisms from motor mechanisms (see Borden, 1979, for a review) and have argued that deficits could

be specific to either component (Sonies, Stone, & Shawker, 1984), we contend that aging effects on speech production can best be understood within a *sensorimotor* framework. This is consistent with contemporary ideas in the neurophysiology literature which state that the separation of sensory and motor mechanisms for the understanding of motor control is artificial.

It should be expected that the changes we have noted will manifest themselves in the articulatory behavior of older speakers. Support for this idea can be derived from perceptual studies in which listeners have identified the age of speakers from recorded utterances with high accuracy (e.g., Hartman & Danhauer, 1976; Ryan & Burke, 1974). The potential contributions of each of the supraglottal structures to the articulatory pattern of aged speakers will be summarized next.

Because of degenerative changes in pharyngeal muscles and nerves (Kiuchi, Sasaki, Arai, & Suzuki, 1969; Zaino & Benventano, 1977), the ability to change the dimensions of the pharyngeal tube is probably less efficient in older speakers. A decreased ability to change the dimensions of the pharyngeal tube could influence resonance quality, velopharyngeal closure, and vowel and consonant articulation. The dilation of the pharynx consequent to age-related changes could account for the unique resonant quality present in some older speakers (Ryan & Burke, 1974). The contribution of the lateral pharyngeal walls (LPW) in velopharyngeal closure has been well documented (Kelsey, Woodhouse, & Minifie, 1969; Skolnick, McCall, & Barnes, 1973). A demonstration of age-related deficits in LPW movement could explain the observation of greater nasalance in older versus younger speakers (Hutchinson, Robinson, & Nerbonne, 1978). It has also been demonstrated that the cross-sectional area of the pharyngeal lumen varies as a function of vowel height (Minifie, Hixon, Kelsey, & Woodhouse, 1970). Although it is not known how these variations bear on the acoustic distinctiveness of vowel articulations, it is conceivable that the attenuation of these changes in older speakers could affect precision of vowel articulation. An appropriate test of this hypothesis would involve an ultrasonic study of LPW movement for vowels in older and younger speakers, with corresponding acoustic measurements of vowel formant frequencies. It is also known that the volume of the pharynx is larger for voiced stops than it is for voiceless stops (Bell-Berti, 1975; Kent & Moll, 1969; Westbury, 1983). Presumably, the volume expansion and accompanying increase in surface area over time (Muller & Brown, 1980) for voiced stops serves the purpose of maintaining airflow through the vocal folds, and thus vibration of the vocal folds, to satisfy the phonological requirements of voicing (Rothenberg, 1968). Most investigators feel that the mechanism for this volume expansion is an active one (Bell-Berti, 1975; Minifie et al., 1970; Westbury, 1983), so the issue of muscle atrophy and weakness in the geriatric speaker is important. Specifically, if the geriatric speaker cannot produce the rapid muscular changes

that cause pharyngeal expansion, it is conceivable that the conditions for maintaining vocal fold vibration during a stop closure interval would not be met. This idea could be tested by examining the maintenance of vocal fold vibration during stop closure for voiced stops. The prediction that would follow from these considerations is that the duration of vocal fold vibration throughout a closure interval would be *shorter* for geriatric, as compared to young adult, speakers (see Smith, 1978, for an experiment with relevant methodology).

As noted above, some geriatric speakers have been characterized as having hypernasal speech (Hutchinson et al., 1978; Ryan & Burke, 1974). To fully characterize the velopharyngeal mechanism in geriatric speakers, the coordination of velar elevation and LPW displacement should be studied. Relevant studies would include cinefluoroscopic tracking of points on the velum, nasendoscopic examination of the velopharyngeal port, and electromyographic evaluation of activity of the levator veli palatini and superior constrictor muscles. Studies using these methods with young adult speakers have been reported by Kent, Carney, and Severeid (1974), Skolnick et al. (1973), and Bell-Berti (1976), among others.

The kinds of measures that could provide insight into age effects on lingual articulation include kinematics (displacement, velocity, acceleration), vowel formant frequencies, formant trajectory extents and rates, and spirantization. In addition, inferences regarding lingual function in the elderly have been based on diadochokinesis (e.g., Ptacek, Sander, Maloney, & Jackson, 1966; but compare Shanks, 1970). To our knowledge, there are no kinematic studies that directly compare lingual behavior for speech in old and young subjects. It might be predicted, however, that lingual movements in the elderly would be less extensive and slower than corresponding movements in young speakers. Such a comparison might be confounded by the fact that the extent and rate of lingual movements seem to be partially determined by the size of the vocal tract (Kuehn & Moll,

1976), and the size of the vocal tract may increase with age (Israel, 1971). One way to infer the nature of lingual behavior during speech is to make measurements of formant frequencies associated with vowel production (Fant, 1970). Linville (1987) has summarized her work by claiming that the first and second formant frequencies of the vowel /ae/ produced by women *decrease* with age. She suggests that this decrease reflects either changing articulatory patterns with age (see Sonies, Baum, & Shawker, 1984) or the increasing size of the vocal tract with age reported by Israel (1971). A decrease in vowel formant frequencies with age was also reported by Endres, Bambach, and Flosser (1971), who followed the same male subjects over a period of 29 years; these authors also argue that such trends are due to enlargement of the vocal tract with age. Liss et al. (1990) plotted the F1/F2 space for the point vowels produced by male speakers aged 87–93 years and compared these data to previously reported data for young adults. This comparison suggested that the vowel space of the very old speakers was somewhat compressed relative to the younger speakers, suggesting a slight reduction in the "phonetic working space" among the old speakers.

Acoustic techniques can also be used to compare across groups the rates at which various articulatory gestures are made. The rate of frequency change along a formant transition serves as an index of articulatory rate; higher transition rates suggest faster changes within the vocal tract. Liss et al. (1990) showed that their very old speakers tended to produce lower transition rates than young adult and "younger" geriatric speakers (aged 65–80) (see Figure 12.2). At least one of the transition rates examined by Liss et al. can be interpreted more or less unambiguously in terms of tongue movement, so these data suggest slower tongue movements among very old speakers. These findings should be supported by direct kinematic measures of lingual performance.

The implication that older speakers have less extensive lingual movements for vocalic segments can be extended to the efficiency of constrictive sound production (as in the case of stops and fricatives), where there is a requirement of complete or nearly complete obstruction of the vocal tract. For stop consonant production, inefficiency of the constrictive effort is revealed by *spirantization,* or the occurrence of a leaky (incomplete) constriction during the closure interval. This is evidenced acoustically by the presence of noise energy in the closure interval, which contrasts with the normal case of a silent closure interval (see Figure 12.3). It has been demonstrated by Liss et al. (1990) that the very old males produced spirantization of stop closures at a strikingly high rate of occurrence for both lingual and labial stops. In fact, the very old males spirantized stop closure intervals at a rate that was considerably higher than that of Weismer's (1984) young adults and younger geriatrics, and even higher than that of the Parkinson's disease patients, who typically produce a great number of spirantized stop closure intervals in their speech (Logemann & Fisher, 1981).

As noted above, lingual behavior in the speech production of elderly individuals can be studied most directly using kinematic techniques. Such observations would be especially useful in the evaluation of *compound* lingual movements (Kent, 1986), where the tongue postures for successive sound requirements are integrated into a smooth, continuously evolving gesture. Because coordination of complex movements has often been shown to be deficient in older individuals (e.g., Inglin & Woollacott, 1988), it might be expected that compound tongue movements would be less efficient in the elderly. Whereas the underlying mechanisms for a potential deficit of compound movements or for the spirantization phenomenon are unknown, it should be kept in mind that any such deficit must reflect the integrated sensorimotor functioning of the nervous system. When techniques for the evaluation of orofacial sensory function (Schneider, Diamond, & Markham, 1986) are combined with low-risk techniques for tracking tongue movement

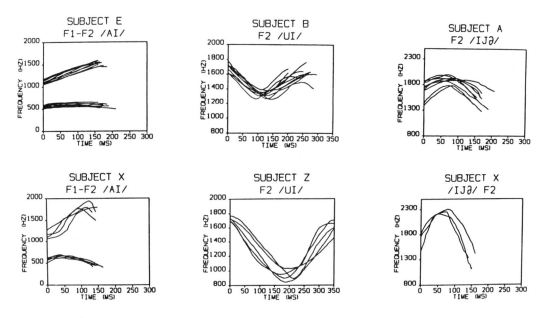

FIGURE 12.2. Comparisons of formant trajectories for three male speakers aged 87–93 (top panels) and three male speakers aged 65–80 (bottom panels). Multiple traces in each panel represent separate trials of the same utterance. Note that for all comparisons, both the frequency range covered by the trajectories and the slopes of the frequency changes are greater for the younger speakers. The trajectories were extracted from sentence materials spoken at preferred (conversational) speaking rates. *Note.* From "Selected Acoustic Characteristics of Speech Production in Very Old Males" by J. M. Liss, G. Weismer, and J. C. Rosenbek, 1990, *Journal of Gerontology: Psychological Sciences, 45,* pp. 35–45. Copyright 1990 by the Gerontological Society of America. Reprinted by permission.

during speech, these mechanisms may be elucidated.

Labial function may be inferred using the same kinds of measures that have been discussed for lingual behavior. In principle, it might be expected that labial articulation would be less affected by aging, because lip function for speech is relatively gross. For example, the lips must close and open for bilabial stop and nasal production and must round and spread for vocalic events. In addition, the lower lip must be retracted against the lower teeth for labiodental productions. There are no data on lip rounding/ spreading or retraction as a function of aging; however, there is evidence (Liss et al., 1990) that very old speakers spirantize bilabial stops to a much greater degree than younger geriatrics or Parkinson's patients. This would seem to suggest that

closing movements of the lips are less extensive in older, as compared to younger, speakers.

Although there are no direct comparisons of closing displacements for bilabial stops across age groups, when the small amount of relevant data from older subjects (Forrest, Weismer, & Turner, 1989) is compared to similar data from younger subjects (e.g., Kelso, Vatikiotis-Bateson, Saltzman, & Kay, 1985; Sussman, MacNeilage, & Hanson, 1973), there do not appear to be differences. However, comparisons of displacement across age groups do not lead to simple statements about underlying mechanisms. Displacement of the lips for adequate bilabial stop production requires appropriate motor programming, proprioception, traction, and mandibular function. It could be, for example that the spirantiza-

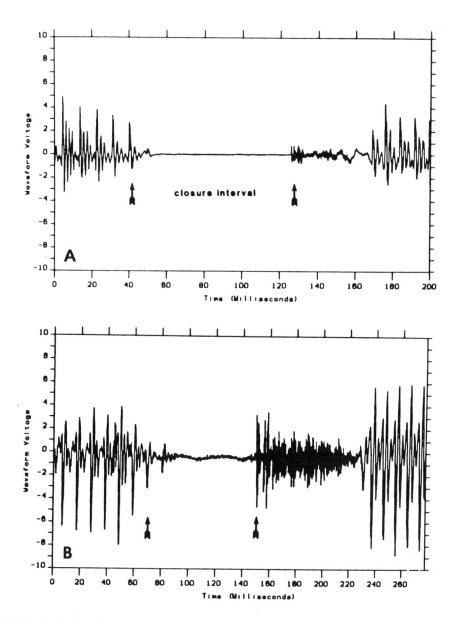

FIGURE 12.3. Waveform analysis of spirantization. Stop consonants produced without spirantization should have quiet closure intervals, as in the interval between the arrows in "A"; stops produced with spirantization will have "noisy" closure intervals, as depicted in the corresponding interval in "B."

tion of bilabial stops in the old speakers studied by Liss et al. (1990) occurred because of impaired sensory function in the lips and/or temporomandibular joint. This reinforces the need for studies of sensory function that go past the available information on sensory thresholds in orofacial structures (e.g., Curtis & Fucci, 1983) and link specific sensory deficits with observed kinematic deficits.

There are no age comparison data on jaw function for speech. We would expect, however, to find aging effects on the articulatory behavior of the mandible because of the documented changes in bony structure, muscles that move the jaw and their associated sensory structures, and the biomechanical and sensory integrity of the temporomandibular joint. The interplay of these several influences of age on jaw function make this a likely structure to reveal the effects of age on articulatory behavior.

To this point the potential effects on articulation in older speakers have been discussed in terms of single articulators. It is obvious, however, that speech production involves the intricate coordination of all articulators to produce an acceptable acoustic output. Investigators have studied this issue by observing patterns of "interarticulator coordination," and measuring temporal and/or spatial regularities between the movements of two or more articulators or between a single articulator and events in the acoustic waveform (Kelso, Saltzman, & Tuller, 1986; Lubker, McAllister, & Lindblom, 1977; Perkell, 1986). Issues of articulatory coordination can also be inferred by studying the acoustic waveform, especially in the case of glottal-supraglottal coordination. It has been shown that when a voiceless stop is preceded by a vowel, supraglottal closure and cessation of vocal fold vibration occur nearly simultaneously (see Lofqvist & Yoshioka, 1984, for a review). Acoustically, this is reflected by the cessation of the voicing pulses at the boundary of the vocalic formant pattern and the silent interval, as shown in Figure 12.4. Weismer (1984) has shown by means of acoustic techniques that geriatric speakers tend to continue vocal fold vibration into a voiceless closure interval, suggesting that there is a loss of coordination between glottal and supraglottal gestures. These kinds of observations should be extended to other articulatory pairings or groupings, because they may reveal subtle effects of aging that cannot be obtained from studies of single articulators. A similar claim has been made for the understanding of postural deficits in the elderly (Inglin & Woollacott, 1988).

The Nervous System

The potential effects of age-related changes in the peripheral nervous system on speech motor control have been introduced in the previous sections of this chapter. The current section provides a more detailed account of changes in the nervous system with age, and the possible ways in which these might affect speech production. Table 12.4 provides a synopsis of these changes.

In general, any reduction in the neural drive to muscles will be associated with a loss of the normal trophic influences on the metabolic activity of muscle cells. The result of this, as has been demonstrated in Parkinson's disease and spasticity (Dietz & Berger, 1983; Dietz, Quintern, & Berger, 1981; Edstrom, 1970), is that the muscles become more fibrotic and thus stiffer. In fact, Dietz et al. (1981) and Dietz and Berger (1983) have argued that a large part of the *movement* deficit in spasticity and Parkinsonism is probably due to changes in the peripheral composition of muscle, as well as to the disordered neural drive. As we have seen, these kinds of muscular changes are known to occur in the larynx and supraglottal musculature. It should be kept in mind, therefore, that the potential influence of age-related changes in the nervous system on speech motor control should include changes that affect the structure of the peripheral plant.

A pervasive finding in the peripheral nervous system of elderly people is that their nerve conduction velocities are slower than those of young individuals (Kenney, 1982). This might lead to the expectation of general slowing of speech motor behaviors, as well as disruption of interarticulator coordination. However, it is not even clear if conduction velocities are correlated with articulatory behavior within a given age group (or within a given person). One approach to linking the molecular aspects of the central nervous system—such as nerve conduction velocities—with a more molar behavior, such as articulatory function, would be to measure and compare conduction velocities and speech timing across age groups. The results of such a study would bear on the speculation of Smith et al. (1987) that the similarity in percentage reductions of conduction velocities

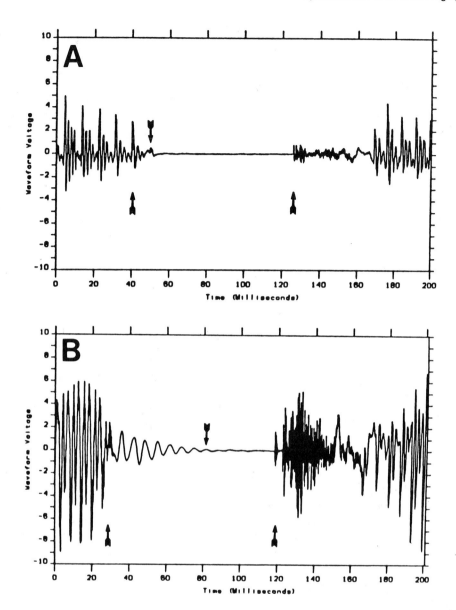

FIGURE 12.4. Waveform analysis of dyscoordination between supraglottal and glottal gestures. For voiceless stops, vocal fold vibrations usually cease roughly at the instant of supraglottal closure, as indicated by the downward-pointing arrow in "A"; loss of coordination between glottal and supraglottal gestures is shown in "B," where vocal fold vibrations continue well into the voiceless closure interval (see the sinusoidal-like pulses between the first upward- and downward-pointing arrows).

and speech segment duration across age suggests a fairly simple explanation for the slowing of the speaking rate in the elderly.

Another possible explanation for the slow speaking rate in elderly speakers (see also Mysak, 1959; Weismer, 1984) is that age-related changes in central neurotransmitters result in a generalized slowing of all sensorimotor processes. There is evidence of progressive degeneration of the dopaminergic system with age (see Morgan & Finch, 1988), as well as some behavioral

TABLE 12.4
Synopsis of Age-Related Anatomical and Functional Changes in the Nervous System and Their Implications for Speech Production

Anatomical Changes	Functional Changes	Implications for Speech
Decreased brain weight; gyral atrophy; vascular anomalies	Diminished/slowed cognitive function	Slowed lexical access; failures of prearticulatory editors; dysfluencies
Decreased conduction velocities	Slowness of movement	Slow articulatory movements; slow speaking rate
Changes in neurotransmitter levels	Bradykinesia/akinesia	Reduced phonetic working space; slow articulatory movements; slow speaking rate

findings that are consistent with a dopamine-poor brain (McNeill, Koek, Brown, & Rafols, 1988; Mortimer, 1988). These neurotransmitter changes are qualitatively similar to those seen in Parkinson's disease, but are less extensive. This fact has led researchers (Mortimer, 1988) to speculate that Parkinson's disease may be considered partly as a form of accelerated aging. Although Mortimer did not find strong support for this notion when the classic limb symptoms of Parkinson's disease were studied in normally aging individuals, Liss et al. (1990) noted striking similarities between certain features of speech production in very old males and in persons with Parkinson's disease. The features in the Liss et al. study that were similar in the two groups of subjects generally required fine control and coordination, whereas Mortimer's study was concerned with nonfunctional symptoms such as rigidity and tremor. In addition, Liss et al.'s subjects were older than those studied by Mortimer, increasing the potential for subtle aging effects to be detected. This latter consideration emphasizes the need for studies of speech motor control in aged individuals to include very old subjects.

There is an abundance of evidence that indicates additional degenerative changes with age in the brain. Gross changes include decreased brain weight, gyral

atrophy, and ventricular dilation; microscopic changes include neuroglial cell loss, myelin loss, senile plaques, and amyloid deposits (see Peach, 1987, for a review). Vascular changes and neurotransmitter changes such as declines in norepinephrine and serotonin also occur, in addition to the decreases in dopamine that have been described. The fact that these changes influence brain function is supported by the observations of electroencephalographic, metabolic, and evoked response changes with age (Peach, 1987). It is therefore not surprising that there is evidence of deterioration of cognition, memory, and language functions with age.

Most models of speech motor control (e.g., Daniloff & Hammarberg, 1973; Perkell, 1980) do not typically include components that account for language behaviors such as lexical access and syntactic issues (see Fowler, 1985, for an exception). In line with our earlier statements concerning the scope of speech motor control issues, we believe that it is not useful to separate classic language behaviors from motor control behaviors. For example, impaired lexical access in elderly people (see Obler & Albert, 1987; Peach, 1987) might contribute to the pervasive phenomenon of slow speaking rate among this population. This contribution could be quantified by establishing experimental conditions that differed in the amount of formulation required of subjects. The prediction would be that speaking rate would decrease disproportionately for elderly speakers, as compared to young speakers, under conditions in which lexical access demands were increased. To our knowledge, such an experiment has not been reported in the literature. The results of Yairi and Clifton (1972), showing that geriatric speakers have more dysfluencies than young adults in spontaneous speech, support the notion that lexical access difficulties affect speech motor control in the elderly. Other aspects of language behavior, such as syntactic complexity in the speech production of geriatric individuals, should be studied to understand interactions between the linguistic and execution components of speech motor control. One approach to this problem is to study repairs in the spontaneous speech of older and younger individuals. Recent models of interactions between "prearticulatory editors" and syntactic and semantic components of language (Garnsey & Dell, 1984) are likely to be of use in this regard.

Theories of Speech Production

One way in which research on speech motor control in aging speakers can make an important contribution is by addressing general issues in the theory of speech production. To date, no extant theories of speech production have addressed aging effects, probably because of the absence of relevant data, especially on supraglottal articulatory function in the aged.

Most of the major theories of speech production (Daniloff & Hammarberg, 1973; Kelso et al., 1986; Perkell, 1980) seek to explain the phenomena of coarticulation

and interarticulator coordination[3] in young adult speakers. Because more is known about articulatory behavior than about the underlying mechanisms, the bases of most of these theories are inductive, in that their development has been driven by extant databases; action theory (Kelso et al., 1986) is somewhat different in that general notions of coordinative behavior have been used to predict new experimental observations. As we have emphasized throughout this chapter, the speech characteristics of elderly speakers have yet to be clearly delineated. Relatively more is known about the age-related anatomical and physiological changes that may or may not have an influence on speech production. Thus, the inductive nature of current theories (i.e., inferring underlying mechanisms from articulatory behavior) is probably not the best approach for explaining those age-related speech changes. Rather, a deductive approach would allow our current knowledge of speech mechanism changes with aging to be applied to predictions about the resulting articulatory behavior. This deductive approach can be used to explain slowed speaking rate, the influences of this rate change on coarticulatory and coordinative patterns, and the reduction of phonetic working space that occurs with aging. We believe that the best deductive premises will be those that synthesize knowledge of the mechanism changes that result from aging and of important speech production phenomena such as coarticulation.

Conclusions

We know from perceptual studies that listeners are able to identify age from speech samples. We also know that the speech mechanism undergoes various changes with aging. What is not known, however,

---

[3]It should be understood that coarticulation (or coproduction—see Fowler, 1985) and interarticulator coordination are not mutually exclusive phenomena. In some ways, these two phenomena are different reflections of the same vocal tract behavior, whereby multiple structures move synchronously and asynchronously to produce changing area functions.

is the relationship between these two phenomena. Within the framework of our definition of speech motor control, we have attempted to identify the available knowledge and to direct future research efforts that will illuminate this relationship. We believe that studies employing multiple levels of analysis across systems will prove to be the most lucrative.

References

Baum, B. J. (1981). Research on aging and oral health: An assessment of current status and future needs. *Special Care in Dentistry, 1,* 156–165.

Baum, B. J., & Bodner, L. (1983). Aging and oral motor function: Evidence for altered performance among older persons. *Journal of Dental Research, 62,* 2–6.

Bell-Berti, F. (1975). Control of pharyngeal cavity size for English voiced and voiceless stops. *Journal of the Acoustical Society of America, 57,* 456–461.

Bell-Berti, F. (1976). An electromyographic study of velopharyngeal function in speech. *Journal of Speech and Hearing Research, 19,* 225–240.

Benjamin, B. J. (1981). Frequency variability in the aged voice. *Journal of Gerontology, 36,* 722–726.

Benjamin, B. J. (1986). Dimensions of the older female voice. *Language and Communication, 6,* 35–45.

Birren, J. E., & Cunningham, W. R. (1985). Research on the psychology of aging: Principles, concepts and theory. In J. E. Birren & K. W. Schaie (Eds.), *Handbook of the psychology of aging* (Vol. 2, pp. 3–34). New York: Von Nostrand Reinhold.

Blackwood, H. J. J. (1969). Pathology of the temporomandibular joint. *Journal of the American Dental Association, 30,* 1501–1507.

Borden, G. J. (1979). An interpretation of research on feedback interruption in speech. *Brain and Language, 7,* 307–319.

Bunge, M. (1977). Levels and reductions. *American Journal of Physiology, 233,* R75–R82.

Cerella, J. (1985). Information processing rates in the elderly. *Psychological Bulletin, 98,* 67–83.

Cohen, T., & Gitman, L. (1959). Oral complaints and taste perception in the aged. *Journal of Gerontology, 14,* 294–298.

Curtis, A. P., & Fucci, D. (1983). Sensory and motor changes during development and aging. In N. J. Lass (Ed.), *Speech and language: Advances in basic research and practice* (pp. 153–248). New York: Academic Press.

Daniloff, R. G., & Hammarberg, R. E. (1973). On defining coarticulation. *Journal of Phonetics, 1,* 239–248.

Dietz, V., & Berger, W. (1983). Normal and impaired regulation of muscle stiffness in gait: A new hypothesis about muscle hypertonia. *Experimental Neurology, 79,* 680–687.

Dietz, V., Quintern, J., & Berger, W. (1981). Electrophysiological studies of gait in spasticity and rigidity. Evidence that altered mechanical properties of muscle contribute to hypertonia. *Brain, 104,* 431–449.

Edstrom, L. (1970). Selective changes in the sizes of red and white muscle fibres in upper motor lesions and Parkinsonism. *Journal of the Neurological Sciences, 11,* 537–550.

Endres, W., Bambach, W., & Flosser, G. (1971). Voice spectrograms as a function of age, voice disguise, and voice imitation. *Journal of the Acoustical Society of America, 49,* 1842–1848.

Fant, C. G. M. (1970). *Acoustic theory of speech production.* The Hague: Mouton.

Forrest, K., Weismer, G., & Turner, G. S. (1989). Kinematic, acoustic, and perceptual analyses of connected speech produced by Parkinsonian and normal geriatric adults. *Journal of the Acoustical Society of America, 85,* 2608–2622.

Fowler, C. A. (1985). Current perspectives on language and speech production: A critical review. In R. G. Daniloff (Ed.), *Speech science* (pp. 192–278). San Diego, CA: College Hill Press.

Gardner, H. (1985). *The mind's new science.* New York: Basic Books.

Garnsey, S. M., & Dell, G. S. (1984). Some neurolinguistic implications of prearticulatory editing in production. *Brain and Language, 23,* 64–73.

Gracco, L. C. (1988). *Age related changes in the human vestibular fold of the larynx: A histomorphometric study.* Unpublished doctoral dissertation, University of Wisconsin–Madison.

Grillner, S., Lindblom, B., Lubker, J., & Persson, A. (1982). *Speech motor control.* Oxford, England: Pergamon Press.

Hartman, D. E. (1979). The perceptual identity and characteristics of aging in normal male adult speakers. *Journal of Communication Disorders, 12*, 53–61.

Hartman, D. E., & Danhauer, J. L. (1976). Perceptual features of speech for males in four perceived age decades. *Journal of the Acoustical Society of America, 59*, 713–715.

Hirose, H. (1976). Posterior cricoarytenoid as a speech muscle. *Annals of Otology, Rhinology, and Laryngology, 85*, 334–343.

Hixon, T. J. (1982). Speech breathing kinematics and mechanism inferences therefrom. In S. Grillner, B. Lindblom, J. Lubker, & A. Persson (Eds.), *Speech motor control* (pp. 75–93). Oxford, England: Pergamon Press.

Hixon, T. J., Goldman, M., & Mead, J. (1973). Kinematics of the chest wall during speech production: Volume displacements of the rib cage, abdomen, and lung. *Journal of Speech and Hearing Research, 16*, 78–115.

Hixon, T. J., Mead, J., & Goldman, M. (1976). Dynamics of the chest wall during speech: Function of the thorax, rib cage, diaphragm, and abdomen. *Journal of Speech and Hearing Research, 19*, 297–356.

Hoit, J., & Hixon, T. J. (1987). Age and speech breathing. *Journal of Speech and Hearing Research, 30*, 351–366.

Hollien, H. (1987). ''Old voices'': What do we really know about them? *Journal of Voice, 1*, 2–17.

Hollien, H., & Shipp, T. (1972). Speaking fundamental frequency and chronologic age in males. *Journal of Speech and Hearing Research, 15*, 155–159.

Honjo, I., & Isshiki, N. (1980). Laryngoscopic and voice characteristics of aged persons. *Archives of Otolaryngology, 106*, 149–150.

Hutchinson, J. M., Robinson, K. L., & Nerbonne, M. A. (1978). Patterns of nasalance in a sample of normal gerontologic subjects. *Journal of Communication Disorders, 11*, 469–481.

Inglin, B., & Woollacott, M. (1988). Age-related changes in anticipatory postural adjustments associated with arm movements. *Journal of Gerontology: Medical Sciences, 43*, M105–M113.

Israel, H. (1971). Age factor and the pattern of change in craniofacial structures. *American Journal of Physical Anthropology, 39*, 111–128.

Kahane, J. C. (1981). Anatomic and physiologic changes in the aging peripheral speech mechanism. In D. S. Beasley & G. A. Davis (Eds.), *Aging: Communication processes and disorders* (pp. 21–45). New York: Grune & Stratton.

Kahane, J. C. (1987). Connective tissue changes in the larynx and their effects on voice. *Journal of Voice, 1*, 27–30.

Kahn, A., & Kahane, J. C. (1986). India ink pin prick assessment of age-related changes in the cricoarytenoid joint (CAJ) articular surfaces. *Journal of Speech and Hearing Research, 29*, 536–543.

Kelsey, C., Woodhouse, R., & Minifie, F. (1969). Ultrasonic observations of coarticulation in the pharynx. *Journal of the Acoustical Society of America, 46*, 1016–1018.

Kelso, J. A. S., Saltzman, E. L., & Tuller, B. (1986). The dynamical perspective on speech production: Data and theory. *Journal of Phonetics, 14*, 29–59.

Kelso, J. A. S., Vatikiotis-Bateson, E., Saltzman, E. L., & Kay, B. (1985). A qualitative dynamic analysis of reiterant speech production: Phase portraits, kinematics, and dynamic modeling. *Journal of the Acoustical Society of America, 77*, 266–280.

Kenney, R. A. (1982). *Physiology of aging: A synopsis.* Chicago: Year Book Medical Publishers.

Kent, R. D. (1986). The iceberg hypothesis: The temporal assembly of speech movements. In J. S. Perkell & D. H. Klatt (Eds.), *Invariance and variability in speech processes* (pp. 234–242). Hillsdale, NJ: Lawrence Erlbaum.

Kent, R. D., Carney, P. J., & Severeid, L. R. (1974). Velar movement and timing: Evaluation of a model for binary control. *Journal of Speech and Hearing Research, 17*, 470–488.

Kent, R. D., & Moll, K. L. (1969). Vocal tract characteristics of the stop cognates. *Journal of the Acoustical Society of America, 46*, 1549–1555.

Kiuchi, S., Sasaki, J., Arai, T., & Suzuki, T. (1969). Functional disorders of the pharynx and esophagus. *Acta Otolaryngologica* (Suppl. 256).

Knudson, R. J. (1989). Aging in the respiratory system. *Current Pulmonology, 10*, 1–24.

Kuehn, D. P., & Moll, K. L. (1976). A cineradiographic study of VC and CV articulatory velocities. *Journal of Phonetics, 4*, 303–320.

Langer, A. (1976). Oral signs of aging and their clinical significance. *Geriatrics, 31*, 63–69.

Lehiste, I. (1970). *Suprasegmentals.* Cambridge, MA: MIT Press.

Linville, S. E. (1987). Acoustic-perceptual studies of aging voice in women. *Journal of Voice, 1,* 44–48.

Linville, S. E. (1988). Intraspeaker variability in fundamental frequency stability: An age-related phenomenon. *Journal of the Acoustical Society of America, 83,* 741–745.

Liss, J. M., Weismer, G., & Rosenbek, J. C. (1990). Selected acoustic characteristics of speech production in very old males. *Journal of Gerontology: Psychological Sciences, 45,* P35–P45.

Lofqvist, A., & Yoshioka, H. (1984). Intrasegmental timing: Laryngeal-oral coordination in voiceless consonant production. *Speech Communication, 3,* 279–289.

Logemann, J. A., & Fisher, H. B. (1981). Vocal tract control in Parkinson's disease: Phonetic feature analysis of misarticulations. *Journal of Speech and Hearing Disorders, 46,* 348–352.

Lubker, J., McAllister, R., & Lindblom, B. (1977). On the notion of inter-articulator programming. *Journal of Phonetics, 5,* 213–226.

Massler, M. (1971). Oral aspects of aging. *Postgraduate Medicine, 25,* 179–183.

McGlone, R. E., & Hollien, H. (1963). Vocal pitch characteristics of aged women. *Journal of Speech and Hearing Research, 6,* 164–170.

McNeill, T. H., Koek, L. L., Brown, S. A., & Rafols, J. A. (1988). Age related changes in the nigrostriatal system. In J. A. Joseph (Ed.), General determinants of age-related declines in motor function. *Annals of the New York Academy of Sciences, 515,* 239–248.

Minifie, F., Hixon, T. J., Kelsey, C., & Woodhouse, R. (1970). Lateral pharyngeal wall movement during speech production. *Journal of Speech and Hearing Research, 13,* 584–595.

Mittman, C., Edelman, N. H., Morris, A. H., & Shock, N. W. (1965). Relationship between chest wall and pulmonary compliance and age. *Journal of Applied Physiology, 20,* 1211–1216.

Moffett, B. C., Jr., Johnson, L. C., McCabe, J. B., & Askew, H. C. (1964). Articular remodeling in the adult human temporomandibular joint. *American Journal of Anatomy, 115,* 119–142.

Morgan, D. G., & Finch, C. E. (1988). Dopaminergic changes in the basal ganglia: A generalized phenomenon of aging in mammals. In J. A. Joseph (Ed.), General determinants of age-related declines in motor function. *Annals of the New York Academy of Sciences, 515,* 145–159.

Morgan, E. E., & Rastatter, M. (1986). Variability of voice fundamental frequency in elderly female speakers. *Perceptual and Motor Skills, 63,* 215–218.

Morrison, M. D., & Gore-Hickman, P. (1986). Voice disorders in the elderly. *Journal of Otolaryngology, 15,* 231–234.

Mortimer, J. A. (1988). Human motor behavior and aging. In J. A. Joseph (Ed.), General determinants of age-related declines in motor function. *Annals of the New York Academy of Sciences, 515,* 54–65.

Muller, E. M., & Brown, W. S., Jr. (1980). Variations in the supraglottal air pressure waveform and their articulatory interpretation. In N. J. Lass (Ed.), *Speech and language: Advances in basic research and practice* (Vol. 4, pp. 317–389). New York: Academic Press.

Mysak, E. D. (1959). Pitch and duration characteristics of older males. *Journal of Speech and Hearing Research, 2,* 46–54.

Neiman, G. S., Klich, R. J., & Shuey, E. M. (1983). Voice onset time in young and 70-year-old women. *Journal of Speech and Hearing Research, 26,* 118–123.

Obler, L. K., & Albert, M. L. (1987). Language skills across adulthood. In J. E. Birren and K. W. Schaie (Eds.), *Handbook of the psychology of aging* (2nd ed., pp. 463–473). New York: Von Nostrand Reinhold.

Peach, R. K. (1987). Language functioning. In H. G. Mueller and V. C. Geoffrey (Eds.), *Communication disorders in aging assessment and management* (pp. 238–270). Washington, DC: Gallaudet University Press.

Perkell, J. S. (1980). Phonetic features and the physiology of speech production. In B. Butterworth (Ed.), *Language production* (Vol. 1, pp. 337–372). New York: Academic Press.

Perkell, J. S. (1986). Coarticulation strategies: Preliminary implications of a detailed analysis of lower lip protrusion movements. *Speech Communication, 5,* 47–68.

Priestly, T. M. S. (1976). A note on the glottal stop. *Phonetica, 33,* 268–274.

Ptacek, P. H., Sander, E. K., Maloney, W. H., & Jackson, C. C. R. (1966). Phonatory and related changes with advancing age. *Journal of Speech and Hearing Research, 9,* 353–360.

Ramig, L. A. (1986). Aging speech: Physiological and sociological aspects. *Language and Communication, 6,* 25–34.

Ramig, L. A., Scherer, R. C., & Titze, I. R. (1986). The aging voice. In V. Lawrence (Ed.), *Care of the professional voice* (pp. 31–38). New York: Voice Foundation.

Rothenberg, M. (1968). The breath-stream dynamics of simple-released-plosive production. *Bibliotheca Phonetica, 6,* 1–117.

Ryan, W. J., & Burke, K. W. (1974). Perceptual and acoustic correlates of aging in the speech of males. *Journal of Communication Disorders, 7,* 181–192.

Schneider, J. S., Diamond, S. G., & Markham, C. H. (1986). Deficits in orofacial sensorimotor function in Parkinson's disease. *Annals of Neurology, 19,* 275–282.

Shanks, S. J. (1970). Effect of aging upon rapid syllable repetition. *Perceptual Motor Skills, 30,* 687–690.

Skolnick, M. C., McCall, G. N., & Barnes, M. (1973). The sphincteric mechanism of velopharyngeal closure. *Cleft Palate Journal, 10,* 286–305.

Smith, B. L. (1978). Effects of place of articulation and vowel environment on ''voiced'' stop consonant production. *Glossa, 12,* 163–175.

Smith, B. L., Wasowicz, J., & Preston, J. (1987). Temporal characteristics of the speech of normal elderly adults. *Journal of Speech and Hearing Research, 30,* 522–529.

Smitheran, J. R., & Hixon, T. J. (1981). A clinical method for estimating laryngeal airway resistance during vowel production. *Journal of Speech and Hearing Research, 46,* 138–146.

Sonies, B. C., Baum, B. J., & Shawker, T. (1984). Tongue motions in elderly adults: Initial in situ observations. *Journal of Gerontology, 39,* 279–283.

Sonies, B. C., Stone, M., & Shawker, T. (1984). Speech and swallowing in the elderly. *Gerontology, 3,* 115–123.

Sussman, H. M., MacNeilage, P. F., & Hanson, R. J. (1973). Labial and mandibular dynamics during the production of bilabial consonants: Preliminary observations. *Journal of Speech and Hearing Research, 16,* 397–420.

Sweeting, P. M., & Baken, R. J. (1982). Voice onset time in a normal aged population. *Journal of Speech and Hearing Research, 25,* 129–134.

Umeda, N. (1982). Boundary: Perceptual and acoustic properties and syntactic and statistical determinants. In N. J. Lass (Ed.), *Speech and language: Advances in basic research and practice* (Vol. 7, pp. 333–371). New York: Academic Press.

Weismer, G. (1980). Control of the voicing distinction for intervocalic stops and fricatives: Some data and theoretical considerations. *Journal of Phonetics, 8,* 417–428.

Weismer, G. (1984). Articulatory characteristics of Parkinsonian dysarthria: Segmental and phrase-level timing, spirantization, and glottal-supraglottal coordination. In M. R. McNeil, J. C. Rosenbek, & A. E. Aronson (Eds.), *The dysarthrias* (pp. 101–130). San Diego, CA: College Hill Press.

Weismer, G. (1985). Speech breathing. In R. G. Daniloff (Ed.), *Speech science* (pp. 47–74). San Diego, CA: College Hill Press.

Weismer, G., & Fromm, D. (1983). Acoustic analysis of geriatric utterances: Segmental and nonsegmental characteristics that relate to laryngeal function. In D. M. Bless and J. H. Abbs (Eds.), *Vocal fold physiology: Contemporary research and clinical issues* (pp. 317–332). San Diego, CA: College Hill Press.

Westbury, J. R. (1983). Enlargement of the supraglottal cavity and its relation to stop consonant voicing. *Journal of the Acoustical Society of America, 73,* 1322–1336.

Wilcox, K. A., & Horii, Y. (1980). Age and changes in vocal jitter. *Journal of Gerontology, 35,* 184–198.

Yairi, E., & Clifton, N. (1972). Dysfluent speech behavior of preschool children, high school seniors, and geriatric persons. *Journal of Speech and Hearing Research, 15,* 714–719.

Zaino, C., & Benventano, T. C. (1977). Functional, involutional, and degenerative disorders. In C. Zaino & T. C. Benventano (Eds.), *Radiologic examination of the oropharynx and esophagus.* New York: Springer-Verlag.

Fluency, Dysfluency, and Aging

13

CHAPTER

David B. Rosenfield, MD,
and Harvey B. Nudelman, PhD ■

Speech, a priori, is motor output. This statement does not deny the importance of other elements of language such as phonology, semantics, and syntax. Rather, it addresses what speech is, at the level of production: a very complex motor output. This motor output is programmed and controlled by the central nervous system.

The central nervous system regulates the activity of the respiratory and laryngeal muscles to produce sound. This sound is subsequently sculpted by articulators to produce the meaningful components of language. The vocal cords (vocal folds) are composed of striated muscles and connective tissue, and are covered by mucosa. Vocal fold muscles, all but one of which are adductors, control the position of the vocal folds and the shape of the vocal fold edge, as well as the distribution of muscle mass within that fold, thus altering the quality of the sound waves produced (Abbs & Rosen-

field, 1986; Borden & Harris, 1980; Hirano, 1981; Rosenfield, Miller, Sessions, & Patten, 1982; Wyke & Kirchner, 1976).

Phonation (the production of sound) requires appropriate stiffness/slackness of laryngeal vocal folds, an appropriate opening (glottal chink) between the vocal folds, and an appropriate air stream through that opening. The air stream is affected by changes in the pressure below the vocal folds (subglottic pressure) and by supraglottic pressure, which is controlled by contraction of the supraglottic musculature (pharyngeal and supralaryngeal articulatory movements). A narrow but specific range of values for these three variables markedly affects phonation. Compromise of any of these variables can drastically alter sound output and cause it to cease (Stevens & Klatt, 1974); compromise of the sound source can produce dysphonia; and articulator compromise can produce slurred

This work was supported by the Kitty M. Perkins, M. R. Bauer, and Ariel-Benjamin-Gideon-Abigail Maida Lowin Medical Research Foundations.

speech. There is considerable research that addresses clinical disturbances in these realms (reviewed by Rosenfield & Barroso, in press).

Although there is an increasing corpus of knowledge pertaining to dysphonia, dysarthria, and, certainly, the aphasias, there is not a great deal known about how the timing of speech production affects these and other disturbances. This is most unfortunate. Speech, as motor output, varies as a function of time. Any complete model of speech and language must address the domain of time in language, as well as the actual motor control system subtending speech. An understanding of brain function pertaining to language and speech output that incorporates time should allow the inclusion of all bona fide findings, no matter how seemingly disparate they are. The road to this goal requires different types of thinking as well as further experimentation.

The classical approach to cerebral modeling of language, sectoring it into semantics, phonology, and syntax, certainly provides interesting data and commentary on language structure and on clinical findings, but far too frequently it falls short of explaining why some patients have perseveration, echolalia, or stuttered dysfluencies. Also, it frequently fails to take into account the incredible variability seen in patients, both normal and brain damaged. Anyone who has examined an aphasic patient well knows that the findings produced at 9:00 in the morning are not necessarily the same as those produced at 10:30 in the morning, let alone the following day. Behavioral performance, such as language output, is highly variable.

There is an expanding body of knowledge pertaining to the role of language compromise in patients with diseased brains. To date, models derived from this information have failed to explain why cerebral lesions can cause fluent people to stutter (reviewed in Rosenfield, 1984) or why stuttering exists in the first place. It is easier to derive what happens to a diseased brain from a model of a normal brain than to extrapolate how a normal brain functions from a model derived from a diseased brain. Understanding the biology of normal fluency may provide understanding of the biology of dysfluency. Therefore, it is important to investigate the speech motor control system.

The Speech Motor Control System

Modeling the speech motor control system will promote understanding of fluency and, therefore, of dysfluency. In the discussion that follows, we paraphrase work that is elsewhere described in greater detail (Nudelman, Herbrich, Hoyt, & Rosenfield, 1987, 1989).

Speech production is a most complex task. The structure of models currently used to investigate the neural basis of motor control (Brooks, 1986) is a good starting point for the study of dysfluency. This is because dysfluency is a disruption of speech motor production, and the measures used for studying the neural basis of motor control cross many disciplines, as do the measures pertaining to investigations of dysfluency (Bloodstein, 1987). Measures used in the study of motor control range from data collected on learning complex motor skills, such as typing and throwing a ball, to interactions of the molecular components subserving muscle contraction.

Motor control models successfully incorporate this wide range of measures by employing classical reductionist thinking. This type of thinking employs a multilayered modeling that relates the wide range of measures heretofore made of the motor system. This approach permits explicit relation of the wide range of measurements and theories that have been applied to the moment of stuttering as well as to the etiology of stuttering.

The reductionist approach views each investigation according to the level of organization (and size, or both) at which one makes the measures. Thus, subatomic particles are organized into atoms and atoms are organized into chemicals. The chemicals are organized into organelles (subcellular components such as the endoplasmic reticulum or mitochondria) and these organelles, in turn, organize into cells. The cells are organized into tissues; the tissues are organized into organs (such as liver or lungs or spleen) and the organs are organized into organ systems (e.g., the respiratory system). Organ systems, in turn, are organized into "coordinated groups of organ systems" (e.g., the speech motor control system). These coordinated organ systems are organized into animals. We stop our level of organization here, although we could continue up through societies and ecologies. At the whole animal level, one can choose to study the animal's behavior and model the psychology proposed to drive it.

In this context, the co-contraction of antagonistic laryngeal muscles observed during some stuttered dysfluencies (Freeman & Ushijima, 1978) is at the organ system level. However, the actual motor programming of the speech signal is at the level of coordinated organ systems, involving respiratory, laryngeal, and articulatory systems. The behavior-motivating theories of stuttering, as well as psychiatric theories of the etiology of stuttering, are at the whole animal level. They address the psychological models of stuttering and its development.

Using a reductionist structure to place the experimental observations at their appropriate level of organization helps define what models of organization must be developed, and hence what experiments must be performed in order to understand the relationships between experiments on stuttering that are performed at different levels.

The reductionist approach can be applied from the top down (from psychology to cells to chemistry to physics) or from the bottom up (from physics to chemistry to cells to psychology). Each approach has limitations. In the top-down approach, measurements of behavior on one level can never produce a unique model of how that observed behavior is accomplished by the components of that level. This can only be done by dissecting the level into its component parts. The bottom-up approach does do this, seeking to calculate the behavior of a level from its structure, its function, its connectivity, and the current conditions of its component parts. This calculation requires simultaneous measurement of current conditions, as well as knowledge of the input-output properties of the component parts. These requirements are not attainable at most levels in biological systems.

The top-down approach usually provides a description that has fewer variables (it produces an input-output model) than does the bottom-up description (which produces a complete model) at the same level. The questions to be asked and the measurements that can be made determine which approach is most appropriate. An analogy amplifies this point.

The behavior of a gas in a bell jar can be described at a macroscopic level (top-down) by the perfect gas law ($PV = nRT$), which relates the pressure, volume, temperature, and number of molecules in the bell jar. This can also be described at a microscopic level (bottom-up), applying Newton's second law ($F = ma$) to each molecule within the bell jar. The second description has far more variables, because calculations are needed for each molecule. The macroscopic (top-down) description is adequate to relate the pressure in the bell jar to its temperature; however, to calculate the relationship between the mean free path of a molecule and the velocity of sound in the gas, a microscopic (bottom-up) description (the kinetic theory of gases) must be used. The level of description employed for the gas depends upon the questions being asked. The top-down approach ($PV = nRT$) does not describe the relationship between the mean path of the molecule and the velocity of sound in the gas; however, it describes well the relationship between pressure, volume, temperature, and the number of molecules within the gas. A unique model of the relationship between sound within the gas and movement of the molecules cannot be produced by analyzing the gas from the $PV = nRT$ top-down approach. Many models can be developed, but none of them will be unique. It is possible to answer questions regarding sound, speed of molecules, pressure, volume, and temperature by using the bottom-up ($F = ma$) approach, but this implies knowing where all molecules are and having more information available than at the $PV = nRT$ level.

The bottom-up approach yields a unique model but, as was commented upon earlier, a wide range of knowledge is needed pertaining to the input-output properties of the component parts and the initial conditions. This level of knowledge, which allows production of a unique model, is not attainable in studying most biological systems. Biological systems inherently have great variability, as witnessed not only by multiple variable clinical findings, but also by virtue of the fact that there are many unobserved inputs and outputs and loops of control for each biological task at hand.

The development of "simple" state variable descriptions ($PV = nRT's$) for a behavior at each level can provide the necessary link for relating studies performed at adjacent levels if the state variable description captures the critical properties that are utilized by the next higher level of organization within that total system. One seeks the relationship between reductionist levels by trying to derive the critical state variables at one level from the state variables of the components of the level below. Thus, in the example just cited, $PV = nRT$ (higher level) is derived from the average velocity of gas molecules calculated at the lower level.

Using this analogy, Nudelman et al. (1987, 1989) contend that a stuttering event (whole animal behavior level) can be linked to a simple state variable model of the adjacent lower "coordinated groups of organ systems" level (e.g., speech motor system) by a control theory approach. Having discussed this approach to the complex problem of speech motor output, we will now look at dysfluency per se to determine whether one can model dysfluent output and what happens to fluency in aging.

Stuttering

What do we know about the speech motor control system and fluency? In some instances, acquired cerebral lesions produce dysfluent behavior (reviewed in Rosenfield, 1984; reviewed in Bloodstein, 1987, pp. 85–87). In other cases, such as that of the developmental stutterer, dysfluency is produced without any apparent cerebral lesions. No investigator has proven that anything is "broken" in the brains of stutterers.

Stuttering is a disturbance of speech motor output, characterized by repetitions, lengthening, and inappropriate pauses in the generation of consonants, vowels, and words. These disturbances are nonrandom, occurring primarily at the beginning of sentences and phrases (Bloodstein, 1987; Rosenfield, 1984).

The stutterer's speech is composed of sounds improperly patterned in time. It is difficult to pinpoint the exact location of the stutterer's dysfluencies. Thus, when a stutterer says "s-s-sound," where is the actual dysfluency? At one time, researchers contended that the dysfluency was on the *s*. Most investigators now concur that the deficit is on the transition from one sound to the next. Indeed, the stutterer can say the *s*, but not the *ound*. The stutterer copes with the motor output difficulty by repeating the *s* until the following *ound* is secured (Rosenfield, 1984). It is in this context that we contend, along with others (Freeman, 1979; see Bloodstein, 1987, for a review), that the stutterer's dysfluency is not the problem but, rather, the response to the problem. Nudelman et al. (1987, 1989) contend that the stuttered dysfluency is the response to a motor instability in the speech motor control system.

Stuttering occurs in all cultures and all civilizations and is mentioned in all languages. It is referred to on Mesopotamian clay tablets, in the Old Testament, and in the Koran (reviewed in Rosenfield, 1984). One percent of the world's adult population stutters. There is a higher concordance of stuttering among identical and fraternal twins, suggesting a strong genetic component. The prevalence among males is considerably higher than among females (Porfert & Rosenfield, 1978; Rosenfield, 1984; Rosenfield & Boller, 1985). Stuttering appears to be a part of the human genome.

The location of stuttered dysfluencies is not random. Stutterers' dysfluencies occur where fluent speakers' occasional dysfluencies occur, at the beginning of sentences and phrases. A stutterer seldom says, "See you in the morning-g-g-g," but rather, "S-S-See you in the morning." Stuttering is worse under stress, although it has never been proven to be psychogenic. Psychotherapy does not cure stuttering, although stuttering is affect sensitive (Rosenfield, 1984).

Several maneuvers evoke fluency in stutterers, the most potent of which is singing. Others include speaking in cadence with a metronome, oral reading, white noise, broadband noise, delayed auditory feedback, speaking during inhalation, and repetition of the same passage (known as the adaptation effect) (Bloodstein, 1987; Rosenfield, 1984).

To date no one has found any focal brain lesions in stutterers that account for their dysfluencies. It appears as though there have always been individuals, over thousands of years, who have been dysfluent. Yet, during most of their speech output they are fluent. Stutterers do talk. Thus, these individuals can be fluent as well as dysfluent, without any definite hole in the brain. How can we model their dysfluencies?

Dysfluency: Reductionism and Control Theory

Dysfluency Resulting from Instability

The complex task of speaking requires the accomplishment of several functions. The generation of an idea is linguistically formulated into some type of message. The speech motor system must somehow encode this message into a signal that produces a coordinated sequence of movements in the laryngeal, respiratory, and articulatory motor systems (Borden & Harris, 1980). The combined actions of these muscle groups, in turn, produce the acoustic temporal patterns of speech. This process is formalized by speech production modelers (refer to Borden & Harris, 1980, pp. 138–156, for an overview) into hierarchical model structures containing various combinations of these four functions or stages: ideation, linguistic programming, motor programming, and motor output. Where do these four functions or stages fit into a reductionist structure?

Different speech production models offer differing schemes for executing and linking these four stages. Regardless of the model chosen, they all must eventually engage neural processing on the "coordinated groups of organ systems" level. We use the term *functional control loops* to refer to loops that perform functions that we *hypothesize* must be accomplished before the animal can produce the observed behavior. These "loops" may involve inputs and outputs from the cortex, basal ganglia, and various other structures. Further, they may involve hundreds of thousands of synaptic connections. We are not addressing which parts of the brain are involved; this may be unanswerable at this time. However, we hypothesize that certain functions must be accomplished before the animal can produce the observed behavior. When we have a way to measure these loops, we can then model brain function to incorporate data from lesion experiments and can model anatomical findings to make sense out of what the brain is doing in terms of speech motor output.

It is in this setting that speech production is modeled as a collection of functional control loops that perform and monitor the specified function (e.g., linguistic programming). At the reductionist structure level of "coordinated groups of organ systems," the top-down approach is employed. In the bottom-up approach, each functional loop is divided into its many subloop components. In the absence of measurements confirming the uniqueness and specification of these subloops (MacNeilage, 1980), the top-down approach is used, because the requirements of the bottom-up approach are not met.

The hypothesized structure of the functional control loop models ranges from a simple sequential process connecting the stages, with no feedback between them, to a temporally overlapping, parallel execution of the stages with feedback (Borden & Harris, 1980). This latter model is the most general, since other models can be represented as a subset of it. (In more formal terms, the output of a sequential model can be derived from the output of a feedback model by setting the feedback parameters equal to zero.) Note that the opposite is not true: There are properties of a temporally overlapping parallel execution model with feedback that cannot be derived from the sequential model (Nudelman et al., 1987, 1989).

These hierarchical speech production models represent a proposed model of the "coordinated groups of organ systems" level and can be formally represented by a functional, nested, multiloop control system. This is also the structure used in the study of the neural basis of motor control (Brooks, 1986).

The concept of loops in this type of modeling is very important. From a control theory viewpoint, Grimm and Nashner (1978) contend that the human motor system is a very complex multiloop system. It consists of feedback loops within loops, all of which interconnect. The multiloop system can be tuned from the simple regulation of myotatic reflex gain to the complex cognitive work that links speech and thought. According to Grimm and Nashner, this multiloop system is dependent on an anatomical substrate; this substrate is used for the flexible creation and re-creation of loops by various physiological mechanisms. In a multiloop system, to an unknown extent, loops are physiological transients set up by stimuli, experience, and conscious control.

Nudelman et al. (1989) elaborate on this, in generic terms, in order to prevent misunderstanding:

1. The nervous system contains *anatomical loops*, that is, possible neural polysynaptic pathways from the input of a cell back to the same input of that cell.

2. Actual active loops are not currently observable in human experiments. They are a subset of anatomical loops that are transiently active before and during movements such as speaking (Brooks, 1986).

3. Functional control loops perform functions that we *hypothesize* must be accomplished before the body can achieve the observed performance. Recall that in the speech modeling previously discussed, four proposed functions are needed for speech production: ideation, linguistic programming, motor programming, and motor performance.

4. Last, the body has control loops that are completed ("closed" in engineering terms) by the sensory monitoring (feedback) of the controlled (output) performance (Grimm & Nashner, 1978). As an example, a firing alpha motor neuron that causes muscle contraction (performance) receives sensory feedback through muscle spindles and Golgi tendon organs. We term these loops *performance control loops*. These are the loops with which one interacts experimentally in order to measure performance. Alternatively stated, performance measures are the output for an input-output analysis of the top-down approach.

In the top-down approach, not all of these proposed functional loops are observable. It is impossible to measure all of the parameters necessary to define them uniquely. Indeed, one measures the behavior of a performance control loop triggered by a group of functional control loops that, at a particular time, are composed of a group of *actual active loops* that are only a subset of a possible anatomical loop. At the behavioral (performance) level, it is possible to observe only the actions of these loops acting together (in engineering terms, the "lumped" action of all these loops). On the behavioral level, only the input-output of these lumped loops can be measured and quantified. The contribution of each proposed component loop to the behavior cannot be uniquely specified.

Nudelman et al. (1987, 1989) describe the speech motor control system as being lumped into two nested functional control loops. They describe an outer loop, consisting of all the loops that decide which sounds are to be produced (a lumped model of the ideational and linguistic functional loops of the speech production models) and an inner phonatory loop (consisting of a lumped model of the motor programming functional loop and performance loop) that controls the vocal apparatus. Using a laryngeal tracking paradigm, they demonstrate that the lower loop is stable in stutterers and that time delays in the outer loop can render the speech motor system unstable. When the system is unstable, stuttered dysfluencies evolve. The outer loop consists of multiple nested loops and multiple anatomical loops, all of which involve, in all likelihood, multiple connections between the cortex, basal ganglia, thalamus, and brainstem structures. The following example illustrates the lumped action of loops.

The ringing of a public address system (microphone, amplifier, speaker, and microphone) in an auditorium is caused by positive feedback from the loudspeaker to a microphone; if the positive feedback is large enough, the system becomes unstable and produces ringing. Whether or not this occurs is a function of the combined properties of the system components: the sensitivity of the microphone, the gain setting of the amplifier, the sensitivity of the speaker, and the proximity of the speaker to the microphone. There is a region of component settings for which the system becomes unstable; in this setting, it will ring. In one instance, the microphone may be too sensitive even though the amplifier

gain is low. In another, the amplifier gain may be too high, and even though the microphone's sensitivity is not very high, ringing will occur.

How the public address system is analyzed will not only depend upon the questions being asked; even if only the ringing is being investigated, the whole system must be studied. Individually analyzing the structure and the integrity of the components of the loudspeaker system will not explain why the system becomes unstable. The instability can be explained only by realizing that the ringing is an emergent property of the system and not of the components by themselves. On the other hand, analyzing how a loudspeaker system becomes unstable and produces ringing will not explain how a microphone works. Asking how a microphone works involves not only asking different questions, but sometimes pursuing different modes of investigation. The instability (ringing) can be understood only in terms of the combined properties and connectivity of the components of the system. Instability is an important emergent property of complex feedback systems. Systems can become unstable even though all of the components are still functioning properly.

This example demonstrates the need for positive feedback. Physiological control systems normally have negative feedback. As reviewed by Nudelman et al. (1989), there are conditions under which negative feedback effectively becomes positive feedback, causing the system to become unstable. As discussed by Anand (1974), the Nyquist stability criteria provide us with the conditions under which the system becomes unstable. We provide an intuitive grasp of this.

A negative feedback control system compares the measured actual output to the desired output by subtracting the former signal from the latter, forming what is known as an *error signal*. The system, having earlier decided what its desired output is to be, selects appropriate action, depending upon the properties of the error signal, such as its sign and magnitude. The error signal is a function of time and can be broken down into its various sine wave components. Any signal over time, no matter how complex, can be broken down into a mathematical sum of sine wave components.

Consider what happens when a given frequency component has a phase shift of $-180°$. When a system subtracts to find the error signal, negative feedback becomes effectively positive (because $\sin(a - 180) = -\sin(a)$ and subtracting a negative number is the same as adding a positive number). If the gain is greater than 1, the error signal increases with each traverse of the loop until the physical limits of the system are reached. Employing engineering terms, the system becomes unstable. This instability of the speech motor control system is momentary, making intended speech motor output impossible. Repetitions, prolongations, and other outputs characteristic of the stuttering event are the system's response to the momentary instabilities of the speech motor control system.

These issues are complicated. Intuitively, it makes sense that investigators studying motor disturbances in speech output must address what causes the motor system to become unstable. Control theory (Anand, 1974; Nudelman et al., in press) provides the formalism to do this. Dysfluencies, at least in stutterers, appear to be an emergent system property. Therefore, attempts to find out what lesions in the brain produce dysfluencies will not be effective. If we are going to make sense out of why dysfluent people are not dysfluent all the time (i.e., why the motor system is not unstable all the time) and why there is such variability of findings, we cannot ignore control theory and the motor control literature.

Stutterers do not stutter all the time. Nudelman et al. (1987, 1989) posit that stutterers stutter only when an instability occurs in the speech motor control system. In their model, instability (stuttering) arises from the interaction of two lumped loops on the "coordinated group of organ systems" level. All possible functional loops on the "coordinated group of organ systems" level

should be lumped according to the observation being made. In their experiments, they lumped them into two loops, an outer functional loop that decides and monitors what sounds are to be made and an inner performance loop that programs, performs, and monitors the production of these sounds. An instability occurs when time delays in the outer loop equal the phase margin of the inner loop. The phase margin measures the dynamic properties of the inner loop (Anand, 1974; see Nudelman et al., in press, for further explanation) that predict where instabilities will occur.

Dysfluency Resulting from Injury

Having presented a model that presents stuttering as the response to a motor instability where nothing is broken, we can now ask what happens when something actually is broken. In this setting, it is conceivable that cerebral lesions can cause time delays and, therefore, instabilities, or that distorted speech output can occur because of disruption in the system components. The system can no longer do what it was programmed to do. The dysfluencies observed may reflect the system trying to compensate for the disruption of its components.

It is rare for a previously fluent individual to become a stutterer. However, an increasing number of investigators report fluent individuals who become nonaphasic stutterers following cerebral insult. The insult usually involves cortical or subcortical damage in either hemisphere; it is usually mild, but can be severe. These patients are distinguished from developmental stutterers in that the acquired stutterers have dysfluencies scattered throughout the sentence, and fluency-evoking maneuvers are usually ineffective. Further, they are seldom distraught over their altered speech output, as opposed to the developmental stutterers (Bloodstein, 1987, pp. 85–87; Rosenfield, 1972, 1984).

Palilalics are another group of acquired dysfluents. These individuals compulsively repeat phrases and words, the reiterations occurring at increasing speed with an associated phonatory volume decrescendo. Palilalia is usually seen in postencephalitic Parkinson's disease, pseudobulbar palsy, and idiopathic Parkinson's disease. At one time it was frequently associated with syphilis (Boller, Albert, & Denes, 1975; Rosenfield & Barroso, in press). Most palilalics have basal ganglia compromise.

Thus far, it is apparent that cerebral lesions compromising fluency can involve the basal ganglia (palilalics) but can also extend to multiple cortical and subcortical structures (acquired stutterers). There is no specified cerebral pathway that, when compromised, always produces dysfluent behavior. Rather, there are multiple inputs to the speech output system that can cause dysfluent (output) behavior.

Compromise of the brain from stroke and tumor can render a fluent person dysfluent. How do cerebral changes associated with aging alter fluency? How do the cerebral changes associated with Alzheimer's disease alter fluency in fluent subjects and in dysfluent subjects?

Fluency and Aging

There are not many investigations of fluency in the aging process. The definition of fluency is yet to be resolved, as is a definition of the "normal" cerebral changes in aging, discussed elsewhere in this volume. Some researchers have investigated stutterers, examining what happens to their speech output over time. Others have investigated nonstutterers to determine what happens to their fluent production over time.

Manning and Shirkey (1980) nicely review these issues. They note that although considerable effort has been expended on the study of the onset and development of stuttering in children, stutterers in middle- and late-adult years receive little investigative attention. Yairi and Clifton (1972) examined three 15-person groups of nonstuttering subjects: preschool

children, high school seniors, and geriatric individuals. The latter group was composed of 7 females and 8 males, ranging in age from 69 years, 7 months, to 87 years, 11 months, the mean age being 78 years, 1 month. All but one were above the age of 70. None of these patients had any known pathologies. The authors analyzed spontaneous speech samples, obtained from presenting three picture cards selected from the *Children's Apperception Test*, to their subjects. Subjects also were asked to tell a "Once Upon a Time" story for each picture. Manning and Shirkey analyzed speech output in terms of interjections of sounds, syllables, words, or phrases; part-word repetition; word repetition; phrase repetition; revisions or incomplete phrases; dysrhythmic phonation; and tensions (tense pauses). They then calculated the mean total of dysfluencies per 100 words spoken. The score was 7.65 ($\pm$2.60) for the preschool children, 3.83 ($\pm$2.19) for the high school seniors, and 6.29 ($\pm$3.15) for the geriatric subjects. Statistical evaluation revealed a significant difference between the preschool group and the high school group, and between the geriatric group and the high school group. However, there was no significant difference between preschool children and geriatric persons. It is apparent from the relatively large standard deviations that there is considerable overlap between groups.

The relative distributions of each dysfluency type indicated that the category of "interjections" was the main factor differentiating the three groups. Although the preschool and geriatric groups did not differ significantly in the total number of dysfluencies, the geriatric subjects demonstrated nearly twice as many interjections as did the preschool children. The high school subjects had fewer total dysfluencies than the geriatric subjects, but a similar proportion of interjections. The dysfluency types most often produced by the geriatric speakers were interjections (2.92 per 100 words) and revision/incomplete phrases (1.47 per 100 words). The dysfluency type produced least often by the geriatric subjects was the "tense pause" (0.02 per 100 words).

Yairi and Clifton's findings support the concept that fluency increases concomitant with chronological age through the early adult years. They suggest that the number of fluency breaks increases during adulthood, noting that these fluency breaks are not characteristic of the dysfluencies of stutterers; rather, their fluency breaks (interjections and revision/incomplete phrases) are among the dysfluencies that other investigators (Johnson, 1961; Williams & Kent, 1958; Wingate, 1962) have shown to be characteristic of normal adult speakers.

There is some evidence that stutterers' fluencies improve over the years. However, this is difficult to determine. It may well be that many stutterers find better coping strategies, employ therapeutic techniques that they have learned from speech-language pathologists or have discovered themselves, or have less tension about their speech output and therefore improve this output. It is not known for certain whether stutterers become more dysfluent or less dysfluent as they age (Bloodstein, 1987; Manning & Shirkey, 1980).

Fluent individuals may develop dysfluencies as they age. Some investigators have addressed this issue in the course of evaluating age-matched controls for various investigations of diseases associated with aging. Thus, Illes (1989) investigates the neurolinguistic features of spontaneous language production in Alzheimer's disease, Huntington's chorea, and Parkinson's disease. She notes that temporal interruptions of varying types are frequent in Alzheimer's and Huntington's patients; only long-duration silent hesitations are frequent in Parkinson's language samples. Syntactic complexity is reduced in Huntington's chorea. Illes contends that there is a unique neurolinguistic profile for spontaneous language production in each of these neurodegenerative diseases and that, perhaps, the pathology involving the neostriatum disrupts syntactic organization. She comments that phonemic approximations, modalizations, interjections, and filled hesitations (all types of dysfluent output) fail to differentiate any of her groups, including

their comparison to controls, in that there was considerable variability for these measures.

Several investigators contend that Alzheimer's patients do not have significant speech motor dysfluencies. Powell, Cummings, Hill, and Benson (1988) observe that Alzheimer's patients have relative sparing of motor speech functions and, when compared to multi-infarct dementia patients, have minimally disturbed mechanical speech components, such as pitch, melody, articulation, and rate. Cummings, Darkins, Mendez, Hill, and Benson (1988) found that Alzheimer's patients have minimal compromise of what the authors term ''reiterative speech abnormalities'' (echolalia, palilalia, logoclonia, and stuttering). Cummings, Benson, Hill, and Read (1985), comparing Alzheimer's patients to 70 controls, had found earlier not only that reiterative disturbances were minimal in Alzheimer's patients, but that age-matched controls did not have any deficits whatsoever in this realm.

The experimental setting in which an individual is tested for dysfluency is certainly important, and what is considered to be a dysfluency is even more important. No one doubts that fluent speakers can have dysfluent output, but it is not clear how this is truly affected by aging. What is clear is that Alzheimer's patients do not have marked disturbances in speech motor output. Rather, their problem pertains more to anomia and other aspects of language dysfunction, reviewed elsewhere in this volume. Alzheimer's patients, although they are aging and compromising their language output, fail to develop significant dysfluent speech output.

Why does Alzheimer's disease compromise language but not speech motor output? Why are there no stuttered dysfluencies in Alzheimer's patients? They simply may not have any damage in the part of the brain that can cause dysfluency. However, as we expand our body of knowledge regarding anatomical and pathological findings in Alzheimer's disease (see Ripich, chapter 15 of this volume), we may determine what parts of the brain can be damaged without compromising the anatomical loops involved in fluency production. When this knowledge is coupled with a knowledge of which anatomical loops are compromised in acquired stuttering, we will have acquired more information regarding the biological perspective of fluency changes in aging.

References

Abbs, J. H., & Rosenfield, D. B. (1986). Motor impairments of speech: Nonaphasic disorders of communication. In S. H. Appel (Ed.), *Current neurology* (pp. 177–206). Chicago: Yearbook Medical Publishers.

Anand, D. K. (1974). *Introduction to control systems.* Oxford, England: Pergamon Press.

Bloodstein, O. (1987). *A handbook on stuttering.* Chicago: National Easter Seal Society.

Boller, F., Albert, M., & Denes, F. (1975). Palilalia. *British Journal of Disorders of Communication, 10,* 92–97.

Borden, G. J., & Harris, K. S. (1980). *Speech science primer: Physiology, acoustics, and perception of speech.* Baltimore, MD: Williams & Wilkens.

Brooks, B. B. (1986). *The neural basis of motor control.* New York: Oxford University Press.

Cummings, J. L., Benson, D. F., Hill, M. A., & Read, S. (1985). Aphasia and dementia of the Alzheimer type. *Neurology, 35,* 394–397.

Cummings, J. L., Darkins, A., Mendez, M., Hill, M. A., & Benson, D. F. (1988). Alzheimer's disease and Parkinson's disease: Comparison of speech and language alterations. *Neurology, 38,* 680–684.

Freeman, F. (1979). Phonation and stuttering: A review of current research. *Journal of Fluency Disorders, 4,* 78–89.

Freeman, F., & Ushijima, T. (1978). Laryngeal muscle activity during stuttering. *Journal of Speech and Hearing Research, 21,* 538–562.

Grimm, R. J., & Nashner, L. N. (1978). Long loop dyscontrol. In J. E. Desmedt (Ed.), *Progress in clinical neurology: Vol. 4. Cerebral motor control in man: Long loop mechanisms* (pp. 70–84). Basel: Karger.

Hirano, M. (1981). *Clinical examination of voice* (pp. 7–9). New York: Springer-Verlag.

Illes, J. (1989). Neurolinguistic features of spontaneous language production dissociate three forms of neurodegenerative disease: Alzheimer's, Huntington's, and Parkinson's. *Brain and Language, 37,* 628–642.

Johnson, W. (Ed.). (1961). Measurements of oral reading and speaking rate and dysfluency of adult male and female stutterers and nonstutterers. *Journal of Speech and Hearing Disorders* (Monograph Suppl.), *7,* 1–20.

MacNeilage, P. F. (1980). Distinctive properties of speech motor control. In G. E. Stelmach & J. Requin (Eds.), *Tutorials in motor behavior.* Amsterdam: North Holland Publishing Company.

Manning, W. H., & Shirkey, E. A. (1980). Fluency and the aging process. In D. Beasley & G. A. Davis (Eds.), *Aging: Communication processes and disorders* (pp. 175–189). New York: Grune & Stratton.

Nudelman, H. B., Herbrich, K. E., Hoyt, B. D., & Rosenfield, D. B. (1987). Dynamic characteristics of vocal frequency tracking in stutterers and nonstutterers. In H. F. M. Peters & W. Hulstijn (Eds.), *Speech motor dynamics in stuttering* (pp. 161–169). Vienna, Austria: Springer-Verlag.

Nudelman, H. B., Herbrich, K. E., Hoyt, B. D., & Rosenfield, D. B. (1989). A neuroscience model of stuttering. *Journal of Fluency Disorders, 14,* 399–427.

Porfert, A. R., & Rosenfield, D. B. (1978). Prevalence of stuttering. *Journal of Neurology, Neurosurgery and Psychiatry, 41,* 954–956.

Powell, A. L., Cummings, J. L., Hill, M. A., & Benson, D. F. (1988). Speech and language alterations in multi-infarct dementia. *Neurology, 38,* 717–719.

Rosenfield, D. B. (1972). Stuttering and cerebral ischemia. *New England Journal of Medicine, 287,* 991.

Rosenfield, D. B. (1984). Scientific approaches to stuttering. *CRC Critical Reviews in Clinical Neurobiology, 1,* 117–139.

Rosenfield, D. B., & Barroso, A. B. (in press). Dysarthria, dysfluency and dysphagia. In W. G. Bradley, R. B. Daroff, G. M. Fenichel, & C. D. Marsden (Eds.), *Neurology in clinical practice.* Stoneham, MA: Butterworth.

Rosenfield, D. B., & Boller, F. (1985). Stuttering. In P. J. Vinkin, G. W. Bruyn, & H. L. Klawans (Eds.), *Handbook of clinical neurology* (Vol. 46, pp. 169–173). Amsterdam: Elsevier.

Rosenfield, D. B., Miller, R. H., Sessions, R. B., & Patten, B. M. (1982). Morphologic and histochemical characteristics of laryngeal muscles. *Archives of Otolaryngology, 108,* 662–666.

Stevens, K. N., & Klatt, D. H. (1974). Current models of sound sources for speech. In B. Wyke (Ed.), *Ventilatory and phonatory control systems: An international symposium* (pp. 279–292). Oxford, England: Oxford University Press.

Williams, D. E., & Kent, L. R. (1958). Listener evaluation of speech interruptions. *Journal of Speech and Hearing Research, 1,* 124–131.

Wingate, M. E. (1962). Evaluation and stuttering: III. Identification of stuttering and the use of a label. *Journal of Speech and Hearing Disorders, 27,* 368–377.

Wyke, B. D., & Kirchner, J. A. (1976). Neurology of the larynx. In R. Hinchcliffe & D. Harrison (Eds.), *Scientific foundation of otolaryngology* (pp. 546–574). London: William Heinemann Medical Books.

Yairi, E., & Clifton, N. F. (1972). Disfluent speech behavior of preschool children, high school seniors, and geriatric persons. *Journal of Speech and Hearing Research, 15,* 714–719.

Language and Aging

SECTION

Audrey L. Holland, PhD ■

Until recently, developmental psycholinguistics and its application to speech-language pathology have been considered to be within the domain of child language. As our interest in aging has increased generally, developmental psycholinguistics has necessarily broadened to cover the whole age span. This section of the handbook reflects this broadened concern.

The six chapters represent state-of-the-art coverage of language issues as they relate to older individuals, and are thus quite comprehensive in scope. The first three chapters of this section relate to pathologies of language in aging. They are united in facing the challenges of integrating studies of disorders with findings concerning normal aging. Chapman and Ulatowska comprehensively summarize the unique problems of aphasia and aging and make clear the point that aphasia probably is not validly studied unless reference is made to where in the life-span it was incurred. It is almost a truism that one cannot truly understand any language disorder, or the person who suffers from it, unless one studies the broader context in which the language disorder occurs. But aphasia is the disorder that is most affected by its physical, psychological, and sociological context. Chapman and Ulatowska have forcefully focused on these factors here.

In addition to having conceptualized this entire project, Ripich has illustrated her conceptualization with her thorough introduction to the problems of differential diagnosis and assessment of dementing disorders. More than for any other condition, the recent nationwide concern with dementia has galvanized the profession to become responsive to issues in aging. The issues are all spelled out here, including the many unanswered questions concerning research needs, the plausibility of intervention, and some potential directions for the future.

The section includes a brief chapter on head injury in the elderly, a topic that has been little studied but is of surprising importance. Forbes and I have attempted to summarize the scant literature, but also, more importantly, to sensitize readers to the subtlety of some of the issues and to make them aware that the topic is worthy of further study.

This section of the handbook includes a unique and very important chapter by Au and Bowles describing the influence of memory on language in aging. Although the cognitive-linguistic interface is an important issue generally in speech-language pathology, it is perhaps nowhere more important than in its relation to aging, and memory is the most significant aspect of cognitive function for the study of language and aging. Au and Bowles provide a solid overview of current approaches to the study of memory and demonstrate their understanding of its unique relevance to clinical issues in language. Although the focus of their work is on normal aging, the chapter also has striking implications for work on disordered language in the elderly.

Hooper and Johnson have presented a comprehensive overview of assessment and intervention issues concerning the aging segment of the language population. Not only do these authors present a thorough survey of available and appropriate instruments for testing, but they are also careful to describe adjustments to standard procedures that might be necessary for the valid assessment of aging individuals. They provide a humanistic framework within which to plan treatment and to determine when and for whom intervention is appropriate.

De Santi and Obler provide a review of some of the special methodological issues that concern research on the language of aging individuals. Not only are the research issues presented here, but some of the rigors and pitfalls of conducting research with the elderly are forthrightly considered. Because research in aging language is new and still covers relatively uncharted territory, these issues are timely and important; when they are considered carefully, they have the potential for speeding along the process of collecting knowledge of aging language.

It is perhaps the case that these chapters raise more questions than they answer. Nevertheless, they provide a rudimentary map for the territory. This map should become more richly detailed as future research and experience with the special problems of language in the elderly are investigated. As the graying of America (and the rest of the planet) continues, the issues raised here will continue to ferment and grow in importance, and new answers will be found. Perhaps my fondest hope for this area of study is that we learn enough in the next 10 years to make this work obsolete by the turn of the century.

Aphasia and Aging

Sandra B. Chapman, PhD, and
Hanna K. Ulatowska, PhD ■

The evidence for extension of the life-span in recent years is impressive. Unfortunately, a longer life expectancy does not ensure well-being for the added years of life. Rather, the prevalence of disease processes, such as cerebrovascular disease and degenerative brain diseases, multiplies with age. These disease processes alter not only medical status, but also aspects of cognitive functions such as language functioning. The primary challenge for professionals in neurology, neuropsychology, neurolinguistics, and aphasiology is to seek answers for questions concerning age-related changes versus disease-related changes.

The purpose of this chapter is fourfold. First, literature characterizing language in the older aphasic patient is reviewed. One fundamental question raised is whether language in elderly aphasic patients differs from that observed in younger patients. If so, how does language disruption differ and what explanations might account for these differences as a function of age? Second,

methodological guidelines are offered for investigations in geriatric aphasiology regarding ways to distinguish aphasia-related changes from both age-related changes and changes related to other, non-aphasic conditions. The information necessary for making a differential diagnosis will be derived from contrastive studies of relevant populations, for example, (a) young versus old aphasic subjects, (b) young versus old Wernicke's and Broca's aphasic subjects, (c) older aphasic patients versus normal elderly adults, and (d) older aphasic patients versus patients with different dementia types. These particular contrasts are important in order to detect similarities and differences across elderly populations that may identify co-occurring processes. Third, considerations for selection of appropriate tests and tasks to measure language and communicative function in older aphasic patients are discussed. Finally, clinical implications of the relevant issues in aphasia and aging are offered.

Characterization of Aphasia in Elderly Aphasic Patients

Unfortunately, when compared to the profile of language in younger aphasic patients, the profile in elderly aphasic patients is not favorable. Older aphasic individuals tend to exhibit a more debilitating aphasia than younger patients do. The severity of aphasia tends to increase with age because the risk of confounding factors is greater for elderly patients. Finally, while the evidence is equivocal, recovery appears to be slower and less pronounced in elderly aphasic patients. These three issues will be discussed in this chapter and explanations for the discrepancies as a function of age will be considered.

Age-Related Patterns in Aphasia Type

Language Differences

In general, classification for both younger and older aphasic patients has been established by using aphasia batteries, including the *Boston Diagnostic Aphasia Examination* (Goodglass & Kaplan, 1983; Harasymiw, Halper, & Sutherland, 1981; Obler, Albert, Goodglass, & Benson, 1978) and the *Western Aphasia Battery* (Holland & Bartlett, 1985; Kertesz, 1982). Despite the considerable controversy over the use of these diagnostic tools in classifying aphasia type, an age-related pattern of aphasia type has been replicated by both retrospective and prospective studies using different aphasia batteries. The findings appear to be quite robust.

The evidence for language differences in older aphasic subjects as compared to younger aphasic subjects is overwhelming. Older aphasic patients are more likely to manifest language reflective of Wernicke's aphasia, whereas Broca's aphasia is more prevalent in younger aphasic patients

(Brown & Grober, 1983; Harasymiw et al., 1981; Holland & Bartlett, 1985; Obler et al., 1978). The mean age difference between the two aphasia types is nearly 10 years. The incidence of Broca's aphasia peaks at ages 40 and 50, whereas the incidence of Wernicke's aphasia continues to increase with age until 70 years of age.

The major studies describe patients according to type of aphasia (e.g., Wernicke's and Broca's aphasia), rather than according to specific linguistic disruptions. Therefore, the language characteristics must be inferred from the widely held view of the aphasia types. As it is classically defined, Wernicke's aphasia is correlated with damage to the left posterior region of the perisylvian cortex or primary language area. Impairment to this region frequently produces disturbances of language characterized by impairments of auditory comprehension, repetition, and naming with relative preservation of fluency. Paraphasic errors and empty terms such as indefinite pronouns pervade the expressive language of Wernicke's aphasic patients. In contrast, Broca's aphasia is classically associated with lesions localized to the left anterior region of the perisylvian cortex. Broca's aphasia is characterized by relative preservation of auditory comprehension with marked impairment of fluency. Furthermore, the language of Broca's aphasic patients is characterized by primarily information-bearing terms as opposed to the empty language frequently expressed by Wernicke's aphasic patients. Naming and repetition are impaired in both Broca's and Wernicke's aphasia. In sum, the greater prevalence of Wernicke's aphasia in older patients implies that older aphasic patients are more likely to exhibit relatively fluent speech, paraphasic errors, and impaired comprehension and content than younger patients are.

Explanations of Age-Related Changes

Several explanations have been offered to account for differences in speech and language disturbances as a function of age

(Carter, 1978; Eslinger & Damasio, 1981; Holland & Bartlett, 1985; Obler et al., 1978). Three hypotheses relate to (a) vascular changes with age, (b) generalized neuro-pathophysiological changes with age, and (c) continuing lateralization of language function into later adulthood.

Perhaps the most frequently proposed hypothesis is that the age-related shift in aphasia type from an anteriorly based aphasia to a posteriorly based aphasia represents a probable shift in the location of the cerebral damage to a more posterior focus with advancing age. The presumed shift in focus could be due either to changes with age in arterial configuration, changes in blood flow, or etiologic changes. The assumptions underlying an etiologic basis are that embolic, thrombotic, and hemorrhagic foci change over the life-span. Kertesz and Sheppard (1981) suggested that younger patients may be more likely to throw off embolisms from cardiac or carotid disease that cause more anteriorly based lesions, whereas elderly patients may be more prone to suffer cerebral thrombosis in the posterior branches of the middle cerebral artery.

Currently, there is no evidence to support the etiologic hypothesis and, in fact, research counter to this pattern has been reported. The age of Wernicke's aphasics continues to be greater than for other types of aphasia even when the etiology is neoplasm (Micheli, Caltagirone, Gainotti, Masullo, Silveri, & Villa, 1981). Moreover, a retrospective study of 200 patients also failed to confirm a relationship between age and stroke location as identified by computerized tomography (Habib, Ali-Cherif, Poncet, & Salamon, 1987). Although there was a tendency for lesions to become more posterior with age, this tendency was only significant up to age 45. No relation between age and posterior location for stroke was observed beyond the age of 45. Habib and colleagues concluded that a posterior shift of stroke location, as assessed by anatomical measures, did not occur with age. The researchers suggested that measures of brain function may provide more

insight into the mechanisms underlying the behavioral differences. Functional abnormalities in posterior regions of the brain may contribute to the language differences, because behavior can be altered as a consequence of changes in brain function in the absence of any measurable structural abnormality. Future research in this area should help to clarify this possibility.

A second possible explanation is that "normal" neurological changes that accompany aging give rise to the age-related differences in aphasia. Changes in both brain anatomy and brain function have been reported with age. These normal changes may contribute to altered cognitive-linguistic function, manifested as different aphasia types. In regard to structure, there is evidence of a decline in neuronal density in the superior temporal gyrus, the region where Wernicke's area lies (Brody, 1955). Since this posterior region is specifically associated with comprehension and fluent language, the reduction of neural tissue in this area may contribute to the behavioral manifestations of a Wernicke's-type aphasia in older patients. In regard to brain function, blood flow studies suggest that anterior brain regions tend to manifest greater reduction of blood flow with increased age. Since anterior brain regions are associated with inhibition, dysfunction to this region may yield increased output or verbosity. These data are by no means exhaustive. Other regions of the brain are also reportedly altered with aging. However, these isolated findings support a possible interaction between age-related neurological changes and stroke, resulting in a different type of aphasia in older patients than in younger patients.

A third potential explanation is that developmental changes occur in brain specificity for language as manifested by a continuous evolution of the neural organization of the language area (Brown & Grober, 1983). Brown and Jaffe (1975) reported that lesions to similar brain regions produced distinct behavioral manifestations and aphasia types at different ages. Specifically, a lesion to Wernicke's area resulted in motor aphasia in a child, conduction aphasia in middle age, and jargon aphasia in later life. This explanation presupposes that the nervous system and its special functions continue to change throughout life. The possibility of neural plasticity in the normal aging brain is consistent with recent anatomical evidence of dendritic growth in aging animal brains (Diamond, 1983; Diamond, Rosenzweig, Bennett, Lindner, & Lyon, 1972).

At present, the explanation does not appear to be a simple one. Whether the differences between younger and older aphasic patients are strictly the result of linguistic deficits is unresolved. Obler et al. (1978) postulated that the increased incidence of Wernicke's aphasia in older patients may be due to the interaction of age-related neurological and behavioral changes overlaid on the effects of focal brain damage in the left hemisphere. Despite the uncertainty, there is general agreement that older patients manifest different linguistic profiles than younger patients.

Severity of Aphasia in Aging

Evidence indicates that the severity of linguistic deficits in aphasia increases with advancing age (Holland & Bartlett, 1985). At onset, severity ratings indicate greater impairment for elderly patients than for younger aphasic patients. The documentation of greater deficits as a function of age is not surprising, given the inherent differences between Broca's and Wernicke's types of aphasia. Wernicke's aphasic patients typically manifest greater involvement of all language modalities, such as listening, speaking, reading, and writing, than do Broca's patients. The greater involvement of all modalities observed in Wernicke's aphasia may emanate from the presence of a more profound comprehension impairment, because other modalities, such as expression, are intrinsically tied to comprehension.

Furthermore, the severity of aphasia in older patients is compromised by the pres-

ence of a more generalized cognitive impairment. Holland and Bartlett (1985) found a greater reduction in both linguistic and other cognitive functions in older aphasic patients as compared to younger patients. Specifically, patients in the older age group performed more poorly on the *Raven's Coloured Progressive Matrices*.

Interestingly, the likelihood of a global aphasia is increased, or is at least as likely, for younger aphasic patients (Holland & Bartlett, 1985). At first glance, evidence of a greater prevalence of global aphasia in younger patients seems to contradict the greater impairment in older patients. It is important to note, however, that this higher incidence of global aphasia in younger patients was found only for the acute stages. Holland and Bartlett (1985) found that as early as 3 months after onset, all the younger patients had resolved to a less severe aphasia. This degree of resolution did not occur in the population of older, global aphasic patients.

Aphasia Recovery in Aging

The findings supporting a relationship between age and patterns of recovery in aphasia are equivocal. While no study argues against some degree of improvement in elderly patients, several studies suggest that the gains in language recovery of older patients are not as pronounced as those of younger patients. The improvements are smaller and the rate of recovery is slower (Holland & Bartlett, 1985; Holland, Greenhouse, Fromm, & Swindell, 1989; Mitchell, 1958; Sands, Sarno, & Shankweiler, 1969; Schow, Christensen, Hutchinson, & Nerbonne, 1978; Vignolo, 1964). The investigators conclude that age is an important predictor of recovery in aphasia. In contrast, evidence from other studies indicates that age is not a significant factor in predicting recovery (Basso, Capitani, & Vignolo, 1979; Culton, 1971; Keenan & Brassell, 1974; Kertesz & McCabe, 1977; Sarno, 1980; Sarno & Levita, 1971). Recovery with treatment appears to be essentially the same for patients of all age groups if confounding variables such as education, medical condition, medication, or living environment are controlled.

Several explanations are offered to account for the disparity in findings. First, studies that control the complicating variables may eliminate patients who are representative of the "typical" geriatric population. As Holland and Bartlett (1985) point out, rarely is all else equal in elderly- and younger-patient populations. Second, the trends observed in large-group studies obscure individual recovery patterns (Chapman, 1988; Holland & Bartlett, 1985). Some elderly patients recover remarkably well. Most recent evidence supports the notion that the potential for recovery is not determined by the patient's age but rather by how well the patient has aged. Prognosis should be based on individual patterns of recovery and not on whether the patient is regaining a functional level commensurate with that of a younger person.

Recovery is more complicated in elderly individuals because of the heterogeneity in biological, sociological, and psychological factors. The view that aging affects the body much like a disease process, reducing the body's ability to maintain, repair, and improve itself, is inaccurate. Despite the evidence that older patients are likely to experience a decline on anatomical, physiological, and metabolic measures, the aging brain shows a capacity to restructure and change (Buell & Coleman, 1979; Greenough & Green, 1981). Sociologically, older individuals undergo the most dramatic changes in their social status since early adulthood. They often experience an abrupt change in employment, family constellation, social network, financial resources, and living environment. The shrinking social network reduces opportunities for interaction and eventually leads to modification of communication style. For example, efficient transfer of information may become less important than opportunities to interact for

extended intervals (Ulatowska, Cannito, Hayashi, & Fleming, 1985). Psychological factors also interact with recovery. For instance, the more involved the person has been in challenging mental abilities preceding a stroke, the better the prognosis. Older individuals tend to be less involved in daily activities that require memory and problem solving (Schaie, 1983). Recent evidence indicates that new learning is possible in very old persons, although it takes more time and effort to acquire new information than it did in younger years.

Thus, it is not so much chronological age that predicts recovery, but rather intactness of biological, sociological, and psychological systems. Furthermore, the desire to improve and to receive treatment is important to the recovery process. Isolating the factors that affect recovery is essential to treatment decisions. In the section that follows, contrasts between different clinical populations are discussed as they relate to older aphasic patients. These contrasts are requisite for identifying confounding factors in the older aphasic individual.

Relevant Contrasts to Aphasia and Aging

Comparisons of Young and Elderly Aphasic Patients

A number of studies have compared younger aphasic patients with older aphasic patients. From these studies, three empirical facts were documented regarding aphasia in elderly patient populations. First, as discussed above, differences in type and severity of aphasia as a function of age were identified. Second, anatomical evidence was not consistent with hypothesized focus as predicted by classical brain/behavior theory. According to classical brain/behavior principles of aphasia, older aphasic patients were expected to manifest a left posterior lesion focus consistent with the focus commonly associated with Wernicke's aphasia. Third, in general, the amount of recovery in both young and older aphasic patients was found to be similar when confounding factors were eliminated.

Although previous studies identified important behavioral and neuropathological aspects in the elderly aphasic patient, their primary merit was in providing impetus and direction for future research with the older aphasic patient. These studies laid the groundwork for different avenues of investigation that were motivated by the need to confirm or refute possible explanations for the age-related differences in aphasia type. Three issues warrant attention: (a) the influence of normal age-related changes; (b) the influence of age within aphasia type, for example, young versus old Wernicke's patients; and (c) the influence of concomitant diseases other than the aphasia. Normal age-related changes should be established by longitudinal studies of language changes across the lifespan. The changes of language performance in normal elderly can then be matched against the language disruption of older aphasic patients. Comparisons of young Wernicke's patients with older Wernicke's aphasic patients could further clarify the added effects of aging on stroke. Finally, it is important to consider disease-related changes other than those attributable to aphasia through comparisons of older aphasic patients with other elderly, clinical populations. Disorders common to aging include different types of dementia, hypertension, and diabetes, to mention a few. In this chapter, we will restrict our discussion to elderly individuals with aphasia and a dementing disorder, either dementia of the Alzheimer's type (DAT) or multi-infarct dementia (MID).

Comparisons of Normal Elderly and Elderly Aphasic Individuals

An understanding of normal language and neuropathophysiological correlates in the elderly is essential to understanding lan-guage differences in elderly aphasic patients. This fact is underscored by the recent evidence that certain language patterns commonly found in Wernicke's aphasic patients also appear in the language of the normal elderly (Cannito, Hayashi, & Ulatowska, 1988; North, Ulatowska, Macaluso-Haynes, & Bell, 1986; Ulatowska, Hayashi, Cannito, & Fleming, 1986). Such findings imply that the presence of normal changes may impede sorting out age-related changes from pathological changes. Unfortunately, norms for changes in language with age are extremely limited, restricting the ability to delineate specific criteria for differential diagnosis. In this section, an overview of the language changes relevant to language in older aphasic patients is presented. The neurological findings in aging are specified by Civil and Whitehouse in chapter 1 of this book. Thus, only selected neurological correlates of language are mentioned here.

Language

As previously described, language in older aphasic patients is characterized by impaired naming and auditory comprehension. In addition, their speech is described as fluent, with reduced content relative to the amount of language expressed. How pervasive are these problems in the language of the normal elderly? As the following information indicates, these same behaviors are found in both populations, although the degree of impairment is greater in aphasic patients.

Naming

Considerable evidence exists to suggest that naming ability declines with advancing age. One common complaint of elderly people is increased difficulty in finding words in everyday speaking and writing. While word recognition is maintained or even increased with age, the ability to access vocabulary appears to decrease with increasing age (Bowles & Poon, 1985). Furthermore, some evidence suggests that object naming, naming latency, and word fluency decline with age (Obler & Albert, 1981; Schow et al., 1978). Some discrepancy in the literature exists in characterization of naming abilities in elderly subjects, probably as a consequence of the nature of the task assessing lexicon. In contrast to lowered performance on word-generation tasks, elderly adult speakers demonstrated higher performance in conversational speech as measured by type-token ratios than did younger speakers (Walker, Hardiman, Hedrick, & Holbrook, 1981). Older adults may display a more varied vocabulary in conversation than they demonstrate on more artificial naming tasks. While incongruity exists in characterization of naming ability in the elderly with advancing age, the difficulty in lexical access appears to be real.

Comprehension

Among other findings, deficits in language comprehension in the normal elderly population have also been reported (Cohen, 1979; Feier & Gerstman, 1980; Obler & Albert, 1984; Peach, 1987). Comprehension deficits in the elderly have been attributed to (a) decline in hearing acuity; (b) general cognitive concomitants of aging such as longer response time, attentional deficits, difficulty in changing tasks, memory deficits, and distractibility; and (c) a general slowness of neurological response (Obler & Albert, 1984; Peach, 1987). Comprehension of inference is particularly problematic for elderly patients (Cohen, 1979). This latter deficit may reflect an inefficiency in the language processing system in simultaneously interpreting surface meaning and integrating the information.

In addition to the naming and comprehension deficits, changes in flow of speech have been reported with age. Evidence suggests that older adults become somewhat "hyperfluent" and are described as verbose or loquacious (Obler & Albert, 1981). In sharp contrast, taciturnity has also been described (Critchley, 1984). The most frequent hypothesis for the increased verbosity is a general tendency toward disinhibition secondary to age-dependent changes in the frontolimbic system. The decreased quantity, on the other hand, could be the consequence of subcortical deterioration. In addition, an increase in the use of vague and indefinite words has been reported with age, along with reduced clarity of language (North et al., 1986; Obler & Albert, 1984).

Neurological Aspects

The neuropathophysiological correlates of aging are far from conclusive. Some evidence from both structural and functional brain imaging studies (computed tomography and positron emission tomography) supports changes to frontal regions of the brain (Kuhl, Metter, Riege, & Hawkins, 1984; Kuhl, Metter, Riege, & Phelps, 1982; Metter, 1988; Sandor, LeMay, Kido, & Rumbaugh, 1981). It has been hypothesized that regional changes underlie the increased fluency with advancing age. If so, this may help explain why a fluent aphasia is more likely with advancing age. In addition, electrophysiological changes on electroencephalography have been described over the left anterior temporal regions in adults over 60 years of age (Finitzo, Bartlett, & Pool, 1989; Kooi, Guvener, Tupper, & Bagchi, 1964; Silverman, Busse, & Barnes, 1955). Other researchers identified more right hemispheric changes in electrophysiology with age (Duffy, Albert, McAnulty, & Garvey, 1984). The changes over the right hemisphere may explain reduced recovery in older patients.

In summary, reports of age-related deficits in language have identified deficits similar to those observed in Wernicke's aphasia. These deficits include changes in naming, auditory comprehension, content, and fluency of speech. Although it is highly unlikely that normal elderly individuals would be misdiagnosed as having aphasia, some deficits observed in older aphasic patients may be the consequence of normal aging processes rather than of the aphasia itself. Comparisons between normal elderly and older aphasic individuals on both standardized aphasia batteries and experimental tasks is critical to differentiation of the confounding effects of aging. While some advancements have been achieved in altering evaluation procedures for older aphasia patients, such as modifying cutoff scores, considerably more attention to this dilemma is required to distinguish age-related changes from aphasia-related changes (Davis & Holland, 1981).

Comparisons of Young and Elderly Wernicke's and Broca's Aphasic Patients

Distinguishing the effects of aging in aphasia is not easily achieved. Contrasting younger and elderly patients with Wernicke's type of aphasia may help to elucidate some factors of aging alone. Despite the fact that Wernicke's aphasia increases with age, approximately 25% of the Wernicke's patients are younger than 50 years of age (Harasymiw et al., 1981). The comparison of younger and older Wernicke's patients should include not only group studies but also longitudinal studies of patients. Longitudinal studies would clarify how Wernicke's patients evolve over time as aging factors come into play.

Comparisons of younger and elderly patients with Broca's type of aphasia would also be of interest in addressing the question of how a nonfluent aphasia might be influenced by the aging process. Perhaps the conflicting perspective of comprehension deficits in Broca's aphasia may be complicated by the inclusion of patients at all age levels. The Broca's patients with the most difficulty on comprehension tasks may be the older patients.

Comparisons of Elderly Aphasic Patients with Demented Patients

The possibility of dementia co-occurring with aphasia is increased for older patients as compared to younger aphasic patients.

Holland and Bartlett (1985) found that 23% of the aphasic patients they studied who were over 70 years of age showed signs of dementia. In contrast, none of their aphasic patients under 60 years of age manifested such clinical signs. All dementia appeared subsequent to a stroke, because patients with a premorbid history of dementia were excluded from their study. The behavioral manifestations were characterized by naming difficulties, digressive and pragmatically inappropriate conversation, and family reports of further deterioration in cognitive abilities. The risk of dementia in elderly aphasic patients makes it necessary to determine the presence of dementia. The dilemma of distinguishing aphasic symptomatology from dementing or normal aging is further emphasized by recent evidence that discourse in patients with mild-stage dementia resembles that of normal old-elderly adults over 85 years of age (Ulatowska & Chapman, in press). Dementia of the Alzheimer's type and multi-infarct dementia, the most common dementias in elderly populations, are discussed next. These two dementia types are described in detail in chapter 15 of this text.

Alzheimer's Dementia

The language observed in patients with DAT is frequently compared with the language of Wernicke's aphasic patients. The similarities are of particular relevance to this chapter, because Wernicke's aphasia is more common to elderly aphasic patients. Both clinical populations exhibit auditory comprehension impairments, verbal deficits in naming, and spontaneous language and memory problems (Bayles, 1985; Kaszniak & Wilson, 1985). Despite what appear to be considerable similarities, there are marked differences between patients with DAT and Wernicke's aphasia (Bayles & Kaszniak, 1987; Ulatowska & Chapman, in press). In general, the deficits observed in DAT are primarily in communicative functions rather than being primarily linguistic deficits. Moreover, language abilities in DAT are preserved relative to cognitive abilities. In contrast, the communicative deficits in Wernicke's aphasia are mainly the result of linguistic deficits. Furthermore, in aphasia, cognitive abilities tend to be preserved relative to linguistic abilities. It is likely that the similarities between the two populations are parallel on the surface only. The similar disruptions are likely to be the result of different underlying mechanisms.

Unfortunately, the gap in performance between Wernicke's aphasic patients and DAT patients may diminish as the age of the aphasic patient increases. This premise is based upon the evidence that normal old-elderly (older than 85 years of age) performed similarly to DAT patients on cognitive and linguistic measures relevant to communicative function (Ulatowska & Chapman, in press). Thus, age interacts with aphasia to produce some of the same behavioral changes as those observed in DAT, complicating the differential diagnostic process.

Multi-infarct Dementia

Comparisons between elderly aphasic and MID patients are necessary to disentangle important factors related to differentiation of an ongoing disease process from a more static process. In MID, new symptoms appear episodically and suddenly, as they do in the onset of symptoms in aphasia, but distinct from the slow insidious process observed in DAT. MID may not be easily differentiated from aphasia, particularly in elderly adults, because the risk of repeated cerebrovascular accidents or one major stroke with multiple transient ischemic attacks increases with age. Powell, Cummings, Hill, and Benson (1988) suggested that MID may represent a collection of dissimilar clinical presentations linked only by a common cerebrovascular etiology.

Summary

This overview has served to delineate the facts concerning aphasia in the elderly and to illustrate the complexity of distinguishing aphasia-related deficits from disease-related and age-related changes in language function. In general, there is a consensus regarding several issues of aphasia and aging. The most widely accepted premise is that the incidence of Wernicke's aphasia increases with advancing age. In addition, there is general agreement that when all other factors (e.g., health, education, and social status) are held constant, chronological age alone is not a good predictor of either severity or prognosis in aphasia. Some very elderly patients improve and recover remarkably well. Unfortunately, the risk of concomitant problems is greater with increasing age. Thus, what is needed is an improved methodology for distinguishing aphasia-related factors from other factors.

There is considerable evidence of behavioral overlap in language dissolution among elderly aphasic, normal elderly, and dementing individuals. The overlap illustrates the factors that complicate the process of answering the pertinent questions relevant to aphasia and age. At this stage, we offer some suggestions for addressing the question of whether the language deficits reflect aphasia alone or whether some additional process is taking place. As has been indicated, contrastive studies of the populations are necessary. The issue of concern now is what methods should be implemented to address the relevant issues. Our particular bias is that discourse provides a promising behavioral measure to aid in differential diagnosis. Furthermore, single-case studies are required to elucidate the critical features of distinction.

Methodological Considerations in Investigations of Aphasia and Aging

Use of Aphasia Batteries

For the most part, language in elderly aphasic patients has been assessed using aphasia batteries. Although these batteries are useful, there are certain limitations of which the speech-language pathologist should be aware. The usefulness of comprehensive aphasia batteries is seen in their ability to identify the language disruptions common to aphasia. Test construction is based upon empirical information about aphasic deficits and thus is designed to measure different language modalities and different levels of language. Batteries have also been useful in profiling aphasia symptomatology and establishing level of severity.

On the other hand, the aphasia batteries have certain limitations when they are used with elderly patients; therefore, the results obtained should be interpreted cautiously. One limitation is that the tests have not been validated on sizable elderly populations, either normal or aphasic. Recent evidence suggests that normal elderly individuals may exhibit difficulty on certain subtests such as object description, generative naming, and measures of reading and writing (Davis & Baggs, 1985). The question raised is whether lowered performance on these specific measures implies pathological behavior or simply represents "normal" age-related behavioral differences. Thus, the tests are somewhat limited in distinguishing aphasia-related deficits from age-related deficits. This insensitivity is not restricted to aging factors but extends to factors of dementing disorders (Bayles, Boone, Tomoeda, Slauson, & Kaszniak, 1989). Furthermore, aphasia tests may be negatively biased toward elderly patients because of the artificiality of the testing situation. Elderly adults tend to be more anxious than younger adults during testing conditions. This increased anxiety is probably due to the fact that they have not been participants in testing situations for a considerably longer period of time (Whitbourne, 1976). Anxiety arises from fear of failure, contributed to by the lack of saliency and familiarity of the tasks.

Discourse Measures

At present, aphasia batteries are beneficial in diagnosing language impairment in older aphasic patients. However, the aphasia tests alone are inadequate for purposes of differential diagnosis because they tap primarily linguistic behavior. Linguistic measures are necessary but insufficient to distinguish between aphasia-related deficits and other potential factors at risk in elderly patients. Supplemental tasks that measure cognitive abilities are also necessary, because cognitive disabilities are more prominent and less equivocal than linguistic function in both normal elderly and dementing populations. Different elderly populations may exhibit similar language deficits for different reasons. For example, deficits in language comprehension have been identified for normal elderly adults and aphasic patients on measures of complex syntactic structures and integration of inferential meaning from paragraph-length material. In aphasic patients, the primary deficit appears to be linguistic. For elderly and dementing populations, comprehension may be compromised more by underlying cognitive impairments, such as attention, memory, and reasoning impairments, than by primary linguistic deficits.

A fundamental question concerns measurement of both linguistic and cognitive abilities. Tasks in which cognitive and linguistic processing are intricately related will provide the most promising approach. Discourse measures may prove beneficial for two reasons. First, considerable information is now available on discourse processing in aphasia, old-elderly, and dementia (Bayles & Kaszniak, 1987; Bond, Ulatowska, Macaluso-Haynes, & May, 1983; Cannito et al., 1988; Nicholas, Obler, Albert, & Helm-Estabrooks, 1985; North et al., 1986; Obler & Albert, 1981; Ulatowska, Freedman-Stern, Weiss Doyel, Macaluso-Haynes, & North, 1983; Ulatowska, North, & Macaluso-Haynes, 1981; Ulatowska et al., 1985). Second, discourse represents the level of communicative function wherein the interaction between linguistic and cognitive abilities is most clearly manifested (Ulatowska et al., 1985). Discourse provides a vehicle for examining both organization of information and facility with language. Thus, discourse may provide an optimal measure for differentiating linguistically related disorders from more cognitively based disorders. Potentially, discourse measures could help to sort out aphasia-related deficits from certain concomitant problems inherent to the aging process.

Language abilities should be evaluated at multiple levels of usage—the word, sentential, and discourse levels. A multilevel analysis of language will provide the most valuable information in terms of identification of (a) similarities and differences and (b) spared and impaired abilities across clinical populations (Ulatowska & Chapman, 1989). In the diagnostic process, it is imperative to identify not only the losses but also the preserved abilities. Spared abilities may be as significant to the differential diagnosis as deficits, because clinical populations manifest similar impairments. It is possible that the appearance of similar impairments results from the limited number of ways in which language structure can break down; however, the potential mechanisms underlying similar disruptions may be quite different.

Longitudinal and Single-Case Studies

Using aphasia batteries to evaluate elderly populations is problematic, because normal declines in language with age and with dementia confound our results (Bayles et al., 1989; Davis & Baggs, 1985). The most important issue to be addressed is how to measure and identify the effects of normal aging on language performance. Most of the evidence regarding differences with age have been derived from cross-sectional studies (Albert, 1988). Although such an approach has provided interesting findings, it is difficult to interpret the results because people at various ages differ along a number of dimensions other than age, such as health care, nutrition, education, and sociocultural opportunities. What is greatly needed is longitudinal testing in which the same individuals are repeatedly assessed as they continue to age. The inherent methodological problem in longitudinal studies is

patient dropout. Despite this drawback, longitudinal studies are necessary in order to determine the changes that occur with the progressive behavioral decline observed in normal aging and dementing processes. Furthermore, longitudinal studies will be useful in addressing the presence of continuous or stepwise progressions of symptoms in different elderly populations. Longitudinal single-case studies will fill a notable void in the normative aging data; in addition, single-case studies allow for greater in-depth evaluations from multiple disciplines. Evaluation of coexisting processes and their potential interactive effects is feasible with single patients.

Clinical Implications

This chapter has focused on the relevant issues in geriatric aphasiology in terms of aphasia characteristics and dilemmas in differential diagnosis. Addressing the diagnostic problems has implications not only for future research, but also for clinical management. Until recently, it was felt that deficits resulting from stroke warranted intervention, but those resulting from normal aging and from dementia did not, because they were thought to be more resistive to treatment. More recently, the increased recognition of communication impairment in DAT and in normal elderly has motivated speech-language pathologists to reexamine their role in management of the various elderly populations.

The older aphasic patient provides the most vivid illustration of the vital need for a holistic approach to the study of aging. To view language disturbances without regard for other potentially debilitating factors would do considerable disservice to the patient. Losses must be viewed within the total conceptual framework of the aging process.

The clinical framework for managing older patients with aphasia requires that neurological, psychological, and sociological processes intrinsic to aging be considered in relation to the effect they have on aphasia. Identification of the factors that may hinder improvement is essential to clinical management. Whereas most elderly patients benefit from therapeutic intervention, intervention is not warranted for many others, either because the patients do not desire treatment or because the prognosis is guarded. A number of factors may reduce motivation; some are inherent to the disease process and others may be alleviated. For instance, aphasic patients with a coexisting dementia may lack the motivation to participate in therapy. In dementia, apathy may arise from intrinsic neurological alterations. Lack of desire may also be traceable to the side effects of medication, depression, or dramatic alteration in support systems. These factors are presumably more responsive to modification than the first.

Communicative competence in geriatric populations offers an ideal vantage point for viewing age- and disease-related deficits. Since communicative adequacy, as measured by discourse, reflects both linguistic and cognitive abilities, the speech-language pathologist should be instrumental in establishing criteria for differential diagnosis. Older aphasic patients provide an important comparison group because more is known about communication and language changes in aphasia than in any other population. The older aphasic patient will teach us so that we may, in turn, manage the individual patient more effectively.

References

Albert, M. S. (1988). General issues in geriatric neuropsychology. In M. S. Albert & M. B. Moss (Eds.), *Geriatric neuropsychology* (Vol. 1, pp. 3–10). New York: Guilford Press.

Basso, A., Capitani, E., & Vignolo, L. (1979). Influence of rehabilitation on language skills in aphasic patients. *Archives of Neurology, 36,* 190–196.

Bayles, K. (1985). Communication in dementia. In H. K. Ulatowska (Ed.), *The aging brain* (pp. 157–174). Austin, TX: PRO-ED.

Bayles, K., Boone, D., Tomoeda, C., Slauson, T., & Kaszniak, A. (1989). Differentiating Alzheimer's patients from the normal elderly and stroke patients with aphasia. *Journal of Speech and Hearing Disorders, 54,* 74–87.

Bayles, K., & Kaszniak, A. (1987). *Communication and cognition in normal aging and dementia.* Austin, TX: PRO-ED.

Bond, S., Ulatowska, H., Macaluso-Haynes, S., & May E. (1983). Discourse production in aphasia: Relationship to severity of impairment. In R. H. Brookshire (Ed.), *Proceedings of the Clinical Aphasiology Conference.* Minneapolis: BRK Publishers.

Bowles, N., & Poon, L. (1985). Aging and retrieval of words in semantic memory. *Journal of Gerontology, 40,* 71–77.

Brody, H. (1955). Organization of the cerebral cortex: Study of aging in the human cerebral cortex. *Journal of Comparative Neurology, 102,* 511–556.

Brown, J. W., & Grober, E. (1983). Age, sex and aphasia type. *Journal of Nervous and Mental Diseases, 171,* 431–434.

Brown, J., & Jaffe, J. (1975). Hypothesis on cerebral dominance. *Neuropsychologia, 13,* 107–110.

Buell, S., & Coleman, P. (1979). Dendritic growth in the aged brain and failure of growth in senile dementia. *Science, 206,* 854–856.

Cannito, M. P., Hayashi, M. M., & Ulatowska, H. K. (1988). Discourse in normal and pathologic aging: Background and assessment strategies. *Seminars in Speech and Language, 2,* 117–134.

Carter, J. E. (1978). Age, aphasia, and stroke localization [Letter to the editor]. *Archives of Neurology, 35,* 619.

Chapman, S. B. (1988). The older aphasic patient: The problems and the potential. *Seminars in Speech and Language, 2,* 135–147.

Cohen, G. (1979). Language comprehension in old age. *Cognitive Psychology, 11,* 412–429.

Critchley, M. (1984). And all the daughters of music shall be brought low: Language function in the elderly. *Archives of Neurology, 41,* 1135–1139.

Culton, G. (1971). Reaction to age as a factor in chronic aphasia in stroke patients. *Journal of Speech and Hearing Disorders, 36,* 563.

Davis, A., & Baggs, T. (1985). Rehabilitation of speech and language disorders. In L. Jacobs-Condit (Ed.), *Gerontology and communication disorders.* Rockville, MD: American Speech-Language-Hearing Association.

Davis, G., & Holland, A. (1981). Age in understanding aphasia. In D. S. Beasley & G. A. Davis (Eds.), *Aging, communication processes, and disorders*. New York: Grune & Stratton.

Diamond, M. (1983). The aging rat forebrain: Male-female left-right environment and lipofuscin. In D. Samuel, S. Algeri, S. Gershon, V. Grimm, & G. Toffano (Eds.), *Aging of the brain* (pp. 93–98). New York: Raven Press.

Diamond, M., Rosenzweig, M., Bennett, E., Lindner, B., & Lyon, L. (1972). Effects of environmental enrichment and impoverishment on the rat cerebral cortex. *Journal of Neurology, 3,* 47–64.

Duffy, F., Albert, M., McAnulty, G., & Garvey, A. (1984). Age-related differences in brain electrical activity of healthy subjects. *Annals of Neurology, 16,* 430–438.

Eslinger, P., & Damasio, A. (1981). Age and type of aphasia in patients with stroke. *Journal of Neurology, Neurosurgery and Psychiatry, 44,* 377–381.

Feier, C., & Gerstman, L. (1980). Sentence comprehension abilities throughout the adult lifespan. *Journal of Gerontology, 35,* 729–735.

Finitzo, T., Bartlett, J., & Pool, K. (1989). The role of topographic and quantitative electrophysiology in cognitive issues in aging. In A. Small (Ed.), *Communication sciences and disorders and aging.* ASHA Report. Rockville, MD: American Speech-Language-Hearing Association.

Goodglass, H., & Kaplan, E. (1983). *The assessment of aphasia and related disorders* (2nd ed.). Philadelphia: Lea & Febiger.

Greenough, W. T., & Green, E. J. (1981). Experience and changing brain. In J. McGaugh & S. Kiesler (Eds.), *Aging: Biology and behavior.* New York: Academic Press.

Habib, M., Ali-Cherif, A., Poncet, M., & Salamon, G. (1987). Age-related changes in aphasia type and stroke location. *Brain and Language, 31,* 245–251.

Harasymiw, S. J., Halper, A., & Sutherland, B. (1981). Sex, age and aphasia type. *Brain and Language, 12,* 190–198.

Holland, A. L., & Bartlett, C. L. (1985). Some differential effects of age on stroke-produced aphasia. In H. K. Ulatowska (Ed.), *The aging brain: Communication in the elderly.* Austin, TX: PRO-ED.

Holland, A. L., Greenhouse, J. B., Fromm, D., & Swindell, C. S. (1989). Predictors of language restitution following stroke: A multivariate analysis. *Journal of Speech and Hearing Research, 32,* 232–238.

Kaszniak, A., & Wilson, R. (1985). *Longitudinal deterioration of language and cognition in dementia of the Alzheimer's type.* Paper presented as part of a symposium at the International Neuropsychological Society meeting, San Diego, CA.

Keenan, J. S., & Brassell, E. G. (1974). A study of the factors related to prognosis for individual aphasic patients. *Journal of Speech and Hearing Disorders, 39,* 257–269.

Kertesz, A. (1982). Western Aphasia Battery. New York: Grune & Stratton.

Kertesz, A., & McCabe, P. (1977). Recovery patterns and prognosis in aphasia. *Brain, 100,* 1–18.

Kertesz, A., & Sheppard, A. (1981). The epidemiology of aphasic and cognitive impairment in stroke: Age, sex, aphasia type and laterality differences. *Brain, 104,* 117–128.

Kooi, K., Guvener, A., Tupper, C., & Bagchi, B. K. (1964). Electroencephalographic patterns of the temporal region in normal adults. *Neurology, 14,* 1029–1035.

Kuhl, D. E., Metter, E. J., Riege, W. H., & Hawkins, R. A. (1984). The effect of normal aging on patterns of local cerebral glucose utilization. *Annals of Neurology, 15* (Suppl.), 133–137.

Kuhl, D. E., Metter, E. J., Riege, W. H., & Phelps, M. (1982). Effects of human aging on patterns of local cerebral glucose utilization determined by the (18F) fluorodeoxyglucose method. *Journal of Cerebral Blood Flow and Metabolism, 2,* 163–171.

Metter, E. J. (1988). Positron emission tomography and cerebral blood flow studies. In M. S. Albert & M. B. Moss (Eds.), *Geriatric Neuropsychology.* New York: Guilford Press.

Micheli, B., Caltagirone, C., Gainotti, G., Masullo, C., Silveri, M., & Villa, G. (1981). Influence of age, sex, literacy and pathologic lesion on incidence, severity and type of aphasia. *Acta Neurologica Scandinavica, 64,* 370–382.

Mitchell, J. (1958). Speech and language impairment in the older patient. *Geriatrics, 13,* 467–476.

Nicholas, M., Obler, L., Albert, M., & Helm-Estabrooks, N. (1985). Empty speech and Alzheimer's disease and fluent aphasia. *Journal of Speech and Hearing Research, 28,* 405–410.

North, A. J., Ulatowska, H. K., Macaluso-Haynes, S., & Bell, H. (1986). Discourse performance in older adults. *International Journal of Aging and Human Development, 23,* 267–283.

Obler, L. K., & Albert, M. L. (1981). *Language in the elderly aphasic and in the dementing patient.* New York: Academic Press.

Obler, L. K., & Albert, M. (1984). Language in aging. In M. L. Albert (Ed.), *Clinical neurology of aging* (pp. 245–253). New York: Oxford University Press.

Obler, L., Albert, M., Goodglass, H., & Benson, F. (1978). Aphasia type and aging. *Brain and Language, 6,* 318–322.

Peach, R. (1987). Language functioning. In H. Mueller & V. Geoffrey (Eds.), *Communication disorders in aging.* Washington, DC: Gallaudet University Press.

Powell, M. D., Cummings, J. L., Hill, M. A., & Benson, D. F. (1988). Speech and language alterations in multi-infarct dementia. *Neurology, 38,* 717–719.

Sandor, T., LeMay, M., Kido, D. K., & Rumbaugh, C. (1981). Automated tissue analysis from computerized axial tomographic scans. *Computers and Biomedical Research, 14,* 125–130.

Sands, E., Sarno, M., & Shankweiler, D. (1969). Long-term assessment of language function in aphasia due to stroke. *Archives of Physical Medicine and Rehabilitation, 50,* 202–207.

Sarno, M. (1980). Language rehabilitation outcome in the elderly aphasic patient. In L. Obler & M. Albert (Eds.), *Language and communication in the elderly.* Lexington, MA: Heath.

Sarno, M. T., & Levita, E. (1971). Natural course of recovery in severe aphasia. *Archives of Physical Medicine and Rehabilitation, 52,* 175–179.

Schaie, K. (1983). The Seattle Longitudinal Study: A 21 year exploration of psychometric intelligence in adulthood. In D. Schaie (Ed.), *Longitudinal studies of adult psychological development* (pp. 64–135). New York: Guilford Press.

Schow, R. L., Christensen, J. M., Hutchinson, J. M., & Nerbonne, M. A. (1978). *Communication disorders of the aged: A guide for health professionals.* Baltimore, MD: University Park Press.

Silverman, A., Busse, E., & Barnes, R. (1955). Studies in the process of aging: Electroencephalographic findings in 400 elderly subjects. *Electroencephalography and Clinical Neurophysiology, 7,* 67–74.

Ulatowska, H. K., Cannito, M. P., Hayashi, M. M., & Fleming, S. G. (1985). Language abilities in the elderly. In H. K. Ulatowska (Ed.), *The aging brain: Communication in the elderly.* Austin, TX: PRO-ED.

Ulatowska, H. K., & Chapman, S. B. (1989). Discourse considerations for aphasia management. In R. Pierce (Ed.), *Seminars in speech and language* (pp. 298–314). New York: Thieme.

Ulatowska, H. K., & Chapman, S. B. (in press). Discourse changes in dementia. In R. Lubinski (Ed.), *Dementia and communication: Research and clinical implications.* Toronto: B. C. Decker.

Ulatowska, H. K., Freedman-Stern, R., Weiss Doyel, A., Macaluso-Haynes, S., & North, A. J. (1983). Production of narrative discourse in aphasia. *Brain and Language, 19,* 317–334.

Ulatowska, H. K., Hayashi, M. M., Cannito, M. P., & Fleming, S. G. (1986). Disruption of reference in aging. *Brain and Language, 28,* 24–41.

Ulatowska, H. K., North, A. J., & Macaluso-Haynes, S. (1981). Production of narrative and procedural discourse in aphasia. *Brain and Language, 13,* 345–371.

Vignolo, L. (1964). Evolution of aphasia and language rehabilitation: A retrospective study. *Cortex, 1,* 344–367.

Walker, V., Hardiman, C., Hedrick, D., & Holbrook, A. (1981). Speech and language characteristics of an aging population. In N. Lass (Ed.), *Speech and language: Advances in basic research and practice.* New York: Academic Press.

Whitbourne, S. K. (1976). Test anxiety in elderly and young adults. *International Journal of Aging and Human Development, 7,* 201–210.

Language and Communication in Dementia

Danielle N. Ripich, PhD ∎

Dementia is not a disease but rather a symptom complex that is said to affect as much as 10% of the population over 65 years of age (Wells, 1979). Despite our rapidly accumulating knowledge base on dementia, much remains unclear. Two main challenges exist in clinical work in dementia. The complexities of these challenges are reflected in the literature discussed in this chapter. The initial challenge is the area of diagnosis. Many dementias occur secondarily to other disorders, so that the dementia may initially be masked. There are also disorders whose symptoms resemble those of dementia and in some ways are perhaps related. The co-occurrence and/or occurrence of these disorders can provide confusion in the diagnostic process. A confirmed diagnosis of dementia of the Alzheimer's type (DAT), the most frequently occurring kind of dementia, can only be made on the basis of histopathological evidence of plaques and tangles found in brain tissue upon autopsy. Therefore, assessment and intervention in DAT must

proceed based on a diagnosis of probable or possible dementia. For all of these reasons, neat, clean diagnoses are often not obtainable.

The second area of challenge in clinical work in dementia is in the realm of assessment and intervention. The absence of standardized measures requires clinicians to rely on subjective judgments and behavioral rating scales in determining the extent of the dementia. Although the literature on language and dementia has grown in the past 10 years, prior to that time little research was conducted (Au, Albert, & Obler, 1988; Hart, 1988). Therefore, the patterns of language dissolution in the various dementing illnesses are only beginning to be documented. There are currently no standardized tests of language in dementia. A variety of tools developed primarily for assessment of other language disorders must be employed as measures. Using these measures, subtypes of DAT are now being identified. The heterogeneity of the symptom presentation in these subtypes further complicates the assessment and intervention process.

The primary goal of this chapter is to provide organizing schemas that can be used clinically to meet the problematic challenges of diagnosis, assessment, and intervention in dementia. For more comprehensive examination of dementia, readers are referred to Bayles and Kaszniak (1987) and Lubinski (1991). Initially, a framework for organizing the dementias and related disorders is presented to provide a basis for differential diagnosis. Various classification systems, their theoretical bases, and their relevance are included in the discussion of this framework. Next, patterns of language and communication in dementia are presented and organized by levels of language processing: pragmatics, semantics, syntax, and phonology. Reading and writing are also examined. Language symptoms that are generally found in each of the three stages of dementia are summarized. Finally, a plan for assessment and intervention is proposed that is consistent with the perspective of a comprehensive model of brain-language behavior (Au et al., 1988; Ulatowska & Chapman, chapter 2 of this text; Whitehouse, 1986).

Dementia Types and Associated Disorders

The term *dementia* is used here to refer to impairment in short- and long-term memory, associated with impairment in abstract thinking, impaired judgment, other disturbances of higher cortical function, or personality change. The disturbance is severe enough to interfere significantly with work, usual social activities, or relationships with others (American Psychiatric Association, 1987, p. 103).

There are both reversible and irreversible dementias. All possible causes of reversible dementias must be ruled out in the diagnostic process before moving to an identification of irreversible dementia. Reversible or treatable dementias include

those that result from drug toxicity, metabolic imbalances, infections, tumors, normal-pressure hydrocephalus, alcohol abuse, neurosyphilis, and epilepsy. Geriatric depression (pseudodementia) is classified as a reversible dementia in some diagnostic models (Tonkovich, 1988). Irreversible dementias include DAT, multi-infarct dementia (MID), Pick's disease, and those associated with Parkinson's disease, Huntington's chorea, Wilson's disease, supranuclear palsy, Creutzfeldt-Jakob disease, and Korsakoff's disease.

One dichotomy used to distinguish dementia types is the cortical versus subcortical distinction. This classification system is controversial and even its advocates acknowledge that the terms may be inappropriate and the concept of the dichotomy of functioning has yet to be documented (Whitehouse, 1986). The distinction made between cortical dementias (DAT and Pick's disease), the subcortical dementias (Huntington's chorea, Parkinson's disease, Wilson's disease, and supranuclear palsy), and mixed or vascular dementias (MID, Creutzfeldt-Jakob disease, and Korsakoff's disease) emphasizes the separation of these anatomical regions but fails to account for neurochemical and neuropathological relationships between areas (Whitehouse, 1986). Nevertheless, the cortical and subcortical distinction provides a neuroanatomical organization that is useful in sorting out the syndromes that cause dementia. In the cortical dementias the dementia is the primary dysfunction, whereas in the subcortical dementias the dementia occurs as a secondary feature of the symptom complex. Appendix 15.A presents a chart outlining the characteristics of cortical, subcortical, and mixed dementias, as well as related disorders.

Cortical Dementias

Alzheimer's Disease

Of the irreversible dementias, Alzheimer's disease is by far the most common, accounting for 65% of all dementias (Moss & Albert, 1988). DAT refers to a classical clinical syndrome with gradual and steady onset and course, accompanied by characteristic neuropathological changes: helical neurofibrillary tangles (Wisniewski, Narang, & Terry, 1976), senile plaques (Wisniewski & Merz, 1985), and granulovascular degeneration (Woodward, 1962). Further, recent research has pointed to losses of neurons (Terry, Peck, De Teresa, Schechter, & Horoupian, 1981), neurotransmitters (Bartus, Dean, Beer, & Lippa, 1983) and neuropeptides (Bissette, Reynold, Kilts, Widerlov, & Nemeroff, 1985) as significant indicators of DAT (Hollander, Mohs, & Davis, 1986).

In addition to the basic criteria of dementia previously described, DAT, or primary degenerative dementia as labeled by the *Diagnostic and Statistical Manual of Mental Disorders* (*DSM III-R*), has two *DSM III-R* diagnostic criteria (American Psychiatric Association, 1987):

1. Insidious onset with a generally progressive deteriorating course

2. Exclusion of all other specific causes of dementia by history, physical examination, and laboratory studies

This syndrome involves the loss of intellectual abilities such as memory, judgment, abstract thought, and other higher cortical functions, and causes personality and behavioral changes. DAT may be accompanied by depression, delusions, and, more rarely, delirium. First-degree biological relatives of others with presenile DAT are more likely to develop the disease, because it is believed to be inherited as an autosomal dominant trait (Heyman et al., 1983). Presently, a confirmed diagnosis of DAT can only be made upon autopsy.

Pick's Disease

This relatively rare progressive neurological disease is characterized by marked frontotemporal lobe atrophy as well as Pick bodies within the neurons and inflated and swollen neurons. The pattern of neuronal degeneration (primarily frontal lobe atrophy, including the inferior motor area and anterior temporal lobes and sparing of the posterior cingulate gyrus and parietal lobes) differs from the diffuse pattern found in DAT. However, the amygdaloid nucleus and hippocampus are involved in both disorders (Brun & Englude, 1981). Dementia of the frontal lobe type has been identified by Neary, Snoden, Northern, and Goulding (1988) as possibly representing a form of Pick's disease. These authors contend that this form of dementia may be more common than is presently recognized. Pick's disease occurs between 40 and 60 years of age, more often in women than men. As it proceeds, cognition, language, and memory decline; patients become mute near the end of the disease course (Cummings & Duchen, 1981).

Subcortical Dementias

Parkinson's Disease

The dementia syndrome occurs in approximately 40% of all Parkinson's disease patients; however, changes in mental status are ubiquitous as in other subcortical dementias (Cummings, 1988). The changes include depression (Mayeux, Stern, Rosen, & Leventhal, 1981), bradyphrenia (Rogers, 1986), visuospatial disturbances (Boller et al., 1984), executive functioning deficits (Cummings & Duchen, 1981), and impaired recall (with other memory aspects relatively spared) (Flowers, Pearce, & Pearce, 1984).

Results of a recent study by Cummings, Darkins, Mendez, Hill, and Benson (1988) suggest that in Parkinson's disease the loss of speech and language abilities is a reflection of the overall cognitive loss, whereas the loss of language in DAT correlates less strongly with severity of dementia and may result from pathological changes specific to language areas of the cortex. Specifically, this study found four distinctions between speech and language in DAT and Parkinson's disease. First, DAT patients exhibit more language disturbances than equally demented Parkinson's disease dementia patients on the current assessment battery. Second, Parkinson's disease patients with and without overt dementia have more prominent speech and writing abnormalities than DAT patients. Third, Parkinson's disease patients with overt dementia have more prominent abnormalities of the motor aspects of speech and writing, as well as of select aspects of language function, than Parkinson's disease patients without dementia. Finally, Parkinson's disease patients with dementia may be distinguished from DAT patients on the basis of speech and language characteristics. These findings confirm earlier studies suggesting that language is relatively spared in this subcortical dementia.

Huntington's Chorea

Although choreic motor disturbances are the major characteristic of this autosomal dominant progressive disease, cognitive and psychiatric disturbances are early manifestations (Mayeux, 1984). Huntington's patients generally experience equally impaired recent and remote memory (Albert, Butters, & Brandt, 1981), as well as problems in language organization and naming problems (Kennedy, Fisher, Shoulson, & Caine, 1981). A case study by Moss, Mastri, and Schut (1988), of a patient with coexisting late-onset Huntington's chorea and DAT, showed verbal skills relatively well preserved compared to other areas of cognitive functioning.

Supranuclear Palsy and Wilson's Disease

These rarely occurring dementias have symptoms common to the other subcortical dementias previously described (Cummings & Benson, 1984). These symptoms are attributable to dysfunction of the basal ganglia and frontal subcortical connections (Cummings et al., 1988).

Mixed Dementias

Multi-Infarct Dementia

The *DSM III-R* criteria (American Psychiatric Association, 1987) for MID include the basic dementia criteria with the addition of the following characteristics:

1. Stepwise deteriorating course with "patchy" distribution of deficits (i.e., affecting some functions, but not others) early in the course

2. Focal neurological signs and symptoms (e.g., exaggeration of deep tendon reflexes, extensor plantar response, pseudobulbar palsy, gait abnormalities, or weakness of an extremity)

3. Evidence from history, physical examination, or laboratory tests of significant cerebrovascular disease that is judged to be etiologically related to the disturbance

MID is the second most common subtype of dementia but occurs much less frequently than DAT. It accounts for approximately 20% of all dementia patients and occurs concurrently with DAT in another 15% (Tomlinson, 1977). This dementia, with its abrupt onset and stepwise course of "patchy" losses of function depending on the areas damaged by the infarcts, is presumed to result from vascular disease and is sometimes termed *vascular dementia*. MID results from multiple cerebral vascular accidents occurring over time. The neurological characteristics are multiple areas of softening of brain tissue and may possibly include pathological alterations in cerebral blood vessels (Tomlinson, 1977). In addition to the focal neurological signs listed above, cognitive functions such as memory, abstract thinking, judgment, impulse control, and personality are nearly always affected (Tonkovich, 1988). This disorder is more common in males (Butler & Lewis, 1982) and is without a documented familial pattern. It appears to have arterial hypertension, extracranial vascular disease, and valvular disease of the heart as predisposing factors (Cohen & Eisdorfer, 1984).

Clinical evaluation may be the only means of distinguishing MID from DAT. There are no *Wechsler Adult Intelligence Scale–Revised* (Wechsler, 1981) data that serve to distinguish the two groups, nor is there a standard battery of psychometric tests for differentiation. Hachinski et al. (1975) developed ischemic scoring systems of 13 items designed to create two distinct nonoverlapping groups. A study by Wagner, Oesterreich, and Hoyer (1985) evaluated the validity of the ischemic score as a differential diagnostic tool. Results indicate that the ischemic score was of major importance in differentiating vascular-type dementia (MID) from DAT and depression. Molsa, Paljarvi, Rinne, Rinne, and Sako (1985) also found good discrimination (70% accuracy) between DAT and MID patients using the Hachinski scoring method.

Perhaps because of the heterogeneity of the language problems and the "patchy" nature of the loss of cognitive functioning in MID patients, there have been no large-scale studies of language loss in MID (Bayles & Kaszniak, 1987). A recent comparison study of speech and language alterations between DAT and MID patients (Powell, Cummings, Hill, & Benson, 1988) revealed that the verbal output of these two subject groups differed in several ways. The MID patients demonstrated greater motor speech disruption, whereas the DAT patients showed more difficulty in language, such as empty speech and marked anomia. These results are noteworthy in that they revealed differences in these two syndromes despite the heterogeneity of the symptom complexes of DAT and especially of MID. MID is a subtype of dementia that warrants additional research and documentation of patterns of loss as well as comparisons to other forms of dementia.

Creutzfeldt-Jakob Disease and Korsakoff's Disease

Dementia occurs in the syndromes of Creutzfeldt-Jakob disease, a rare viral degenerative disorder, and Korsakoff's disease, a disorder resulting from chronic alcohol abuse. Creutzfeldt-Jakob disease is fairly stereotypic and moves rapidly through three identifiable stages. First, symptoms of neurological decline emerge. Second, these diverse and widespread neurological disturbances become evident and aphasia, apraxia, and agnosia appear. Finally, the patient moves to a terminal vegetative state and is mute (Cummings & Benson, 1983). Korsakoff's disease is thought by some researchers, but not all (Tonkovich, 1988), to result in generalized dementia.

Related Disorders

Aphasia

The relation between aphasia and dementia has been debated in the literature. Cummings, Benson, Hill, and Read (1985) reported that all 30 DAT subjects they tested demonstrated aphasia and that aphasia should be included as a diagnostic criterion for DAT. However, Bayles, Tomoeda, and Caffrey (1983) listed five criteria to differentiate aphasia and dementia. First, the rate of onset is sudden in aphasia and slow in DAT. Second, decline is continuous in DAT but not in aphasia. Next, DAT results in diffuse brain atrophy, whereas aphasia results from focal lesions. Further, they contend that dementia affects a range of cognitive abilities and aphasia does not. Finally, aphasic patients' performance on verbal and nonverbal tasks is dissociated but dementia patients show simultaneous decline in these performances. More recently, Bayles and Kaszniak (1987) have acknowledged that it is difficult to develop strict criteria for this differentiation.

Au et al. (1988) hold that studying all language function impairments in ways that lead toward the development of a comprehensive model of brain-language relationships is more useful than using a differential approach. These authors, in contrast to Bayles and Kaszniak (1987), Wertz (1978), Horner (1985), and others, propose that the language breakdown in dementia be viewed as a variation of the classical aphasia syndrome. This view appears to come from the same broad theoretical basis as Whitehouse's (1986) argument against separating cortical and subcortical dementia. In both cases the argument is that there is more to be gained from examining commonalities than from developing a differentiating perspective.

Faber-Langendoen et al. (1988) studied aphasia in demented patients and concluded that aphasia is a common feature of DAT and identifies a subgroup with a more rapid progression of dementia. Furthermore, they contend that aphasia represents a specific dysfunction beyond the global cognitive impairment of DAT. Both the differentiating and commonality perspectives are valid and depend on whether aphasia is defined as a result of "focal" or generalized brain damage. Shut (1988) reports cases in which a single vascular infarct, a homorganic stroke, produced part or all of the symptoms of the dementia complex. The etiologic relationship between cerebrovascular disease and dementia warrants further study.

Bayles, Boone, Tomoeda, Slauson, and Kaszniak (1989) reported on a group of neuropsychological tests that differentiated DAT patients (early and middle stages) from fluent and nonfluent aphasics (classified on the basis of word fluency measures). Memory tasks such as delayed spatial recognition, delayed verbal recognition, and delayed story retelling showed significant differences between DAT patients and both groups of aphasics, with aphasics performing better. Mild DAT patients performed better than nonfluent aphasics on the word fluency measure. Possibly the most difficult language differentiations among these language impairments are between early-stage DAT and the empty language of fluent and anomic aphasia (Nicholas, Obler, Albert, & Helm-Estabrooks, 1985). Evaluation of memory performance can assist in this differentiation.

Slowly Progressive Aphasia

Mesulam (1982) identified a group of six patients who presented a slowly progressive aphasic disorder (SPA) without the additional intellectual and behavioral disturbances of dementia. The pattern of symptoms in these patients suggested the presence of a selective degeneration of the perisylvian region of the left hemisphere, distinct from Alzheimer's or Pick's diseases.

Mesulam's patients were all right-handed. Heath, Kennedy, and Kapur (1983) confirmed the clinical entity of SPA in a left-handed patient.

As researchers began to study progressive aphasia, a variety of theoretical and methodological questions were raised. Wechsler, Verity, Rosenschein, Fried, and Scheibel (1982) reported that a patient who was previously described as manifesting a focal aphasic syndrome as the primary symptom of presenile dementia (Wechsler, 1977) was found at autopsy to have pathologically confirmed Pick's disease and an apparently unique basilar dendritic pattern consisting of unusually long unbranched basilar dendrites. These findings suggested that progressive aphasia may be an unusual presentation of Pick's disease.

Concern regarding the comprehensiveness of Mesulam's assessment was voiced by Foster and Chase (1983). These authors stated that a more quantifiable neuropsychological assessment would provide convincing evidence that the progressive aphasia patients were not cognitively impaired. Related to this line of thinking was a position taken by Kirshner, Webb, Kelly, and Wells (1984). They pointed out that, in at least a subset of SPA patients, the language disturbance may be only an initial (if quite isolated) manifestation of a more generalized syndrome of cognitive deterioration. Although this view of progressive aphasia as a precursor to dementia has been upheld by other researchers (Assal, Favre, & Regli, 1984; Poeck & Luzzatti, 1988; Sapin, Anderson, & Pulaski, 1989), Kirshner and colleagues (Kirshner, Tanridag, Thurman, & Whetsell, 1987) disputed the original report in a subsequent article that revealed postmortem autopsy results from the cases reported in the 1984 paper. Two patients from the 1984 study were reclassified as having SPA with no evidence of associated dementia. Mesulam (1987) redefined SPA as primary progressive aphasia (PPA). This syndrome is characterized by aphasia with a relative or total sparing of activities of daily living, judgment, insight, and overall comportment.

This aphasia does not fit neatly into existing classification schemes; however, anomia is the most common feature.

The focus of research in progressive aphasia to date has been in determining the presence of neuropathologies that may precipitate SPA and PPA (Mandell, Alexander, & Carpenter, 1989; Morris, Cole, Banker, & Wright, 1984) and in assuring that subtle cognitive deficits found in dementia and other syndromes are noted in neuropsychological testing (Kirshner et al., 1984; Poeck & Luzzatti, 1988). Relatively little attention has been given to the careful and comprehensive examination of the dissolution of language in this syndrome. Reports of language deficits are often anecdotal (Assal et al., 1984; Wechsler, 1977). A comprehensive protocol that includes a measure of functional communication as well as linguistic evaluation has not been used with SPA or PPA patients. The confusion surrounding the basis and manifestation of progressive aphasia has contributed to the unsystematic measurement of language decline in this syndrome.

Right-Hemisphere Damage

Right-hemisphere damage often results in a loss of orientation and in thought disorders. These disturbances are evident in tasks of conversation (Myers, 1986). The communication impairments associated with right-hemisphere damage are described as disorders of "expression and reception of complex contextually based communicative events resulting from disturbance of the attentional and perceptual mechanisms underlying nonsymbolic, experiential processing" (Myers, 1986, p. 446). These characteristics are found in DAT patients as well, and their presence can complicate a diagnosis of DAT. However, right-hemisphere-damaged patients do not exhibit the auditory comprehension problems found in dementia patients (Bayles & Kaszniak, 1987).

Dementia and Depression

Geriatric depression often co-occurs with dementia and is sometimes termed *pseudo-*dementia (Wells, 1979) or *dementia syndrome of depression* (Folstein & McHugh, 1978) because the symptoms exhibited are quite similar; differential diagnosis of these two disorders is sometimes difficult. A comprehensive history is useful in discriminating between these disorders.

Based on a review of available literature, Wells (1980) developed a method of comparing and contrasting dementia and pseudodementia based on (a) the medical history, (b) clinical behavior and complaints, and (c) memory and cognitive and intellectual performance. The following contrasts illustrate discernable differences in these disorders. In pseudodementia there is a definitive onset with rapid occurrence of most symptoms. This is in contrast to true dementia, with its gradual onset and slow progression of symptoms. Patients with pseudodementia make little effort to perform clinical tasks, whereas dementia patients in the early stages often make every effort to prove themselves adequate. Although the pseudodementia patient's performance is highly variable on tasks of similar difficulty, the dementia patient's poor performance is consistent across similar tasks.

In summary, DAT is the most frequently occurring type of dementia. It is classified as a cortical dementia along with Pick's disease. Subcortical dementias (Parkinson's disease, Huntington's chorea, Wilson's disease, and supranuclear palsy) occur as a part of a more extensive symptom complex. This cortical-subcortical distinction is not universally recognized, but serves to organize the syndromes. *Mixed* or *vascular dementia* is a designation for MID. The relationship of aphasia and slowly progressive aphasia with the communication features of dementia is an area of contention among researchers. The basis of disagreement appears to be whether aphasia is defined as resulting from focal brain damage, or more broadly as resulting from any brain damage. Slowly progressive aphasia patients and patients with right-hemisphere damage have some language and spatial memory symptoms in common with dementia patients. It is important to note that these related disorders may co-occur with dementia. Careful comparisons across neuropsychological and language measures are necessary for accurate diagnosis and assessment.

Language and Communication Deficits in Dementia

The relationship between thought and language has long been debated by researchers and various theoretical positions have been developed. This debate has fostered numerous recent investigations into language breakdown in dementia. In addition, theoretical views of language have shown a dramatic move from a formalist linguistic perspective to a functionalist pragmatic perspective (Bates & MacWhinney, 1979; Bayles & Kaszniak, 1987; Terrell & Ripich, 1989). The shift to a functional perspective requires that we view pragmatics, rather than syntax, as central to and regulative of the language system (Prutting & Kirchner, 1983). When we view pragmatics as central to the language system we must also view communicative competence as more basic than linguistic competence and structure our models accordingly. This perspective is particularly relevant to investigation of DAT in that decline in pragmatics appears to be critical to the loss of functional communication in these patients.

There are in the literature numerous investigations of aspects of language in dementia. However, to date no comprehensive examination of communication deficits in Alzheimer's disease has been conducted (Bayles & Kaszniak, 1987). Additionally, minimal normative data are available for evaluating the performance of individuals with DAT on functional communication tasks (Fromm & Holland, 1987, 1989; Holland, 1984). Although declines in phonology, syntax, and semantics have been well documented (Bayles, 1982; Bayles et al.,

1989; Murdoch, Chenery, Wilks, & Boyle, 1987; Schwartz, Marin, & Saffran, 1979), the degree of decline in communication abilities seems to exceed the decline in these specific language areas (Fromm & Holland, 1987; Ripich & Terrell, 1988; Ulatowska et al., 1986). Therefore, a complete description of communication competence rather than linguistic knowledge is necessary for assessment in dementia. This broadened perspective requires analysis of communication units beyond the sentence level.

Existing data describe the linguistic abilities of demented subjects on selected tasks for one of three purposes: (a) identification of dementia when it may be in question as a diagnosis (Bayles & Boone, 1982), (b) differentiation of dementia and other neurogenic communication disorders (Bayles, 1986; Deal, Wertz, & Spring, 1981; Halpern, Darley, & Brown, 1973; Holland, McBurney, Mossy, & Reinmouth, 1985; Horner & Heyman, 1982; Rochford, 1971; Watson & Records, 1978), and (c) descriptions of the unique features of the language of dementia (Appell, Kertesz, & Fisman, 1982; Barker & Lawson, 1968; Obler, 1983; Pick, 1892; Schwartz et al., 1979; Whitaker, 1976).

Language Processing Levels

The following is a summary of the information gleaned from previous research on the four levels of language processing.

Pragmatics

Although this area appears to contribute most to the communicative deficit in DAT and measures of pragmatics appear to be the most sensitive to interetiologic discrimination (Bayles, 1986), documentation of the pragmatic deficits is limited (Kempler, in press). In the early stage of dementia these deficits take the form of poor topic maintenance, briefer but more frequent turns, more directives, and breakdowns in cohesion and coherence (Hutchinson & Jensen, 1980; Irigaray, 1973; Ripich, Terrell, & Spinelli, 1983; Ripich, Vertes, Whitehouse,

& Fulton, 1988; Terrell & Ripich, 1986); in the middle stage as vague speech; and in the final stage as difficulty in maintaining eye contact and conversational turns.

In addition, the discourse of DAT speakers is described as confusing, lacking coherence (Appell et al., 1982), and less cohesive than the speech of normal elderly speakers (Ripich & Terrell, 1988). Bayles (1984) anecdotally reports that requests are often missing in the early to middle stages of the disease. However, confirmation and clarification requests have been reported to occur more frequently in early DAT patients' speech when compared to normal elderly (Ripich et al., 1988). Other discourse differences identified in DAT include high use of indefinite references (Irigaray, 1973; Kempler, 1988; Obler, 1983; Ripich & Terrell, 1988) and disordered and diminished content (Bayles, 1982; Kirshner et al., 1984).

The *Discourse Ability Profile* (Ripich & Terrell, in preparation; Terrell & Ripich, 1989) was used to examine and organize the discourse of early- to middle-stage Alzheimer's patients on a variety of discourse tasks. Results showed significantly poorer overall discourse performance by Alzheimer's patients. The procedural discourse task, requiring the giving of instructions, was the poorest and narrative abilities were somewhat poorer than those of age- and education-matched cohorts. However, conversational skills showed no differences. These results suggest that the pragmatic deficits noted in DAT patients may be dependent on the nature of the discourse genre and task (Kimbarow & Ripich, 1989). Further systematic examination of discourse as an aspect of communicative functioning may lead to a better understanding of the relative contribution of linguistic and discourse impairments to the dissolution of communication in Alzheimer's disease.

Nicholas et al. (1985) examined the relationship in Alzheimer's subjects' performances between the linguistic impairment of anomia assessed by the *Boston Naming Test* and the discourse impairment measured by the Cookie Theft picture on the *Boston Diagnostic Aphasia Examination*. They concluded that the naming deficits did not underlie the emptiness of the discourse content. However, some of the referential errors may have resulted from anomic difficulties. Methodologically, we are beginning to develop creative ways of systematically tapping natural language in ecologically valid contexts. These methodologies will allow us to determine the reliability and validity of what to date must be viewed as tentative findings in pragmatic communication.

Semantics

Semantics is thought to be at a highly disordered linguistic level in DAT. Deficits are characterized by limited vocabulary (de Ajuriaguerra & Tissot, 1975; Ernest, Dalby, & Dalby, 1970) and naming difficulty (Bayles & Tomoeda, 1983; Huff, Corkin, & Growdon, 1986; Kaszniak & Wilson, 1985; Neils, Boller, Cole, & Gerdeman, 1987), both of which are likely to be caused by breakdown in cognitive processing, perhaps at the prespeech level (Allison, 1962; Appell et al., 1982; Grossman, 1978; Irigaray, 1967; Obler, 1981; Schwartz et al., 1979; Warrington, 1975). Anomia has been the subject of the most research in language and dementia (Appell et al., 1982; Bayles & Boone, 1982; Bayles & Tomoeda, 1983; Kirchner et al., 1984; Skelton-Robinson & Jones, 1984). Even so, the nature of the anomic disorder in DAT and the impact of perceptual and linguistic factors on it remain controversial (Hart, 1988). The majority of researchers appear to support the view that the primary breakdown in the anomia is cognitively based as opposed to perceptual. However, there remains a dispute regarding the nature of the cognitive deficit as being a processing limitation or degradation or as being a failure of the underlying lexical representation (Grober, Buschke, Kawas, & Fuld, 1985; Schwartz et al., 1979).

Syntax

Many investigators report relatively intact syntax in dementia (Appell et al., 1982; Bayles & Boone, 1982; Obler, 1983; Schwartz et al., 1979; Whitaker, 1976). However, Constantinidis (1978) reported missing phrases and sentences, as well as a breakdown in phrase markers and grammatical agreement. Irigaray (1967) described poor noun choice and incorrect verb tense in DAT patients. This discrepancy has not yet been resolved. However, it appears that comprehension of syntax is relatively more impaired than production (Emery, 1988; Linebarger, Schwartz, & Saffran, 1983). One theory for the presence of this disparity is that syntax is a relatively automatic cognitive function that does not require a great deal of attention by the speaker and so is preserved in the midst of a more general cognitive decline (Kempler, Curtiss, & Jackson, 1987). Further support for this view comes from Whitaker's (1976) case study of a demented woman (not DAT) who spontaneously corrected errors of syntax and phonology when repeating sentences even though her language was restricted to echolalia and she was unresponsive to commands.

Phonology

Although phoneme errors have been reported in several investigations (Constantinidis, 1978; Ernest et al., 1970), these appear to be indicative of a "higher" semantic or syntactic problem and not a problem with the individual "speech sounds" or morphophonemics (individual language units signaling a change in meaning). However, there have been no firm findings to support this possibility.

Diagnosis and Assessment

Conceptual Model and Rationale

Correct diagnosis and comprehensive assessment of DAT and other forms of dementia are critical for prognosis, treatment, and case management. The initial diagnostic workup and assessment pre-

cedes intervention; however, assessment must be viewed as a dynamic and ongoing process (Sohlberg & Mateer, 1989). Because the rate of change is variable and the symptom complex heterogeneous, systematic reassessment is required. Dementia is a symptom complex that includes physical, social, cognitive, and communication features; therefore, multiple perspectives are required for adequate diagnosis and assessment. These perspectives can only be provided by an interdisciplinary team of professionals from medicine, nursing, social work, psychology, speech-language pathology, and audiology. An overview of the appropriate case history, medical laboratory studies, and neuropsychological test and behavioral ratings, as well as language and communication measures, will be presented based on this collaborative perspective. Although the results of the communication assessment may be used for differential diagnosis, it is more likely that results will be used to evaluate the patient's progression in the course of the dementia. To this end, the communication assessment must be viewed in terms of other measures of psychological, cognitive, and medical status.

A communication assessment of dementia must be broadly based and move beyond traditional linguistic measures. Communication is considered to be the most complex organizational and interactive behavior of human beings. Breakdowns in the ability to use language successfully and appropriately offer insight into the underlying cognitive decline of persons with dementia (Ripich et al., 1983; Ulatowska, Cannito, Hayashi, & Fleming, 1985). A recommended battery for communication assessment that includes measures of language and functional communication abilities will be presented and its rationale discussed.

Diagnosis and Initial Evaluation

A complete, exhaustive evaluation for dementia should include (a) a careful and thorough case history, (b) neurological and medical diagnostic studies and examinations, (c) behavioral assessment, and (d) a language and communication assessment. The next sections detail important considerations in the first three of these areas of assessment, followed by a comprehensive examination of language and communication assessment. Readers are directed to Ripich (1991) for further elaboration of the diagnostic/assessment process.

Case History Interview

No peripheral marker for DAT is presently known; diagnosis depends on a variety of different kinds of information that exclude other possible causes for the presenting symptoms. Therefore, it is crucial that the history be fully developed because of the role the information plays in the diagnosis. Historical data are important to the speech-language pathologist in the assessment process in that they provide information describing the communication contexts and communicative demands encountered by the patient on a daily basis. Taking the history of a demented patient is difficult because of the memory, attention, and language problems associated with this disorder. A family member, the caregiver, or a close friend must serve as the informant or coinformant along with the patient. It may be helpful to have additional family members corroborate or expand on the essential information (Albert, 1988). Burnside (1980) provides a full discussion of environmental factors to be considered in interviews with older adults.

A complete history should include information in the areas of health, psychological and cognitive status, and social and communication status as well as any special problems that may be occurring. The *Alzheimer Dementia Risk Questionnaire* developed by Breitner and Folstein (1984) is a useful guide for conducting a full history of education, work, family, course of DAT, and present symptoms. The interview segment dealing with communication status involves questions regarding hearing,

communication environment, speech and language abilities, and functional communication. The basic questions asked in speech and language adult case histories are appropriate for these patients (See Chapey, 1986).

Neurological and Medical Evaluation

In combination with a careful history, a physical and neurological examination should be completed by the patient's primary physician or geriatrician, or a neurologist. The examination should include a series of diagnostic laboratory studies with certain ancillary studies when appropriate (National Institutes of Health Consensus Conference, 1987; National Institute on Aging Task Force, 1980). These recommended studies are listed in Figure 15.1.

This list should serve as a guide to the SLP for the sorts of tests required to initially identify dementia and to differentiate among its various disease bases. Interpretation of these test results can only lead to a presumptive clinical diagnosis (McKhann et al., 1984). However, the results serve to rule out a variety of systemic diseases and disorders, as well as cerebrovascular diseases and other conditions that may produce symptoms similar to those associated with DAT.

Behavioral Assessment

Behavioral assessment can best be completed using three approaches: (a) performance on neuropsychological tests; (b) observation of behavior in naturalistic contexts; and (c) reports from family members, friends, and caregivers regarding the patient's behavior. These three approaches provide a multimodal perspective of behavior. They allow for a comprehensive assessment as well as providing data for cross-checking performance by looking for confirming evidence across several behavioral assessment methods.

Behavioral assessments conducted by neuropsychologists normally generate considerable direct information concerning memory, attention, orientation, and so on

A. Blood Studies

  1. Complete blood cell count

  2. Sedimentation rate

  3. Glucose

  4. Urea nitrogen

  5. Electrolytes

  6. Calcium and phosphorus

  7. Bilirubin

  8. Thyroid function

  9. Vitamin B_{12} and folate

  10. Tests for syphilis

  11. Tests for AIDS (optional)

B. Radiographic Studies

  1. Chest X ray

  2. Computerized axial tomography of the brain

  3. Magnetic resonance imaging

  4. Regional cerebral blood flow—positron emission tomography (optional)

C. Other Studies

  1. Electrocardiogram (possibly Holter monitor)

  2. Urinalysis

  3. Lumbar puncture (optional)

  4. Electroencephalogram

FIGURE 15.1. Medical and neurological diagnostic studies. *Note.* Adapted from "Senility Reconsidered: Treatment Possibilities for Mental Impairment in the Elderly" by the National Institute on Aging Task Force, 1980, *Journal of the American Medical Association, 244,* pp. 259–263. Also adapted from the National Institutes of Health Consensus Conference, 1987, *Journal of the American Medical Association, 258*(23), pp. 3411–3416.

and more cursory information regarding communication, language, and speech. In contrast, SLPs comprehensively assess communication, language, and speech functions and more generally examine the domains of overall cognitive status. The overlap and separation of assessment domains should be acknowledged and discussed by the professionals and a working alliance developed to optimize patient care (Schear & Skenes, chapter 4 of this book). Figure 15.2 lists the behavioral assessment

tools recommended for use with dementia patients.

Mental status. Mental status assessment may be completed using the *Blessed Orientation and Memory Examination* (Blessed, Tomlinson, & Roth, 1968; Fuld's (1978) modification of this examination, the *Mini-Mental State Examination* (Folstein, Folstein, & McHugh, 1975); or the *Mental Status Questionnaire* (Goldfarb, 1975). In addition to mental status assessment, a series of cognitive functioning rating scales provide sys-

Mental Status

Blessed Orientation and Memory Examination (Blessed, Tomlinson, & Roth, 1968)
Mental Status Questionnaire (Kahn, Goldfarb, Pollack, & Peck, 1960)
Mini-Mental State Examination (Folstein, Folstein, & McHugh, 1975)

Behavior Rating Scales

Brief Cognitive Rating Scale (Reisberg, 1983)
Clinical Dementia Rating (Hughes, Berg, Danzinger, Coben, & Martin, 1982)
Functional Assessment Stages (Reisberg et al., 1984)
Global Deterioration Scale for Age Related Cognitive Decline and Alzheimer's Disease (Reisberg, Ferris, DeLeon, & Crook, 1982)
Mattis Dementia Rating Scale (Mattis, 1976)

Intelligence

Wechsler Adult Intelligence Scale–Revised (Wechsler, 1981)

Memory

Benton Visual Retention Test (Benton, 1974)
California Verbal Learning Test (Delis, Kramer, & Kaplan, 1987)
Fuld Object Memory Test (Fuld, 1980)
Wechsler Memory Scale–Revised (Russell, 1975)

FIGURE 15.2.   Behavioral assessment tools for dementia patients.

tematic guides for measuring loss and/or maintenance of abilities.

Behavioral rating. The *Brief Cognitive Rating Scale (BCRS)* (Reisberg, 1983) is a rapid structured instrument for use in assessing cognitive decline regardless of etiology. There are several observational rating scales designed specifically to evaluate the status of dementia patients. The *Mattis Dementia Rating Scale* (Mattis, 1976) is a widely used tool. Although it is not useful for differential diagnosis, it has the advantage of measurement through the late stages of the disease when patients often become untestable by other instruments. The *Global Deterioration Scale (GDS) for Age Related Cognitive Decline and Alzheimer's Disease* (Reisberg, Ferris, DeLeon, & Crook, 1982) is a scale of seven stages designed to parallel the seven levels within each of the five Axis categories of the *BCRS*.

Although there is a great variability in the presentation and progression of DAT, as well as difficulty in differentiating the latter stages of symptoms, developing distinct stages of the illness has utility (Moss &

Albert, 1988). The *Functional Assessment Stages (FAST)* distinguishes 15 distinct progressive characteristics of the disease (Reisberg et al., 1984). These characteristics can be related to the seven stages within the *GDS* and levels within the Functioning and Self Care section of the *BCRS*. *FAST* is particularly useful in the later stages of the disease when other measures may not carefully identify the magnitude of the breakdown.

The *Clinical Dementia Rating* (Hughes, Berg, Danzinger, Coben, & Martin, 1982) offers ratings from 0 (healthy), 0.5 (questionable), 1 (mild dementia), and 2 (moderate dementia) to 3 (severe dementia) across six categories: Memory, Orientation, Judgment, Community Affairs, Home and Hobbies, and Personal Care. This scale is frequently used to stage patients for subject groups in dementia research. However, it is interesting to note that the scale does not include communication as a domain to be rated.

Intelligence. Given the complex and diverse nature of cognitive disturbances in dementia, intelligence and memory should be assessed. At present there are no specific standardized comprehensive psychometric tests for dementia or DAT, so batteries of tests designed to assess cognitive functioning are most often used. A neuropsychological test battery should include assessments of all the domains of intelligence and memory with additional assessments of abstraction abilities. The *Wechsler Adult Intelligence Scale–Revised (WAIS-R)* (Wechsler, 1981) is the most frequently used instrument for documenting intellectual functioning. Breakdown between verbally based abilities (Verbal scale) and visuospatial and visuomotor skills (Performance scale) may reflect lateralized versus diffuse brain dysfunction (Sohlberg & Mateer, 1989). Individual subtest scores may reveal discrete areas of impairment such as construction (Block Design subtest) and cognitive flexibility (Similarities and Comprehension subtests) (Bayles, 1986).

Memory. Both the *Wechsler Memory Scale (WMS)* (Wechsler, 1945) and the *Revised Wechsler Memory Scale (WMS-R)* (Russell, 1975) are used for the assessment of memory functioning. The *WMS-R* has been shown to differentiate normal and demented persons (Logue & Wyrick, 1979). Haaland, Linn, Hunt, and Goodwin (1983) developed norms for ages 65–80 years for the *WMS-R*. Although there are certain limitations to the application of these norms in that the volunteer subjects were better educated than the general population (Bayles & Kaszniak, 1987, p. 312), they provide much needed age-appropriate data for interpretation of memory performances. Other commonly used memory assessments are shown in Figure 15.2.

In addition to the assessment of intelligence and memory, a neuropsychological battery should include tests to examine skills of abstraction, such as comprehension of proverbs and picture absurdities. Both DAT and Pick's disease demonstrate problems in this area of cognitive functioning early in their course (Moss & Albert, 1988). A complete neuropsychological assessment should also evaluate visual acuity field and

perception, fine motor skills, hearing acuity and discrimination, and written and oral language skills.

Language and Communication Assessment

Conceptual Model and Rationale

The assessment battery presented in Table 15.1 is designed to address the communication abilities of dementia patients based on conceptual models of language processing that include "top-down" (knowledge-driven) and "bottom-up" (data-driven) organization (Danks & Glucksberg, 1979; Lemme & Danes, 1982). These models are relevant to the study of dementia because they consider the language features that are more vulnerable to cognitive dissolution (i.e., knowledge-based pragmatics and semantics) as well as those that are better maintained (i.e., data-driven syntax and phonology).

A comprehensive evaluation of communication in dementia should include (a) a standardized test of linguistic competence that assesses oral and written language production and comprehension; (b) additional tests for specific language problems in pragmatics, semantics, syntax, and phonology; and, finally, (c) a language memory task. Table 15.1 lists recommended assessment tools for measuring these communication abilities.

This language and communication assessment battery is designed to be administered in approximately 2 hours. It may be completed across several sessions if necessary. It is critical that a supportive test atmosphere be developed for dementia patients.

Comprehensive Language Tests

Although no standardized battery of measures of communication is presently avail-

TABLE 15.1
Language and Communication Assessment Measures for Use with Dementia Patients

Level	Behavior	Measure
I. Comprehensive	Receptive and expressive oral and written language	*Arizona Battery for Communication Disorders of Dementia* (Bayles & Kaszniak, 1987) *Boston Diagnostic Aphasia Examination* (Goodglass & Kaplan, 1983) *Western Aphasia Battery* (Kertesz, 1982) *Porch Index of Communicative Ability* (Porch, 1967)
II. Pragmatics and Discourse	Schemata Turn taking Topic management Conversational repair Speech act use Paralinguistic features Nonlinguistic features Cohesion and coherence	*Discourse Abilities Profile* (Terrell & Ripich, 1989)
III. Semantics	Lexical comprehension	*Peabody Picture Vocabulary Test* (Dunn & Dunn, 1981)
	Confrontation naming	*Boston Naming Test* (Kaplan, Goodglass, & Weintraub, 1983)
	Word fluency	*FAS Word Fluency Measure* (Borkowski, Benton, & Spreen, 1967)
IV. Syntax	Sentence comprehension	*Auditory Comprehension Test for Sentences* (Shewan, 1979) *Token Test* (DeRenzi & Faglioni, 1978)
	Sentence formulation	*Reporter's Test* (DeRenzi & Ferrari, 1978)
V. Phonology	Word production	*Boston Diagnostic Aphasia Examination* (subtest III) (Goodglass & Kaplan, 1983)
VI. Memory and Language	Delayed story retelling	Completeness of novel story retold after 1 hour

able, the *Arizona Battery for Communication Disorders of Dementia (ABCD)* (Bayles & Kaszniak, 1987) is in the process of being standardized. This battery of linguistic- and nonlinguistic-based subtests examines communication problems in dementia. The *ABCD* expands the language measures of most standardized aphasia tests by evaluating memory, linguistic reasoning, and visuospatial abilities. The relationship of these tasks to those of primarily linguistic tasks offers valuable information regarding language and cognitive status.

Standardized tests of aphasia such as the *Boston Diagnostic Aphasia Examination (BDAE)* (Goodglass & Kaplan, 1983), the *Western Aphasia Battery* (Kertesz, 1982), and the *Porch Index of Communicative Ability* (Porch, 1967) provide an evaluation of breakdowns in linguistic functioning across domains in receptive and expressive contexts. A discussion of patterns of performance of DAT patients on these tests is found in Bayles and Kaszniak (1987). Figure 15.3 describes communication patterns across the early, middle, and late stages of DAT.

Pragmatics

The *Discourse Abilities Profile* (*DAP*) (Terrell & Ripich, 1989) serves as a format for organizing and recording observations of patients during various discourse interactions. A comprehensive discussion of the administration and interpretation of the *DAP* can be found in Terrell and Ripich

(1989) and Ripich and Terrell (in preparation).

The *DAP* is divided into four sections. Three of these sections correspond to the three genres of discourse: narrative, procedures, and spontaneous conversation. In each of these sections specific discourse features of the genre are tallied. In addition, the examiner indicates an overall rating of the patient's performance within the genre (excellent, good, adequate, fair, poor). The fourth section of the *DAP* corresponds to three general discourse features (paralinguistic behavior, nonlinguistic behavior, and coherence) that are required for successful discourse regardless of genre. Per-

Early Stages

Pragmatics: Able to maintain conversations. Some difficulty with giving instructions and storytelling. Some breakdown in pronominal referencing. Frequent requests for clarification and confirmation.

Semantics: Word fluency and word finding compromised. Difficulty with comprehension of abstract and/or complex concepts.

Syntax: No errors generally.

Phonology: No errors.

Middle Stages

Pragmatics: Poor topic maintenance, poor use of pronominal reference and other cohesion devices.

Semantics: Poor word fluency, confrontation naming, diminished vocabulary, circumlocutions and empty speech frequently used.

Syntax: Occasional grammatical errors. Some difficulty with comprehension of complex structures.

Phonology: No errors.

Late Stages

Pragmatics: Lack of coherence, mutism in final stage, prosody intact.

Semantics: Paraphasia, echolalia, palilalia, comprehension poor.

Syntax: Grammar generally preserved with some use of elliptical clauses. Poor comprehension of grammatical structures.

Phonology: May have occasional errors, but no non-native language sound combinations.

FIGURE 15.3. Communication patterns in dementia of the Alzheimer's type.

formances within these domains are also rated as excellent, good, adequate, fair, or poor.

Semantics

Assessment of semantic abilities using the *Peabody Picture Vocabulary Test* (*PPVT*) (Dunn & Dunn, 1981), the *Boston Naming Test* (*BNT*) (Kaplan, Goodglass, & Weintraub, 1983), and/or the *FAS Word Fluency Measure* (Borkowski, Benton, & Spreen, 1967) is recommended. The *PPVT* is a word recognition test and is sensitive to the kinds of recognition difficulties DAT patients experience. Bayles and associates (1989) found the *PPVT* to be one of the most discriminating measures between normal and mild DAT patients. Although this recognition task is less active than the word fluency/generative naming task in the *FAS Word Fluency Measure* (Bayles, 1986), it has value as a diagnostic and assessment tool. The *FAS Word Fluency Measure* assesses generative naming of words beginning with the letters "F," "A," and "S." Expressive naming difficulties are an early presenting and persistent problem in DAT (Bayles & Kaszniak, 1987). However, the heterogeneity of DAT patients' performances suggests that it is important to examine individual as well as group patterns of error types (Shuttleworth & Huber, 1988; Stevens, 1989). Confrontation naming as examined by the *BNT* necessitates recognition of the stimulus, recall of its linguistic elements, and production of the target item. Research shows that confrontation naming errors result from disruptions in the semantic network (Smith, Murdoch, & Chenery, 1989). DAT patients demonstrate poor generative naming early in the course of their illness (Nebes & Brady, 1988), poorer than their confrontation naming ability (Bayles & Tomoeda, 1983).

Syntax and Phonology

Although syntax and phonology are relatively well preserved in the early stages of dementia, additional information regarding expression and comprehension perform-ance on these levels may be useful for some patients (Constantinidis, 1978). DAT patients' comprehension at the syntactic level shows a greater deficit on the *BDAE* subtests and the *Auditory Comprehension Test of Sentences* (*ACTS*), both initially and over time, as compared to single-word comprehension scores on the *PPVT* (Bayles & Kaszniak, 1987). The *ACTS* systematically varies word frequency, sentence length, and syntactic complexity. The short version of the *Token Test* (DeRenzi & Faglioni, 1978; Spellacy & Spreen, 1969), also a measure of sentence comprehension, allows for assessment of mild syntactic errors and can be administered quickly. The *Token Test* is sensitive to the mild auditory comprehension problems demonstrated in early dementia. The *Reporter's Test* (short version) (DeRenzi & Ferrari, 1978), an expressive language task, is a measure of language formulation abilities. This test uses the test stimuli from the *Token Test* and can elicit mild syntactic errors. Phonology can be assessed in the context of the words and sentences from subtest III on the *BDAE*.

Memory and Language

A delayed recall task is an excellent way to assess the extent to which memory problems are impinging on language functioning. Across a period of approximately 1 hour patients can be asked to retell a 70- to 100-word story as a way of assessing functional memory. Bayles et al. (1989) found that after a lapse of 1 hour DAT subjects remembered only 2% of a story compared to 96% of story features recalled by normal elderly during a delayed story-retelling task. It is beyond the scope of this chapter to address the complex area of memory and language. However, both Moss and Albert (1988) and Bayles and Kaszniak (1987) provide extensive discussions of this area.

Intervention

Intervention in all types of dementia reflects the premises discussed previously under diagnosis and assessment. First, continual reassessment is a part of the intervention process in this highly variable and heterogeneous symptom complex. Evaluation at 6-month intervals provides information regarding change and/or maintenance of competencies. Results of minimal or no change can be a very encouraging factor for many patients and families. Identification of further decline in an area can focus and structure case management. Second, the intervention process must ideally be multidisciplinary to address the scope of problems arising from this disorder. A collaborative perspective on patient, caregiver, and family counseling; education; and communication treatment provides the optimal opportunity for comprehensive support of all aspects of intervention.

Finally, intervention must be viewed in the broadest possible terms and include education and counseling for all those in the communicative environment. In this way, creative programs can be designed to assist patients to ''stay in the communication game'' as long as possible. For example, if we view the Alzheimer's patient as being a weak player in the tennis match, we can help the patient to ''stay in the game'' by hitting the ball directly to him or her. Using these premises to guide our intervention, we can explore the complex challenge of case management with DAT patients.

Developing the communication skills of professionals such as nurses, social workers, and physicians as well as direct caregivers can enhance the quality of life for the demented patient. As a result of the degenerative nature of DAT, these patients are initially cared for by family and eventually need institutionalization for long-term care. It is important that all those who care for this increasing population of patients have adequate training to communicate effectively with them. Primary caregivers of Alzheimer's patients report a gradual erosion of sociability and maintain that communication is the single most distressing problem they face (Carroll, 1989; Poulshock & Deimling, 1984). The goal of quality caregiving, therefore, should clearly be to prolong and promote communication between these patients and their primary caregivers for as long as we can and on as high a level as possible (Clark, 1989; chapter 8 of this book).

Conclusions

The diagnosis, assessment, and intervention challenges in dementia have been addressed and organizing schemas to be used in meeting these challenges presented. The primary goal of this chapter, then, has been met. However, there remains the larger goal of continuing to expand our knowledge base and our perspective on dementia. This chapter challenges professionals working with dementia patients to continue, through research and expanded clinical services, to meet the complex needs of these persons.

References

Albert, M. S. (1988). Assessment of cognitive dysfunction. In M. S. Albert & M. B. Moss (Eds.), *Geriatric neuropsychology* (pp. 57–81). New York: Guilford Press.

Albert, M. S., Butters, N., & Brandt, J. (1981). Patterns of remote memory in amnesic and demented patients. *Archives of Neurology, 38*, 495–500.

Allison, R. S. (1962). *The senile brain.* London: Edward Arnold.

American Psychiatric Association. (1987). *Diagnostic and statistical manual of mental disorders* (3rd ed. rev.). Washington, DC: American Psychiatric Association.

Appell, J., Kertesz, A., & Fisman, M. (1982). A study of language functioning in Alzheimer's patients. *Brain and Language, 17,* 73–91.

Assal, G., Favre, C., & Regli, F. (1984). Aphasia as a first sign of dementia. In J. Wertheimer & M. Marois (Eds.), *Senile dementia: Outlook for the future.* New York: Alan R. Liss.

Au, R., Albert, M. L., & Obler, L. K. (1988). The relationship of aphasia to dementia. *Aphasiology, 2*(2), 161–173.

Barker, M. G., & Lawson, J. S. (1968). Nominal aphasia in dementia. *British Journal of Psychiatry, 114,* 1351–1356.

Bartus, R. T., Dean, R. L., Beer, B., & Lippa, A. S. (1983). The cholinergic hypothesis of geriatric memory dysfunction. *Science, 217,* 408–417.

Bates, E., & MacWhinney, B. (1979). A functionalist approach to the acquisition of grammar. In E. Ochs & B. Schiefflin (Eds.), *Developmental pragmatics.* New York: Academic Press.

Bayles, K. A. (1982). Language function in senile dementia. *Brain and Language, 16,* 265–280.

Bayles, K. A. (1984). Language and dementia. In A. Holland (Ed.), *Language disorders in adults.* Austin, TX: PRO-ED.

Bayles, K. A. (1986). Management of neurogenic communication disorders associated with dementia. In R. Chapey (Ed.), *Language intervention strategies in adult aphasia* (2nd ed., pp. 462–473). Baltimore, MD: Williams & Wilkins.

Bayles, K. A., & Boone, D. R. (1982). The potential of language tasks for identifying senile dementia. *Journal of Speech and Hearing Disorders, 47,* 210–217.

Bayles, K. A., Boone, D. R., Tomoeda, C. A., Slauson, T. J, & Kaszniak, A. W. (1989). Differentiating Alzheimer's patients from the normal elderly and stroke patients with aphasia. *Journal of Speech and Hearing Disorders, 54*(1), 74–87.

Bayles, K. A., & Kaszniak, A. W. (1987). *Communication and cognition in normal aging and dementia.* Austin, TX: PRO-ED.

Bayles, K. A., & Tomoeda, C. K. (1983). Confrontation and generative naming abilities of dementia patients. In R. H. Brookshire (Ed.), *Clinical Aphasiology Conference proceedings.* Minneapolis: BRK Publishers.

Bayles, K. A., Tomoeda, C. K., & Caffrey, J. T. (1983). Language in dementia producing diseases. *Communication Disorders, 7,* 131–146.

Benton, A. L. (1974). *Revised Visual Retention Test: Clinical and experimental application* (4th ed.). New York: Psychological Corporation.

Bissette, G., Reynold, G. P., Kilts, C. D., Widerlov, E., & Nemeroff, C. B. (1985). Corticotropin-releasing factor-like immunoreactivity in senile dementia of the Alzheimer's type: Reduced cortical and striatal concentrations. *Journal of the American Medical Association, 254,* 3067–3069.

Blessed, G., Tomlinson, B. E., & Roth, M. (1968). The association between quantitative measures of dementia and of senile changes in the cerebral grey matter of elderly subjects. *Journal of Psychiatry, 114,* 797–811.

Boller, F., Passafiume, D., Keefe, N. C., Rogers, K., Morrow, L., & Kim, Y. (1984). Visuospatial impairment in Parkinson's disease: Role of perceptual and motor factors. *Archives of Neurology, 41,* 485–490.

Borkowski, J. G., Benton, A. L., & Spreen, O. (1967). Word fluency and brain damage. *Neuropsychologia, 5,* 135–140.

Breitner, J. C., & Folstein, M. (1984). A prevalent disorder with specific clinical features. *Psychological Medicine, 14,* 63–80.

Brun, A., & Englude, E. (1981). Regional pattern of degeneration in Alzheimer's disease: Neuronal loss and histopathological grading. *Histopathology, 5,* 549–564.

Butler, R. N., & Lewis, M. I. (1982). *Aging and mental health.* St. Louis, MO: C. V. Mosby.

Burnside, I. M. (1980). *Psychological nursing care of the aged.* New York: McGraw-Hill.

Carroll, D. (1989). *When your loved one has Alzheimer's.* New York: Harper & Row.

Chapey, R. (1986). The assessment of language disorders in adults. In R. Chapey (Ed.), *Language intervention strategies in adult aphasia* (2nd ed., pp. 126–136). Baltimore, MD: Williams & Wilkins.

Clark, L. (1989). Improving communication with Alzheimer disease patients. In D. Carroll (Ed.), *When your loved one has Alzheimer's.* New York: Harper & Row.

Cohen, D., & Eisdorfer, C. (1984). Risk factors in late life dementias. In J. Wertheimer & M. Marois (Eds.), *Senile dementia: Outlook for the future* (pp. 221–237). New York: Alan R. Liss.

Constantinidis, J. (1978). Is Alzheimer's disease a major form of senile dementia? Clinical, anatomical, and genetic data. In R. Katzman, R. D. Terry, & K. L. Bick (Eds.), *Alzheimer's disease: Senile dementia and related disorders* (pp. 15–25). New York: Raven Press.

Cummings, J. L. (1988). The dementias of Parkinson's disease: Prevalence, characteristics, neurobiology, and comparison with dementia of the Alzheimer type. *European Neurology, 28*(1), 15–23.

Cummings, J. L., & Benson, D. F. (1983). *Dementia: A clinical approach.* Stoneham, MA: Butterworth.

Cummings, J. L., & Benson, D. F. (1984). Subcortical dementia: Review of an emerging concept. *Archives of Neurology, 41,* 874–879.

Cummings, J. L., Benson, D. F., Hill, M. A., & Read, S. (1985). Aphasia and dementia of the Alzheimer type. *Neurology, 35,* 394-397.

Cummings, J. L., Darkins, A., Mendez, M., Hill, M. A., & Benson, D. F. (1988). Alzheimer's disease and Parkinson's disease: Comparison of speech and language alterations. *Neurology, 38,* 680-684.

Cummings, J. L., & Duchen, L. (1981). Kliver-Bucy syndrome in Pick's disease: Clinical and pathologic correlations. *Neurology, 31,* 1415-1422.

Danks, J., & Glucksberg, S. (1979). Experimental psycholinguistics. *Annual Review of Psychology,* 313-339.

de Ajuriaguerra, J., & Tissot, R. (1975). Some aspects of language in various forms of senile dementia (comparisons with language in childhood). In E. H. Lenneberg & E. Lenneberg (Eds.), *Foundations of language development* (Vol. 1, pp. 323-339). New York: Academic Press.

Deal, J., Wertz, R., & Spring, C. (1981). Differentiating aphasia and the language of generalized intellectual impairment. In *Clinical Aphasiology Conference proceedings.* Minneapolis: BRK Publishers.

Delis, D. C., Kramer, J. H., & Kaplan, E. (1987). *California Verbal Learning Test.* New York: Psychological Corporation.

DeRenzi, E., & Faglioni, P. (1978). Normative data and screening power of a shortened version of the Token Test. *Cortex, 14,* 41-49.

DeRenzi, E., & Ferrari, C. (1978). The Reporter's Test: A sensitive test to detect expressive disturbances in aphasics. *Cortex, 14,* 279-293.

Dunn, L. M., & Dunn, L. M. (1981). *Peabody Picture Vocabulary Test–Revised.* Circle Pines, MN: American Guidance Service.

Emery, O. B. (1988). Language and memory processing in senile dementia of the Alzheimer's type. In L. L. Light & D. M. Burke (Eds.), *Language, memory, and aging* (pp. 221-243). New York: Cambridge University Press.

Ernest, B., Dalby, M., & Dalby, A. (1970). Aphasic disturbances in presenile dementia. *Acta Neurologica Scandinavica, 46* (Suppl. 43), 99-100.

Faber-Langendoen, K., Morris, J. C., Knesevich, J. W., La Barge, E., Miller, J. P., & Berg, L. (1988). Aphasia in senile dementia of the Alzheimer type. *Annals of Neurology, 23*(4), 365-370.

Flowers, K. A., Pearce, I., & Pearce, J. M. S. (1984). Recognition memory in Parkinson's disease. *Journal of Neurology, Neurosurgery, and Psychiatry, 47,* 1174-1181.

Folstein, M. F., Folstein, S. E., & McHugh, P. R. (1975). Mini-Mental State: A practical method for grading the cognitive state of patients for the clinician. *Journal of Psychiatric Research, 12,* 189-198.

Folstein, M. F., & McHugh, P. R. (1978). Dementia syndrome of depression. In R. Katzman, R. D. Terry, & K. Bick (Eds.), *Alzheimer's disease: Senile dementia and related disorders.* New York: Raven Press.

Foster, N. L., & Chase, T. N. (1983). Diffuse involvement in progressive aphasia. *Annals of Neurology, 13*(2), 224-225.

Fromm, D., & Holland, A. (1987, November). *Functional communication in Alzheimer's disease.* Paper presented at the annual convention of the American Speech-Language-Hearing Association, New Orleans, LA.

Fromm, D., & Holland, A. (1989). Functional communication in Alzheimer's disease. *Journal of Speech and Hearing Disorders, 54,* 535-540.

Fuld, P. A. (1978). Psychological testing in differential diagnosis of dementias. In R. Katzman, R. D. Terry, & K. L. Bick (Eds.), *Alzheimer's disease: Senile dementia and related disorders* (pp. 185-193). New York: Raven Press.

Fuld, P. A. (1980). Guaranteed stimulus processing in the evaluation of memory and learning. *Cortex, 16,* 255-271.

Goldfarb, A. I. (1975). Memory and aging. In R. Goldman & M. Rockstein (Eds.), *The physiology and pathology of human aging.* New York: Academic Press.

Goodglass, H., & Kaplan, E. (1983). *The assessment of aphasia and related disorders* (2nd ed.). Philadelphia: Lea & Febiger.

Grober, H., Buschke, H., Kawas, C., & Fuld, P. (1985). Impaired ranking of semantic attributes in dementia. *Brain and Language, 26,* 276-286.

Grossman, M. (1978). The game of the name: An examination of linguistic reference after brain damage. *Brain and Language, 6,* 112-119.

Haaland, K. Y., Linn, R. T., Hunt, W. C., & Goodwin, J. S. (1983). A normative study of Russell's variant of the Wechsler Memory Scale in healthy elderly population. *Journal* of Consulting and Clinical Psychology, 51, 878–881.

Hachinski, V. C., Iliff, L. D., Zilhka, E., duBoulay, G. H. D., McAllister, V. L., Marshall, J., Russell, R. W. R., & Symon, L. (1975). Cerebral blood flow in dementia. Archives of Neurology, 32, 632–637.

Halpern, H., Darley, F., & Brown, J. (1973). Differential language and neurological characteristics in cerebral involvement. Journal of Speech and Hearing Disorders, 38, 162–173.

Hart, S. (1988). Language and dementia: A review. Psychological Medicine, 18, 99–112.

Heath, P. D., Kennedy, P., & Kapur, N. (1983). Slowly progressive aphasia without generalized dementia. Annals of Neurology, 13(6), 687–688.

Heyman, A., Wilkinson, W. E., Hurwitz, B. J., Schmechel, D., Sigmon, A. H., Weinberg, T., Helms, M. J., & Swift, M. (1983). Alzheimer's disease: Genetic aspects and associated clinical disorders. Annals of Neurology, 14, 507–515.

Holland, A. (1984). Language disorders in adults. Austin, TX: PRO-ED.

Holland, A., McBurney, D. H., Mossy, J., & Reinmouth, O. M. (1985). The dissolution of language in Ack's disease with neurofibrillary tangles: A case study. Brain and Language, 24, 36–58.

Hollander, E., Mohs, R. C., & Davis, K. L. (1986). Antemortem markers of Alzheimer's disease. Neurobiology of Aging, 7, 367–387.

Horner, J. (1985). Language disorder associated with Alzheimer's dementia, left hemisphere stroke, and progressive illness of uncertain etiology. In R. H. Brookshire (Ed.), Clinical Aphasiology Conference proceedings (pp. 149–158). Minneapolis: BRK Publishers.

Horner, J., & Heyman, A. (1982). Language changes associated with Alzheimer's dementia: A discussion session. In R. H. Brookshire (Ed.), Clinical Aphasiology Conference proceedings. Minneapolis: BRK Publishers.

Huff, F. J., Corkin, S., & Growdon, J. H. (1986). Semantic impairment and anomia in Alzheimer's disease. Brain and Language, 28, 235–249.

Hughes, C. P., Berg, L., Danzinger, W. L., Coben, L. A., & Martin, R. L. (1982). A new clinical scale for staging of dementia. British Journal of Psychiatry, 140, 566–572.

Hutchinson, J. M., & Jensen, M. A. (1980). A pragmatic evaluation of discourse communication in normal and senile elderly in a nursing home. In L. Obler & M. Albert (Eds.), Language and communication in the elderly (pp. 59–74). Lexington, MA: D. C. Heath.

Irigaray, L. (1967). Approche psycholinguistique de langage des déments. Neuropsychologia, 5, 25–52.

Irigaray, L. (1973). Le langage des déments. The Hague: Mouton.

Kahn, R., Goldfarb, A., Pollack, M., & Peck, A. (1960). Brief objective measures for the determination of mental status in the aged. American Journal of Psychiatry, 117, 326–328.

Kaplan, E., Goodglass, H., & Weintraub, S. (1983). Boston Naming Test. Philadelphia: Lea & Febiger.

Kaszniak, A. W., Fox, J., Gandell, D. L., Garron, D. C., Huckman, M. S., & Ramsey, R. G. (1978). Predictors of mortality in presenile and senile dementia. Annals of Neurology, 3, 246–252.

Kaszniak, A. W., & Wilson, R. S. (1985). Longitudinal deterioration of language and cognition in dementia of the Alzheimer's type. Symposium: Communication and Cognition in Dementia: Longitudinal Perspectives. International Neuropsychological Society, San Diego, CA.

Kempler, D. (1988). Lexical and pantomime abilities of Alzheimer's disease. Aphasiology, 2, 147–159.

Kempler, D. (in press). Language changes in dementia of the Alzheimer type. In R. Lubinski (Ed.), Dementia and communication research and clinical implications. Toronto: B. C. Decker.

Kempler, D., Curtiss, S., & Jackson, C. (1987). Syntactic preservation in Alzheimer's disease. Journal of Speech and Hearing Research, 30, 343–350.

Kennedy, J., Fisher, J., Shoulson, I., & Caine, E. (1981). Language impairment in Huntington's disease. Neurology, 31(2), 81–82.

Kertesz, A. (1982). Western Aphasia Battery. New York: Grune & Stratton.

Kimbarow, M. L., & Ripich, D. N. (1989). Task influences on discourse production in adults. Paper presented at the annual conference of the American Speech-Language-Hearing Association, St. Louis, MO.

Kirshner, H. S., Tanridag, O., Thurman, L., & Whetsell, W. O. (1987). Progressive aphasia without dementia: Two cases with focal spongiform degeneration. *Annals of Neurology, 22,* 527–532.

Kirshner, H. S., Webb, W. G., Kelly, M. P., & Wells, C. E. (1984). Language disturbance: An initial symptom of cortical degenerations and dementia. *Archives of Neurology, 41,* 491–496.

Lemme, M., & Danes, N. (1982). Models of auditory linguistic processing. In N. Lass, L. McReynolds, J. Northern, & D. Yoder (Eds.), *Speech, language and hearing: Vol. I. Normal processes.* Philadelphia: Saunders.

Linebarger, M., Schwartz, M., & Saffran, E. (1983). Sensitivity to grammatical structure in so-called agrammatic aphasics. *Cognition, 13,* 361–392.

Logue, P., & Wyrick, L. (1979). Initial validation of Russell's revised Weschler Memory Scale: A comparison of normal aging versus dementia. *Journal of Consulting and Clinical Psychology, 47,* 176–178.

Lubinski, R. (1991). *Dementia and communication research and clinical implications.* Toronto: B. C. Decker.

Mandell, A. M., Alexander, M. P., & Carpenter, S. (1989). Creutzfeldt-Jakob disease presenting as isolated aphasia. *Neurology, 39,* 55–58.

Mattis, S. (1976). Mental status examination for organic mental syndrome in the elderly patient. In R. Bellack & B. Karasu (Eds.), *Geriatric psychiatry* (pp. 77–121). New York: Grune & Stratton.

Mayeux, R. (1984). Behavioral manifestations of movement disorders: Parkinson's and Huntington's disease. *Neurologica Clinics, 2*(3), 527–540.

Mayeux, R., Stern, Y., Rosen, J., & Leventhal, J. (1981). Depression, intellectual impairment, and Parkinson disease. *Neurology, 31,* 645–650.

McKhann, G., Drachman, D., Folstein, M., Katzman, R., Price, D., & Stadlan, E. M. (1984). Clinical diagnosis of Alzheimer's disease: Report of the NINCDS-ADRDA Work Group under the auspices of the Department of Health and Human Services Task Force on Alzheimer's Disease. *Neurology, 34,* 939–944.

Mesulam, M. M. (1982). Slowly progressive aphasia without generalized dementia. *Annals of Neurology, 22*(4), 533–534.

Mesulam, M. M. (1987). Primary progressive aphasia—Differentiation from Alzheimer's disease. *Annals of Neurology, 22*(4), 533–534.

Molsa, P. K., Paljarvi, L., Rinne, J. O., Rinne, U. K., & Sako, E. (1985). Validity of clinical diagnosis in dementia: A prospective clinicopathological study. *Journal of Neurology, Neurosurgery, and Psychiatry, 48,* 1085–1090.

Morris, J. C., Cole, M., Banker, B. Q., & Wright, D. (1984). Hereditary dysphasic dementia and the Pick-Alzheimer spectrum. *Annals of Neurology, 16,* 455–466.

Moss, M. B., & Albert, M. S. (1988). Alzheimer's disease and other dementing disorders. In M. S. Albert & M. B. Moss (Eds.), *Geriatric neuropsychology* (pp. 145–178). New York: Guilford Press.

Moss, R. J., Mastri, A. R., & Schut, L. J. (1988). The coexistence and differentiation of late onset Huntington's disease and Alzheimer's disease. *Journal of the American Geriatric Society, 36,* 237–241.

Murdoch, B. E., Chenery, H. J., Wilks, V., & Boyle, R. S. (1987). Language disorders in dementia of the Alzheimer's type. *Brain and Language, 31,* 122–137.

Myers, P. S. (1986). Right hemisphere communication impairment. In R. Chapey (Ed.), *Language intervention strategies in adult aphasia* (2nd ed., pp. 444–461). Baltimore, MD: Williams & Wilkins.

National Institute of Health Consensus Conference. (1987). *Journal of the American Medical Association, 258*(23), 3411–3416.

National Institute on Aging Task Force. (1980). Senility reconsidered: Treatment possibilities for mental impairment in the elderly. *Journal of the American Medical Association, 244,* 259–263.

Neary, D., Snoden, J. S., Northern, B., & Goulding, P. (1988). Dementia of frontal lobe type. *Journal of Neurology, Neurosurgery, and Psychiatry, 51,* 353–361.

Nebes, R. D., & Brady, C. B. (1988). Integrity of semantic fields in Alzheimer's disease. *Cortex, 24,* 291–299.

Neils, J., Boller, F., Cole, M., & Gerdeman, B. (1987). *Naming ability in mild Alzheimer's disease subjects.* Paper presented at the annual convention of the American Speech-Language-Hearing Association, New Orleans, LA.

Nicholas, M., Obler, L. K., Albert, M. L., & Helm-Estabrooks, N. (1985). Empty speech in Alzheimer's disease and fluent aphasia. *Journal of Speech and Hearing Research, 28,* 405–410.

Obler, L. K. (1981). [Review of *Le langage des déments*, by L. Irigaray, 1973. The Hague: Mouton]. *Brain and Language, 12*, 375–386.

Obler, L. K. (1983). Language and brain dysfunction in dementia. In S. Segalowitz (Ed.), *Language functions and brain organization* (pp. 267–282). New York: Academic Press.

Pick, A. (1892). Über die beziehungen der senilen hernatrophie zur aphasie. *Prager Medizinishe Wochenschrift, 17*, 165–167.

Poeck, K., & Luzzatti, C. (1988). Slowly progressive aphasia in three patients: The problem of accompanying neuropsychological deficit. *Brain, 111*, 151–168.

Porch, B. E. (1967). *Porch Index of Communicative Abilities*. Palo Alto, CA: Consulting Psychologists Press.

Poulshock, S. W., & Deimling, G. T. (1984). Families caring for elders in residence: Issues in the measurement of burden. *Journal of Gerontology, 39*(2), 230–239.

Powell, A. L., Cummings, J. L., Hill, M. A., & Benson, D. F. (1988). Speech and language alterations in multi-infarct dementia. *Neurology, 38*, 717–719.

Prutting, C., & Kirchner, D. (1983). Applied pragmatics. In T. Gallagher & C. Prutting (Eds.), *Pragmatic assessment and intervention issues in language*. Austin, TX: PRO-ED.

Reisberg, B. (1983). *Alzheimer's disease: The standard reference* (pp. 178–179). New York: Free Press.

Reisberg, B., Ferris, S. H., Anand, R., DeLeon, M. J., Schneck, M. K., Buttinger, C., & Borenstein, J. (1984). Functional staging of dementia of the Alzheimer's type. *Annals of the New York Academy of Science, 435*, 481–486.

Reisberg, B., Ferris, S. H., DeLeon, M. J., & Crook, T. (1982). The Global Deterioration Scale for assessment of primary degenerative dementia. *American Journal of Psychiatry, 139*, 1136–1139.

Ripich, D. N. (1991). Differential diagnosis and assessment. In R. Lubinski (Ed.), *Dementia and communication research and clinical implications.* (pp. 188–233). Toronto: B. C. Decker.

Ripich, D., & Terrell, B. (1988). Patterns of discourse cohesion and coherence in Alzheimer's disease. *Journal of Speech and Hearing Disorders, 53*, 8–15.

Ripich, D. N., & Terrell, B. Y. (in preparation). Discourse abilities profile: Clinical evaluation of communication in Alzheimer's patients. *Aphasiology.*

Ripich, D., Terrell, B., & Spinelli, F. (1983). Discourse cohesion in senile dementia of the Alzheimer's type. In R. H. Brookshire (Ed.), *Clinical aphasiology: Conference proceedings* (pp. 316–321). Minneapolis: BRK Publishers.

Ripich, D. N., Vertes, D. R., Whitehouse, P., & Fulton, S. (1988). *Conversational discourse patterns in senile dementia of the Alzheimer's type.* Paper presented at the annual convention of the American Speech-Language-Hearing Association, Boston, MA.

Rogers, D. (1986). Bradyphrenia in Parkinsonian patients. *Neurology, 45*, 447–450.

Russell, E. W. (1975). A multiple scoring method for the assessment of complex memory functions. *Journal of Consulting and Clinical Psychology, 43*, 800–809.

Sapin, L. R., Anderson, F. H., & Pulaski, P. D. (1989). Progressive aphasia without dementia: Further documentation. *Annals of Neurology, 25*, 411–413.

Schwartz, M., Marin, O., & Saffran, E. (1979). Dissociations of language function in dementia: A case study. *Brain and Language, 7*, 277–306.

Shewan, C. M. (1979). *Auditory Comprehension Test for Sentences*. Chicago: Linguistics Clinical Institutes.

Shut, L. J. (1988). Dementia following stroke. *Clinics in Geriatric Medicine, 4*(4), 767–784.

Shuttleworth, E. C., & Huber, S. J. (1988). The naming disorder of dementia of the Alzheimer type. *Brain and Language, 34*, 222–234.

Skelton-Robinson, M., & Jones, S. (1984). Nominal dysphasia and the severity of senile dementia. *British Journal of Psychiatry, 145*, 168–171.

Smith, S. R., Murdoch, B. E., & Chenery, H. J. (1989). Semantic abilities in dementia of the Alzheimer type. *Brain and Language, 36*, 314–324.

Sohlberg, M. M., & Mateer, C. A. (1989). *Introduction to cognitive rehabilitation: Theory and practice*. New York: Guilford Press.

Spellacy, F. J., & Spreen, O. (1969). A short form of the Token Test. *Cortex, 5*, 390–397.

Stevens, S. J. (1989). Differential naming difficulties in elderly dysphasic subjects with senile dementia of the Alzheimer type. *British Journal of Disorders of Communication, 24*, 77–92.

Terrell, B. Y., & Ripich, D. N. (1986). *Conversational discourse in senile dementia of the Alzheimer's type.* Presented to the annual convention of the American Speech-Language-Hearing Association, Detroit, MI.

Terrell, B., & Ripich, D. (1989). Discourse competence as a variable in intervention. *Seminars in Speech and Language Disorders, 24,* 77–92.

Terry, R. D., Peck, A., De Teresa, R., Schechter, R., & Horoupian, D. S. (1981). Some morphometric aspects of the brain in senile dementia of the Alzheimer's type. *Annals of Neurology, 10,* 184–192.

Tomlinson, B. E. (1977). The pathology of dementia. In C. E. Wells (Ed.), *Dementia.* Philadelphia: F. A. Davis.

Tonkovich, J. D. (1988). Communication disorders in the elderly. In B. B. Shadden (Ed.), *Communication behavior and aging: A sourcebook for clinicians* (pp. 197–215). Baltimore, MD: Williams & Wilkins.

Ulatowska, H. K., Cannito, M. P., Hayashi, M. M., & Fleming, S. G. (1985). Language abilities in the elderly. In H. K. Ulatowska (Ed.), *The aging brain: Communication in the elderly* (pp. 125–139). Austin, TX: PRO-ED.

Ulatowska, H. K., Haynes, S. M., Donnell, A. J., Bristow, J. M., Allard, L. R., & Flower, A. A. (1986, November). *Discourse abilities in dementia.* Paper presented at the American Speech-Language-Hearing Association Conference, Detroit, MI.

Wagner, O., Oesterreich, K., & Hoyer, S. (1985). Validity of the ischemic score in degenerative and vascular dementia and depression in old age. *Archives of Gerontology and Geriatrics, 4,* 333–345.

Warrington, E. K. (1975). The selective impairment of semantic memory. *Quarterly Journal of Experimental Psychology, 27,* 635–657.

Watson, J., & Records, L. (1978). The effectiveness of the Porch Index of Communicative Abilities as a diagnostic tool in assessing specific behaviors of senile dementia. *Clinical Aphasiology Conference proceedings.* Minneapolis: BRK Publishers.

Wechsler, A. F. (1977). Presenile dementia presenting as aphasia. *Journal of Neurology, Neurosurgery, and Psychiatry, 40,* 303–305.

Wechsler, A. F., Verity, M. A., Rosenschein, S., Fried, I., & Scheibel, A. B. (1982). Pick's disease: A clinical, computed tomographic, and histologic study with Golgi impregnation observations. *Archives of Neurology, 39,* 287–290.

Wechsler, D. (1945). A standardized memory scale for clinical use. *Journal of Psychology, 19,* 87–95.

Wechsler, D. (1981). *Wechsler Adult Intelligence Scale–Revised manual.* New York: Psychological Corporation.

Wells, C. E. (1979). Pseudodementia. *American Journal of Psychiatry, 36,* 895–899.

Wells, C. E. (1980). The differential diagnosis of psychiatric disorders in the elderly. In J. Cole & J. Barrett (Eds.), *Psychopathology in the aged.* New York: Raven Press.

Wertz, R. T. (1978). Neuropathologies of speech and language: An introduction to patient management. In D. F. Johns (Ed.), *Evaluation of appraisal techniques in speech and language pathology.* Reading, MA: Addison-Wesley.

Whitaker, H. A. (1976). A case of the isolation of language function. In H. Whitaker & H. Whitaker (Eds.), *Studies in neurolinguistics* (Vol. 2). New York: Academic Press.

Whitehouse, P. J. (1986). The concept of subcortical and cortical dementia: Another look. *Annals of Neurology, 19,* 1–6.

Wisniewski, H. M., & Merz, G. S. (1985). Neuropathology of the aging brain and dementia of the Alzheimer's type. In C. M. Gaitz & T. Samorajski (Eds.), *Aging 2000: Our health care destiny: Vol. 1. Biomedical issues* (pp. 231–243). New York: Springer-Verlag.

Wisniewski, H. M., Narang, H. K., & Terry, R. D. (1976). Neurofibrillary tangles of paired helical filaments. *Journal of Neurological Sciences, 17,* 173–181.

Woodward, J. (1962). Clinico-pathological significance of granulovascular degeneration in Alzheimer's disease. *Journal of Neuropathology and Experimental Neurology, 21,* 85–91.

Appendix 15.A
Characteristics of Cortical, Subcortical, and Mixed Dementias

	Cortical Dementias	
	Dementia of the Alzheimer's Type	Pick's Disease
Onset	Gradual	Gradual
Etiology	Diffuse damage: Neurofibrillary tangles Senile plaque Granulovascular degeneration	Pick bodies Inflated neurons Atrophy of the anterior portions of the frontal and temporal lobes
Course	Progressive Irreversible	Progressive Irreversible
Language and Speech	Semantics and pragmatics impaired early Syntax and phonology impaired later Speech impaired very late	Slow, deliberate speech Anomia Breakdowns in syntax Defect in auditory comprehension
Memory	Impaired early Worse for recent events	Impaired—recent memory
Performance Characteristics	Tries to perform Alert Consistent level of performance	Emotional lability and apathy Loss of tact and judgment
Physical Characteristics Gait Movement	Normal (some pacing)	Motor involvement in later stages

	Subcortical Dementias	
	Parkinson's Disease	Huntington's Chorea
Onset	Sporadic	Insidious

Etiology	Autosomal dominant Degenerative disease of the nervous system, especially in the substantia nigra	Variety of causes: Autosomal dominant trait Idiopathic Drug induced Postencephalitic Arteriosclerotic Loss of Golgi cells in corpus striatum
Course	Progressive Irreversible	Progressive Irreversible
Language and Speech	Language minimally impaired Speech impaired Weak breathy voice Abnormal pitch rate and loudness Inappropriate silences	Dysarthria worsens Language organization, sequencing, and naming abilities impaired as the disease progresses
Memory	Forgetful Impaired recall Slowed response	Impaired, especially for remote events early in the disease
Performance Characteristics	Slowness of responses	Early stages: Irritability Apathy Untidiness Impulsiveness
Physical Characteristics Gait Movement	Abnormal Slow Tremor Rigidity Bradykinesia	Abnormal Shuffling gait Jerky gait Festinating Choreic

Subcortical Dementias		
	Supranuclear Palsy	Wilson's Disease
Onset	Gradual	Gradual
Etiology	Related to changes in the reticular formation, thalamus, or hypothalamus	Inherited autosomal recessive trait Basal ganglia Excessive levels of copper in the brain and liver
Course	Progressive	Progressive Rapid progression if untreated/ undiagnosed

Language and Speech	Dysarthria Speech becomes inaudible and unintelligible with gurgling, harsh guttural sounds	Dysarthria Irregular articulatory breakdown Hypernasality Inappropriate silences
Memory	Impaired	Impaired
Performance Characteristics		
Physical Characteristics	Pseudobulbar palsy, dystonia, and severe rigidity of head/neck producing a backward retracted head position	Slowness Tremors Rigidity Bradykinesia or involuntary movements Later stages—severe ataxia Dysphagia Masklike face

Mixed Dementias		
	Korsakoff's Disease	Creutzfeldt-Jakob Disease
Onset	Gradual	Variable: gradual/sudden
Etiology	Cortical atrophy resulting from chronic alcohol abuse	Infectious, transmissible, unconventional virus Results in degenerative cortical tissue, i.e., songiform encephalopathy and nonspecific atrophy
Course	Stable or minimally progressive	Rapidly progressive
Language and Speech		In stage 2: Aphasia Apraxia Agnosia In stage 3: Mutism
Memory	Decreased skills Poor attention Amnesia	Forgetfulness in initial phase
Performance Characteristics	Affective lability	Apathetic

Physical Characteristics	May show disturbances	Sensory and visual impairments Cranial nerve palsies, rigidity, myoclonus, tremor Cerebellar disturbances

---

Mixed Dementias

Multi-Infarct Dementia

Onset	Sudden
Etiology	Multiple lesions Softening of brain tissue Alteration in cerebral blood vessels
Course	Stepwise Irreversible
Language and Speech	Impaired pattern dependent on site of lesion
Memory	Impaired—depends on site of lesion
Performance Characteristics	Variable performance based on focal lesions
Physical Characteristics Gait Movement	May be abnormal, dependent on site of lesion

---

Related Disorders

	Aphasia	Slowly Progressive Aphasia	Depression (Pseudodementia)
Onset	Sudden	Gradual	Can be dated with some precision
Etiology	CVA Tumor Trauma	Perisylvian region, left-hemisphere degenera-tion	Unknown
Course	Reversible Spontaneous recovery	Progressive Irreversible	Rapid progression of symptoms Reversible

Language and Speech	Impaired across all levels of language Speech not impaired	Anomia and pure word deafness Speech not impaired	Word-finding problems Speech slowed Reduced intonation, contour, and intensity
Memory	Not impaired	Not impaired	Impaired equally for remote and recent events
Performance Characteristics	Poorer on language-based than nonlanguage tasks	Poorer on language-based than nonlanguage tasks	No effort to perform Uneven performance May do better on harder tasks
Physical Characteristics Gait Movement	May show right hemiparesis, hemiplegia	Not impaired	Gait slowed and shuffling Movement slowed

Head Injury in the Elderly: Implications for Speech-Language Pathology

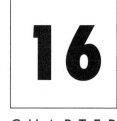

CHAPTER

Audrey L. Holland, PhD,

and Margaret M. Forbes, MA ■

Typically, head injury is thought to occur among the young, and indeed it is most common between the ages of 15 and 30 (Anderson, Miller, & Kalsbeek, 1983; Galbraith, 1987; Jennett & MacMillan, 1981). Yet no age group, from infancy onward, is free of it, and the literature suggests that after gradually declining from age 30 on, there is a second, albeit lesser peak in the incidence of head injury after age 70 (Annegers, Grabow, Kurland, & Laws, 1980; Klauber, Barrett-Connor, Marshall, & Bowers, 1981). In addition, the sparse literature indicates that elderly victims of head injury are quite different from younger victims.

The main thrust of the difference is that the consequences of head injury for the elderly may well be more dismal than at any other point in the life-span. Along the continuum from apparently minor to severe head trauma, diagnosis and management of brain injury present a different and more complex set of problems in the elderly than in the young. Only a few studies of head

injury in the elderly have been conducted, and reports have been chiefly concerned with the broad issues of survival rates, resumption of independent living, and degree of overall impairment. Studies of communication impairments and other neuropsychological deficits in the head-injured elderly are notably lacking, as are studies of the appropriate rehabilitation techniques and their efficacy. This chapter will first summarize some of the available data that provide a picture of the ways in which head injury differs in the elderly and will then discuss some of the implications of these differences.

Two recent studies, one in Scotland by Pentland, Roy, and Miller (1986), and one in the United States by Amacher and Bybee (1987), are particularly relevant. The Pentland et al. study is a retrospective comparison of more than 1,500 patients under age 65 with 449 patients over 65 who were hospitalized at the Edinburgh Head and Spinal Injury Unit over 2 years. The Amacher and Bybee work is also a retrospective study; it concerns the "old-old," or those 80 years old and above. This study provides a more detailed follow-up of the course subsequent to head injury for the 56 patients over age 80 who were admitted to Hartford Hospital from 1981 to 1985. Both studies report on such factors as sex ratios, mechanisms of injury, length of stay, and outcomes. It is important to summarize and compare the two studies briefly, in order to highlight some of the differences in causes, consequences, and outcomes of head injury in the elderly.

Causes, Consequences, and Outcomes

Gender Differences

Most epidemiologic studies of head injury report approximately a 4:1 ratio of males to females. These two studies suggest that the ratio becomes more nearly equal in the older age groups. In the Pentland study, the sex distribution among the over-65 sample was in line with general admissions to the hospital, or a ratio of approximately 1:1, males to females. Among Amacher and Bybee's old-old patients (80–96 years of age), the ratio had climbed to 3:2 in favor of women. Others report somewhat different male-female ratios (Klauber et al., 1981, report that rates of head injury increase more in men than in women after age 60), but the trend toward a more nearly even distribution of head injuries between males and females with increasing age has been noted in a number of studies (Galbraith, 1987; Hernesniemi, 1979). Given that survival rates are higher among females in the 8th decade of life, the apparent shift in ratio is not surprising.

Causes

Falls

The shift in ratio with age may also be related to another distinguishing charac-

teristic of head injury in the elderly. In the overall population of the head injured, the predominant cause of injury is motor vehicle accidents. This is not true for those over 70, and it is motor vehicle accidents (including motorcycle accidents) that have traditionally put males at greater risk for head injury. Rather, in the Pentland et al. study, as well as in others (e.g., Hernesniemi, 1979; Klauber et al., 1981), falls take over as the major cause. In those over 65 in the Pentland et al. study, alcohol ingestion was judged to have been a likely contributor to falls causing head injury in 54% of the males (compared to 44% of the younger males) and in 12% of the females (compared to 25% of the younger females). Overall, falls in the Pentland et al. study account for about 60% of head injuries, whereas in the Amacher and Bybee study of those over 80, falls account for nearly 80% of head injuries. It should be noted that falls are the single greatest cause of accidental deaths among the elderly; they are responsible for more than 50% of all accidental deaths in individuals over the age of 65. More elderly people die from falls than from all other accidents combined (Grigsby, 1984). Amacher and Bybee list medical factors that are likely to contribute to head-injury-producing falls, including previous stroke, postural dizziness, antihypertensive medicine, hyponatremia, hip disease, Parkinsonism, myocardial infarct, diabetic neuropathy, and organic brain syndrome. They note than in a high percentage of their cases one of these problems, which all tend to be more common with increasing age, was listed as contributing to the fall. Amacher and Bybee point out that among the 56 patients they followed, 9 had fallen on staircases and 4 had slipped on icy sidewalks. Five more had fallen after standing up quickly; one 80-year-old woman slipped while climbing a ladder; and, finally, an 84-year-old man fell off a ladder while painting his house. The authors state, "One cannot escape the conclusion, on reading through the case histories of these events, that common sense home safety measures for older people could help reduce their incidence of head injury" (pp. 956–957).

Motor Vehicle Accidents

Motor vehicle accidents are the second most frequent mechanism of head injury in the elderly, but here it is of interest that at least in the larger of the two studies, pedestrian accidents predominated, whereas in younger groups those who are injured in motor vehicle accidents are more likely to be drivers or passengers than pedestrians. In addition, in Amacher and Bybee's old-old group, of the six (10.7%) who were injured in motor vehicle accidents, only three (all male) were driving, and the other three (all female) were passengers. According to this study, although motor vehicle accidents are still the second most common source of head injury in those over 80, they are a very distant second place indeed.

Abuse and Attacks

It seems appropriate to discuss briefly a somewhat different topic related to the causes of head injury in the elderly. The topic concerns assault against the elderly. Abuse is typically perpetrated on elderly individuals who have chronic multiple diseases ranging from congestive heart failure and carcinoma to a much more frequent incidence of dementia, and who live with their abusers in situations of high dependency and resultant stress (Koin, 1984). It is likely that a significant number of elderly individuals who appear to have fallen or to have been assaulted have been the victims of abuse, and those who see these patients must be aware of this possibility. Abuse and assault of the elderly have an additional, also chilling component. That is, the elderly are disproportionately frequent victims of criminal attacks. (For example, both muggings reported in Amacher and Bybee's research involved elderly women who were attacked on their way to church.)

As a poignant example, the grandfather of a friend recently died at the age of 75. The death of this man's wife and a subsequent financial problem had previously forced him to move away from his old neighborhood, where he was well known and more likely to be protected by neighbors. A frail-looking man, he was walking down an unfamiliar street when he was attacked by two youths, who robbed him of a few dollars and a watch. He was found a few hours later, was hospitalized, and died a few days later of his head injury. This is not an uncommon story. It is just the elderly version of the drunken-driver tragedy of head injury in younger adults, with similar sociological significance.

Consequences and Degree of Injury

Across the rest of the life-span, mild head injuries predominate. So, too, at first glance, is this true of the elderly. Both Amacher and Bybee and Pentland et al. report that the great majority of patients studied had mild head injuries. Pentland et al. reported 84% to have *Glasgow Coma Scale (GCS)* scores between 13 and 15; Amacher and Bybee reported 75% in this range. The Pentland study had a slightly higher percentage of moderate injuries and a slightly lower percentage of severe injuries, which may be accounted for in part by the fact that the Amacher and Bybee study was limited to those over 80, and the Pentland et al. study also included some of the "younger-old," between 65 and 80 years of age.

A very important difference between the young and old groups concerns intracranial hematomas, which were a significant feature not only in the severely head-injured elderly groups and severely injured younger patients, but in the older moderately and mildly injured groups as well. For Pentland et al., intracranial hematomas were roughly three times more common in patients over age 65 than they were in their younger group, with an overall incidence of 9.4% as opposed to 2.7%. For Amacher and Bybee, with their still older subjects, the overall incidence rose to 29%. Further difficulty results from the fact that in the elderly, intracranial hematomas may resemble other neurological disorders, such as stroke or seizure, and thus may cause difficulties and delays in correct diagnosis and treatment (Lehman, 1988). What these figures presage is that even mild and moderate degrees of head injury have the potential for very grave outcomes in elderly patients.

In Pentland's survey, 55% of the moderately injured group over age 65 suffered severe disability or death, compared to 15% of the moderately injured younger group. Of the 42 elderly patients followed by Amacher and Bybee who had "minor" injuries in addition to the intracranial hematomas mentioned previously, 6 patients required craniotomies and 5 died. Those with severe head injuries in both older groups had vastly higher percentages of poorer outcomes than would be predicted for younger patients.

Some authorities suggest that head trauma is more serious in the elderly than in the young because the elderly brain is shrunken and the tamponade effect is minimized. Galbraith (1987) says that the difficulty is that the elderly have "a reduced cerebral reserve," and thus cannot recover from even a mild head injury as easily as the young. It is also suggested that old neurons do not withstand insult as well, possibly as a result of metabolic changes (Grigsby, 1984). This is a complex issue, not yet totally understood. Nevertheless, poorer prognosis is clearly another way in which head injury in the elderly differs from head injury in younger people.

This contrast in prognosis is vividly illustrated when we compare the data we have collected in our study of recovery in children ages 5–16 with mild and moderate head injury to the data on elderly brain-injured patients. Although age and severity must be taken into account to predict recovery from closed head injury, most of our mildly injured children have recovered by 1 month, and most of the severely injured children in our sample demonstrated normal neuropsychological profiles by 1 year post-injury (Leahy & Holland, 1985). It is clear that this would not be the case for elderly subjects studied in similar detail.

Other features of Amacher and Bybee and Pentland et al., including length of stay in the hospital, noncerebral causes of death in the elderly patient, and medically complicating features of recovery, also converge to suggest that head injury in the elderly is probably always a serious condition. In addition, there is some suggestion that outcome deteriorates in each decade between the ages of 60 and 80, with the worst outcome for those over 80 (Hernesniemi, 1979).

That there is probably no such thing as the "mildly head-injured elderly" is illustrated by a study by Roy, Pentland, and Miller (1986) in which the subjects are 146 patients 65 years of age or more admitted to the Edinburgh Royal Infirmary neurotrauma unit with minor head injuries. Although 73% were discharged to their former homes, their hospital stays were twice as long as those of younger patients, 34 of them were transferred elsewhere for additional treatment, and 6 required a change of domicile. While the outcome is far from catastrophic, it is also far worse than would be expected for minor head injury in a younger group. Roy et al. recommend that a larger proportion of the elderly with minor head injuries be admitted to the hospital because of the possible complications of such injuries.

Having described some of the ways in which the elderly head injured are unique, it is appropriate to discuss a few of the implications of these observations and to provide examples of problems in the diagnosis and management of elderly survivors of head injury.

Differential Diagnosis and Case Management

The following is a pertinent, if apocryphal, example. A 72-year-old inpatient of a geriatric psychiatry unit had retired some years previously from his job in a factory and had a history of depression. He had been admitted to the unit because he had recently become aggressive to his wife and family and was complaining of severe headaches that he said were responsible for his aggression. He did not appear particularly responsive to others' speech, and the staff wanted to know if he was malingering or aphasic, or if he really had a significant hearing loss. A speech-language pathologist with interest in geriatric problems was consulted. As the consultant interviewed the patient, it became apparent from his history that he had sustained a fall a few months previously. This fall had produced no obvious effects, and he was not seen by a physician. However, within a few weeks after his fall, his headaches began. Second, his "factory" job was actually in a foundry. Third, his language comprehension was essentially normal, but commensurate with long-term compromised auditory function. As an inpatient, he had not been seen by a neurologist, and the psychiatrist in charge felt that his headaches were part of his depression. Here, then, is the list of this patient's possible problems, as compiled by our astute consultant:

1. Genuine hearing loss, related to a 40-year history of working in noise

2. Possible reactions to toxins in the foundry, including changes in his neuropsychological and affective status

3. Possible head injury

The consultant recommended that he be evaluated by a neurologist for his possible head injury and by an audiologist for his hearing loss. The result was that the man was diagnosed as having a subdural hematoma. Following its evacuation, he returned to his pre-head-injury level of functioning and was fitted with a hearing aid.

This patient illustrates many of the implications that stem from the data presented here. Although the consultant may have been a good detective in suggesting head injury, the medical staff and social workers were particularly poor ones. A geriatric facility should be so attuned to falls in the elderly that they are among the first lines of investigation. It is well known that hematomas are insidious medical conditions that are much more common among the elderly brain injured than among the young. Once it became known that this patient had suffered a fall some weeks before, appropriate neurological, neuroradiological, and neurosurgical consultations should have been undertaken. Why had these things not occurred? Why was the staff more interested in his apparent hearing status than in his questionable neurological status? Part of the answer may lie in the documented tendency for physicians to spend less time interviewing and obtaining medical histories from their elderly patients than from their younger ones (Koin, 1984). Part of the story in this man's case may well have been the blind man and elephant phenomenon, with psychiatrists examining with their psychiatric biases. This approach is especially likely in the case of an apparently aggressive patient.

Whatever the reasons for this failure in diagnosis, increasing the sensitivity of medical and paramedical personnel to the importance and complexity of head injury in the elderly should be a priority for those interested in geriatric medicine.

Another possibility for confusion exists in the differential diagnosis of head injury and early dementia. The cognitive parallels and similarities between early dementia and head injury have often been noted in the literature. We know that the effects of closed head injury can defy visualization by computerized tomography, and it seems reasonable that, for example, a fall producing a mild head injury could go unreported. In no group of patients is there a higher risk of confusing two conditions, and misdiagnosing a head-injured patient as demented could have dire medical and surgical consequences. In addition, there are some available therapeutic techniques for lessening the effects of head injury, but few for lessening dementia.

In addition to receiving a meticulous medical workup, it is critical for the elderly patient who suddenly develops dementing-like behavior to be observed carefully by clinicians who understand both dementia and head injury. If the behavior in question does not worsen, but stabilizes, there is every reason to suggest that cognitive rehabilitation might be appropriate.

Rehabilitation and Recovery

For speech-language pathologists involved in rehabilitation, the question of how well the elderly head-injured patient can recover has important implications. It is hard to justify using scarce rehabilitative resources on this population if they do not improve the patients' outcome. Unfortunately, we found no published reports documenting the effectiveness of formal intensive rehabilitation programs in improving the language or other neuropsychological deficits of elderly brain-injured patients. The one study we located that addressed outcome following rehabilitation was conducted at Gaylord Hospital, Wallingford, CT (Davis & Acton, 1988). The authors make clear their concern that elderly patients are routinely assigned to expensive rehabilitation in the absence of any efficacy data.

This retrospective study compared 26 patients over 50 years old with no prior debilitating illness, who were admitted to the hospital with closed head injury, to a control group of head-injured patients under the age of 25, matched to the elderly group for length of post-traumatic amnesia, which is widely considered to be a measure of severity of head injury.

Through a chart review, information for both groups was obtained on duration of post-traumatic amnesia, cognitive level upon admission and at discharge, length of stay in the traumatic-brain-injury unit, and disposition. Information about the subjects' premorbid status and their treatment during the acute stage of their care was obtained through chart review and interviews with patients and their families.

All subjects participated in a formal, intensive, multidisciplinary rehabilitation program. The younger group clearly made a fuller recovery. One hundred percent were living at home and were independent in the activities of daily living by the time of follow-up. Thirteen were employed at least part-time. Nineteen of the 26 still reported some difficulties, such as balance problems, deficits in short-term memory, and tremor. The average *Rancho Los Amigos* (*RLA*) level, a general rating of cognitive functioning, improved from 6 at admission to 7 at discharge.

Although recovery in the elderly group did not match that of the younger group, 85% eventually returned home, and more than half were independent in activities of daily living. All reported continuing difficulties, ranging from mild short-term memory loss to a need for total care. The average *RLA* increased from 5 at admission to 6 at discharge. There was no significant difference in the change of *RLA* levels between the young group and the elderly group.

This study indicates that many older people can make a good recovery from traumatic brain injury, even though they may not recover as fully as younger patients. The recovery in these patients occurred following a formal rehabilitation program, but Davis and Acton correctly note the need for further studies to confirm the effectiveness of such programs for the elderly.

It remains for those involved in rehabilitation to identify the impairments in language and other neuropsychological functions that are characteristic of brain-injured elderly patients and to devise and test the efficacy of techniques for their remediation. The need for such efforts will only increase as the population continues to grow older.

Conclusions

The goal of this chapter has been to sensitize the reader to the unique world of head injury in the elderly, as well as to point out what happens when the aged experience what is usually considered to be a young person's problem. As we have just seen, while head injury can create serious problems for the elderly, a significant proportion of elderly head-injured patients achieve a very good outcome. Some, such as an individual described by Amacher and Bybee, make extraordinary recoveries:

. . . an 87 year-old active man who enjoyed folk-dancing and driving to his children's homes was involved in a car accident in which his head struck the driver's side window. His admission GCS was 15, but within 3 hours the GCS fell to 8. At craniotomy, a single artery on the left parietal operculum was discovered to be the source of the hematoma. He responded slowly postoperatively, began speaking his native Italian at 2 weeks, and went home at 4 weeks without deficit and speaking English well. By 3 months after injury, he had returned to dancing and driving. (1987, p. 955)

References

Amacher, A. L., & Bybee, D. E. (1987). Toleration of head injury by the elderly. *Neurosurgery, 20*(6), 954–957.

Anderson, D. W., Miller, J. D., & Kalsbeek, W. D. (1983). Findings from a major U. S. survey of persons hospitalised with head injuries. *Public Health Report, 98,* 475.

Annegers, J. F., Grabow, J. D., Kurland, L. T., & Laws, E. R. (1980). The incidence, causes, and secular trends of head trauma in Olmstead County, Minnesota. *Neurology, 30,* 912–919.

Davis, C. S., & Acton, P. (1988). Treatment of the elderly brain-injured patient. *Journal of the American Geriatrics Society, 36,* 225–229.

Galbraith, S. (1987). Head injuries in the elderly. *British Medical Journal, 294,* 325.

Grigsby, J. (1984). Surgical and traumatic emergencies. In G. Schwartz, G. Bosker, & J. Grigsby (Eds.), *Geriatric emergencies* (pp. 179–187). Baltimore, MD: Robert J. Brody.

Hernesniemi, J. (1979). Outcome following head injuries in the aged. *Acta Neurochirurgica, 49,* 67–79.

Jennett, B., & MacMillan, R. (1981). Epidemiology of head injury. *British Medical Journal, 282,* 101.

Klauber, M. R., Barrett-Connor, E., Marshall, L. F., & Bowers, S. A. (1981). The epidemiology of head injury. *American Journal of Epidemiology, 113,* 500–509.

Koin, D. (1984). Abuse and neglect in the aged. In G. Schwartz, G. Bosker, & J. Grigsby (Eds.), *Geriatric emergencies* (pp. 171–178). Baltimore, MD: Robert J. Brody.

Leahy, L. F., & Holland, A. L. (1985). *Age-at-onset of pediatric closed head injury: Recovery of function.* Paper presented at the Annual Convention of the American Speech-Language-Hearing Association, Washington, DC.

Lehman, L. B. (1988). Head trauma in the elderly. *Postgraduate Medicine, 83,* 140–142, 145–147.

Pentland, B., Roy, C. W., & Miller, J. D. (1986). Head injury in the elderly. *Age and Ageing, 15,* 193–202.

Roy, C. W., Pentland, B., & Miller, J. D. (1986). The causes and consequences of minor head injury in the elderly. *Injury, 17,* 220–223.

Memory Influences on Language in Normal Aging

17

CHAPTER

Rhoda Au, PhD, and Nancy Bowles, PhD ■

I t has been well established that memory deficits accompany the aging process even in relatively healthy older adults (see Burke & Light, 1981; Craik, 1977, for reviews). At the same time, tests used to assess language competence often make demands on memory processing (Hasher & Zacks, 1988; Light, 1988; Ulatowska, Cannito, Hayashi, & Fleming, 1985). It is, therefore, important in assessing the language of older adults to be aware of how memory deficits may influence the outcome of tests of language competence.

We will begin the first section with a brief overview of the types of memory processes that show deficits in healthy older adults as well as those that are typically spared. The second section will discuss how these deficits might be expected to influence measures of language production and comprehension. We will also present data from language tasks and consider how older adults may use compensatory strategies to reduce demands on memory.

Episodic Memory in Normal Aging

Tulving (1972) distinguished between two different types of memory, episodic and semantic. *Episodic memory* encompasses representations of events that have been experienced by an individual and are tagged with respect to time and place of occurrence. Standard tests of short- and long-term recall and recognition involve episodic memory. *Semantic memory* refers to the store of knowledge about one's language: words, their meanings and interrelationships, and the rules necessary for their use. A broad definition of semantic memory also includes the store of general world knowledge (Hintzman, 1978).

In tests involving episodic memory, a distinction is made between measures of primary (or short-term) memory and secondary (or long-term) memory. A test involving primary memory is one that requires recall or recognition of items immediately after they have been presented for study, without any intervening activity. One such test is the digit span test from the *Wechsler Adult Intelligence Scale–Revised* (Wechsler, 1981). In a primary memory task, information is maintained in memory only as long as conscious attention is directed to the items to be remembered. Age differences have been shown to be minimal in tests of primary memory (see Craik, 1977, for a review).

Baddeley and Hitch (1974) distinguished between primary memory and working memory functions. Primary memory is invoked for tasks that involve memory for a small set of items with no additional attention-demanding task requirements; working memory is implicated when tasks require some manipulation of the items to be remembered. If a memory test requires any manipulation of the information that is temporarily stored or any additional processing while information is held in memory, an age-related deficit is typically observed; elderly subjects do worse than young subjects (Craik & Rabinowitz, 1984).

There is also impairment with age on tests of secondary (long-term) memory, which is involved when more permanent representations of to-be-remembered items have been encoded and stored. Such representations are required when the time between study and test precludes maintenance of the items in working memory because of intervening processing. In laboratory tests involving secondary memory, lists of words or text materials are presented for study and the task is to recall the studied items. Typically, young adults recall more items than older adults (Hultsch & Dixon, 1984; Perlmutter, 1979; Schonfield & Robertson, 1966). The magnitude of the deficits can be reduced by providing cues for retrieval of the to-be-remembered items (Laurence, 1967). The more complete a retrieval cue is, the smaller any age-related deficit will be.

In tests of recognition involving secondary memory, old items that were previously presented for study are displayed along with new, distractor items. The task is to identify the old items. In this kind of test, in which the complete target item is provided as a cue, age deficits are minimal (Erber, 1974; Perlmutter, 1979) and, under some circumstances, are virtually eliminated (Bowles & Poon, 1982; Schoenfield & Robertson, 1966). Such results suggest that newly learned items are available to older adults but that there is some reduction in the ability to access those items, because of inefficiencies in either the storage of new items or their retrieval.

In summary, age-related deficits in episodic memory tests are widely observed. They are particularly noteworthy in tests that involve working memory, in which attention is required both to hold items in memory and to perform additional processing on those or other items. Deficits are also consistently observed in recall tasks that depend on secondary memory, but these age differences can be reduced by providing cues to aid in retrieval.

Semantic Memory in Normal Aging

It was long believed that, although there were age-related deficits in episodic memory, semantic memory was spared with age. However, recent data challenge this notion and suggest that under some conditions elderly adults suffer from retrieval deficits in semantic memory as well as in episodic memory.

Semantic memory is commonly viewed as a richly connected network involving at least three levels of representation: a perceptual level, consisting of structural features (e.g., visual features of a visual stimulus); a semantic level, comprising conceptual features of a stimulus; and a lexical level, including the phonological and orthographic features of the word name associated with the stimulus.

Vocabulary test scores have been widely used as a measure of semantic memory integrity. In a standard vocabulary test the stimulus consists of a word that supplies the complete phonological features (for an auditory presentation) or orthographic features (for a visual presentation) that are necessary to access its representation at the lexical level of semantic memory. The task is to provide the conceptual features (from the semantic level) in the form of a definition. Typically there are no age-related differences in vocabulary scores (see Kramer & Jarvik, 1979; Schaie, 1980, for reviews). The equivalence of young and elderly adults on vocabulary tests has been taken as evidence that semantic memory was unchanged in normal aging, because vocabulary performance requires access to conceptual information in semantic memory.

Another semantic memory measure that is widely used in the laboratory setting is lexical decision, which is thought to require access to words at the lexical level. In this task a string of letters is displayed and the subject is asked to indicate whether or not the letter string forms a real word. Although older adults are slower than young adults in making lexical decisions, as they are in virtually all tasks, there is typically no age difference in the ability to identify words and nonwords (Bowles & Poon, 1982, 1988; Howard, 1983; Howard, McAndrews, & Lasaga, 1981). That is, there appears to be no significant age difference in lexical access, at least as measured in the lexical decision task in which lexical features (orthographic or phonological) are provided in the stimulus.

Organization of semantic memory also appears to be unaffected by age. This is seen in tests such as word and category association that are thought to reflect the connections that make up semantic memory. In a word association test the stimulus is a word and the task is to name the first word that comes to mind; in a category association test, which is simply a restricted word association test, the stimulus is a category name and the task is to name the first exemplar of the category that comes to mind. Typically there are no age-related differences in first responses given on association tests (e.g., Bowles, Williams, & Poon, 1983; Burke & Peters, 1986; Howard, 1980), leading to the conclusion that organization

within the semantic network does not change with increasing age.

The assumption that semantic memory processes do not change with age finds further support from primed lexical decision experiments. In the primed lexical decision task, each target letter string is preceded by a priming word. In the case where the letter string forms a word, the priming word is either semantically related or unrelated to the target word. For both young and elderly adults, the lexical decision is more rapid following a semantically related priming word than an unrelated priming word, and the magnitude of this effect is comparable for the two age groups (Burke, White, & Diaz, 1987; Cerella & Fozard, 1984; Howard et al., 1981). These results show that young and elderly adults respond to the same semantic relationships; that is, semantic relatedness and its effect on processing do not vary across age groups.

There is considerable support for the notion that the content and organization of semantic memory are well maintained in healthy older adults. Further, the ability to access conceptual information, such as the definition of a word in semantic memory, is typically unimpaired well into old age. And finally, lexical access appears to be unimpaired when the stimulus is at the lexical level, such as the letter string in a lexical decision task. Recently, however, a semantic memory task has been identified that does reveal an age-related deficit, even in healthy older adults, and that is confrontation naming. This is a task that requires the subject to provide lexical information (a word name) when given conceptual information (such as the definition of a word or the picture of an object; this is the mirror image of the vocabulary task. An age-related deficit is often observed in tasks of this type, with elderly subjects consistently producing fewer names than young subjects.

Naming in Normal Aging

Confrontation naming tests typically consist of the presentation of pictured objects that subjects are asked to name. In these tasks, the picture stimulus is thought to directly activate its semantic representation, then to indirectly activate the word name at the lexical level (Carr, McCauley, Sperber, & Parmelee, 1982).

The *Boston Naming Test* (Kaplan, Goodglass, & Weintraub, 1976) is commonly used in testing naming abilities. It consists of simple line drawings of 69 common and less common objects. When Borod, Goodglass, and Kaplan (1980) administered this test to normal young and elderly adults, they found that subjects over 70 years of age named significantly fewer items than younger subjects. Nicholas, Obler, Albert, and Goodglass (1985) reported similar results for the naming of action pictures. They also found that older subjects more often required phonological cues (the initial sound of the target name) to elicit a correct response than did younger subjects. However, young and elderly subjects were equally likely to produce a correct response when they were given a phonological cue (information at the lexical level). In other words, in the absence of any phonological information, older subjects had more difficulty in spontaneously retrieving the target word than did younger subjects. When partial phonological information was provided, elderly subjects were just as likely as younger subjects to correctly retrieve the target word.

Bowles and Poon (1985) obtained similar results in a naming-to-definition experiment with orthographic priming. In this paradigm the stimulus was the definition of a target word of relatively low normative frequency and the task was to name the word that was defined. Each definition was preceded by a priming stimulus that was orthographically related, semantically related, unrelated, or neutral with respect to the target word or was the correct target word itself. Elderly adults retrieved fewer target words than young adults in every condition, except when the prime was the correct target word or the initial two letters of the target word. In those two conditions the older subjects were as accurate as the

young subjects. These results again demonstrate that when partial or complete orthographic/phonological information was provided, no age differences in naming were found.

These laboratory results have been confirmed in a more natural setting using structured diary recordings. Burke, Worthley, and Martin (1988) asked participants to report tip-of-the-tongue experiences in the course of daily living. Older subjects reported more such experiences than did young subjects. In another study of everyday memory, Cohen and Faulkner (1986) reported a questionnaire study of memory blocks for proper names. Participants filled out a questionnaire each time a name block occurred in their lives. They found that partial phonological information about a blocked target name was significantly less available for the older adults than for the young adults. Both results support the laboratory data and suggest again that there is difficulty at the lexical level in activating the phonological information necessary to produce a desired word name.

In summary, semantic memory organization and processing, which are inextricably linked to language processing, are for the most part well preserved throughout the life-span. It has been shown, however, that retrieval of less frequently used word names, in the absence of any phonological or orthographic cues, is somewhat impaired in older adults. This is seen in a greater number of word retrieval failures and in longer retrieval times.

The next section addresses how the memory deficits that have been discussed, both episodic and semantic, might be expected to influence measures of comprehension and language production.

The Role of Episodic and Semantic Memory in Tests of Language Competence

Language competence is generally measured by tests of *comprehension*, the ability to understand the meaning of messages that are received from a speaker or writer, and *discourse,* the ability to produce meaningful messages orally or in writing. In terms of semantic memory processing, comprehension requires access to word meanings when the word names are given as input. If comprehension required only access to word meanings, no age differences would be expected. However, it requires more than accessing definitions; current and previous words and concepts must be temporarily held in memory at the same time that processing leading to their integration and interpretation is carried out. These processes are widely thought to make demands on working memory (Chafe, 1972; Cohen, 1979; Davis & Ball, 1989; Hasher & Zacks, 1988; Light & Burke, 1988; Ulatowska et al., 1985). These constructive processes include a combination of simultaneous on-line encoding, storage, manipulation, integration, and reorganization of stimulus information. To the extent that such processes make demands on working memory, older adults would be expected to exhibit deficits on comprehension tasks; age-related deficits in comprehension would be found for tests that ask for recall of implicit information as opposed to explicit information. Implicit recall requires constructive processing, which takes place in working memory, whereas explicit recall involves retrieval of previously presented information. Age-related differences would also occur if the syntactic structures of the test stimuli are complex, since processing these sentences would place greater demands on working memory. The working-memory hypothesis would also predict greater age-related differences for oral comprehension versus written comprehension, because oral comprehension involves storage processes that are not needed in written comprehension.

Spontaneous discourse also involves working memory. On an oral discourse task, a subject is required to simultaneously construct the intended message, store what has just been said, and retrieve from semantic memory the word to be said. On a writ-ten discourse task, the demands on working memory are minimized by the constant availability of the previously emitted information; however, the task still requires retrieval of lexical information in the absence of lexical cues.

As in naming tests, spontaneous discourse tasks rely on word retrieval in the absence of orthographic and phonological cues. However, it is possible to compensate for semantic retrieval deficits more easily in discourse tasks than in naming tests. A discourse task typically requires subjects to produce a spontaneous output that has a directed message. The same message can be represented by many unique strings of words. Hence, if a subject has difficulty retrieving a specific word, it is possible to compensate by choosing another word or words in its place. Word retrieval difficulties in discourse may be revealed by the use of indefinite terms, more general or more common words that give up some precision, and circumlocutions. Additional compensatory strategies, such as generating unnecessary comments or questions in the middle of the task, using filler phrases, or pausing, may also be used to "cover up" or "stall for more time" to retrieve words.

The hypothesis that memory changes associated with normal aging influence language performance is consistent with research results. We now turn our discussion toward a review of studies of language comprehension and production, interpreted with respect to their degree of involvement of working memory and semantic retrieval.

Comprehension in Normal Aging

Comprehension is often assessed using tests of inferential reasoning. Subjects are typically asked to read sentences or short paragraphs and then respond to a question or set of questions that asks for explicit or implicit information. These tests can vary in the demands they make on working memory. If the question asks for recall of explicit information, the amount of constructive processing that involves working memory will be minimal. If the question calls for the recall of implicit information, and thereby requires integration of information from earlier sentences, there will be significant involvement of working memory. Age differences in these tasks would be expected to reflect the amount of such constructive processing that is required. Elderly subjects will do significantly worse than young subjects on tasks that involve substantial constructive processing.

Cohen (1979) reported age differences on a test of comprehension that involved integrative and constructive processing. Subjects were asked to listen to messages that contained several sentences. After each message, subjects were asked to respond to two questions about the presented material, one that required recall of facts and another that required an inference. Age differences were found for the inferential question, which required active construction and integration of presented information; elderly subjects made significantly fewer correct inferences than younger subjects. In contrast, no significant age differences were found in the factual question, which only required retrieval of verbatim information. Cohen suggested that when demands on memory were great, age-related differences were found; when memory requirements were reduced, differences between young and older subjects were minimal. Other studies of inferential reasoning have led to similar conclusions (Hasher & Zacks, 1988; Light & Albertson, 1988; Light & Capps, 1986).

Another paradigm used to test comprehension involves the manipulation of sentence syntax. Subjects are presented with sentences that vary in syntactic structure. Although sentence syntax conditions vary across studies, typically, sentence structures that evoke longer response times or more errors are considered to be more complex than sentences that lead to shorter reaction times or fewer errors. Another measure of syntactic complexity is based on Chomsky's theory of language acquisition (1979). Chomsky suggested that the pattern of language acquisition reflects linguistic complexity. Certain syntactic structures do not emerge until later stages of language acquisition; these types of sentences are considered more complex than sentence structures that appear in the early stages of language development. Regardless of which measure of syntactic complexity is chosen, it is generally thought that different sentence structures place different demands on working memory (Emery, 1985, 1986; Davis & Ball, 1989; Kynette & Kemper, 1986; Light & Burke, 1988). Age-related differences should occur when sentence stimuli require multiple processes such as storage, manipulation, and integration. Age-related differences would also be predicted for sentence stimuli whose syntactic structures are considered developmentally complex.

Kynette and Kemper (1986) presented young and elderly subjects with sentences that had left- or right-branching clauses. Left-branching sentences place greater demand on working memory than right-branching sentences because the left-branching clause cannot be integrated until additional information is provided by the remainder of the sentence (e.g., left-branching sentence: "Although it was difficult, Sally was able to finish the job"; right-branching sentence: "Sally was able to finish the job, although it was difficult"). Subjects were asked to listen to grammatical and ungrammatical sentences and to either repeat the grammatical sentences or correct the ungrammatical sentences. Consistent with the working-memory hypothesis, elderly subjects had greater difficulty correcting ungrammatical sentences with left-branching clauses than with right-branching clauses. In contrast, young subjects had no difficulty correcting either left- or right-branching ungrammatical sentences.

Emery (1986) adopted Chomsky's definition of linguistic complexity and suggested a direct relationship between linguistic complexity and performance deficits. She administered several tests of comprehension, among which were included two tests that manipulated sentence syntax—for example, using active versus passive voice or right-branching versus left-branching sentences. She reported no age-related differences on tasks that involved simple linguistic components (those that emerge in the early stages of language development). Age differences were found when test stimuli involved complex linguistic components. Emery concluded that age-related differences are likely to occur when the comprehension task places greater demands on working memory. Other studies that manipulated sentence syntax reported similar findings. Elderly subjects do worse than younger adults if the syntactic manipulation leads to significant involvement of working memory (Davis & Ball, 1989; Feier & Gerstman, 1980).

In laboratory tests of comprehension that involved inferential reasoning and syntactic manipulations, elderly subjects demonstrated deficits in performance when compared to young adults. It is suggested here that this decline in comprehension is at least in part a consequence of age-related changes in working memory. Yet in normal conversation, these comprehension deficits are not often apparent. Why are comprehension deficits less evident in these contexts than they are in research studies? It is possible that older subjects develop compensatory strategies to accommodate working-memory limits. For example, a conversation may draw on a person's semantic knowledge, which can be used to help interpret and integrate the verbal input. Familiar topics of conversation, which involve information already stored in semantic memory, may reduce the amount of new information that must be held in working memory. If one already knows that the winning response in chess is "Checkmate," there is less new information to store from the sentence "The chess champion triumphantly said 'Checkmate' as he made his final move." Unfamiliar topics, which have minimal semantic representation, must rely on more demanding processing to store new information, processing that is more susceptible to the influence of age-related deficits in working memory.

There is evidence that older adults can make use of prior knowledge to reduce the effects of their working-memory deficit. Smith, Rebok, Smith, Hall, and Alvin (1983) asked young and elderly subjects to read three different paragraphs. One of the three paragraphs contained information that was familiar to both groups of subjects, the second contained information that was unfamiliar, and the third contained sentences that were scrambled so that they formed a nonsense story. Smith et al. found that elderly subjects recalled significantly less information than young subjects when the topics were unfamiliar. However, elderly subjects did just as well as young subjects in recalling stories that contained familiar information. Furthermore, both groups did equally poorly on nonsense stories. Smith et al. suggested that elderly adults relied on prior knowledge to facilitate story processing in the familiar-story condition. In the unfamiliar condition, this strategy could not apply, and elderly subjects had to rely solely on memory. In the nonsense condition, working memory was equally strained in both groups, not unlike the demands of a typical test of working-memory capacity. This interpretation gained further support from Smith et al.'s analysis of recall errors. Although the number of items correctly recalled from the stories on familiar topics was comparable for the two age groups, elderly subjects made more story additions and distortions. These kinds of errors are consistent with the notion that older adults are more likely to draw on knowledge stored in semantic memory when interpreting stories about familiar topics rather than holding all of the incoming information in episodic working memory. Addition and distortion errors could reflect imprecision in selecting the appropriate semantic information.

There is evidence from semantic memory tasks that older adults are more likely to make use of contextual information under some conditions than are young adults. A number of investigators have interpreted the greater reliance on context as a compensatory device for inefficient processing (see Stanovich, 1980, for a review). This strategy serves to reduce the demand on working memory by decreasing the amount of processing required to access and integrate the input. Cohen and Faulkner (1983) found that older subjects showed greater contextual facilitation in a lexical decision task than did young subjects. Similarly, Bowles and Poon (1988) reported that older adults were more likely than young adults to make use of context in a lexical decision task in which the context was of limited value in predicting the target word. Wingfield, Poon, Lombardi, and Lowe (1985) manipulated linguistic structures in a speech processing task and showed that elderly subjects benefited more than young adults from the semantic and syntactic context. All of these investigators concluded that older subjects use context effectively to compensate for processing deficits.

Further support for the working-memory hypothesis comes from the comparison of comprehension performance on oral versus written tasks. Clearly, oral comprehension places greater demands on working memory than written comprehension. Unlike written comprehension, oral comprehension requires that the information be held in working memory. Given this added ''burden'' on working memory, it would be predicted that age-related deficits on oral comprehension tasks would be greater than those found on written comprehension tasks. Hasher, Zacks, and colleagues tested this hypothesis in a series of studies (Hasher & Zacks, 1988; Zacks & Hasher, 1988; Zacks, Hasher, Doren, Hamm, & Attig, 1987). They asked subjects to listen to or read three different types of passages: explicit, expected, and unexpected. The explicit passage condition required subjects to retrieve information that was stated explicitly in the paragraph. The expected passage condition required subjects to make an inference that was expected, given the context of the paragraph. The unexpected passage condition required subjects to make an inference that was not predicted, given the context. In this condition, subjects had to reevaluate the information in the paragraph to make the inference.

Across all presentation modalities, young and old subjects were equally able to retrieve the explicit information. Age differences emerged when additional processing demands necessary to make inferences became involved. When information was presented orally, elderly subjects had difficulty drawing inferences in the expected and unexpected conditions as compared to young subjects. Since oral presentation places the greatest demands on working memory, these results coincide with the working-memory hypothesis. Results from the written passages were more complex. Hasher, Zacks, and colleagues devised two written presentation procedures: cumulative and noncumulative. In the cumulative condition, sentences appeared one at a time so that the passage in its entirety was present when the last sentence appeared. In the noncumulative condition, sentences appeared one at a time; however, as each sentence was read, it would disappear and be replaced by the following sentence. Thus, the noncumulative condition imposed working-memory demands that were not present in the cumulative condition. No age-related differences in making inferences were reported in the cumulative condition. Age-related differences were found, however, in making inferences from the unexpected passages in the noncumulative condition. It is important to note that elderly subjects were able to make inferences in the expected, noncumulative condition. They only demonstrated difficulty in making an inference when working-memory demands were maximized because both storage and constructive processes were engaged. When the working-memory demand was reduced in the cumulative condition and the expected, noncumulative condition, elderly subjects were able to draw inferences as well as young subjects. Hasher and Zacks (1988) concluded that the absence or presence of age-related deficits in comprehension depended on the extent of working-memory demands.

In summary, it has been argued that working-memory constraints associated with normal aging contribute to reduced performance on comprehension tests. Inferential reasoning performance, commonly used as an indicator of adult comprehension, is impaired in older adults to the degree that the reasoning task relies on working memory. Similarly, comprehension of sentences that vary in syntax will be impaired with age if processing requires significant involvement of working memory. It is possible that older adults compensate, to some extent, for age-related decline in working memory by using semantic knowledge and context to reduce the demands on working memory.

Discourse in Normal Aging

Competence in language production is generally measured by evaluating oral or written samples of language generated in response to some stimulus. Like language comprehension tasks, language production tasks are also thought to involve working-memory processing (Kemper, 1988; Kynette & Kemper, 1986). The role of working memory in discourse can be inferred by comparing performance on oral and written discourse tasks. In oral discourse, working-memory demands are maximized because the speaker must simultaneously remember what has just been said and plan what is to be said next. Written discourse minimizes working-memory involvement because the writer can refer back to previously written responses. It would be expected, then, that older adults would be less handicapped by their working-memory limitations in written discourse than in oral discourse. There is considerable evidence to support this expectation.

Obler (1980) reported a study of oral discourse in which subjects were presented with the logical memory passages from the Wechsler Memory scale, form II. She found that older subjects produced sentences of shorter length than did younger subjects. In addition, elderly subjects' stories were marked by increased use of indefinite terms and additions. Obler concluded that the oral discourse performance of elderly subjects was poor compared to that of young subjects. In contrast, Sandson, Obler, and Albert (1987) reported on the written descriptions of the Cookie Theft picture from the *Boston Diagnostic Aphasia Examination* (Goodglass & Kaplan, 1972), produced by young and elderly subjects. They found that the written samples of elderly adults were marked by well-structured, complex, embedded sentences. The discrepancy in results between the Sandson et al. study and the Obler study may reflect different demands on working memory in written versus oral discourse.

Kynette and Kemper (1986) investigated both oral and written discourse in young versus elderly subjects. They found that elderly subjects produced oral responses that were consistently less syntactically complex (as determined by the mean number of clauses per utterance) than their corresponding written samples. They also reported a significant correlation between memory capacity and length of utterance. Subjects who demonstrated greater memory capacity tended to produce longer utterances.

Chafe (1982) and Kroll (1977) reported results that parallel those of Kynette and Kemper (1986). Chafe (1982) noted in her study that the oral discourse of older adults was characterized by numerous fragmented utterances, which were integrated during the course of conversation. In contrast, written samples of these same subjects contained complete, complex sentences with embedded and subordinate clauses. Chafe suggested that the difference between oral and written language stems from (working) memory demands rather than linguistic factors.

Older adults may be at an additional disadvantage in producing discourse because of their deficit in retrieval of words from semantic memory. There is suggestive evidence from discourse studies that is consistent with this interpretation. Obler (1980) recorded discourse samples from subjects who were asked to describe the Cookie Theft picture. She reported that the oral descriptions by elderly subjects were distinguished from those by younger subjects by the presence of more "elaborated empty speech." Elaboration referred to the use of more modifiers, interjections, and prepositional phrases. Empty speech was the label for a reduced number of themes and a greater number of words produced relative to the number of content units. Obler found that measures of empty speech correlated negatively with performances on the *Boston Naming Test:* poorer naming (word retrieval) performance was associated with a greater amount of empty speech. In an oral discourse test similar to that of Obler (1980), Sandson et al. (1987) found that discourse samples from elderly subjects included more comments, questions, indefinite terms, and filler phrases than did those of young adults. In an oral vocabulary test, Botwinick, West, and Storandt (1975) reported that older subjects gave longer, more elaborate definitions than younger subjects, who produced superior synonyms and more concise definitions. All of these results can be interpreted as reflecting word retrieval deficits of older adults. Empty speech can be seen as a stalling device to hold the listener's attention while retrieval is attempted (Obler, personal communication). Elaboration may result from the need to use a number of words to express an idea or describe an object (circumlocution) when its name cannot be retrieved.

There is some evidence that the act of word retrieval itself may involve working memory for older adults. Ulatowska et al. (1985) reported age-related differences in complex spoken discourse. Older adults' discourse samples that were syntactically complex contained fewer proper nouns and more high-frequency general nouns when compared to discourse samples from middle-aged persons. These results suggest a possible interaction between our two major memory factors: working memory and word retrieval in semantic memory. When working memory demands increased, as indicated by increased syntactic complexity, spontaneous word retrieval decreased, as seen in the decreased number of nouns generated.

In summary, elderly adults produce written and oral discourse that is different from that of young adults. We attribute this difference at least in part to age-related changes in word retrieval and in working memory. Circumlocutions, increased elaboration, greater reliance on high-frequency words, less variety in word choice, and increased use of filler phrases and indefinite terms suggest difficulty in semantic retrieval processes. Reduced syntactic complexity in oral discourse, as compared to written discourse, may reflect working-memory deficits.

Conclusions

In this chapter we have addressed the ways in which normal age-related changes in episodic and semantic memory may affect language performance. There is evidence that even healthy older adults show deficits in processing in working memory and in retrieval of words from semantic memory in the absence of lexical cues. Both kinds of processes are inextricably linked to language performance. Comprehension and discourse tasks, used to evaluate language competence, make demands on working memory. Therefore, some of the age differences observed in language performance can be attributed to changes in working-memory processes rather than to changes in language competence. In addition to its involvement with working memory, discourse requires retrieval of words from semantic memory. Age differences in discourse, such as elaboration, empty speech, and settling for more common, less precise words, may result from the inability to retrieve the best word, reflecting a memory rather than a linguistic source.

It may not be possible to separate age-related changes in memory processes from age-related changes in linguistic processes. However, it is important to be aware that measures of language performance are influenced by the memory demands of the task. The influence of working-memory deficits on language testing can be minimized by the use of written materials, and knowledge of an individual's memory status can aid in the interpretation of language tests.

References

Baddeley, A. D., & Hitch, G. (1974). Working memory. In G. H. Bower (Ed.), *The psychology of learning and motivation* (Vol. 8, pp. 47–89). New York: Academic Press.

Borod, J., Goodglass, H., & Kaplan, E. (1980). Normative data on the Boston Diagnostic Aphasia Examination, Parietal Lobe Battery, and the Boston Naming Test. *Journal of Clinical Neuropsychology, 2,* 209–215.

Botwinick, J., West, R., & Storandt, M. (1975). Qualitative vocabulary test responses and age. *Journal of Gerontology, 30,* 574–577.

Bowles, N. L., & Poon, L. W. (1982). An analysis of the effect of aging on recognition memory. *Journal of Gerontology, 37,* 212–219.

Bowles, N. L., & Poon, L. W. (1985). Aging and retrieval of words in semantic memory. *Journal of Gerontology, 40,* 71–77.

Bowles, N. L., & Poon, L. W. (1988). Age and context effects in lexical decision: An age by context interaction. *Experimental Aging Research, 14,* 201–205.

Bowles, N. L., Williams, D., & Poon, L. W. (1983). On the use of word association norms in aging research. *Experimental Aging Research, 9,* 175–177.

Burke, D. M., & Light, L. L. (1981). Memory and aging: The role of retrieval processes. *Psychological Bulletin, 90,* 513–546.

Burke, D. M., & Peters, L. J. (1986). Word associations in old age: Evidence for consistency in semantic encoding during adulthood. *Psychology and Aging, 1,* 283–292.

Burke, D. M., White, H., & Diaz, D. L. (1987). Semantic priming in young and older adults: Evidence for age-constancy in automatic and attentional processes. *Journal of Experimental Psychology: Human Perception and Performance, 13,* 79–88.

Burke, D., Worthley, J., & Martin, J. (1988). I'll never forget what's-her-name: Aging and tip of the tongue experiences in everyday life. In M. M. Gruenberg, P. E. Morris, & R. N. Sykes (Eds.), *Practical aspects of memory* (Vol. 2, pp. 113–118). New York: Wiley.

Carr, T. H., McCauley, C., Sperber, R. D., & Parmelee, C. M. (1982). Words, pictures, and priming: On semantic activation, conscious identification, and the automaticity of information processing. *Journal of Experimental Psychology: Human Perception and Performance, 8,* 757–777.

Cerella, J., & Fozard, J. L. (1984). Lexical access and age. *Developmental Psychology, 20,* 235–243.

Chafe, W. L. (1972). Discourse structure and human knowledge. In J. Carroll & R. Freedle (Eds.), *Language comprehension and the acquisition of knowledge* (pp. 41–69). Washington, DC: V. W. Winston.

Chafe, W. L. (1982). Integration and involvement in speaking, writing, and oral literature. In D. Tannen (Ed.), *Spoken and written language: Exploring orality and literacy* (pp. 35–54). Norwood, NJ: Ablex.

Chomsky, C. (1979). *The acquisition of syntax in children from 5 to 10.* Cambridge, MA: MIT Press.

Cohen, G. (1979). Language comprehension in old age. *Cognitive Psychology, 11,* 412–429.

Cohen, G., & Faulkner, D. (1983). Word recognition: Age differences in contextual facilitation effects. *British Journal of Psychology, 74,* 239–251.

Cohen, G., & Faulkner, D. (1986). Memory for proper names: Age differences in retrieval. *British Journal of Developmental Psychology, 4,* 187–197.

Craik, F. I. M. (1977). Age differences in human memory. In J. E. Birren & K. W. Schaie (Eds.), *Handbook of the psychology of aging* (pp. 384–420). New York: Van Nostrand Reinhold.

Craik, F. I. M., & Rabinowitz, J. C. (1984). Age differences in the acquisition and use of verbal information: A tutorial review. In H. Bouma & D. G. Bouwhuis (Eds.), *Attention and performance X. Control of language processes* (pp. 471–499). Hillsdale, NJ: Lawrence Erlbaum.

Davis, G. A., & Ball, H. (1989). Effects of age on comprehension of complex sentences in adulthood. *Journal of Speech and Hearing Research, 32,* 143–150.

Emery, O. (1985). Language and aging. *Experimental Aging Research* (Monograph). Mount Desert, ME: Beech Hill.

Emery, O. (1986). Linguistic decrement in normal aging. *Language and Communication, 6,* 47–64.

Erber, J. T. (1974). Age differences in recognition. *Journal of Gerontology, 29,* 177–181.

Feier, C. D., & Gerstman, L. J. (1980). Sentence comprehension abilities throughout the adult life span. *Journal of Gerontology, 35,* 722–728.

Goodglass, H., & Kaplan, E. (1972). *Boston Diagnostic Aphasia Examination.* Philadelphia: Lea & Febiger.

Hasher, L., & Zacks, R. T. (1988). Working memory, comprehension, and aging: A review and a new view. In G. Bauer (Ed.), *Advances in research and theory: The psychology of learning and motivation* (Vol. 22, pp. 193–225). New York: Academic Press.

Hintzman, D. L. (1978). *The psychology of learning and memory.* San Francisco: W. H. Freeman.

Howard, D. V. (1980). Category norms: A comparison of the Battig and Montague (1969) norms with the responses of adults between the ages of 20 and 80. *Journal of Gerontology, 35,* 225–231.

Howard, D. V. (1983). The effects of aging and degree of association on the semantic priming of lexical decisions in young and old adults. *Experimental Aging Research, 9,* 145–151.

Howard, D. V., McAndrews, M. P., & Lasaga, M. I. (1981). Semantic priming of lexical decisions in young and old adults. *Journal of Gerontology, 36,* 707–714.

Hultsch, D. F., & Dixon, R. A. (1984). Memory for text materials in adulthood. In P. B. Baltes & O. G. Brim (Eds.), *Life-span development and behavior* (Vol. 6). New York: Academic Press.

Kaplan, E., Goodglass, H., & Weintraub, S. (1976). *The Boston Naming Test.* Experimental edition.

Kemper, S. (1988). Geriatric psycholinguistics: Syntactic limitations of oral and written language. In L. L. Light & D. M. Burke (Eds.), *Language, memory, and aging.* New York: Cambridge University Press.

Kramer, N., & Jarvik, L. F. (1979). Assessment of intellectual changes in the elderly. In A. Raskin and L. F. Jarvik (Eds.), *Psychiatric symptoms and cognitive loss in the elderly* (pp. 221–271). Washington, DC: Hemisphere.

Kroll, B. (1977). Combining ideas in written and spoken English: A look at subordination and coordination. In E. Keenan & T. Bennett (Eds.), *Discourse across time and space* (Vol. 5). Los Angeles: U.S.C. Occasional Papers in Linguistics.

Kynette, D., & Kemper, S. (1986). Aging and the loss of grammatical forms: A cross-sectional study of language performance. *Language and Communication, 6,* 65–72.

Laurence, M. W. (1967). A developmental look at the usefulness of list categorization as an aid to free recall. *Canadian Journal of Psychology, 21,* 153–165.

Light, L. (1988). Language and aging: Competence versus performance. In J. E. Birren & V. L. Bengtson (Eds.), *Emergent theories of aging* (pp. 177–213). New York: Springer.

Light, L. L., & Albertson, S. A. (1988). Aging and comprehension of pragmatic implications. In L. L. Light & D. M. Burke (Eds.), *Language, memory, and aging.* New York: Cambridge University Press.

Light, L. L., & Burke, D. M. (1988). Patterns of language and memory in old age. In L. L. Light & D. M. Burke (Eds.), *Language, memory, and aging.* New York: Cambridge University Press.

Light, L. L., & Capps, J. L. (1986). Comprehension of pronouns in young and older adults. *Developmental Psychology, 22,* 580–585.

Nicholas, N., Obler, L., Albert, M., & Goodglass, H. (1985). Lexical retrieval in healthy aging. *Cortex, 21,* 595–606.

Obler, L. K. (1980). Narrative discourse style in the elderly. In L. K. Obler & M. L. Albert (Eds.), *Language and communication in the elderly.* Lexington, MA: D. C. Heath.

Perlmutter, M. (1979). Age differences in the consistency of adults' associative responses. *Experimental Aging Research, 5,* 549–553.

Sandson, J., Obler, L. K., & Albert, M. L. (1987). Language changes in healthy aging and dementia. In S. Rosenberg (Ed.), *Advances in applied psycholinguistics* (Vol. 1). New York: Cambridge University Press.

Schaie, K. W. (1980). Cognitive development in aging. In L. K. Obler & M. L. Albert (Eds.), *Language and communication in the elderly* (pp. 7–25). Lexington, MA: Lexington Books.

Schonfield, D., & Robertson, B. A. (1966). Memory storage and aging. *Canadian Journal of Psychology, 20,* 228–236.

Smith, S. W., Rebok, G. W., Smith, W. R., Hall, S. E., & Alvin, M. (1983). Adult age differences in the use of story structure in delayed free recall. *Experimental Aging Research, 9,* 191–195.

Stanovich, K. (1980). Toward an interactive model of reading. In S. Dornic (Ed.), *Attention and performance VI.* Hillsdale, NJ: Lawrence Erlbaum.

Tulving, E. (1972). Episodic and semantic memory. In E. Tulving & W. Donaldson (Eds.), *Organization and memory.* New York: Academic Press.

Ulatowska, H. K., Cannito, M. P., Hayashi, M. M., & Fleming, S. G. (1985). Language abilities in the elderly. In H. K. Ulatowska (Ed.), *The aging brain: Communication in the elderly.* Austin, TX: PRO-ED.

Wechsler, D. (1981). *Manual for the Wechsler Adult Intelligence Scale–Revised.* New York: Psychological Corporation.

Wingfield, A., Poon, L. W., Lombardi, L., & Lowe, D. (1985). Speed of processing in normal aging: Effects of speech rate, linguistic structure, and processing time. *Journal of Gerontology, 40,* 579–585.

Zacks, R. T., & Hasher, L. (1988). Capacity theory and the processing of inferences. In L. L. Light & D. M. Burke (Eds.), *Language, memory, and aging* (pp. 154–170). New York: Cambridge University Press.

Zacks, R. T., Hasher, L., Doren, B., Hamm, V., & Attig, M. S. (1987). Encoding and memory of explicit and implicit information. *Journal of Gerontology, 42,* 418–422.

Assessment and Intervention Issues

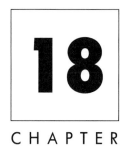

18

CHAPTER

Celia R. Hooper, PhD, and Alex F. Johnson, PhD ■

Health care delivery systems have dramatically changed since the days of the British almshouse for poor and aged citizens. In the United States, since World War II, there has been a slow but steady attempt to plan health care services for the aged segment of our population as a separate demographic group (Pegels, 1981). Traditionally, rehabilitation services such as speech-language pathology have been placed in the category of supportive medical services (Brody, 1974). These services have been viewed by many as a means for reducing the number of hospital days rather than as being methods for the enhancement of the quality of life for the older adult. With the move to more home health care delivery, rehabilitative services have been selected to reduce the effects of a disability and maintain or promote an adequate lifestyle (Council of Home Health Agencies and Community Health Services, 1981). Accompanying an increase in home health care services, there has been a logical move to family management models, involving home-based rehabilitation and assessment of the total family for intervention decisions.

This shift to issues of quality of life and health promotion has affected assessment and rehabilitation of the older adult. This chapter will review the special adjustments in assessment of the older adult, meaningful areas of assessment and treatment, and a decision-making model for management. Although some of the topics covered in this chapter may apply to patients of any age, the authors have attempted to focus specifically on the older patient. This focus has taken into account the shift from inpatient acute care settings to home health and in- and outpatient rehabilitation settings, as well as the shift to the home health setting. Throughout the chapter special emphasis is given to the role of the family and/or other caregivers, as well as to the specific individual with a communication disability.

Assessment

The goals of clinical assessment in the older adult with a suspected speech or language disorder may be varied. Usually the clinician has a primary goal of diagnosis accompanied by other goals, such as patient or family counseling, treatment planning, prognosis, and referral. As Groher (1988) pointed out, decompensation of communication may be the result of a lifetime of cumulative effects or the product of a new, difficult-to-detect pathology. The usual procedure in assessment of older adults by clinicians is to select tests or protocols developed for younger adults and apply them to geriatric assessment. Recently, new items and procedures have been developed for use with speech and language assessment of the older adult, and normative data are emerging for use with more traditional speech and language measures. The last frontier will be to change the clinician or clinical observer to a geriatric thinker—one who adapts perceptions and expectations during the assessment of the older adult.

Adjusting Procedures to the Needs of the Older Adult

Four main procedural changes in assessment of the older adult will make the results more valid and meaningful. Adjusting the ''test'' and the instructions; adjusting the examiner's expectations; adjusting the goals of the assessment; and adjusting the listening, speaking, and observing skills of the examiner will all lend more meaning to the results.

Adjusting the Test and Instructions

Helpful adjustments of the test and instructions include an explanation of the test item's purpose to the older adult and an adjustment of the test item's time constraints, if these exist. Groher (1988), in an excellent review of time variables in the testing procedures of older persons, pointed out that older adults perform better without the pressure of time. These adults perform more slowly, particularly with more items, and they value accuracy over speed. As Groher reminded aphasiologists, in language testing and language learning, the use of meaningful materials, complemented by adequate time to observe, will help the patient perform optimally in language activities. If it is necessary to put the patient under the pressure of time or item complexity to observe the effects of that pressure, it will be necessary to give the patient an explanation and reassurance before or after the pressured event, particularly if more testing is to follow. Instructions may have to be repeated, adapted, given more slowly, or followed by an explanation or example.

Adjusting the Examiner's Expectations

In addition to test procedure adjustment, examiner adjustment may be required as well. Expectations that a patient will sit in his or her chair, respond immediately, find the task interesting, and react in a manner exactly like the example in the test manual are usually unrealistic. The examiner can expect the older adult to be unfamiliar with, or many years removed from, the teacher/pupil model of information exchange. Indeed, it may be considered insulting. The examiner may discover that the patient tires very quickly or objects to a particular task. This requires preparation to increase flexibility in the assessment session. The examiner may expect to gain more information in the assessment when it more closely resembles natural conversation or when it takes place in a more ''natural'' setting. Most hospitals and speech clinics are very unnatural or frightening places for older adults. The examiner should also be prepared for the possible reaction of an older adult who does not view the often younger clinician as all-knowing and wise.

Adjusting the Goals of Assessment

The clinician facing the older adult needs to know why the patient is being assessed. What are the goals of this assessment? Was the patient referred by another professional or a family member, or is this a self-referral? Is the assessment being performed with a chronically ill older adult or someone in the acute stages of a health crisis? Does the referral source, the patient, or the family caregiver have a philosophy of rehabilitation whose aim is "back to normal"? Is this assessment being used for some decision-making process in patient or family management, such as nursing home placement, medical diagnosis, or insurance determination, and are the patient and family aware of this decision making? Are there any hidden agendas that may be revealed during the assessment on the part of the patient, the family, or other professionals? All of these questions will affect the assessment, and particularly the counseling process, for the patient, family, and caregiver.

Responses to referral sources should match requests, accurate information should be given to families regarding realistic recovery, and assessment protocols should be designed to match the goal of any particular assessment. McNeil (1984) reviewed general test batteries in aphasia and their assessment purpose. He commented that most aphasiologists use a battery of tests determined by the purpose of the assessment. Too often, particularly in health care settings, speech-language pathologists and other professionals have set protocols for patients according to the probable disorder label. For example, there may be a "dementia protocol" or a "laryngectomy protocol." While there may be some justification for these sets of procedures, such as research projects, time efficiency, or test-retest comparisons, adjustments must fit the goal or purpose of the assessment in order to achieve counseling and management after the assessment.

Adjusting the Listening, Speaking, and Observing Skills of the Examiner

Textbooks in communication disorders and many other clinical professions are full of information about good listening skills, particularly in the diagnostic process and history taking. The examiner should consider the following suggestions that result from this knowledge base:

1. Give instructions several times, slowly if necessary, and speak at a loudness level that is comfortable for the patient. If you are not certain of the comfortable loudness level, ask!

2. Allow time for "visiting" (Newton, 1988) during the assessment, either at the beginning, or interspersed between subtests. Use information gained from informal conversation in the language or speech sample analysis if that is needed in the assessment.

3. Remind the older patient continually of the purpose of each task and the purpose of the assessment in general.

4. Pay very careful attention to your nonverbal behavior, particularly to behaviors that may indicate impatience, boredom, fatigue, or hurriedness and that may cause stress and time pressure for the older patient.

5. Allow for pauses and engage in thoughtful listening when the patient reveals personal information.

6. When the patient exhibits a problem with topic maintenance or discourse organization, provide a written list of items, such as "Things We Are Going to Talk About Now" or "Tasks We Will Do Today," and then check off the items as they are completed.

Jones and Williams (1988) use a task for the assessment of older adults that they designed for training medical students in observation. In questioning the use of standard mental status examinations to examine the very dynamic process of mental functioning, they suggest that more careful observations be made of older adults in clinical Gestalt. They outline observations to make when talking with an older adult. Although some of the items apply to observation of an adult of any age, they are particularly useful when observing an older adult who may not be able to tell the examiner much about his or her personal life or personal history. Jones and Williams suggest observations in the categories of general appearance, grooming, behavior, and language. This observational task adds much valuable information to the assessment and imparts an almost investigative excitement to the assessment. Such excitement can only add to the patient's self-esteem and feeling that the examiner has a genuine interest in accurate history taking.

Meaningful Assessment: What and How to Test

The speech-language assessment has a number of purposes: description of the disorder, if it exists; relation of the disorder to causation; and provision of information for clinical management. Nation and Aram (1984) suggest that the effective diagnostician is able to make periodic "shifts of focus" during the assessment session in order to meet the various purposes of the evaluation.

The examiner must undergo careful preparation to accomplish the multiple purposes of diagnosis. Following are some suggestions for preparation:

- Request reports from other professionals.

- Collect pre-intake questionnaires well before the assessment session.

- Conduct preliminary family interviews before the assessment.

- Structure the patient interview process to make maximum use of available time.

- Become familiar with the patient's environment (home, nursing home, etc.).

- Request that the patient bring family photographs, newspaper clippings, or personal memorabilia to the evaluation in order to collect an optimal speech/language sample.

Such preparation helps the examiner select from all speech and language behaviors those most critical for assessment, based on an analysis of the medical/physical, social, emotional, occupational, and communication background of the patient.

Following is a review of the behaviors that are most commonly assessed in the geriatric patient with a suspected communication disorder.

Speech

Any disorder or disease process affecting the central or peripheral processes for speech programming, initiation, transmission, or production can cause the speech behaviors of voice, resonance, phonetic structure, or prosody to be different or disordered as compared to normal. As discussed in section 3 of this text, one must acknowledge that normative data for all of the speech behaviors of older adults do not exist. However, the chapters in section 3 review the current state of the art in knowledge of speech production and aging, thus giving the examiner clues for important speech behaviors to assess.

In any language assessment, the clinician is likely to evaluate or observe speech behavior that may indicate the presence of dysarthria or apraxia. Kearns and Simmons (1988) review the diagnostic protocol in motor speech disorders, including dysarthria, apraxia, and dysprosody. Any adequate oral motor examination, which will include both oral and verbal movement and possibly a mastication/deglutition evaluation, will quickly reveal the presence of dysarthria, a "speech disorder resulting from damage to neural mechanisms that regulate speech movements" (Netsell, 1984).

Beginning with Darley, Aronson, and Brown in 1969 and extending through the 1980s, many investigators have helped to define the types of dysarthria and corresponding lesions in the nervous system in order to achieve a more refined assessment and differential diagnosis. As a result of their work, investigators with a neurophysiological emphasis began to look at measurements that would provide a baseline and would change if treatment was administered. Rating scales for describing articulatory abilities and overall intelligibility have been developed by Darley, Aronson, and Brown (1975) and Enderby (1983). Instrumental measures of speech production in dysarthria have been reviewed by Rosenbek, McNeil, and Aronson (1984). Figure 18.1 lists important observations to make in the assessment of the dysarthric patient, regardless of the test or protocol used.

Apraxia of speech is described as a "neurogenic phonologic disorder caused by sensorimotor impairment of the capacity to program the positioning of the speech musculature and the sequencing of muscle movements for volitional production of phonemes" (Rosenbek & LaPointe, 1981, p. 160). In the assessment of suspected apraxia of speech or oral apraxia, Rosenbek et al. (1984) suggest that the deficiency pattern be assessed by using a commercially available apraxia test or by supplementing a standard articulation test with various speaking tasks. A test such as the *Apraxia Battery for Adults* (Dabul, 1986) tests for both oral apraxia (impaired nonspeech oral movements) and apraxia of speech. Dabul (1986) suggests that performance load tests be utilized, which include tests of phonetic complexity, speaking rate, utterance length, verbal formulation requirements, and word familiarity. Helm-Estabrooks (1989), in the *Boston Assessment of Severe Aphasia*, includes items for apraxia, including limb apraxia, that are particularly sensitive to the prob-lems of the older, more severely impaired patient.

Language

In the previous chapters in this section of the text, language behaviors that are disordered in the older adult, and the protocols to test those behaviors, give the examiner suggestions for assessing the older adult. Typically, the older adult presents with a question regarding the competency of language behavior, which derives from such causal factors as stroke (most common), traumatic brain injury, suspected dementia of the Alzheimer's type (DAT), and other less frequently occurring lesions or degenerative conditions. Although there is recognition that specific linguistic behaviors will differ depending upon the causal factor of the language disorder, there has been some disagreement among aphasiologists about what to call the communication problems of patients with dementia versus those with stroke-induced aphasia. Today, those who are assessing older adults take a much broader view of aphasia than aphasiologists of the past. There is a realization by speech-language pathologists, neuropsychologists, neurologists, and other professionals interested in the brain-language relationship that

History:
    Subjective complaints and information; particular adjustments patients have made to speaking and/or swallowing

Examination of oral structures and function

Speech production assessment:
    Intelligibility (Yorkston & Beukelman, 1981)
    Perceptual observation of voice and resonance (Wilson & Rice, 1977)
    Standard articulation battery
    Respiratory function for speech
    Acoustic measures (fundamental frequency during isolated speech tasks and conversational stress, frequency perturbation, intensity, rate)
    Aerodynamic measures of oral and nasal airflow
    Observation of vocal fold movement (if indicated)

Dysphagia examination (if indicated by history or examination)

FIGURE 18.1. Areas of examination in dysarthria.

language disturbance can represent a specific lesion in the traditional language areas of the brain, or it can represent a more general cognitive disorder that manifests itself through language. Thus, a general aphasia test, such as the *Western Aphasia Battery* (Kertesz & Poole, 1983), has been used with a traditional (stroke) population, as well as with other language-impaired populations.

Similarly, the *Boston Diagnostic Aphasia Examination* (Goodglass & Kaplan, 1972) has been used with patients with cerebral vascular accidents and traumatic brain injury and has also been used to describe the language of normal older adults (Borod, Goodglass, & Kaplan, 1980) as well as those with DAT (Whitworth & Larson, 1989). Table 18.1 summarizes information about many of the aphasia tests and other procedures used with an older language-impaired population. A problem lies, however, in the dilemma of what to call the different language disorders in order to imply differentiation of their causal factors. Bayles and Kaszniak (1987), in their excellent review of this issue, suggested that we not use the term *aphasia* for the language of dementia unless it truly represents the focal lesion of the more traditional stroke patient.

Newton (1988), in her review of communication disorders in aged adults, and Ulatowska, Cannito, Hayashi, and Fleming (1985) have suggested that several special areas are important in assessment of the older language-disordered patient. Several of these tests, or tasks, have been generated from research with normal older adults or suggested from the behavior of control groups in studies of older adult language.

Sentence comprehension and discourse comprehension are examples of tasks that are sensitive to age and very mild language impairment. Tasks of sentence and discourse production, such as picture description, story retelling, interview questions, and procedural description (Fishman, 1987; Hendricks, 1987; Mitchell, 1987; Ripich & Terrell, 1988; Ulatowska et al., 1985), are sensitive to the possible general cognitive-linguistic decline of aging and, more impor-

tantly, to early or mild language impairment characteristic of lesions affecting language processes. North and Ulatowska (1981), in an investigation of competence in independent living, point out that the quality of procedural and narrative discourse was associated with functioning in more demanding environments and in community activities. These authors suggest that the examiner consider taking a language sample of the older adult, much as our colleagues do in child language assessment. This sample can then be evaluated with the use of a variety of formal systems, including computerized language analysis as well as rating scales of communication behavior.

Psychological Status

Some investigators remind us that whenever we are assessing an older adult with a language disorder, particularly a post-stroke patient, we must remember the potential component of depression of mood (Adams, 1963; Bleuler, 1924; Dunkle & Hooper, 1983; Folstein, Maiberger, & McHugh, 1977; Hooper & Dunkle, 1984; Post, 1961). Any existing depression can affect the amount and quality of language that is exhibited. In addition, existing depression can limit cognitive activity, which will be reflected in a poorer score on an aphasia test. The depression may be directly attributable to central nervous system changes. Robinson and Benson (1981) suggest that depression appears to be common in hospitalized aphasic patients, with nonfluent aphasic patients being the most depressed group, possibly from a disruption of the catecholamine pathways of anterior lesion. On the other hand, there may be a reactive depression component to the life stresses of living with aphasia and the concomitant physical and social changes. Perhaps the greatest adjustment the older aphasic person may have to face is that of a disability that externally resembles dementia. By virtue of their age, the older aphasic patients may be assumed to be demented by those in the social environment who are less familiar with the behaviors of aphasia.

Full assessment of the presence and degree of depression can be made by a mental health professional, preferably one skilled in geriatric assessment. However, the speech-language pathologist may be in the position of needing screening or referral tools to provide information to the psychiatrist, psychologist, or social worker. Traditional tests or scales, such as the *Mini-Mental State Examination* (Folstein, Folstein, & McHugh, 1975), the *Present State Examination* (Luria & McHugh, 1974), the *Zung Self-Rating Depression Scale* (Zung, 1965; Zung & Wonnacott, 1970); and the *Hamilton Depression Scale* (Hamilton, 1960), which screen mood or depression directly or indirectly, are linguistically bound and extremely difficult to administer to a language-impaired population. Some potentially useful items that are being tested with language-impaired adults include the *Nurses' Rating Scale for Depression* (Robinson & Szetela, 1981), the *Visual Analog Mood Scale* (Folstein, Maiberger, & McHugh, 1977), and the *Visual Analog Mood Scale* procedure (Stern & Hooper, 1989). These scales rely on persons close to a patient to rate behavior, or they rely on the patient's ability to point to a picture depicting a mood or emotion. Of course, all of these measures have limitations, but there appears to be great potential in nonlinguistic measures of mood and depression. The ability to screen more effectively for depression will improve the assessment and intervention by the speech-language pathologist as well as that of the mental health professional.

Cognition

In section 2 of this text, "Psychological and Social Aspects of Aging," Schear and Skenes (chapter 4) review the neuropsychological issues important in the brain-behavior assessment of an older patient. If a language disorder is the presenting problem to be assessed, a complete neuropsychological evaluation may not be appropriate or requested. However, knowing the dependence of language on adequate cognitive skills in any communicator, the speech-language pathologist would be remiss in not observing and screening for adequate cognition. Some aphasia tests, such as the *Western Aphasia Battery* (Kertesz & Poole, 1983), include sections intended to screen for cognitive abilities. Other tests, such as the *Boston Diagnostic Aphasia Examination* (Goodglass & Kaplan, 1972), indirectly allow the examiner to observe cognitive behavior through timing of tasks, switching of the item set, and suggestions for examiner "comments" on each subtest. Examiners interested in differentiating causal factors of the language disorder may request a complete neuropsychological examination but also may include some very revealing language tasks, such as Ulatowska's (Ulatowska, Macaluso-Haynes, & North, 1980) procedural discourse sequencing task or Ripich and Terrell's (1988) story retelling task for elements of memory and topic shift. Many examiners who are interested in differentiating the language disorder of dementia from that of classical aphasia recommend the use of pragmatic language tasks or conversational/discourse language tasks to reveal subtle differences in the two disorders, as discussed above.

Assessment with Other Disciplines

The various disciplines represented in the authorship of this text reflect the multidisciplinary requirements for assessment and management of the older patient. Geriatric communication disorders may be exhibited in patients who receive the majority of their care in settings where speech-language pathology services are not regularly available. Thus, our efforts in assessment and management must be understood by other professionals in order for adequate referrals to be sent and received. The authors of this chapter believe that a geriatric assessment team with ongoing case management is the most effective and efficient means of ensuring that multidisciplinary advantages accrue for the geriatric patient with communication

TABLE 18.1
Assessment Procedures Used with Older Adults

Test	Speech/Language Areas Tested	Populations for Which Test Was Designed	Populations for Which Test Has Also Been Used
Boston Diagnostic Aphasia Examination (Goodglass & Kaplan, 1972)	Auditory comp., conversational speech, oral expression, writing, repetition	Adult aphasia	Normal dementia
Language Modalities Test for Aphasia (Wepman & Jones, 1961)	Identifying semantic relationships, imitation, transcoding	Adult aphasia	
Porch Index of Communicative Ability (Porch, 1967)	Formulation, conceptualization, expression, detection of subtle deficits	Adult aphasia, right-hemisphere patients	Dementia
Western Aphasia Battery (Kertesz & Poole, 1983)	Spontaneous speech, auditory comp., repetition, naming, reading, writing, praxis	Adult aphasia; dementia	Nonaphasic brain-damaged adults
Communicative Abilities in Daily Living (Holland, 1980)	Content/form, production and comprehension, cognition, used for adult aphasia, related neurogenic disorders	Dementia	
Neurosensory Center Comprehensive Examination for Aphasia (Spreen & Benton, 1977)	Comprehension, production, verbal memory, reading, writing, speech	Adult aphasia	Motor speech disorders
Minnesota Test for Differential Diagnosis of Aphasia (Schuell, 1965b)	Auditory disturbances, vision and reading, speech and language, visuomotor and writing disturbances, numerical relations	Adult aphasia	Dementia

TABLE 18.1 (continued)

Test	Speech/Language Areas Tested	Populations for Which Test Was Designed	Populations for Which Test Has Also Been Used
Apraxia Battery for Adults (Dabul, 1986)	Diadochokinetic rate, increasing word length, limb and oral apraxia, latency and utterance time for polysyllabic words, repetition, articulation	Adult aphasia	
Boston Naming Test (Kaplan, Goodglass, & Weintraub, 1983)	Word finding, naming	Dementia	
Sklar Aphasia Scale (Sklar, 1973)	Auditory, visual, oral, and graphic deficits	Adult aphasia	
Aphasia Language Performance Scales (Keenan & Brassell, 1975)	Listening, talking, reading, writing	Adult aphasia	
Functional Communication Profile (Groher, 1988; Sarno, 1969)	Movement, speaking, understanding, reading, other informal assessments	Adult aphasia	
Token Test (DeRenzi & Vignolo, 1962)	Mild auditory comprehension deficits	Adult aphasia	
Revised Token Test (McNeil & Prescott, 1978)	Auditory comprehension	Adult aphasia	
Auditory Comprehension Test for Sentences (Shewan, 1979)	Auditory comprehension, vocabulary, syntax	Adult aphasia	
Reading Comprehension Battery for Aphasia (LaPointe & Horner, 1979)	Reading deficits	Adult aphasia	
Reporter's Test (DeRenzi & Ferrari, 1978)	Mild and moderate disorders of verbal expression	Adult aphasia	

TABLE 18.1 (continued)

Test	Speech/Language Areas Tested	Populations for Which Test Was Designed	Populations for Which Test Has Also Been Used
Peabody Picture Vocabulary Test–Revised (Dunn & Dunn, 1981)	Receptive vocabulary	All ages, especially children	Aphasia
Examining for Aphasia (Eisenson, 1954)	Recognition, comprehension, expression	Adult aphasia	
Subjective Communication Report (Felix, 1977)	Informal assessment of communication	Adult aphasia	Adults with communication disorders
Arizona Battery for Communication Disorders of Dementia (Bayles & Kaszniak, 1987)	Reading comprehension, memory, orientation, reasoning, repetition, writing	Dementia	Adult aphasia
New England Pantomime Test (Duffy & Duffy, 1985)	Expressive and receptive language	Fluent and nonfluent aphasic patients	

impairments. Some professions that are crucial to the care of such a patient include psychology, psychiatry, social work nursing, geriatric medicine, neurology, otolaryngology, and family medicine. The various rehabilitation specialties should also be a part of the team, including speech-language pathology, audiology, occupational and physical therapy, rehabilitation counseling, and physiatry.

It is especially critical for rehabilitation professionals to interact with mental health professionals. Often the rehabilitationist is the team member who has an ongoing, frequently long-term, relationship with the patient. Many important behaviors may be revealed to the rehabilitationist, such as evidence of cognitive decline or depression, which may need the intervention of other team members. Even if the speech-language pathologist is not directly managing or treating the patient, he or she may need to provide consultation to the assessment team if the patient's communication disorder makes evaluation by other team members difficult.

Formality and Timing of the Assessment

Those who assess patients in any field often refer to *formal* and *informal* testing. There is sometimes a casual assumption that formal testing is better, or more data-based, than informal testing. However, examiners who use these terms frequently fail to define them, nor do they consistently offer support for their preference for formal testing. For the sake of discussion, the authors will assume that formal testing involves the use of a standard test instrument containing good psychometric data in the areas of the standardization group, reliability, validity, and usefulness of patient management. This type of testing is usually dependent upon a test instrument that is purchased or a test battery adopted from a publication. Similarly, the assumption can be made that an informal test does not rely upon these standards and is instead an observation of the behavior of interest. Both forms of assessment are critical. More than one

examiner has stories of having drawn conclusions about communication skill based upon a formal test, only to discover different behavior upon observation of communication in a more natural or informal context. Some researchers, noting the functional value of informal testing, attempt to make the observations more standard, as in Holland's (1980) *Communicative Abilities in Daily Living* (CADL). New, more functional formal tests of aphasia, such as Helm-Estabrooks's (1969) *Boston Assessment of Severe Aphasia*, are designed from a clinical need to find formal instruments to examine behavior that has been neglected in the past by other instruments.

The timing of assessment in the life of the communicatively disordered patient will affect the behaviors assessed, the instruments used, and the conclusions drawn. The issue of acute versus chronic care, important to the whole geriatric team, is critical to rehabilitation. Patients in acute care settings or in the acute stages of a communication disorder may be more likely to receive a screening assessment or shortened version of another, more lengthy test (see Table 18.1). Speech-language pathologists may visit an acute care patient frequently during the day or week to note changes in behavior that may occur quickly. The older patient is likely to be more severely language impaired in the acute stages than a younger patient and is less likely to make improvements quickly. In contrast, the patient who has passed the acute stage of some event that has caused a language disorder may make changes much less quickly. Age as a prognostic variable in aphasia has always been somewhat problematic and has not always been viewed as critical in investigations of recovery in acute and chronic aphasia (Hooper & Dunkle, 1984).

Role of the Family and Others in Assessment

Sedgwick (1981) defined the family as a group of people who share a sense of history and who engage in goal setting for the group, not just for individuals. In that sense, although "families" may be related individuals, such as sons, daughters, husbands, and wives, they may also be close friends, neighbors, and nursing home roommates. Using Satir's (1967) open system view of families with each unit in interaction with every other unit, a communication disorder affecting one family member affects all family members. DeBranconier (1972) points out that family life is never the same following a disorder such as aphasia, because the family faces the loss of language in one family member. Hooper and Dunkle (1984) describe two common reactions of family members when communicating with the language-impaired member: (a) the initial reaction of the familiar response established by the preexisting relationship between them and (b) the realization that this member cannot communicate as before. This recurring sense of loss must be addressed with the family, if possible, at the time of the initial assessment. The earlier that family education and counseling begin, the less frightened the family will be and the more helpful they can be during the assessment, and later during the management of the patient (Rollin, 1987). It is impossible to predict who might be the most helpful family member at the time of assessment. Therefore, it is important to explore the attitudes of all significant others.

The role of the family during the assessment, in an optimal situation, is that of information source, patient support, and geriatric assessment team member. Since the hallmark of difficulty in language assessment with this patient population is an inability to obtain a good history from the patient directly, the family becomes crucial in this endeavor. Frequently, other professional team members, particularly the social worker, can also provide information about the family relationship and the role that each family member plays within the family system. As will be discussed next, an analysis of the previous and future communication environment requires the contributions of the family. The family member can help administer test items or stimulate the patient to communicate when the clinician has not been successful. Sometimes the family member can do something as simple as watch the face of the patient for emotional clues. Family members who know the patient well can interpret feelings, thoughts, and less than intelligible utterances.

Assessment of the Communication Environment

Lubinski (1981) and Lubinski, Morrison, and Rigordsky (1981) can be credited with creating an enthusiasm for evaluation of the communication environment. Reporting on work in long-term care facilities, in which they interviewed patients using a standard scale, they determined that there is very little spoken communication in a long-term care environment. This investigation primarily concerned patient interaction. There has been little investigation of physical environment variables (size of rooms, traffic flow, furniture arrangement, color choices, etc.) that enhance communication. The literature from audiology and aural rehabilitation suggests adjustments in lighting and in furniture arrangements to improve hearing, but the architectural literature has almost completely neglected communication and the older adult. Lawton, in chapter 7 of this text, reviews relevant issues regarding the communication environment of the elderly.

In her *Environmental Language Inventory*, Lubinski (1981) begins with a nonstandardized observation tool that assesses communicative opportunities and barriers to communication. She considers both external and internal factors as well as human and physical environmental factors in this profile. From the profile the clinician can operationally plan environmental treatment in the patient's home, a nursing home, or other institutions, such as a senior citizens' center. Lubinski reminds us that studies of the effectiveness of environmental intervention are lacking and may provide important information for treatment. This point seems particularly crucial with older patients, who may be affected by nonlinguistic changes in their environment as much as or more than linguistic changes.

Barriers to Efficient Assessment

Biological Changes in the Aged

As the authors in section 1 of this text point out in several chapters, even normal older adults may experience sensory and motor control problems that can affect speech, language, and hearing. These changes may directly affect one of the communication processes, such as changes in hearing acuity, or they may indirectly affect communication—for example, by changes in vision that restrict access to the environment. When these normal sensory and motor changes are added to a more severe speech, language, or hearing disorder, the older adult may be quite difficult to assess. The process of transferring information into or out of the system through sensory-motor channels in order to proceed with history taking, counseling, and test administration may be fraught with problems.

Psychosocial Changes in the Aged

Section 2 of this text deals with many psychological and social aspects of aging, some of which may serve as barriers to assessment. A fear of being labeled may inhibit some older adults from visiting a setting (such as a hospital or community clinic) with communication disorder services. Once there, the patient may be reluctant to provide historical information or admit the full extent or impact of the communicative problem through the same fear of being labeled. Older adults who are depressed or feeling a lack of control may not be willing to concentrate on an assessment battery. Anger or uncooperativeness may be exhibited as a way of gaining control in a frightening or unfamiliar situation. Following instructions or answering questions from a much younger clinician may seem ridiculous to the patient if the task is not clearly explained and well understood. The relative

usefulness of "naming as many animals as you can" (Goodglass & Kaplan, 1972) may escape the average older adult.

Shortcomings in the Test or Assessment Task

Many shortcomings in the tests or assessment tasks administered to older adults relate directly to the physical changes associated with aging as well as to the communication disorders that may affect older adults. Visual test items may not be easy to see or may not be legible if they are in written form. Auditory items, taped or live, may not be loud enough. Objects may be small and hard to grasp. Other shortcomings in test items may be their seeming inability to relate to the subject's current communication needs. Clinicians giving a complete speech or language battery, such as those in several of the current aphasia tests, may need to explain to the older adult why some apparently irrelevant items are being administered. The greatest shortcoming of assessment items at the current time is the limited normative data on normal older comparison groups. An examination of Table 18.1 reveals many of the tests and procedures used with adults. Few of the tests listed have normative data available to compare the patient of interest with his or her own disorder group or with normal older adults in the patient's age cohort.

Shortcomings in the Test Environment

For most people there is a time period, usually from age 5 until late adolescence, where the teacher/pupil dyad is a normal phenomenon and each part of the dyad knows the role to play. For some adults, formal academic learning may be a lifetime endeavor, including college, local extension courses, job continuing education, or community college coursework. But for most persons, particularly those in lower socioeconomic groups, the teacher/pupil dyad of information presentation, response, and testing is a long-forgotten role; for these people, a test situation can be anxiety producing and even insulting. In addition to the unfamiliarity of the test situation, the test surroundings themselves may be quite unfamiliar and anxiety-producing. The clinical settings where services are provided may invoke fears of death or disability. Because of these fears and associated anxieties, the setting may not lend itself to collecting a valid sample of speech and language behavior (Hendricks, 1987; Mitchell, 1987); the conversation of the patient therefore may not be typical of his or her discourse at home. Professions involved in home health care have long recognized the increased value of testing in the patient's own familiar environment.

In either the clinical setting or the patient's own home, some shortcomings in the environment may be related to the patient's sensory and motor changes. Illumination may be inadequate for good vision or good communication. Room acoustics may be poor and background noise may be distracting. In the clinic, the area used for the assessment may require so much walking or travel that the patient is exhausted before the assessment begins, and difficulties in parking and finding the clinic also can tax the elderly patient.

The Clinician's Understanding of Aging

The effective clinician will have an understanding of both the process of aging and the speech or language disorder of the older adult in order to provide an adequate assessment and plan for management of the patient. Unfortunately, many currently employed speech-language pathologists do not have any formal classroom background in geriatrics or gerontology (Shadden, 1984). They, like the population in general, may have beliefs and attitudes about older adults that are ageist (Kogan, 1979). On the other hand, Shadden (1988), describing a project in which she interviewed older persons and professionals providing services to those individuals, found that health professionals had a positive response bias against any question that implied a negative view of the elderly. Her concern was that the professional, in an attempt to avoid age-

ism, may be avoiding the difficult realities of aging. A compromise in belief systems could be reached with more information about the current situation of older adults in society today, particularly those in a health care crisis.

In addition to an understanding of aging in today's society, the effective clinician would do well to understand the process of the clinical relationship. The behaviors exhibited by the older adult and the clinician may continue to support a dependency that may not assist the patient in controlling his or her own health care management. Communication behaviors of both the speaker and the listener, which are unique when there is a young-old combination, may lead to a communication environment in which there is poor social and/or therapeutic interaction (Shadden, 1988).

The focus of this section has been to draw attention to the adjustments necessary for valid and clinically useful assessment of communicative disorders in the elderly patient. It is essential that clinicians serving this population recognize the need for the development of specialized approaches and skills. In the next section of this chapter, issues and decision making with regard to speech-language rehabilitation in the geriatric population will be considered.

Concepts of Management and Therapy

The issue of management versus therapy has been addressed in a number of recent publications (Nation, 1982). *Management* refers to all of the clinical decisions made about a patient by a clinician, including the obvious decisions made about the type, frequency, duration, and content of therapy. A number of the decisions proposed by Nation (1982) are outlined in Figure 18.2. Review of this figure makes it clear that the concept of management extends far beyond the decision as to whether or not to treat a patient. It includes all of the collective think-

1. Can the speech and language disorder be changed?

2. Can the speech and language symptoms be changed?

3. How will the causal factors be managed?

4. Can the client change his or her disordered speech and language behavior?

5. Are speech and language therapy needed to change the disorder?

6. What treatment plan would have to be designed?

7. What effect would treatment have on the disorder?

8. How successful would treatment be?

9. Are referrals necessary for management of the disorder?

10. What other professional agencies and services might be required?

11. What adjunct therapies would be required?

12. Are the required services available?

13. Does the client complex desire the treatment?

14. Can the client complex implement the recommendations?

15. What role is expected of the client complex in the management plan?

FIGURE 18.2. Management decisions proposed by Nation (1982). *Note.* Adapted from "Management of Speech and Language Disorders," by J. E. Nation, in *Speech, Language, and Hearing: Pathologies of Speech and Language* (pp. 461–476) by N. Lass, L. McReynolds, J. Northern, and D. Yoder (Eds.), 1982, Philadelphia: W. B. Saunders. Adapted by permission of the author.

ing about a specific patient's needs and focuses on the environment in which the patient operates (and, most importantly, communicates). *Therapy* refers to the application of specific techniques for the benefit of improved communication. Management decisions guide therapy.

Our clinical work with the elderly communicatively disordered patient, if it is done well, makes good use of these types of decisions. For many of these patients our decisions about what to include or not include in treatment may be the last in a series of deliberations that include the patient's physical environment, psychological make-up, and social environment. We are being short-sighted when we fail to consider all of these other variables before beginning "treatment" with a patient.

In the remainder of this chapter we will consider the variables that are important in the management of the speech and language problems of the elderly adult within

a decision-making framework. Rather than deal with the specific characteristics of disorders and their management, we will review the process of clinical decision making with the elderly patient.

Patient Management Decisions

Our interactions with elderly patients, their families, and their health care providers supply us with a rich body of information that serves as the database for the decisions we need to make as we approach the management of their communicative disorders. This information comes to us from a variety of contexts and persons and it is our responsibility to evaluate the relevance of each piece of information to the patient's current communicative needs.

Sources of Information for Decision Making

When a patient comes to us for assistance, two major information sets are available to us for making decisions about subsequent management. The first set of information, which we refer to as *patient-specific data,* includes all of the information from the patient's life history—medical, social, and psychological—that affects his or her current communicative needs and problems. Most valuable, of course, are the results of the diagnostic assessment of speech and language, which provides us with a description of the patient's current communicative strengths and difficulties, considers causation, and quantifies and qualifies the degree of impairment. The second information set we use in intervention decision making is the information from the discipline of speech-language pathology that tells us what to expect (or not expect) and what to do when an individual with a particular diagnosis and particular causative factors presents with specific communicative symptoms. This second information set is referred to as *discipline-specific data.* Decision making in speech-language pathology reflects the constant use of data from both of these sets. The clinician must constantly weigh information provided by the patient, the family, the physician, and the clinician's own behavioral observations against the information available from the discipline. Incomplete knowledge in either data set increases the likelihood of error in decision making. Figures 18.3 and 18.4 summarize the types of information included in each data set, respectively.

Patient-Specific Data for Decision Making

The patients who come to us for assistance are unique in many ways. If this were not so, we would have a much easier task. We could merely consider their diagnosis and this would automatically lead to an appro-

I. Historical Data
Age
Cultural variables
Marital status
Family variables
Vocational/educational histories
Current living situation
Psychological history
Typical daily activities

II. Medical Data
Current medical diagnoses
Medical history
Summary of recent hospitalizations and surgeries
Medications
Physical and sensory limitations
Current rehabilitation therapies
Mental health status

III. Speech and Language Data
Speech and language diagnosis
Duration
Severity
Specific symptoms: speech, language, behavioral
Results of previous therapies
Current communicative needs
Patient's motivation for communication

FIGURE 18.3. Patient-specific data for decision making.

priate treatment strategy. However, the elderly patients we see for clinical services bring a lifetime of experiences and backgrounds, as well as a myriad of complex medical problems, that must be considered as we make plans for clinical intervention. Although the importance of emphasizing the unique backgrounds and interests of our patients in management and treatment decision making cannot be overemphasized, it is useful to consider three general types of variables as we approach patient decision making in speech-language pathology: historical data, medical data, and speech and language data.

Historical Data

The uniqueness of each patient is highlighted as we consider the historical variables, especially those contributing to the

I. Diagnosis

Is it treatable?

What are the limitations of treatment?

Is this a degenerative condition?

How successful have various speech and language treatments been when this diagnosis is present?

Are there contraindications for treatment?

II. Prognosis

What is the prognosis given the patient's age, physical limitations, family support system, current medical status, living arrangements, etc.?

III. Intervention

What are the treatments available to the patient?

Have these treatments been tested on other patients?

What is the rate of success of previously tried therapies?

How will the family be included in the treatment program?

Are there technological supports that would be helpful to the patient?

FIGURE 18.4. Discipline-specific data for decision making.

patient's current and premorbid communicative abilities. Cultural background, family situation, vocational and educational background, current living situation, interests and hobbies, and schedule of daily activities all help us to understand the patient's current needs for communication. Every experienced clinician knows that it is these variables that ultimately provide the backdrop for functionally oriented treatment activities. As we proceed to make decisions about management and treatment, a broad understanding of these factors helps us to understand what the patient will need to communicate in the future and with whom, and what topics may be of vital interest to the patient.

A number of clinical tools have become available for collecting data and for considering historical factors in planning intervention. Chapey (1986) has developed a comprehensive set of forms for collecting relevant social and communicative information from language-impaired adults and

their families. Additionally, Ostruni and Santo Pietro (1986) report on the use of a set of "Life Review Diary" forms (Holland, 1984) for the purpose of gathering historical information with demented elderly patients. For some patients, this approach may be less threatening than traditional interview and questionnaire formats. Written forms such as these assist us in organizing the wealth of information about the patient's communicative history and future needs. In addition to the use of questionnaires for data collection regarding the social, psychological, family, and communication styles and interests of the patient, there are a variety of interview and observation formats that have been proposed for use in interaction with elderly patients.

Lubinski (1981) reported on a model specifically focused on assessing the communicative environment and the factors that affect communication, especially in the institutional settings where many elderly communicatively disordered patients reside. While these tools were developed for purposes other than specific history taking by the clinician, experience suggests that they can be a valuable resource for collecting and organizing information about the patient's background, interests, and needs for communication.

Medical History

The patient's medical history and current medical diagnoses are essential to the clinician engaged in patient management decision making about the elderly individual. This information, which usually is collected from the patient's medical record, the primary physician, and the various medical specialists caring for the patient, is most useful in understanding many of the patient's presenting problems and also in planning intervention. It is important for the speech-language pathologist to understand the patient's medical condition and the implications of this condition for participation in treatment activities. Factors of special importance include knowledge of recent hospitalizations and surgeries, current medications, general physical condition, hearing and vision problems, and other therapies (e.g. physical, psychological, and occupational) in which the patient is currently engaged.

Knowledge of recent hospitalizations and surgeries, essential for the diagnostic decision maker, is also important for the individual who provides subsequent patient management. Frequently, information obtained during the hospital stay provides valuable insights into the individual's current condition as well as the prognosis for improvement and recovery from an existing medical problem. The speech-language pathologist must also be cognizant of the medications being taken by the patient and the effects of these medicines. Finally, information obtained from neuropsychology, psychiatry, audiology, neurology, and other disciplines can all be useful in planning treatment.

Speech and Language Data

The patient's speech and language diagnosis is the most obvious piece of information of importance to the decision maker. If the clinician responsible for treatment/management decision making is not the original diagnostician, it is essential to understand the process by which the diagnosis was made, when it was made, and by whom. The diagnostic statement usually indicates the type of communicative impairment and may reflect one of a number of classification systems in use within speech-language pathology. The diagnosis may be quite general ("Patient has aphasia") or highly specific ("Patient exhibits a moderately severe Broca's aphasia with an accompanying apraxia of speech").

Once the speech-language diagnosis has been obtained, a variety of specific questions related to the condition are of interest. First, the duration of the condition must be established. Experienced aphasiologists are well aware that many neurogenic language disturbances change over time. If there is a significant time lapse between the original assessment and the present contact with

the patient, it may be necessary to reassess to determine if the patient's diagnostic picture has changed. Excellent reviews of the evolution of language disturbance in aphasia (Pashek & Holland, 1988; Kertesz & McCabe, 1977) and dementia (Bayles & Kaszniak, 1987) are found in the literature. Information about the severity of the patient's communication disturbance is essential. The issue of measurement of the severity of specific communication disorders is usually subjective and, again, the clinician decision maker must look at the data that support the reported level of severity. The issue of determination of severity can be quite complicated in the elderly patient. Because severity is a relative descriptor, the question becomes, "What is the comparison group for determination of severity?" or "What is the standard for measuring severity?" A few standard measures such as the *Boston Diagnostic Aphasia Examination* (Goodglass & Kaplan, 1972), *Porch Index of Communicative Ability* (Porch, 1967), and *Boston Assessment of Severe Aphasia* (Helm-Estabrooks, 1989) are standardized on patients of various ages and therefore allow for comparisons with other aged persons. Other tools such as the *CADL* (Holland, 1980) and the *Functional Communication Profile* (Sarno, 1969) indicate severity based on the degree of functional communication impairment. Regardless of the tool or approach used for establishing severity, the clinician planning rehabilitation should be familiar with the methodology used to establish severity as provided by the referring clinician. This piece of information will serve as one way to measure progress in therapy.

The specific communicative and behavioral symptoms exhibited by the patient are of great concern to the clinical decision maker. In most cases it is these specific symptoms that will be addressed in the course of treatment. Thus, an exact inventory of the speech and language behaviors of the patient is essential for planning treatment and decision making. Reviews of possible characteristic behaviors of various disorders known to be seen in elderly patients can be found in earlier chapters of this text and in a variety of articles, book chapters, and textbooks on communicative disorders in aging.

The results obtained from previous therapies make up another important variable to be used in considering patient management. The decision maker is interested in the way in which the patient has responded to treatment previously and, most important, in the differential effects of various types of treatments.

The current communicative needs of the patient and his or her current level of communication motivation and interest are key factors used in determining the patient's candidacy for treatment, as well as providing indications of what should be included in the treatment protocol. This issue is at the heart of communication management with the elderly. Good clinical management dictates that what we provide for the patient is therapy directed at meeting her or his communicative needs. Regardless of the type of disorder exhibited, it is essential that we be able to identify each patient's communicative goals.

Discipline-Specific Data for Management Decision Making

The data available to assist in patient decision making are immense. In the previous section of this chapter a data set was proposed for considering patient-specific information in clinical management decision making with the elderly. A vast, ever-changing body of literature is available to us for consideration. The clinician who is well prepared for managing the older patient with a communicative disorder will also be well versed in the specific information of adult speech-language pathology as well as having relevant information from other fields with an interest in speech-language communication behaviors. In the actual decision-making process, the available individual patient data must be juxtaposed against the relevant information from

the discipline. It is this process that brings the unique characteristics of the patient into the reality of the clinical world.

As revealed in Figure 18.4, there are three broad areas to be considered for inclusion as we consider the data from speech-language pathology in decision making with elderly patients. These are diagnosis, prognosis, and available treatments.

Diagnosis

In the previous section we were concerned with the diagnostic label applied to the patient. We will now discuss the implications of that diagnosis for subsequent management. As noted previously, there are two sets of diagnostic information typically available to the clinician engaged in management and treatment of the adult patient with a communicative disorder—the medical diagnosis and the communicative diagnosis. Medical diagnoses, provided by the patient's physician, and communicative diagnoses, provided by the speech-language pathologist, suggest many implications for management. The scientific literature, case studies, and the clinician's own clinical experience provide the framework for making determinations about the relevance of the specific diagnosis to treatment and management. In Figure 18.4, a series of questions is proposed relevant to the patient's diagnosis. The answers to these questions form the data set for planning treatment.

First and foremost, we need to know whether or not a specific diagnostic condition is treatable for a patient with given historical, psychological, and biological factors. That is, what do the literature and our previous experience with similar types of patients tell us about the potential benefits of investing clinical personnel and resources? For most clinical conditions, a growing body of literature demonstrates that for the majority of elderly patients, certain benefits can be obtained from our efforts. As new treatments and technologies become available, the likelihood is increased that we can be of help to even more patients. New intervention strategies for patients who were previously thought to be poor candidates for speech-language rehabilitation have become available in recent years. For example, Helm-Estabrooks, Fitzpatrick, and Baresi (1982) have provided a variety of treatment regimens for patients with global aphasia and have demonstrated that a significant number of these patients make measurable gains with treatment, a finding that challenges the work of a number of early investigators who used more traditional stimulation approaches (Sarno, Silverman, & Sands, 1970; Schuell, 1965a). In a similar vein, the rapid expansion in the number and types of augmentative communication systems and devices has provided a variety of communication options for patients of all ages, including the elderly, with severe speech production disorders. Even those patients with degenerative conditions, such as the irreversible dementias, are now considered as potential treatment candidates early in their illness when compensatory strategies can be introduced to assist them in using available strengths to maintain communication (Bayles & Kaszniak, 1987; Ostruni & Santo Pietro, 1986).

Prognosis

It must be remembered that not every patient can be helped. Before initiating treatment, the potential benefit given a specific diagnosis must be considered. Although a variety of treatment options may be available for most conditions affecting speech and language, the individual characteristics of the patient, along with the specific diagnosis, determine the degree of benefit that can be expected. Even though the professional literature may suggest that a given patient can benefit from treatment, the decision maker must take into account the host of variables (age, sensory loss, fatigueability, living arrangements, family support system, etc.) that may contribute to the degree of improvement expected. For example, most of the newly developed treatment programs for demented patients

are focused on altered communicative input from caregivers, manipulation of the environment, and stimulus reduction. Although a given patient whose diagnosis would indicate potential benefit from a carefully designed intervention program may be available for treatment, it is obvious that without considerable support from others in the communicative environment there is little hope for improvement. Thus, the clinician who is making decisions about patient management must formulate a reasonable prognosis for improvement based on the patient's diagnosis and the individual factors known to be contributory to that patient's improvement.

Available Treatments

As noted above, a variety of treatments are currently available for the elderly patient with communicative impairment. Unfortunately, only a few of these treatments have been subjected to the careful scrutiny of applied researchers within the field. The question "Do patients with diagnosis X benefit from speech and language rehabilitation?" is considerably different from "Which is the best treatment for patient X?" The majority of research in the field of adult speech and language disorders has been devoted to the potential benefits of rehabilitation for a given group of patients, usually based on diagnosis. Although descriptions of various treatment methodologies abound, only a few have been subjected to carefully controlled experimental or quasi-experimental design. While this approach is exciting in that it offers the clinician valuable information about the benefits of treatment, the issue of selecting the most appropriate treatment for a given patient remains clouded.

The clinician who is planning treatment has a number of resources available for selecting and reviewing available treatments for a given speech- and language-disordered patient: (a) review of the results of large-group studies; (b) review of single-subject investigations; (c) review of current texts and commercially produced treatment programs; and (d) attendance at seminars, workshops, and scientific meetings.

Review of Group Studies

As noted earlier, a number of large-group studies have been completed that attempt to document the efficacy of treatment. The purpose of these investigations has not been to evaluate specific treatments, but rather to determine the benefit of treatment for a large group of carefully selected subjects. For the most part, the content of the treatment has not been well controlled in these investigations. This is understandable; the variables that make up "treatment" are numerous and many are impossible to control in a large research project. Despite the lack of specific treatment details, careful review of these research articles will provide some valuable information for the decision maker's clinical database. For reviews of clinical group design research, the reader is referred to Rosenbek et al. (1984) and Chapey (1986).

Single-Subject Studies

The single-subject methodology is now widely used in speech-language pathology because of its value in studying the effects of a specific treatment on a given individual (Hegde, 1987). Rather than examining comparisons between groups of subjects, decision makers use the single-subject method to consider an individual's response under treatment and no-treatment conditions. When more than one subject is included in a study of a given treatment, the results are not statistically compared; instead, each subject's results are considered separately.

The value of reviewing the results of single-subject studies cannot be overstated. These reports provide the practitioner with precise information about the specific communicative characteristics of the subject, the specific treatments that were employed, and the treatment conditions that produced positive or negative results. The clinician planning therapy has the opportunity to repeat the investigation with his or her own patient and compare results. Excellent examples of the clinical application of the single-subject methodology are found in Robert C. Marshall's text, *Case Studies in Aphasia Rehabilitation* (1986).

The primary limitation in using the results of single-subject studies in treatment of our own patients is obvious—our patient may differ in some significant way from the patient presented in the research report. In general, however, the skilled clinician can glean much helpful information from examination and subsequent replication of methodologies proposed in single-subject research.

Published Texts and Commercially Produced Treatment Programs

An abundance of therapy guides, workbooks, computer software programs, treatment "kits," and textbooks are available to the clinician. In recent years, many of these resources have been specifically designed for use with adults with communicative disorders. It is beyond the scope of this chapter to review these materials, but a few general comments are in order.

Textbooks that review and synthesize the plethora of information about various approaches to managing communication disorders in the elderly can be very helpful to the practicing speech-language pathologist. These books provide the clinician with the benefit of an author's painstaking review of the body of literature on a given clinical condition or topic. Although every clinician specializing in work with the elderly should continually review the information provided in journal articles, the overview and synthesis provided by reviews of major texts is most helpful for those delivering services, especially the new or inexperienced clinician.

Recently, a variety of specific treatment programs and materials for elderly communicatively impaired patients have become available. These materials offer major benefits to the practitioner, but also offer potential risks. The advantages are obvious. Neatly packaged, attractive, and usually well designed, they are geared to the interest level of the elderly patient. When these materials are carefully chosen and appropriately applied, they can be invaluable tools for the busy clinician. Thankfully, most practitioners no longer have to spend hours preparing stimuli to be used in treatment. The risks, however, though somewhat less obvious, must also be considered. Few of the commercially packaged treatment programs have been subjected to scientific evaluation. Clinicians who are making decisions about treatment are obligated to carefully review the content of published treatment programs to be sure that the approach used is consistent with the needs of the patient. Workbooks, treatment kits, and computer software should be used to enhance the treatment session and overall management program. Their successful utilization is dependent on the capabilities of the thoughtful decision maker in developing a theoretically sound treatment approach and then selecting materials that fit the program. In general, clinicians should be wary of published approaches that promise to be the "answer" to the patient's overall communicative needs.

It should be mentioned that materials new to the market are reviewed on a regular basis in professional journals. These reviews can be helpful in making decisions about which items to purchase. In any case, each clinician should carefully review commercially available materials and programs before deciding to use them with a given patient.

Seminars, Workshops, and Conventions

The practicing clinician is obligated to continue her or his education by participating in professional development activities. A variety of programs are available to clinicians who wish to expand their fund of knowledge about clinical issues for dealing with the elderly patient; professional journals provide regular announcements of upcoming programs.

Conclusions

This chapter has been directed toward discussion of the special clinical adjustments and decisions that are typically required in order to provide appropriate services to the elderly patient with a communicative disorder. First, some of the considerations and adaptations that should be made in the diagnostic process were presented. Attention was given to the specific physical, technical, and attitudinal barriers to valid and appropriate assessment. Next, patient management was examined from a decision-making perspective. Patient-specific and discipline-specific data of value to the clinical decision maker were reviewed. The authors have focused on the role of the family and other caregivers in the environment as appropriate extenders of the clinician's service delivery system. Finally, the resources available to the clinician for enhancement of service delivery were considered.

References

Adams, G. F. (1963). Mental barriers to recovery from strokes. *Lancet, 2,* 533–537.

Bayles, K., & Kaszniak, A. (1987). *Communication and cognition in normal aging and dementia.* Austin, TX: PRO-ED.

Bleuler, E. (1924). *Textbook of psychiatry.* New York: Macmillan.

Borod, J. C., Goodglass, H., & Kaplan, E. (1980). Normative data on the Boston Diagnostic Aphasic Examination. *Journal of Clinical Neuropsychology, 2,* 209–215.

Brody, S. J. (1974). Long-term care in the community. In E. M. Brody (Ed.), *Social work guide for long-term care facilities.* Washington, DC: U.S. Government Printing Office, National Institute of Mental Health.

Chapey, R. (1986). The assessment of language disorders in adults. In R. Chapey (Ed.), *Language intervention strategies in adult aphasia* (2nd ed., pp. 81–140). Baltimore, MD: Williams & Wilkins.

Council of Home Health Agencies and Community Health Services, National League for Nursing. (1981). In C. C. Pegels (Ed.), *Health care and the elderly.* Rockville, MD: Aspen.

Dabul, B. L. (1986). *Apraxia Battery for Adults.* Tigard, OR: C. C. Publications.

Darley, F., Aronson, A. E., & Brown, J. (1969). Differential diagnostic patterns of dysarthria. *Journal of Speech and Hearing Research*, 12, 462–496.

Darley, F., Aronson, A., & Brown, J. (1975). *Motor speech disorders*. Philadelphia: Saunders.

DeBranconier, L. (1972). Emotional problems in the aphasic and his environment. *Logopaedie en Foniatrie*, 44, 237–242.

DeRenzi, E., & Ferrari, C. (1978). The Reporter's Test: A sensitive test to detect expressive disturbances in aphasics. *Cortex*, 14, 279–293.

DeRenzi, E., & Vignolo, L. (1962). The Token Test: A sensitive test to detect receptive disturbances in aphasics. *Brain*, 85, 665–678.

Duffy, R. J., & Duffy, J. R. (1985). *The New England Pantomime Tests*. Austin, TX: PRO-ED.

Dunkle, R. E., & Hooper, C. R. (1983). Using language to help depressed elderly aphasic persons. *Social Casework*, 64, 539–545.

Dunn, L. M., & Dunn, L. M. (1981). *Peabody Picture Vocabulary Test–Revised*. Minneapolis: American Guidance Service.

Eisenson, J. (1954). *Examination for aphasia*. New York: Psychological Corporation.

Enderby, P. M. (1983). *The Frenchay Dysarthria Assessment*. Austin, TX: PRO-ED.

Felix, N. (1977). *Subjective Communication Report*. Puyallup, WS: Good Samaritan Hospital.

Fishman, S. L. (1987). *Patterns of procedural discourse in persons with senile dementia of the Alzheimer's type*. Unpublished thesis, University of Kansas, Lawrence, KS.

Folstein, M. F., Folstein, S. E., & McHugh, P. R. (1975). Mini-Mental State: A practical method for grading the cognitive state of patients for the clinician. *Journal of Psychiatric Research*, 12, 189–198.

Folstein, M. F., Maiberger, R., & McHugh, P. (1977). Mood disorder as a specific complication of stroke. *Journal of Neurology, Neurosurgery, and Psychiatry*, 40, 1018–1020.

Goodglass, H., & Kaplan, E. (1972). *The assessment of aphasia and related disorders*. Philadelphia: Lea & Febiger.

Groher, M. E. (1988). Modifications in speech-language assessment procedures for the older adult. In B. Shadden (Ed.), *Communication behavior and aging: A source book for clinicians* (pp. 248–260). Baltimore, MD: Williams & Wilkins.

Hamilton, M. (1960). A rating scale for depression. *Journal of Neurology, Neurosurgery, and Psychiatry*, 23, 56–62.

Hegde, M. N. (1987). *Clinical research in communication disorders: Principles and strategies*. Austin, TX: PRO-ED.

Helm-Estabrooks, N. (1989). *Boston Assessment of Severe Aphasia*. San Antonio, TX: Special Press.

Helm-Estabrooks, N., Fitzpatrick, P. M., & Baresi, B. (1982). Visual action therapy for global aphasia. *Journal of Speech and Hearing Disorders*, 47, 385–389.

Hendricks, J. L. (1987). *Narrative story retelling in dementia*. Unpublished thesis. University of Kansas, Lawrence, KS.

Holland, A. L. (1980). *Communicative Abilities in Daily Living*. Baltimore, MD: University Park Press.

Holland L. (1984). *Reality oriented communication training for senile dementia patients* (Doctoral dissertation). Ann Arbor, MI: University Microfilms.

Hooper, C. R., & Dunkle, R. E. (1984). *The older aphasic person: Strategies in treatment and diagnosis*. Rockville, MD: Aspen.

Jones, T. V., & Williams, M. E. (1988). Rethinking the approach to evaluating mental functioning of older persons. *Journal of the American Geriatric Society*, 36, 1128–1134.

Kaplan, E., Goodglass, H., & Weintraub, S. (1983). *Boston Naming Test*. Philadelphia: Lea & Febiger.

Kearns, K. P., & Simmons, N. N. (1988). Motor speech disorders: The dysarthrias and apraxia of speech. In N. Lass, L. McReynolds, J. Northern, & D. Yoder (Eds.), *Handbook of speech-language pathology and audiology*. Philadelphia: B. C. Decker.

Keenan, J. S., & Brassell, E. G. (1975). *Aphasia Language Performance Scales*. Murphreesboro, TN: Pinnacle Press.

Kertesz, A., & McCabe, P. (1977). Recovery patterns and prognosis in Aphasia. *Brain*, 100, 1–18.

Kertesz, A., & Poole, E. (1983). *Western Aphasia Battery*. New York: Grune & Stratton.

Kogan, N. (1979). Beliefs, attitudes, and stereotypes about old people: A new look at some old issues. *Research in Aging*, 1, 11–36.

LaPointe, L., & Horner, J. (1979). *Reading Comprehension Battery for Aphasia*. Austin, TX: PRO-ED.

Lubinski, R., (1981). Environmental language intervention. In R. Chapey (Ed.), *Language intervention strategies in adult aphasia* (pp. 223–248). Baltimore, MD: Williams & Wilkins.

Lubinski, R., Morrison, E. B., & Rigordsky, S. (1981). Perception of spoken communication by elderly patients in an institutional setting. *Journal of Speech and Hearing Disorders, 46,* 405–412.

Luria, R., & McHugh, P. R. (1974). The reliability and clinical utility of the present state examination. *Archives of General Psychiatry, 30,* 866–875.

Marshall, R. C. (1986). *Case studies in aphasia rehabilitation.* Austin, TX: PRO-ED.

McNeil, M. R. (1984). Current concepts in adult aphasia. *International Rehabilitation Medicine, 6,* 128–134.

McNeil, M. R., & Prescott, T. E. (1978). *Revised Token Test.* Austin, TX: PRO-ED.

Mitchell, M. E. W. (1987). *Communication acts in the language of dementia.* Unpublished thesis. University of Kansas, Lawrence, KS.

Nation, J. E. (1982). Management of speech and language disorders. In N. Lass, L. McReynolds, J. Northern, & D. Yader (Eds.), *Speech, language, and hearing: Pathologies of speech and language* (pp. 461–476). Philadelphia: Saunders.

Nation, J. E., & Aram, D. M. (1984). *Diagnosis of speech and language disorders* (2nd ed.). San Diego, CA: College Hill Press.

Netsell, R. (1984). A neurobiologic view of the dysarthrias. In M. R. McNeil, J. C. Rosenbek, & A. E. Aronson (Eds.), *The dysarthrias.* San Diego, CA: College Hill Press.

Newton, M. (1988). Communication disorders in the aging. In Lass, N. J., et al. (Eds.), *Handbook of speech language pathology and audiology.* Philadelphia: B. C. Decker.

North, A., & Ulatowska, H. (1981). Competence in independently living older adults: Assessment and correlates. *Journal of Gerontology, 36,* 576–582.

Ostruni, E., & Santo Pietro, M. J. (1986). *Getting through: Communicating when someone you care for has Alzheimer's disease.* Princeton, NJ: Speech Bin.

Pashek, G. V., & Holland, A. L. (1988). Evolution of aphasia in the first year post-onset. *Cortex, 24,* 411–423.

Pegels, C. C. (1981). *Health care and the elderly.* Rockville, MD: Aspen.

Porch, B. E. (1967). *Porch Index of Communicative Ability: Vol. I. Theory and development.* Palo Alto, CA: Consulting Psychologists Press.

Post, F. (1961). *The significance of effective symptoms in old age: A follow-up of 100 patients.* Unpub-lished M.D. thesis, University of London, England.

Ripich, D. N., & Terrell, B. Y. (1988). Patterns of discourse cohesion and coherence in Alzheimer's disease. *Journal of Speech and Hearing Disorders, 53,* 8–15.

Robinson, R. G., & Benson, D. F. (1981). Depression in aphasic patients: Frequency, severity, and clinical-pathological correlations. *Brain and Language, 14,* 282–291.

Robinson, R. G., & Szetela, B. (1981). Mood changes following left hemisphere brain injury. *Annals of Neurology, 9,* 447–453.

Rollin, W. J. (1987). *The psychology of communication disorders in individuals and their families.* Englewood Cliffs, NJ: Prentice-Hall.

Rosenbek, J. C., & LaPointe, L. L. (1981). Motor speech disorders and the aging process. In D. S. Beasley & G. A. Davis (Eds.), *Aging: Communication processes and disorders* (pp. 159–174). New York: Grune & Stratton.

Rosenbek, J. C., McNeil, M. R., & Aronson, A. E. (Eds.). (1984). *Apraxia of speech.* San Diego, CA: College Hill Press.

Sarno, M. T. (1969). *The Functional Communication Profile: Manual of directions* (Rehabilitation Monograph No. 42). New York: New York University Medical Center, Institute of Rehabilitation Medicine.

Sarno, M. T., Silverman, M., & Sands, E. (1970). Speech therapy and language recovery in severe aphasia. *Journal of Speech and Hearing Research, 13,* 607–623.

Satir, V. (1967). *Conjoint family therapy.* Palo Alto, CA: Science and Behavior Books.

Schuell, H. (1965a). *Differential diagnosis of aphasia with the Minnesota Test.* Minneapolis: University of Minnesota Press.

Schuell, H. (1965b). *Minnesota Test for the Differential Diagnosis of Aphasia.* Minneapolis: University of Minnesota Press.

Sedgwick, R. (1981). *Family mental health: Theory and practice.* St. Louis, MO: Mosby.

Shadden, B. (1984). Administrative considerations in implementation of service delivery models. In L. Jacobs-Condit (Ed.), *Gerontology and communication disorders* (pp. 280–300). Rockville, MD: American Speech-Language-Hearing Association.

Shadden, B. (1988). *Communication behavior and aging: A source book for clinicians.* Baltimore, MD: Williams & Wilkins.

Shewan, C. M. (1979). *Auditory Comprehension Test for Sentences.* Chicago: Biolinguistics Clinical Institute.

Sklar, M. (1973). *Sklar Aphasia Scale* (rev. ed.). Los Angeles: Western Psychological Services.

Spreen, O., & Benton, A. L. (1977). *Neurosensory Center Comprehensive Examination for Aphasia (NCCEA)* (rev. ed.). Victoria, British Columbia, Canada: Neuropsychology Laboratory, University of Victoria.

Stern, R., & Hooper, C. (1989). *Development of visual analog mood scales: Initial reliability and validity analyses*. Unpublished manuscript, University of North Carolina at Chapel Hill, Chapel Hill, NC.

Ulatowska, H. K., Macaluso-Haynes, S., & North, A. J. (1980). Production of discourse and communication competence in aphasia. In R. H. Brookshire (Ed.), *Clinical Aphasiology Conference proceedings*. Minneapolis: BRK Publishers.

Ulatowska, H. K., Cannito, M. P., Hayashi, M. N., & Fleming, S. G. (1985). Language abilities in the elderly. In H. K. Ulatowska (Ed.), *The aging brain: Communication in the elderly*. Austin, TX: PRO-ED.

Wepman, J., & Jones, L. (1961). *The Language Modalities Test for Aphasia*. Chicago: Education Industry Service.

Whitworth, R. H., & Larson, C. M. (1989). Differential diagnosis and staging of Alzheimer's disease with an aphasia battery. *Neuropsychiatry, Neuropsychology, and Behavioral Neurology, 1*, 255–265.

Wilson, F. B., & Rice, M. (1977). *A programmed approach to voice therapy*. Austin, TX: Learning Concepts.

Yorkston, K. M., & Beukelman, D. R. (1981). *Assessment of intelligibility of dysarthric speech*. Austin, TX: PRO-ED.

Zung, W. W. K. (1965). A self rating depression scale. *Archives of General Psychiatry, 12*, 63–70.

Zung, W. W. K., & Wonnacott, T. H. (1970). Treatment prediction in depression using a self rating scale. *Biological Psychiatry, 2*, 321–329.

Methodological Issues in Research on Aging and Language

Susan de Santi, MS, and Loraine K. Obler, PhD ■

Research involves the dynamic interaction between the research questions addressed, the theory or theories from which it derives, and the techniques that are used to answer the question. In some ways, the results obtained from a given research project are shaped by the way the research question was phrased and studied. The published interpretations of the results, and sometimes the research questions as well, are shaped by the underlying theory. Since theories of language and aging are covered more explicitly in chapter 2, this chapter will treat theory as it relates to the research questions. Various techniques that have been used to study language in the aging population will be examined, as well as issues or problems that arise in applying them. Finally, certain of the ethical issues involved in designing research on communication in the elderly will be discussed.

In writing research papers, it is conventional to avoid mention of the difficulties involved in carrying out the research, their effects, and how decisions made in response to them affect our interpretation of the results. This chapter will address those difficulties and consider them as they relate to issues specific to research on communication in the elderly.

Three populations are generally considered in research on language in the elderly: normal elderly individuals, patients with dementia, and patients with aphasia. Somewhat different research problems arise with each group. Because many of the overarching issues (such as subject selection or the choice of longitudinal as compared to cross-sectional or cross-sequential design) must be considered for each population, all three groups will be discussed within each section.

Loraine K. Obler's thinking about research design issues has benefited greatly from her work with Drs. Martin Albert and Rhoda Au at the Boston Veterans Administration Medical Center, and from discussions over the last 8 years with members of a Feminist Research Methodology group in Boston as well as from more recent discussions with Drs. Mary Parlee and Judy Duchan at the City University of New York Graduate School.

Before turning to the specific research design issues to be addressed (i.e., subject selection and longitudinal, cross-sectional, or cross-sequential design), the kinds of research questions that have been asked about language changes in aging and the ways in which they relate to theory will be examined briefly to provide a context for the following sections.

Language and Normal Aging Research

One focus of research on normal aging has been the description of the components of language that change with aging as compared to those that do not. A basic split is seen between studies of language production and comprehension. Language production includes both naming and discourse, in which changes are seen with aging (e.g., Botwinick & Storandt, 1974; Bowles, Obler, Albert, & Nicholas, 1985; Bowles & Poon, 1981; Kynette & Kemper, 1986; Obler & Albert, 1985). Comprehension studies test comprehension of single sentences or entire paragraphs, utilizing a number of measures (e.g., Bergman, 1971; Cohen, 1979; Davis & Ball, 1989; Obler, Nicholas, Albert, & Woodward, 1985). Other studies have been conducted on more specific areas of language performance. Obler and Albert (1985), for example, considered lexicon, discourse, laterality, and comprehension separately in the healthy elderly, documenting that ''different skills have different lifespans of their own.'' Note that the framing of these research topics assumes a certain modular theory of language with dissociable components, some that change with age and others that do not. Moreover, the components that change with age may change at different rates.

In addition to description of the kinds of changes seen in normal elderly individuals, researchers have asked what causes these age-related changes. For example, Bowles and her colleagues (1985) tested naming abilities in healthy elderly individuals to determine the point in the naming process responsible for the deficit that had been reported. Cognitive nonlanguage factors have also been considered to be the cause of language changes. Davis and Ball (1989), for example, point to the effect of short-term memory deficits on the comprehension of complex sentences. A study like that of Bowles et al. implicitly assumes a theory of language as modular, whereas studies like that of Davis and Ball assume a theory in which there is crucial interaction between language and nonlanguage cognitive abilities.

The strategies elderly individuals use to compensate for their language changes constitute a third area of interest. Obler, Obermann, Samuels, and Albert (1985) considered how compensation through use of face- and lipreading might alleviate some of the comprehension difficulties reported in elderly listeners. Such questions assume that the deficient performance measured does not represent breakdown alone, but rather the interaction of breakdown and the patient's active attempts to overcome it (Heeschen, 1985).

Certain of the research questions that have been asked about language changes in healthy aging have also been asked with respect to changes in the language of demented patients. One theoretical consideration is whether the language changes of dementia, particularly those of Alzheimer's dementia, reflect accelerated aging, or whether there is a qualitative difference in the brain changes (and hence in the language changes) associated with dementia and healthy aging. Thus, one focus of research is an attempt to differentiate the language of dementia from the language of healthy elderly (e.g., Bayles & Kaszniak, 1987; Emery, 1985). A second focus is to distinguish for each group which aspects of language are impaired and which are spared (Bayles & Tomoeda, 1983; Causino, Obler, Knoefel, & Albert, 1990; Kempler, Curtiss, & Jackson, 1987: Nebes, 1985; Rosen, 1980).

Language and Dementia Research

Preliminary descriptive work has been necessary in order to delineate the linguistic changes of dementia of the Alzheimer's type (DAT) at various stages of the disorder (Obler & Albert, 1984), and to distinguish among language changes associated with various types of dementia (Bayles & Kaszniak, 1987; Hier, Hagenlocker, & Shindler, 1985; Holland, McBurney, Mossy, & Reinmouth, 1985). The debate between theorists who see language as modularly organized and those who see it as holistically organized has been carried into the research on the language changes of dementia. Such researchers as Kempler et al. (1987), Schwartz et al. (1979), and Bayles and Kaszniak (1987) have provided evidence for the modular view by showing that certain language areas evidence deficits independent from others. Emery (1985), by contrast, works within a Goldsteinian theory of the holistic brain, in which impairment in dementia reflects the interlinking of linguistic and nonlinguistic cognitive neuropsychological abilities.

As with aphasia, the study of language changes of dementia leads to analysis within the framework of Jakobson's regression hypothesis (1968), where the language changes associated with dementia are compared with those known to occur in childhood. The work of de Ajuriaguerra and Tissot (1975) exemplifies this sort of approach. They used Piaget's developmental paradigm to explain the language changes of the various linguistic levels in dementia and correlated them with Piagetian stages of development.

Another important theoretical question that has been addressed in the scholarship on language changes associated with dementia is whether it is appropriate to use the terminology and diagnostics from the study of aphasia to study the language changes of DAT (Au, Albert, & Obler, 1988; Bayles & Tomoeda, 1988). Au et al. (1988) suggest that dementia should be considered a variation of classical aphasia to provide insight into dementia diagnosis, processes underlying dementia and the brain-behavior relationship. The opposite viewpoint is taken by Bayles and Tomoeda (1988), who argue that the two disorders are dissimilar in many ways. Thus, to call both by the same name is confusing and misleading.

Aphasia Research

Within the literature on aphasia in the elderly, two questions have generated a series of studies. The first is the effect of age on recovery from aphasia (Holland & Bartlett, 1985; Sarno, 1980); the second, a discussion of why fluent aphasics are on average a decade older than nonfluent aphasics (e.g., Brown & Grober, 1983; Miceli et al., 1981; Obler, Albert, Goodglass, & Benson, 1978). Both research questions assume something akin to the hypothesis of Brown and Jaffe (1975) that laterality for language and its organization within the left hemisphere change with increasing age in adulthood.

Research Issues

Subject Selection

The Normal Elderly

The methodological process of subject selection is fraught with difficulty (see also Camp, West, & Poon, 1989). Definitional problems arise with each of the groups treated in this paper: normal elderly individuals, demented patients, and aphasic patients. What, for example, is "normal" in the elderly? By "normal" in our research we rarely mean psychology's norm: a representative sample of the population of elderly individuals in our society. Rather, we may mean normal healthy elderly, testable elderly, or elderly individuals who have the time and interest to participate in our research. We usually choose healthy elderly people with reasonably intact hearing and corrected vision, hardly the true norm. On the other hand, it is rare in the studies of normal aging to use neurological screens to rule out subjects in the early stages of dementia. Thus, we must delimit the extent to which we generalize on data from these subjects to the population of elderly at large.

Our research experience indicates that "normal" elderly who volunteer for research studies are likely not only to be somewhat healthier than the average, but also to have more education and higher IQs, and to be generally more active, with stimulating interests. Of course there are problems with picking "normal" younger subjects as well. The college sophomore typically studied in psychology research is no more the norm for the world's 19-year-olds than our 70-year-olds are norms for the world's 70-year-olds. The difficulties in choosing what is normal change across the life-span, thus compounding the problems inherent in generalizing from a sample. One solution is to solicit as diverse a sample as is practical, taking into account as many factors as possible, and then to report all pertinent variables about the subject pool in the write-up. In this way readers and later researchers can replicate the studies reliably or can modify them as necessary to gain a broader, more representative picture. An alternate solution is to match groups on all pertinent variables and then to be careful not to generalize beyond the population studied.

Dementia

Definitional problems also arise in studying Alzheimer's dementia. Only recently (McKhann et al., 1984) has an operational definition of probable DAT been proposed and accepted by the research community. This definition requires medical exclusion of other possible causes of dementia, as well as neuropsychological and language testing. Nevertheless, some researchers still use older terms, such as "organic brain syndrome."

Patients with DAT may sometimes be confused with healthy elderly, depressed elderly, and patients evidencing fluent aphasia types, especially Wernicke's aphasia. This problem of distinguishing dementia from aphasia is not a new one. Recall that one of the two patients Wernicke (1874) described most fully was demented as well as aphasic. Another had been considered demented although she turned out to be aphasic. More recently, in Irigaray's major study of language in dementia (1973; Obler, 1981), some patients appear more likely to have been aphasic than demented. The differential diagnosis is not easy to make at certain stages of DAT; this is why differential diagnosis has been one focus of research. Obviously, clear reports of how subjects were selected are crucial in evaluating any research on communication in demented patients.

Heterogeneity

An additional subject selection issue that arises in studies of both dementia and aphasia is that of the heterogeneity of populations. There are many diseases that cause dementia, including DAT, Pick's disease, multiple infarction, and Parkinson's disease. If we intermingle these populations in studies of language and dementia, our results may be so varied that no clear pattern will emerge. Moreover, even within DAT, it is now understood that there are several subtypes of patients who display different characteristic behavior patterns. For example, Martin et al. (1986) talk about three types of DAT patients: "typical patients" (globally impaired with problems in word finding and visual constructional tasks of equal magnitude), patients whose disturbances are primarily linguistic, and patients whose disturbances are primarily visuoperceptual. The primary methodological concern is that by choosing nonhomogeneous groups to study, behavioral patterns that might have emerged will be obscured.

The issue of subject population homogeneity arises in the study of aphasia as well and thus is important to consider in the study of elderly aphasics. It has been discussed most in the aphasiological literature with respect to the study of agrammatism. For example, some agrammatic patients may have a long mean length of utterance, while others may not. Comprehension of syntactic items may be more or less impaired in different agrammatic patients. This suggests that to simply collect a sizable group of "agrammatics" for study of sentence length or comprehension can obscure patterns that would emerge if the subgroups were studied separately. Certainly, studies that consider all aphasics without subtyping them run this risk to a great degree.

Age

The problem of controlling across age groups for education must be addressed. It is difficult to solve because within a given culture, fashions in education change over time. It is hard to know how much influence older educational approaches have had on the language behaviors we may be testing today. As we will discuss, a common solution is to balance subject groups by equal years of education, but we must keep in mind the possibility that different cohorts will have had different kinds of education within those equal time periods.

Gender

Gender differences have been reported in our culture on language and nonlanguage tasks, and these appear to occur in the elderly as well (e.g., Obler et al., 1985). Yet there are more women than men among the elderly. In selecting a representative sample we must decide whether to choose equal numbers of men and women in order to explore gender differences in performance, or whether to pick more women than men so that when we report how "the elderly"

perform, we will have tested a more representative sample.

Comparison Subjects

A final subject selection issue confronted by researchers in the study of aging is the number of groups, kinds of comparison, and cohort groups to be studied. Often researchers will choose only a young group and an old group (Botwinick & Storandt, 1974; Bowles & Poon, 1981; Bowles et al., 1985). In some research projects, pentagenarians count as old. In other studies, the "young" are contrasted with septagenarians. Recently researchers have started talking about the "old-old" in their 80s and up who are often less studied. Of course, simply generalizing a statement about 50-year-olds or 90-year-olds to all elderly creates a high risk of overgeneralization. In any event, it is preferable to use more than two groups. It may then be possible to find some linear changes with age that are less likely to reflect cohort effects than those that dichotomously distinguish a young and an old group (e.g., Borod, Obler, Albert, & Stiefel, 1983; Davis & Ball, 1989; Nicholas, Obler, Albert, & Helm-Estabrooks, 1985).

The number and composition of groups studied in research on language changes of elderly demented patients or aphasics is also of concern. Some projects study only one group of patients and describe their behavior. This is appropriate for certain types of research, particularly where one wants to explore or categorize communication patterns occurring in a given population. Experimental studies to discover characteristic behaviors that distinguish groups require a control group of normal healthy elderly individuals, in addition to one or several experimental groups. For example, Emery (1985) took the strategy of studying not only demented individuals and a normal elderly control group, but also a young normal group as a control for the healthy elderly. This permitted her to determine which were normal age-related changes in DAT. Bayles, Tomoeda, Kaszniak, Stern, and Eagans (1985) compared normal subjects, a "near-normal" group, patients with mild and moderate DAT, patients with multi-infarct dementia, patients with Parkinson's disease, and patients with Huntington's chorea. Severity of dementia was documented by neurological examination including a mental status test and, in some cases, neuropsychological tests, and performance on 13 neurolinguistic measures. Such grouping avoids assumptions of homogeneity and enables the researchers to determine which behaviors are shared among or between dementia types and which are peculiar to particular types.

Longitudinal, Cross-Sectional, and Cross-Sequential Studies

Longitudinal Research

In theory, most researchers would prefer to conduct longitudinal studies in which the data are elicited from the same individual or group over an extended period of time in order to report the profiles of changes. The advantage of such research is that each subject serves as his or her own control over time. Thus we can trust that hard-to-measure variables such as education and language use remain relatively constant from one "age group" to the next. There are, however, problems with longitudinal studies. One difficulty is the fact that they are done in "real time," and thus a study to research language changes in aging from ages 30 to 80 would take 50 years to conduct. Another problem that arises in longitudinal work is that the important issues to be studied may change over the course of the project. The experimenter, however, is locked into repeating the exact same tests over time, rather than modifying them if earlier techniques become outdated (Bayles & Kaszniak, 1987). Real-life events such as language education techniques may affect an entire cohort that is being studied longitudinally. In addition, the testing situation itself may change. For example, a new laboratory space or new testers may be

assigned, which may affect the outcome in subtle ways that we usually cannot know.

A further issue in long-term longitudinal studies of normal individuals is attrition of the subject population that can confound the results. This problem occurs in all three populations that we consider in this paper. The health of some elderly subjects will deteriorate, which may cause them to drop out of the research. Demented patients may become institutionalized and harder to locate as well as to test. Aphasic patients who were available for testing while they were institutionalized may start to recover and return to distant homes. One method researchers have used to counter this problem is to consider only the results from those subjects who were available for the duration of the project. This is problematic, since the resultant group is presumably healthier than "normal," and perhaps more cooperative. This also raises issues for generalization to the "normal" elderly population.

Longitudinal testing with demented patients can be done at briefer intervals than with normal elderly individuals because language changes in the demented group can be expected to occur more rapidly. Variability of performance is a related issue: Testing on a given day may or may not be representative of the patient's overall language behavior in the larger interval. Indeed, variability in individual performance is a characteristic of dementia and has been seen to increase with advancing age both within groups and for individuals (e.g., Riegel, 1968).

Cross-Sectional Research

Cross-sectional research has its advantages and disadvantages. Researchers are sometimes confronted with cross-sectional results that show a decline in language performance, contradicting longitudinal results that show an actual increase in performance. This may be due to the attrition issue and/or test learning. The effects of having performed a task before may also influence the results of the study in subtle ways, and this influence may be different for different age groups. However, it is not always the case that retest scores are better because the subject remembers the task. On narrative discourse tasks, for example, the subject may give a more abbreviated version the second time. Indeed, elderly subjects may be particularly careful to avoid full repetition of a story to avoid the stereotypic behavior that the forgetful elderly person retells stories.

Cross-sectional data are not only relatively easy to obtain; they also can be less time consuming to gather than longitudinal data. However, the cross-sectional study runs the particular risk of reflecting cohort effects rather than effects that are truly linked to biological age. These effects are apparent differences between age groups that seem to be related to age but may have other bases. Although education has been mentioned as a subject variable, other life experiences of different cohorts might also influence performance on certain communication tasks. Bayles and Kaszniak (1987) include ''health and medical trends, nutritional habits, environmental toxins, and social customs'' among the phenomena that may influence behavior in different cohorts. Attitudes toward test taking among cohorts also may influence performance on research tasks. Younger adults might perform better simply because they have had more recent experience with test taking, or because they are more compliant in the face of pointless tasks.

Cross-Sequential Research

Schaie (1980) has proposed the cross-sequential approach as the best compromise between the longitudinal and cross-sectional approaches. In this type of research, subjects from several different age groups are followed longitudinally as well as being compared cross-sectionally. Needless to say, this work involves some of the pragmatic difficulties of the longitudinal study and some of the theoretical difficulties of the cross-sectional study. However, it is a valuable compromise because it allows research to be conducted over time while eliminating certain cohort effects that might otherwise pass for age-related changes.

Group Versus Case Studies

Debate among aphasia researchers in the last decade has raised the question of the number of subjects necessary for doing useful research. Studies of aphasia have generally employed smaller groups than those of normal populations, simply because it is difficult to assemble large, relatively homogeneous groups of aphasic patients. The behaviorist psychology tradition contends that large-group studies are much more important than small-group or case studies because they are more generalizable to the population. Yet distortions can also arise in large-group studies. The measuring instrument for group study is of necessity one of central tendency. Although this is extremely effective for suggesting common symptoms and even an approximate range of symptoms, it is a measure that is insensitive to the subtle individual differences that are often found in communication disorders in the elderly.

Case studies, by contrast, provide an in-depth analysis of a single case on many aspects of behavior. These studies can also be useful in supporting or contradicting aspects of theories that have been developed on the basis of larger groups, as well as in generating hypotheses that can be followed up with group studies. A case study is particularly useful when dissociation is seen; we can conclude that this dissociation suggests that the two behaviors are independent in normal subjects. For example, Whitaker (1976) reported on the case of a patient with dementia who was able to detect syntactic and phonological errors, but not semantic errors. We understand this dissociation of semantic breakdown from spared syntactic and phonological abilities to mean that semantic organization and processing are separate from phonological and syntactic organization and processing in normal subjects.

An association between two behaviors in a single-case study, by contrast, bears less meaning than a dissociation, because it may be by chance that two behaviors are spared or impaired together. For example, if we test an aphasic patient whose naming ability for color words and body parts is spared relative to naming ability for other categories, we cannot assume that color and body part words are represented in the same area of the brain or lexicon. The next subject we test may have spared naming for only one of the two categories, which would demonstrate the more likely possibility that in this patient, color and body part words are independently organized.

In summary, case studies are useful for demonstrating dissociations; group studies are useful for demonstrating associations. Of course it is important to determine that the patients studied were relatively normal in terms of brain organization before the language disturbance. Information on language processing in patients with lifelong epilepsy in or near the left-hemisphere language area, for example, cannot be presumed to reflect processes in subjects whose brains have developed without seizures.

For the populations considered in this chapter, it is not unusual to have an interesting case report on a demented patient or an aphasic patient, but a case study of a normal elderly individual would be extremely rare. This may be because we assume that in normals, language breakdown is so subtle that it cannot be isolated from other behaviors. Alternately, it may reflect the issue of heterogeneity versus homogeneity discussed previously, whereby we can assume that two normals are more similar than two aphasics or two demented patients. Of course this is not necessarily the case; particularly with respect to language performance, there is a great variability among normals of any age.

Case studies tend to examine a number of different language abilities in specific detail, whereas group studies are more likely to probe language behaviors in more global ways. Schwartz et al. (1979) studied the language behavior of one demented individual, WLP, over a period of 27 months. They analyzed semantic ability, syntactic ability, and the ability to read aloud in order to report the relative dissociation of these abilities. Curtiss, Kempler, and LaRue (1981) also focused on a single demented patient in order to examine the relationship between various aspects of cognition and syntax. They studied the interaction of cognitive deficits with linguistic and metalinguistic deficits.

Group studies of the language changes of dementia and aphasia have examined various linguistic components such as semantics, syntax, and pragmatics to determine if differential linguistic impairment exists and to discover the linguistic levels at which it occurs. Murdoch, Chenery, Wilks, and Boyle (1987), in a global study, tested language production, auditory comprehension, repetition, reading, and writing in a sizable group of patients with DAT. They determined that semantic abilities were impaired, but syntactic and phonological abilities were spared, reinforcing what Whitaker (1976) had reported on the basis of her case study.

Other studies have focused on one aspect of language in an effort to describe the breakdown of a linguistic component or the sparing of aspects of a linguistic component in dementia. Bayles and Tomoeda (1983), for example, studied the nature of naming deficits in dementia in an effort to determine the cause of this problem. Martin and Fedio (1983) demonstrated that differentiation of items within a semantic category was problematic but that broader semantic knowledge was spared in Alzheimer's patients. Kempler et al. (1987) report on syntactic sparing with impaired lexical use in dementia. Causino et al. (1990) examined pragmatic abilities in late-stage demented patients to show that some spared pragmatic behaviors are maintained even at this stage of the disease. De Santi, Obler, Sabo-Abramson, and Goldberger (1989) examined bilingual behaviors in DAT patients and concluded that pragmatic failure was responsible for bilingual discourse breakdown.

Finally, it should be noted that group studies engender all the problems of subject selection discussed above, but attrition is more devastating for the research in a case study. In conclusion, both case studies and group studies have their advantages and disadvantages and the question to be studied should lead to the subject design. The conclusions from each kind of study should be weighed according to the strengths and weaknesses presented here.

Descriptive Versus Experimental Studies

Descriptive studies are conducted in order to analyze and categorize behaviors observed and to understand the patterns underlying them. These studies may be used to distinguish features of one disorder from another in the populations being investigated. Experimental studies, by contrast, are designed to manipulate variables in order to determine which one affects a given outcome. Some scholars consider descriptive studies to be ''pretheoretical,'' but we prefer to assert that both descriptive and experimental studies relate to theory and employ it in different ways.

For the descriptive research study, it is impossible to escape the theoretical constructs that determine which categories are chosen for analysis, even if the researchers do not consider themselves to be working within a given theory. Experimental work, by contrast, appears to relate to a given theory when it is completed, but not infrequently the research has been designed for more practical reasons (to use a subject population on hand, to use equipment that is available, to use a technique that is somehow appealing). The theory is drawn upon at the end stage of the research to provide some framework for understanding the data.

Descriptive studies may be of several types and may use primarily quantitative data, primarily qualitative data, or both. As an example of both quantitative and qualitative data, consider the study of Emery (1985). She addressed her research toward determining the nature (quality) and order of magnitude (quantity) of changes in ''higher order mental processes during the later part of life.'' She explored language by comparing the performance of normal pre-middle-aged and middle-aged adults, normal elderly adults, and elderly adults with DAT. A variety of semantic, syntactic, cognitive, and memory tasks were used. All responses were transcribed and analyzed in an effort to describe the nature of linguistic and cognitive performance for all subject groups. Qualitative analyses involved interpreting responses to interviews and questionnaires. Objective measures from standardized tests were used to determine both qualitative and quantitative differences between the test groups. Results demonstrated that normal elderly subjects performed quantitatively worse than younger adults on linguistic measures, as well as on measures of cognitive development (within a Piagetian framework) and memory. When they were compared to normals, the DAT patients performed worse (quantitatively) as well as qualitatively differently from the normal elderly on all measures.

As an example of qualitative analysis, consider the work of Ripich and Terrell (1988). They compared the patterns of discourse between healthy elderly subjects and patients with DAT in their use of propositions, cohesion, and coherence. They also used judgments by listeners to evaluate the discourse qualities of DAT and normal elderly subjects. Their results indicated that the DAT patients have an impairment in these discourse abilities and that this problem contributes to their communication impairment. As another example, Obler and Albert (1984) described the distinguishing features of the various stages of language decline in this disease on the basis of their clinical observations. Features of language in elderly with normal aging, subcortical dementias, other dementias, and aphasia were also described in order to distinguish the effects of aging from those of DAT.

Experimental studies tend to focus on quantitative measurement of specific language features. Bowles et al. (1985), for example, examined naming abilities in younger and older adults to determine if differences existed. Their study looked at the ability to name in response to a definition, where the stimulus definition was preceded by one of various types of priming stimuli. Results indicated not only that older adults were slower but also that they had fewer successful name retrievals than younger adults. The priming stimulus condition was also a factor for the older but not for the younger adults, suggesting that orthographic and phonemic information is less available to the elderly.

We may contrast such a study with one from Obler et al. (1985), who investigated the use of written input to enhance comprehension abilities in DAT. The comprehension sections of the *Boston Diagnostic Aphasia Examination* (Goodglass & Kaplan, 1972) were administered in written only, auditory only, and combined conditions to early-middle- to middle-staged DAT patients. The results indicated that written input alone or in combination with auditory input aided comprehension in eight of the nine DAT subjects studied. For this study, sections of previously used language batteries were modified to answer the research question.

Experimental studies of language in aphasic patients are more numerous than those of language in demented patients and perhaps even in healthy elderly individuals. This is due in part to the 100-year history of the study of aphasic patients, and in part to our assumption that aphasic patients do not have cognitive impairments that interact with their performance on experimental tasks. With demented patients certainly, and sometimes with healthy elderly individuals as well, we need to spend more time considering technical as well as theoretical issues that may confound apparent linguistic results, as will be discussed in the next two sections of this chapter.

Interaction of Cognitive and Linguistic Factors

Over the history of the study of aphasia there has been some debate as to whether generalized intellectual deterioration is concomitant with aphasia. Intellectual deterioration in the dementias is much marked and clearly interacts with subjects' performance on many tasks. Thus, researchers spend a fair amount of time designing tasks that involve as few intervening cognitive factors as possible. Kempler, Van Lancker, and Read (1988) attempted to separate language and cognition in their study on proverb and idiom interpretation. They designed a test of familiar and novel language comprehension using a picture-pointing response mode. The novel and familiar phrase (idiom and proverb) subtests were matched for length, grammatical structure, and word frequency. According to Kempler et al., "decoding word meaning and syntactic structure" was necessary to comprehend novel phrases. Comprehension of familiar phrases was improbable using the above strategy and required "inferring an abstract meaning." Thus they were able to isolate a fundamentally cognitive dysfunction as opposed to a primarily linguistic one in comprehending words and phrases in DAT.

Of course, these research issues are embedded in a general theoretical one, namely, the extent to which cognition and language are integrally related to each other. Are the two indeed relatively independent? Is language based on nonlanguage cognition? Or do the two interact in complex ways? Some research projects simply take one of these stances as an assumption and build the research questions on that premise, whereas others focus their research on making distinctions between language and cognition.

Task-Related Issues

Stimulus Selection

Research on the elderly modifies some of our standard experimental concerns. For example, if we want to employ high-frequency and low-frequency words for stimuli, we must consider that certain words change frequency for different cohorts. Moskovitch (personal communication) gives the example of the word *atom*, which was used quite frequently in the 1940s and less frequently today. As a result, older subjects would have had more exposure to it than younger ones. For a second example, consider elicitation of spontaneous discourse. Different topics will be of greater interest to individuals of different ages. For example, 30-year-olds may like to discuss computers, whereas 70-year-olds may find retirement investments most interesting. If we ask everyone to speak on topics of interest to 30-year-olds, the 70-year-olds will naturally look worse; conversely, if we ask everyone to speak on topics of interest to 70-year-olds, it might appear that the 30-year-olds are less competent (Siple, personal communication).

Task Difficulty

Task difficulty issues also must be considered in preparing materials for subjects of different ages or different degrees of cognitive health. On a test of lateralization of brain organization for language, Obler, Woodward, and Albert (1984) used different stimulus presentation intervals in order to assure that subjects in each of the age groups (30s, 50s, 60s, and 70s) would be responding at an 80% correct level, so that task difficulty did not interact and give an apparent laterality effect when there was none.

Pacing of the stimulus presentation is also of concern, since there appears to be a general slowing of response with aging. On one comprehension study (Obler et al., 1985), sentences with relatively complex syntax were presented to 30-, 50-, 60-, and 70-year-olds at a "normal" rate—120 words/min. The only individuals who complained about the pace were the older subjects. Thus, while intending to study only syntactic complexity, the researchers might have been making the task differentially difficult

for the elderly populations by using a single rate of presentation.

Instructions

Instructions present a challenge to the researcher, especially with aphasics and demented patients. It is of particular importance to use nonverbal instructions with the aphasic patient whenever possible, that is, to give examples so that the subjects can comprehend the task even if they do not understand all the words in the instructions. With the demented patient, moreover, continuous instruction must be provided to prevent the subject from losing focus. If instructions are given only when the subject appears to be losing attention, and the study is comparing a demented population with a normal aging population, the stimulus presentations will not be consistent.

Ethical Issues

No discussion of research methodology is complete without consideration of ethical issues. In studies of normal aging, the concerns are not markedly different from those for younger adults. The subjects must be informed in advance of the research plan, allowed to leave at any time without financial penalty or the loss of health care, allowed breaks as they desire, and debriefed (when appropriate) at the end of testing; research results should be shared with them in a comprehensible fashion if they express interest.

With demented and aphasic patients, it is important that the subjects understand the informed consent materials they sign. This often means not only having them read the materials, but spending time explaining the study and informed consent issues to them. It may even be necessary to involve family members in making these decisions. When patients with aphasia or dementia are institutionalized, it becomes particularly important to make them understand that they will still receive the same health care even if they decide not to cooperate in research.

The patient who does not particularly want to participate may be encouraged to; however, a patient's wish to decline must be respected. Of course this causes a skewing in the research; the most cooperative patients are being studied and reported on as if they were characteristic of uncooperative patients as well. This limitation must be noted because it cannot be avoided; ethical respect for the patient's integrity must prevail.

Concerns about the ability of aphasic and demented patients to understand the informed consent forms should not preclude studying them. Research provides these patients with the opportunity to contribute to the further professional knowledge of their condition. Indeed, the attention from the experimenter, and the interaction in testing or conversation or research projects generally, may provide them with useful stimulation and healthy interaction, as well as the feeling that they are contributing to scientific knowledge. With all subjects, it is important to provide feedback and support regarding their performance. Although they may understand that the primary benefits of the research are not to themselves as individuals but rather to future groups of patients with difficulties similar to their own, their contribution should be acknowledged.

Videotapes are crucial for certain types of research (e.g., studies of pragmatic abilities), and audio tapes are preferable to writing down patients' responses on most language tasks, as information can be misinterpreted or lost in on-line transcription. Releases must be obtained to show tapes for professional and educational purposes only; care must be taken not to abuse or misuse this information. The anonymity of the subjects can be further protected on tapes by bleeping out their name and/or covering their face.

Choosing labels to describe subjects has ethical ramifications. The differences between such labels as "senile dementia" or "dementia of the Alzheimer's type" have

theoretical implications. The term "senility" is avoided since it implies that all older people will become demented. The term "elderly" conveys more dignity than "old." The differences between "aphasic," "aphasic patient," "patient with aphasia," and "aphasia victim" reflect attitudes toward the patient. To call a patient an "aphasic" suggests that the aphasia the patient presents sums up the patient—that this is not a person apart from the aphasia. The counter-position is that "aphasic" is simply a shortened, easier-to-use form for "patient with aphasia." "Aphasia victim" implies not only that the patient has been struck by a terrible condition, but also that he or she is helpless to recover from it. The choice of the labels used to describe patients should be made with care and consideration.

Bias Toward Reporting Differences

There is a bias in research toward focusing on differences between groups. Our studies tend not to mention, or to underreport, similarities between younger and older adults. These biases interact with the assumptions of society that aging is a negative condition and that elderly subjects will perform worse than younger subjects. No doubt this bias affects the choice of research topics as well as the reporting of data, in that areas of study are selected where decline is expected. As a result, researchers are less likely to learn about areas of communication that do not change across the life-span, or about ones that improve (see Abeles & White Riley, 1977).

Conclusion

It has been necessary to state the disadvantages alongside the advantages of the various research factors discussed in this chapter to stress the importance of considering both in evaluating research papers on language and communication in the elderly. The issues raised are also of value for researchers who are beginning to conduct investigations with elderly subjects. No research project is perfect, but research can be better and more carefully carried out and more honestly and thoughtfully reported, so that our scientific understanding of the fascinating changes in language that our aging brains bring about can continue to advance.

References

Abeles, R., & White Riley, M. (1976–1977). A life-course perspective on the later years of life: Some implications for research. *Social Science Research Council Annual Report*, 1–16.

Au, R., Albert, M., & Obler, L. K. (1988). The relation of aphasia to dementia. *Aphasiology*, 2, 161–173.

Bayles, K., & Kaszniak, A. (1987). *Communication and cognition in normal aging and dementia*. Austin, TX: PRO-ED.

Bayles, K., & Tomoeda, C. (1983). Confrontation naming in dementia. *Brain and Language*, 19, 98–114.

Bayles, K., & Tomoeda, C. (1988). *Are the communication changes of dementia appropriately characterized as aphasia?* Symposium conducted at American Speech-Language-Hearing Association Convention, Boston, MA.

Bayles, K., Tomoeda, C., Kaszniak, A., Stern, K., & Eagans, K. (1985). Verbal preservation of dementia patients. *Brain and Language*, 25, 102–116.

Bergman, M. (1971). Hearing and aging. *Audiology*, 10, 164–171.

Borod, J., Obler, L. K., Albert, M. L., & Stiefel, S. (1983). Lateralization for pure tone and perception as a function of age and sex. *Cortex*, 19, 281–285.

Botwinick, J., & Storandt, M. (1974). Vocabulary abilities in later life. *Journal of Genetic Psychology*, 125, 303–308.

Bowles, N., Obler, L. K., Albert, M., & Nicholas, M. (1985). *Naming impairment in the elderly*. Paper presented at the annual meeting of the Academy of Aphasia, Pittsburgh, PA.

Bowles, N., & Poon, L. (1981). The effect of age on speed of lexical access. *Experimental Aging Research*, 7, 417–425.

Brown, J., & Grober, E. (1983). Age, sex and aphasia type: Evidence for a regional cerebral growth process underlying lateralization. *Journal of Nervous and Mental Diseases*, 171, 431–434.

Brown, J., & Jaffe, J. (1975). Hypothesis on cerebral dominance. *Neuropsychologia*, 13, 107–110.

Camp, C., West, R., & Poon, L. (1989). Recruitment practices for psychological research in gerontology. In M. P. Lawton & A. Henzog (Eds.), *Special Research Methods for Gerontology*. Amityville, NY: Baywood.

Causino, M., Obler, L. K., Knoefel, J., & Albert, M. (1990). Pragmatic abilities in late-stage SDAT. Manuscript submitted for publication.

Cohen, G. (1979). Language comprehension in old age. *Cognitive Psychology*, 11, 412–429.

Curtiss, S., Kempler, D., & LaRue, M. (1981). *Language and cognition in dementia: A case study* (UCLA Working Papers in Cognitive Linguistics). Los Angeles: University of California at Los Angeles.

Davis, G. A., & Ball, H. (1989). Effects of age on comprehension of complex sentences in adulthood. *Journal of Speech and Hearing Research*, 32, 143–150.

de Ajuriaguerra, J., & Tissot, R. (1975). Some aspects of language in various forms of senile dementia (comparisons with language of children). In E. & E. Lenneberg (Eds.), *Foundations of language development: A multidisciplinary approach*. New York: Academic Press.

De Santi, S., Obler, L. K., Sabo-Abramson, H., & Goldberger, J. (1989). Discourse abilities and deficits in multilingual dementia. In Y. Joanette & H. Brownell (Eds.), *Discourse abilities in brain damage: Theoretical and empirical perspectives*. New York: Springer-Verlag.

Emery, O. (1985). Language and aging. *Experimental Aging Research*, 11, 3–60.

Goodglass, H., & Kaplan, E. (1972). *The assessment of aphasia and related disorders*. Philadelphia: Lea & Febiger.

Heeschen, K. (1985). Agrammatism versus paragrammatism: A fictitious effect. In M.-L. Kean (Ed.), *Agrammatism*. New York: Academic Press.

Hier, D., Hagenlocker, K., & Shindler, A. G. (1985). Language disintegration in dementia: Effects of etiology and severity. *Brain and Language, 25,* 117–133.

Holland, A., & Bartlett, C. (1985). Some differential effects on stroke-produced aphasia. In H. Ulatowska (Ed.), *The aging brain: Communication in the elderly.* Austin, TX: PRO-ED.

Holland, A. L., McBurney, D. H., Mossy, J., & Reinmouth, O. M. (1985). The dissolution of language in Pick's disease with neurofibrillary tangles: A case study. *Brain and Language, 24,* 36–58.

Irigaray, L. (1973). *Le langage des déments.* The Hague: Mouton.

Jakobson, R. (1968). *Child language, aphasia, and phonological universals* (A. Keiler, Trans.). The Hague: Mouton. (Original work published in German, 1941).

Kempler, D., Curtiss, S., & Jackson, C. (1987). Syntactic preservation in Alzheimer's disease. *Journal of Speech and Hearing Disorders, 30,* 343–350.

Kempler, D., Van Lancker, D., & Read, S. (1988). Proverb and idiom comprehension in Alzheimer's disease. *Alzheimer's Disease and Associated Disorders, 2,* 38–49.

Kynette, D., & Kemper, S. (1986). Aging and the loss of grammatical forms. *Language and Communication, 6,* 65–72.

Martin, A., Brouwers, P., Lalonde, F., Cox, C., Teleska, P., Fedio, P., Foster, N., & Chase, T. (1986). Towards a behavioral typology of Alzheimer's patients. *Journal of Clinical and Experimental Neuropsychology, 8,* 594–610.

Martin, A., & Fedio, P. (1983). Word production and comprehension in Alzheimer's disease: The breakdown of semantic knowledge. *Brain and Language, 25,* 124–141.

McKhann, G., Drachman, D., Folstein, M., Katzman, R., Price, D., & Stadlan, E. (1984). Clinical diagnosis of Alzheimer's disease: Report of the NINCDS-ADRDA work group under the auspices of the Department of Health and Human Services task force on Alzheimer's disease. *Neurology, 34,* 934–944.

Miceli, G., Catagirone, C., Gainotti, G., Masullo, C., Silveri, M., & Villa, G. (1981). Influence of sex, age, literacy and pathologic lesion on incidence, severity and type of aphasia. *Acta Neurologica Scandinavica, 64,* 370–383.

Murdoch, B., Chenery, H., Wilks, V., & Boyle, R. (1987). Language disorders in dementia of the Alzheimer type. *Brain and Language, 31,* 122–137.

Nebes, R. (1985). Preservation of semantic structure in dementia. In H. Ulatowska (Ed.), *The aging brain: Communication in the elderly.* Austin, TX: PRO-ED.

Nicholas, M., Obler, L. K., Albert, M. L., & Helm-Estabrooks, N. (1985). Empty speech in Alzheimer's disease and fluent aphasia. *Journal of Speech and Hearing Research, 28,* 405–410.

Obler, L. K. (1981). [Review of *Le langage des déments,* by L. Irigaray]. *Brain and Language, 1,* 375–386.

Obler, L. K., & Albert, M. L. (1984). Language in aging. In M. L. Albert (Ed.), *Clinical neurology of aging.* New York: Oxford University Press.

Obler, L. K., & Albert, M. L. (1985). Language skills across adulthood. In J. Birren & K. W. Schaie (Eds.), *Handbook of the psychology of aging.* New York: Van Nostrand Reinhold.

Obler, L. K., Albert, M. L., Goodglass, H., & Benson, D. F. (1978). Aphasia type and aging. *Brain and Language, 6,* 318–322.

Obler, L. K., Nicholas, M., Albert, M., & Woodward, S. (1985). On comprehension across the adult lifespan. *Cortex, 21,* 273–280.

Obler, L., Obermann, L., Samuels, I., & Albert, M. L. (1985). *Written input to enhance comprehension in Alzheimer's dementia.* Paper presented at American Speech-Language-Hearing Association meeting, Washington, DC.

Obler, L. K., Woodward, S., & Albert, M. (1984). Lateralization in aging? *Neuropsychologia, 22,* 235–240.

Riegel, K. (1968). Changes in psycholinguistic performances with age. In G. Talland (Ed.), *Human aging and behavior.* New York: Academic Press.

Ripich, D., & Terrell, B. (1988). Patterns of discourse cohesion and coherence in Alzheimer's disease. *Journal of Speech and Hearing Research, 53,* 8–15.

Rosen, W. (1980). Verbal fluency in aging and dementia. *Journal of Clinical Neuropsychology, 2,* 135–146.

Sarno, M. T. (1980). Language rehabilitation outcomes in the elderly aphasic patient. In L. K. Obler & M. L. Albert (Eds.), *Language and communication in the elderly* (pp. 191–202). Lexington, MA: D. C. Heath.

Schaie, W. (1980). Cognitive development in aging. In L. K. Obler & M. L. Albert (Eds.), *Language and communication in the elderly.* Lexington, MA: D. C. Heath.

Schwartz, M., Marin, O., & Saffran, E. (1979). Dissociation of language function in dementia: A case study. *Brain and Language, 7,* 277–306.

Wernicke, C. (1874). Der aphasisch Symptomen Complex. Eine psychologische Studie auf anatomischer Basis. Breslau: Cohn & Weigert. [The aphasia symptom-complex: A psychological study on an anatomic basis].

Reprinted in G. Eggert (Trans.), *Wernicke's works on aphasia: A sourcebook and review.* The Hague: Mouton, 1977.

Whitaker, H. A. (1976). A case of isolation of the language function. In H. Whitaker & H. A. Whitaker (Eds.), *Perspectives in neurolinguistics and psycholinguistics: Vol. 2. Studies in neurolinguistics.* New York: Academic Press.

Geriatric Audiology

SECTION

Barbara E. Weinstein, PhD,
and Craig W. Newman, PhD ∎

The theme of the chapter by Lichtenstein, Bess, and Logan is the importance of early identification of older adults with hearing impairment to forestall the onset of its psychosocial consequences. They begin their chapter with an overview of the demographics of hearing loss and move to a discussion of the functional effects of unremediated hearing loss. The fact that hearing loss is associated with decline in cognitive function, depression, functional health status, and psychosocial/communication function underlines the importance of early identification and remediation of the hearing-impaired elderly.

Prior to mounting a screening program, several criteria must be met to assure that the disorder warrants the expenditure of time and money. Hearing loss in older adults satisfies each of the criteria enumerated by the authors, and thus screening efforts are justifiable. Lichtenstein, Bess, and Logan offer a description of the validity of several screening protocols that have been standardized on adults and the elderly. They present the sensitivity, specificity, predictive values, and overall accuracy associated with the protocols to enable clinicians to reach an educated decision regarding the screening procedure that best meets the needs of the population in question. The authors acknowledge that the debate regarding the most valid procedure for identifying the elderly hearing impaired awaits resolution. They conclude the chapter with suggestions for future research that may help to untangle the controversy surrounding screening protocols used with the elderly.

Gordon-Salant's chapter on audiologic assessment provides the reader with a scholarly review of the literature on the test battery used

in assessment of the hearing status of older adults. Her extensive overview of each of the procedures includes a discussion of the audiometric
trends typical of elderly individuals, factors that may influence findings or confound the interpretation of results, and modifications in test
protocols that may minimize the "aging effect." A major theme inherent in the chapter is that the interpretation of audiologic information
on older adults is dependent on the clinician's ability to distinguish
what is considered to be "normal" from what is considered to be
"abnormal/pathological" for a given population. The variability in performance so typical of older adults further confounds the interpretation of findings on routine as well as complex tasks.

The components of the test battery described by Gordon-Salant
include (a) the case history, (b) hearing handicap assessment, (c) air/
bone conduction testing, (d) speech testing, and (e) immittance testing. While Gordon-Salant views these five tests as "routine," she
acknowledges the importance of tests of central auditory nervous system function when certain behaviors or test results are indicative of
possible auditory processing problems. Her review of the behavioral
measures of central auditory nervous system function and their application to elderly people is comprehensive, state-of-the-art, and clinically applicable. The material covered in the chapter should set the stage
for a decision regarding the need for differential testing or for a hearing aid/assistive listening device (ALD) and/or aural rehabilitation.

The chapter by Jacobson and Spitzer offers a comprehensive review
of the literature on the effects of age on the interpretation of electrophysiological measurements of the auditory and vestibular systems.
The emphasis is on quantification, using electrophysiological techniques, of the functional effects of the anatomical changes in the auditory and vestibular pathways. The approach taken by the authors is
to provide a critical review of studies on the effect of aging and hearing loss on interpretation of short-, middle-, and long-latency evoked
potentials to assist the reader in resolving the controversies surrounding clinical and research findings. The extensive review of the effects
of age on endogenous evoked potentials represents a departure from
the bulk of chapters included in texts of this nature.

The second section of their chapter is devoted to balance problems
in aging adults. The prevalence of "falls" is discussed as is the devastating impact of falls on the general well-being of the elderly. This discussion is followed by a state-of-the-art review of available data as they
relate to the effects of aging on vestibular assessment techniques,
including caloric, ocular motility, rotational, and posturographic testing. Practical suggestions for performing vestibulometric procedures
in older adults completes the section. In light of the inadequacies inherent in the research on the effects of aging on tests of auditory and vestibular function, the authors conclude the chapter with suggestions
for research to assist in the resolution of the dilemmas confronting the
clinician.

In their chapter, Stach and Stoner discuss hearing aids, ALDs, and
the impact of audiologic and nonaudiologic factors on hearing aid
benefit and success in older adults. The nonaudiologic variables include
psychosocial factors, physical factors, the hearing health care delivery

system, and the economics of hearing aids. The audiologic factors include senescent changes in the central auditory pathways, speech understanding difficulties in a variety of listening situations, and the electroacoustic characteristics of hearing aids. These audiologic and nonaudiologic factors interact to create a challenge to the audiologist who is fitting older adults and to the consumer in his or her adjustment to amplification. Stach and Stoner offer suggestions for minimizing the effects of the aforementioned variables, including methods for reducing background noise and instrument complexity. It is hoped that their technical suggestions will help to increase the usefulness of personal hearing aids.

Although many older adults derive benefit from amplification, as documented by improvements in word recognition ability and reductions in the perceived handicap associated with hearing loss, it is apparent that not all older adults are candidates for conventional hearing aids. The use of ALDs to supplement hearing aids or to meet individual communication requirements is discussed at length by Stach and Stoner. These alternative technologies, such as hard-wired, frequency-modulated, or infrared light systems, are viewed as "need-specific amplification" by the authors, who offer situational applications of available technologies. The chapter concludes with two case presentations that illustrate how ALDs can be used by older adults to overcome the communication and psychosocial difficulties that accompany hearing loss.

Lesner and Kricos view hearing loss as a disability that interferes with communication in general, and psychosocial function in particular. Hence, audiologic rehabilitation is a holistic process that is client-centered and designed to minimize the social, emotional, and vocational handicap associated with impaired hearing. The definition of audiologic rehabilitation adopted by the authors sets the stage for a process that is multidimensional in its focus and a challenge to professionals who choose to incorporate audiologic rehabilitation into their practice.

The audiologic rehabilitation program described by Lesner and Kricos is derived from the procedural model developed by Stephens and Goldstein. It entails evaluation of receptive communication status including audition, vision, and auditory-visual integration. Assessment of the psychological, sociological, vocational, and educational implications of hearing loss is integral to the assessment protocol. Consideration of physical function including the status of the auditory mechanism, upper limb mobility, mental status, and manual dexterity is imperative, because alterations in any of these areas will influence hearing aid use and benefit. Finally, understanding the individual's amplification status and communicative needs is critical to the assessment process as well.

The authors' comprehensive discussion of factors influencing candidacy is followed by a review of considerations integral to the design of a program of audiologic rehabilitation. This description flows into a detailed review of the components to a rehabilitation program, which includes counseling of the hearing impaired and family members, hearing aid orientation, speechreading training, and auditory-visual communication training. The training model and strategies for reducing the communication handicap characterizing selected older adults is multidimensional in scope, yet client-centered to ensure that the individual needs of the hearing impaired are met.

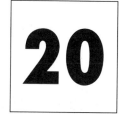

Screening the Elderly for Hearing Impairment

20

CHAPTER

Michael J. Lichtenstein, MD, MSc, Fred H. Bess, PhD, and Susan A. Logan, MSc ■

This chapter focuses on the initial identification (diagnosis) of hearing impairment in the elderly. While final classification of impairment and rehabilitation plans depend on full audiologic assessment, here we are concerned with the initial steps involved in screening. There are two central questions: First, what evidence is there that screening for hearing impairment is effective? Second, what tools are available to accomplish this task?

To answer these questions the chapter considers six areas. First, hearing impairment, disability, and handicap are defined; second, the epidemiology of hearing impairment and handicap is reviewed; third, the principles of assessing the effectiveness of screening programs as they apply to hearing are discussed; fourth, the effectiveness of screening tools for hearing impairment is reviewed; fifth, the need for comparing criteria of hearing impairment with functional scales is discussed; and sixth, future research needs are summarized.

Definitions of Hearing Impairment, Disability, and Handicap

Structural, biochemical, physiological, and psychological changes occur in all humans as they age. These changes, though often measurable, may not constitute a need for recognition and intervention unless they affect an individual's life. In the medical model, a structural change may be recognized as a *disease* or *target disorder*. This structural change may or may not express itself as an *illness*, that is, the cluster of symptoms and signs manifested by an individual in response to having the target disorder. The impact of the target disorder and illness may further be categorized by considering the *predicament*, the social and economic consequences of the condition (Sackett, Haynes, & Tugwell, 1985).

The paradigm is that the structural changes of aging, whatever their source, must not be separated from their functional and psychosocial consequences (World Health Organization, 1980). In considering these consequences there are four steps. First, an abnormality develops within the individual (a pathologically demonstrable entity or disease). Second, someone becomes aware of such an occurrence; the pathological state is exteriorized or measurable (*impairments*). Impairments represent dysfunction at the level of the organ system. Third, the behavior of the individual is altered because of the impairment (*disability* or *illness*). Disabilities represent disturbances at the level of the person. Fourth, the resulting disability places the individual at a disadvantage relative to others (*handicap* or *predicament*). Handicaps reflect the response of society to the individual's impairment and disability.

In this context, levels of hearing dysfunction may be defined as follows:

1. A *hearing impairment* is a change for the worse in auditory anatomical structure or function that produces hearing loss (AAO/ACO, 1979). The terms *hearing impairment* and *hearing loss* are used interchangeably.

2. A *hearing disability* occurs when a hearing impairment is severe enough to interfere with an individual's ability to perceive speech and environmental sounds (Salomon, 1986).

3. A *hearing handicap* occurs when a hearing impairment is severe enough to interfere with an individual's physical and psychosocial functional status (Salomon, 1986).

There is not a perfect one-to-one association between hearing impairment and the degree of disability or handicap produced. For example, a mild high-frequency hearing loss may be completely handicapping to a musical conductor, whereas the same degree of loss may not interfere at all with an architect's ability to perform his or her job. For the conductor, aural rehabilitation may be essential; for the architect, it may be unnecessary. Given this conceptual framework, it becomes clear that in screening for hearing impairment, the audiometric results should be linked with an assessment of disability and handicap.

Epidemiology of Hearing Disorders in the Aged

The prevalence of hearing impairment depends on the criteria used to define it. In the Framingham Study of hearing loss in the elderly the prevalence of impairment was 31% using the criterion of an average loss of 25 dB hearing level (HL) or greater at 0.5, 1, and 2 kHz in the better ear. When the criterion was changed to include the 4-kHz frequency in the average, the prevalence increased to 47% (Moscicki, Elkins, Baum, & McNamara, 1985). As another example, in a clinical study of aged patients screened in primary care practices, the prevalence of hearing impairment ranged from 29% (using the criterion of a 40-dB HL loss or greater at 1 or 2 kHz in both ears, or 1 and 2 kHz in each ear) to 62% (using the criterion of an average loss of 25 dB HL or more at 1, 2, and 4 kHz in the better ear) (Bess, Lichtenstein, Logan, & Burger, 1989).

Regardless of the criteria used, men tend to have greater levels of loss at frequencies greater than 1 kHz than women. Age is by far the major determinant in predicting who is likely to have impaired hearing (Moscicki et al., 1985).

Hearing disability was assessed in the National Health Interview Survey in home interviews by use of a self-rating hearing scale and the Gallaudet scale (National Center for Health Statistics [NCHS], 1982). The self-rating hearing scale asked about deafness, trouble hearing, and tinnitus. The Gallaudet scale asked about hearing and understanding at levels of whispering, normal voice, shouting (across a room), or speaking loudly into an ear. In addition, the Gallaudet scale inquired about speech and noise discrimination. Using these self-reports of hearing ability, hearing disability was the third most common chronic condition in persons over 65 years old in the United States (arthritis and hypertension were more common). The prevalence of hearing disability increased exponentially with age. While it was reported as a problem by 5% of persons 18 to 44 years old, it affects 26% of persons 65 to 74 years old and 38% of those 75 years of age and older (Collins, 1988). In the older age groups, as with hearing impairment, the proportion of persons with hearing disability was greater among men (31%) than women (23%) (NCHS, 1982). Persons with hearing disability were also more likely to be retired, have less than a 12th-grade education, and have family incomes of less than $7,000 annually (NCHS, 1982).

The National Health Interview Survey also documented an association between hearing disability and handicap in all age groups (NCHS, 1982). Persons having no trouble hearing were contrasted with those with all levels of hearing trouble and those who at best could hear shouted speech. The proportion of persons over age 65 who reported handicaps for each of these three groups is given in Table 20.1. For each of the handicaps (limited activity, annual days spent in bed, annual physician contacts, and self-reported health status) there is a gradient where a greater proportion of persons who at best can hear shouted speech have these problems compared to those without hearing trouble. In spite of the association between hearing disability and handicap, 92% of persons with trouble hearing who were interviewed in the National Health Interview Survey did not perceive their hearing impairment as a primary or secondary cause of their limitation in activity (NCHS, 1982).

Clinical studies have also documented associations between hearing impairment and various handicaps. Although not all studies have had consistent findings, hearing impairment has been associated with dementia in both outpatients (Herbst & Humphrey, 1980; Uhlmann, Larson, Rees, Koepsell, & Duckert, 1989) and institutionalized patients (Weinstein & Amsel, 1986). In addition, decline in cognitive function in demented patients has been observed to be more rapid in those who are also hearing impaired (Peters, Potter, & Scholer, 1988; Uhlmann, Larson, & Koepsell, 1986). Depression, another prevalent problem among the aged, has also been associated with hearing impairment in elderly dwelling in the community (Herbst & Humphrey, 1980; Jones, Victor, & Vetter, 1984). Finally, hearing impairment has been associated

TABLE 20.1
Proportion of Persons Aged 65 and Older with Handicaps Stratified by Level of Self-Reported Hearing Disability

Handicap	Hearing Disability		
	No trouble hearing (%)	All levels of hearing trouble (%)	At best, can hear shouted speech (%)
Limited in activity	38	56	66
Eight or more annual days in bed	18	24	30
Six or more annual physician contacts	28	34	37
Fair to poor self-reported health status	27	38	46

Note. From "Hearing Ability of Persons by Sociodemographic and Health Characteristics: United States" by National Center for Health Statistics and P. W. Ries, 1982, in *Vital and Health Statistics*, Series 10, No. 140, DHHS Publication No. PHS 82-1568, Public Health Service, Washington, DC: U.S. Government Printing Office.

with global function and quality of life; the greater the hearing loss, the greater the level of self-reported physical and psychosocial dysfunction (Bess, Lichtenstein, Logan, Burger, & Nelson, 1989) and the poorer the reported quality of life (Mulrow et al., 1990a).

The causal nature of these generally consistent, graded associations between hearing impairment and resulting handicap remained unproven until completion of a recent randomized trial of aural rehabilitation (Mulrow et al., 1990b). One hundred ninety-four aged male subjects with mean high-frequency pure tone averages of 52 dB HL were randomized to receive hearing aids immediately or be placed on a waiting list. In the group receiving hearing aids there was an 85% and 68% improvement in communicative function compared to controls as measured by the *Hearing Handicap Inventory for the Elderly* (Ventry & Weinstein, 1982) and the *Quantified Denver Scale of Communication* (Alpiner, 1978), respectively. A 30% improvement was also observed in cognitive performance as measured by the *Short Portable Mental Status Questionnaire* (Pfeiffer, 1975). Finally, this study found a 26% improvement in depressive symptoms as assessed by the *Geriatrics Depression Scale* (Yesavage et al., 1983). The effect was noted within 6 weeks and sustained at 4 months. Thus, in an experimental study, aural rehabilitation with hearing aids resulted in a substantial improvement in hearing-related disability and handicap, with small to moderate effects in other handicapping domains.

Applicability of Screening Principles to Hearing

Screening in health care is the process of examining asymptomatic persons to determine if they are likely or unlikely to have the target disorder of interest (Morrison, 1985). Once a screening test is positive, the individual is further evaluated with a more definitive test to determine if the condition is truly present. Hearing impairment in the elderly is an accessible disorder for screening: It is common, progressive, and easily detected. The belief is held by audiologists and physicians that early identification and rehabilitation will ameliorate the adverse effects of hearing impairment.

To judge the effectiveness of a screening program, seven questions must be answered (Cadman, Chambers, Feldman, & Sackett, 1984). The data required to answer all seven questions regarding hearing impairment in the aged are not available, but the questions do provide a framework for assessment and future investigation:

1. *Has the effectiveness of the program been demonstrated in a randomized trial?* Yes. It has recently been shown, in a randomized controlled trial, that hearing aid rehabilitation results in improved communication and quality of life (Mulrow et al., 1989). Two thirds of the subjects in this experimental study were screened in general medical clinic settings. The importance of this study was that aural rehabilitation had positive effects on outcomes other than improved hearing, indicating that hearing impairment may have a causal role in broader types of handicap and disability.

2. *Are efficacious treatments available?* Yes. Hearing aids provide the necessary amplification to overcome hearing impairment. Overall efficacy, however, must be judged by the individual recipient's use of and satisfaction with aural rehabilitation.

3. *Does the burden of suffering warrant screening?* Yes. Hearing impairment has consistently been associated with functional deficits and impairments beyond just the ability to communicate. Hearing impairment affects 25 to 40% of persons over 65 years of age and has been associated with depression and dementia (Herbst & Humphrey, 1980; Weinstein

& Amsel, 1986). There is evidence that impaired hearing results in faster cognitive declines in Alzheimer's disease (Uhlmann et al., 1986).

4. *Are there good screening tests?* Yes. Physical diagnostic tests such as the finger rub and whispered voice have been recently validated (MacPhee, Crowther, & McAlpine, 1988; Uhlmann, Rees, Psaty, & Duckert, 1989). Other instruments, a hand-held audioscope, and self-administered questionnaires have also been validated (Lichtenstein, Bess, & Logan, 1988b).

5. *Does the program reach those who could benefit?* Possibly. Most older persons will see a primary care physician on an annual or biannual basis, providing opportunities for hearing tests. The ability of screening programs to reach other aged subjects (homebound and institutionalized) remains to be demonstrated.

6. *Can the health care system cope with the program?* Unknown. When it becomes accepted that aural rehabilitation results in reduced functional disability and improved quality of life, there will be increased pressure to provide and pay for these services. Resource analyses are needed before public policy can be changed to cover the large population segment that would be eligible for rehabilitation.

7. *Do persons with positive screenings comply with advice and interventions?* Unknown. In one study, 59% of persons complied with further hearing assessment with pure tone audiometry, regardless of the outcome of a screening test (Lichtenstein et al., 1988b). This figure may be higher if only persons with positive screens are referred for evaluation. Persons who did not comply with further audiologic assessment were less likely to perceive themselves as having a hearing handicap. In a smaller study of volunteers who were screened, only 52% of those who failed the protocol for hearing impairment subsequently followed up with the

recommendation for audiologic testing (Koike & Johnston, 1989). Further studies are needed on how older persons adapt to and use hearing aids.

Although progress is being made in investigating the effectiveness of screening for hearing impairment, hearing function should be assessed as part of a standard physical examination when an aged person visits his or her primary care physician.

Screening for Presbycusis

The performance of several types of screens for hearing impairment have been assessed: (a) self-assessment measures (*HHIE-S, SAC*), (b) physical diagnostic maneuvers (whispered voice, tuning fork, finger rub), and (c) pure tone measures (an audioscope).

Self-Perception Scales

Hearing Handicap Inventory for the Elderly–Screening Version

The *Hearing Handicap Inventory for the Elderly–Screening Version* (*HHIE-S*) is a self-administered 10-item questionnaire that detects emotional and social problems associated with impaired hearing (Ventry & Weinstein, 1982) (see Figure 20.1). Subjects answer questions about circumstances related to hearing by stating whether the situation presents a problem. A "no" response scores 0, "sometimes" scores 2, and "yes" scores 4. Total *HHIE-S* scores range from 0 to 40.

Test-retest repeatability for the *HHIE-S* as determined using the Pearson Product-Moment correlation is .84 ($p < .0001$), indicating a high degree of repeatability.

The sensitivities and specificities for different *HHIE-S* scores were determined by examining the distributions of test results in those with and without hearing impairment as defined by the audiogram (hearing impairment defined here as missing a 40-dB

Does a hearing problem cause you to feel embarrassed when you meet new people?

Does a hearing problem cause you to feel frustrated when talking to members of your family?

Do you have difficulty hearing when someone speaks in a whisper?

Do you feel handicapped by a hearing problem?

Does a hearing problem cause you difficulty when visiting friends, relatives, or neighbors?

Does a hearing problem cause you to attend religious services less often than you would like?

Does a hearing problem cause you to have arguments with family members?

Does a hearing problem cause you to have difficulty when listening to television or radio?

Do you feel that any difficulty with your hearing limits/hampers your personal or social life?

Does a hearing problem cause you difficulty when in a restaurant with relatives or friends?

FIGURE 20.1. *Hearing Handicap Inventory for the Elderly*–Screening Version. *Note.* From "The Hearing Handicap Inventory for the Elderly: A New Tool" by I. M. Ventry and B. E. Weinstein, 1982, *Ear and Hearing, 3,* pp. 128–134.

HL signal at either 1 or 2 kHz in each ear or 1 and 2 kHz in one ear). The receiver operator characteristics for the *HHIE-S* at the physicians' offices and the hearing center were virtually identical. With a cutoff point of 8, the sensitivity of the *HHIE-S* was 72% and 76% and specificity was 77% and 71% in the hearing center and physicians' offices, respectively. Above a score of 24, the specificity of the *HHIE-S* was 98% in the hearing center and 96% in the physicians' offices. The corresponding sensitivities were 24% and 30%.

Two studies have independently shown the test accuracy of the *HHIE-S* to be in the 74–79% range (Lichtenstein et al., 1988b; Mulrow, Tuley et al., 1990). The *HHIE-S* has been directly compared with the *Quantified Denver Scale of Communication Function* (Alpiner, 1978) and was found to be more accurate in detecting persons with hearing impairment. The *HHIE-S* was also more responsive than the Denver scales for detecting changes in hearing handicap following hearing aid rehabilitation (Mulrow, Tuley, & Aguilar, 1990).

The likelihood ratios for different levels of the *HHIE-S* are given in Table 20.2. In this group the pretest probability of having a hearing impairment was 30%. For those with *HHIE-S* scores of 0–8, the post-test probability of hearing impairment declined to 13%. For those with scores of 26–40, the post-test probability of impairment rose to 84%. The *HHIE-S* shows a similar level of performance against different definitions of hearing impairment as well. Similar likelihood ratios are found for speech-frequency pure tone averages, high-frequency pure tone averages, and speech reception thresholds (all at 25 dB in the better ear) (Lichtenstein et al., 1988a). Thus the *HHIE-S* is a valid repeatable screening test with a robust performance against different definitions of hearing impairment.

Self Assessment of Communication

The *Self Assessment of Communication* (*SAC*) is a 10-item self-administered questionnaire (Schow & Nerbonne, 1982) (see Figure 20.2). Like the *HHIE-S*, subjects respond to 10 questions about communication difficulties. Responses are recorded on a scale ranging from "almost never" (scored as 1) to "practically always" (scored as 5). A percentage score is then calculated by multiplying the raw score by 2, subtracting 20, and multiplying by 1.25.

When tested on a sample of 50 individuals aged 20 to 80 years, the *SAC's* test-retest reliability was .80 (Schow & Nerbonne, 1982).

The sensitivity and specificity of the *SAC* has been tested in a sample of approximately 1,100 volunteers screened at a

TABLE 20.2
Probability of Hearing Impairment Given a
Hearing Handicap Inventory for the Elderly (HHIE-S) **Score**

HHIE-S Score	Pretest Probability of Hearing Impairment (%)	Likelihood Ratio (95% C.I.)[a]		Post-Test Probability of Hearing Impairment (%)
0–8	30	0.4	(0.2– 0.7)	13
10–24	30	2.3	(1.2– 4.3)	50
26–40	30	12.0	(2.6–55.0)	84

Note. Adapted from "Validation of Screening Tools for Identifying Hearing-Impaired Elderly in Primary Care" by M. J. Lichtenstein, F. H. Bess, and S. A. Logan, 1988, *Journal of the American Medical Association, 259,* pp. 2875–2878. The *HHIE-S* was completed at the hearing center. Pure tone was tested at 40 dB at 1000 and 2000 Hz in each ear. Hearing impairment is defined as either (a) inability to hear tone at one frequency in *each* ear or (b) inability to hear both frequencies in one ear.
[a] C.I. = confidence interval.

health fair (Schow, Smedley, & Longhurst, 1990). Of these, 273 were between the ages of 60 and 69 and 133 were 70 years of age and older. Compared against a pure tone definition of a 40-dB loss at 1 and 2 kHz, a *SAC* score of greater than 18 had a sensitivity of 85% and 80% among the 60- to 69-year-old and 70-or-older groups, respectively. The corresponding specificities were 71% and 69%, respectively.

Although it is not specifically studied in aged individuals, the *SAC* has similar diagnostic characteristics when tested against different pure tone criteria for hearing impairment. In the volunteer sample with an average age of 53 years, the best performance was noted against pure tone criteria of 40 dB at 1 and 2 kHz. The optimal cutoff point on the *SAC* was at 18, yielding a sensitivity of 80% with a specificity of 78% (Schow et al., 1990).

At the time of this writing, the two self-assessment questionnaires, the *HHIE-S* and the *SAC*, have not been directly compared against each other in a single study. In different studies, they appear to have similar diagnostic characteristics. The *SAC's* questions are longer and it has not yet been validated in a screened sample of aged individuals (i.e., in a sample that does not consist only of volunteers).

Physical Diagnostic Maneuvers

Recently, several clinical screening measures have been validated against pure tone audiometry as diagnostic aids for detecting the hearing-impaired aged. These include the whispered voice test (MacPhee et al., 1988; Uhlmann, Rees, Psaty, & Duckert, 1989), the finger rub, and tuning fork tests (Uhlmann, Rees, Psaty, & Duckert, 1989).

Two groups have tested the whispered voice test using different administration techniques, in different clinical settings, and comparing the results against different audiometric criteria. MacPhee and colleagues (1988) studied 62 individuals admitted to acute rehabilitation wards in a geriatric inpatient unit. They administered the whispered voice test by standing behind the individual and occluding one of the ears. The patient was asked to repeat a series of three random numbers at four decreasing levels of loudness: a conversational voice at 6 in. and 2 ft from the ear and a whispered voice following complete exhalation at 6 in. and 2 ft. A pass was achieved if the patient correctly repeated all three numbers or achieved a greater than 50% success rate over three triplet sets of numbers. The audiometric criterion for hearing impairment was defined as an average pure tone thresh-

Do you experience communication difficulties in situations when speaking with one other person? (for example, at home, at work, in a social situation, with a waitress, a store clerk, with a spouse, boss, etc.)

Do you experience communication difficulties in situations when conversing with a small group of several persons? (for example, with friends or family, co-workers, in meetings or casual conversations, over dinner or while playing cards, etc.)

Do you experience communication difficulties while listening to someone speak to a large group? (for example, at church or in a civic meeting, in a fraternal or women's club, at an educational lecture, etc.)

Do you experience communication difficulties while participating in various types of entertainment? (for example, movies, TV, radio, plays, night clubs, musical entertainment, etc.)

Do you experience communication difficulties when you are in an unfavorable listening environment? (for example, at a noisy party, where there is background music, when riding in an auto or bus, when someone whispers or talks from across the room, etc.)

Do you experience communication difficulties when using or listening to various communication devices? (for example, telephone, telephone ring, doorbell, public address system, warning signals, alarms, etc.)

Do you feel that any difficulty with your hearing limits or hampers your personal or social life?

Does any problem or difficulty with your hearing upset you?

Do others suggest that you have a hearing problem?

Do others leave you out of conversations or become annoyed because of your hearing?

FIGURE 20.2. *Self Assessment of Communication (SAC). Note.* From ''Communication Screening Profile: Use with Elderly Clients'' by R. L. Schow and M. A. Nerbonne, 1982, *Ear and Hearing, 3,* pp. 135–147.

old of greater than 30 dB at 0.5, 1, and 2 kHz. The concordance between two observers was 88% of all ears. Of the 124 ears tested, 61% were deemed impaired by the audiometric criterion. Judged against this pure tone standard, the sensitivity and specificity of the whispered voice test were 100% and 84% at 2 ft and 73% and 100% at 6 in., respectively. For conversational voice at 2 ft, the sensitivity was 47% and the specificity was 100%.

Uhlmann and colleagues (Uhlmann, Rees, Psaty, & Duckert, 1989) administered the whispered voice test to 34 demented and 31 nondemented aged outpatients. In their study the whispered voice test used spondee words and was first administered face to face to familiarize the patients with the procedure. The examiner then administered six words at a distance of 6 in. from the test ear. With correct identification of 3 out of 6 words (50% criterion), the examiner withdrew at 6-in. increments until the patient failed to meet the 50% correct identification criterion. The pure tone criterion for impaired hearing was a pure tone average of 40 dB or greater at 0.5, 1, 2, and 3 kHz. The inter-rater reliability was .67 in 44 ears of nondemented subjects, and .78 in 38 ears of demented subjects. Among demented patients, in 68 ears, at a distance of 7 in., the whispered voice test had a sensitivity of 90% with a specificity of 78%. For nondemented patients, at a distance of 11 in. and with a sensitivity of 90%, the corresponding specificity was 70%. With the sensitivity level lowered to 80%, the specificities were 89% among demented subjects and 82% among nondemented subjects. The correlation between the whispered voice test and the pure tone averages ranged from .44 (at 0.25 kHz) to .72 (at 2 kHz).

Other physical diagnostic maneuvers for detecting hearing impairment in the aged also have diagnostic utility. Uhlmann and colleagues (Uhlmann, Rees, Psaty, & Duckert, 1989) tested the performance of a 512-Hz tuning fork, a 1024-Hz tuning fork, and the finger rub test; these instruments have also been tested against pure tone audiometry in their demented and nondemented subjects. In the finger rub test, the examiner rubs her or his index finger and thumb successively together 1 in. from the external auditory canal and slowly withdraws until the signal is no longer heard. For the tuning forks, the examiner holds the fork firmly by the stem and strikes the tines gently against the heel of her or his hand. After the examiner briefly checks to confirm that the tuning fork has been properly struck, the vibrating fork is held 1 in. from the external auditory canal. The tuning fork is withdrawn from the ear at a rate of 1 ft/s and the patient is instructed to report when the tone is no longer audible. In this study,

ears were considered hearing impaired if the average loss at 0.5, 1, 2, and 3 kHz was greater than or equal to 40 dB. The results are given in Table 20.3.

In demented patients, at set sensitivities, the observed specificities ranged from 82% to 95%; however, among nondemented subjects, the specificities were lower, 49% to 69%. The tests were also found to be repeatable, with correlation coefficients of .89 and .90 for the finger rub in nondemented and demented patients, .66 and .87 for the 512-Hz tuning fork, but only .38 and .58 for the 1024-Hz tuning fork.

Pure Tone Measures

The Welch-Allyn Audioscope is a hand-held instrument that delivers a 20-, 25-, or 40-dB HL tone at 500, 1000, 2000, and 4000 Hz. To use the audioscope, the largest ear speculum needed to achieve a seal within the external auditory canal is selected. The tym-

TABLE 20.3
Sensitivities and Specificities of Physical Examination Tests in Detecting Hearing Impairment

Test	Distance[a]	Spec.	Distance[a]	Spec.	Test/Retest Reliability
	Demented Patients (68 ears)				
	(Sens. = 90%)		(Sens. = 80%)		(38 ears)
512-Hz tuning fork	40	53%	27	82%	.66
1024-Hz tuning fork	36	63%	23	95%	.38
Finger rub	8	85%	3	95%	.89
	Nondemented Patients (62 ears)				
	(Sens. = 90%)		(Sens. = 80%)		(44 ears)
512-Hz tuning fork	40	56%	34	64%	.87
1024-Hz tuning fork	45	44%	31	69%	.58
Finger rub	21	44%	16	49%	.90

Note. Adapted from ''Validity and Reliability of Auditory Screening Tests in Demented and Non-demented Older Adults'' by R. F. Uhlmann, T. S. Rees, B. M. Psaty, and L. G. Duckert, 1989, *Journal of General Internal Medicine,* *4,* pp. 90–95.
[a] Distance of test from ear in centimeters.

panic membrane is then visualized; if it is obstructed by cerumen, the impaction must be removed before testing. The tonal sequence is then initiated with the subject indicating by raising a finger that he or she hears the tone.

The audioscope has been validated in the aged against pure tone audiometry (Lichtenstein et al., 1988b) using the definition for hearing impairment proposed by Weinstein and Ventry (1983): Subjects were considered hearing impaired if (a) they had a 40-dB loss at either the 1000- *or* 2000-Hz frequencies in both ears or (b) they had a 40-dB loss at 1000 *and* 2000 Hz in one ear. Subjects were tested in physicians' offices and in a hearing center.

The kappa statistic, which is a measure of the observed agreement that is not a result of chance, was used to test between-occasion and between-observer agreement for the audioscope results (Sackett et al., 1985). The between-location agreement of audioscope results is shown in Table 20.4 by frequency and ear. The kappa values ranged from .41 for the left ear at 500 Hz to .74 for the left ear at 2000 Hz.

The performance of the audioscope against the audiogram definition of hearing impairment is shown in Table 20.5. Using this definition, the prevalence of hearing impairment was 30%. The sensitivity of the audioscope in the physicians' offices and the hearing center was identical, 94%. However, the specificity of the audioscope was significantly lower in the physicians' offices compared to the hearing center (72% vs. 90%). The lower specificity in the physicians' offices probably arises from higher ambient background noise levels in these settings. Thus the audioscope is a sensitive, repeatable test for the detection of hearing impairment in the elderly. Its moderate specificity in the primary care setting would have the effect of an increase in false positive identification of hearing impairment.

Both the audioscope and *HHIE-S* were tested and compared in the same study (Lichtenstein et al., 1988b). The audioscope is very sensitive but moderately specific in the physicians' offices. The *HHIE-S* is

TABLE 20.4
Between-Location Agreement of Audioscope Results: Physicians' Offices vs. Hearing Center

Frequency (Hz)	Kappa Statistic[a]	
	Right Ear	Left Ear
500	.50	.41
1000	.50	.51
2000	.71	.74
4000	.65	.62

Note. Adapted from "Validation of Screening Tools for Identifying Hearing-Impaired Elderly in Primary Care" by M. J. Lichtenstein, F. H. Bess, and S. A. Logan, 1988, *Journal of the American Medical Association, 259,* pp. 2875–2878.
[a] All values are statistically significant at *p* < .0001.

moderately sensitive but highly specific at scores greater than 24. The greatest test accuracy (83%) in identifying hearing impairment was found when the two tests were combined. Persons should be considered in need of referral if they fail the audioscope *and* have an *HHIE-S* score greater than 8 *or* they pass the audioscope *and* have an *HHIE-S* score greater than 24.

All the screening tests studied are useful tools in the initial identification of hearing impairment in the elderly; to determine if any one test is better than the others would require direct comparative studies performed under field conditions. Each test has its advantages and disadvantages. The *HHIE-S* and *SAC* questionnaires remove observers from the screening process, rely on self-reporting, and have been validated against different criteria of pure tone loss. They have the disadvantage of being less sensitive and specific than some of the other screening tools, depending on the score chosen as predictive of hearing handicap. The physical examination maneuvers are inexpensive and portable. While the reported interobserver agreement is fairly high, further standardization is necessary (e.g., less variability in intensity of the whispered voice or more accurate measurement of the distance from the ear for the finger

TABLE 20.5
**Sensitivity and Specificity of the Audioscope for Detecting Hearing Impairment
When Compared to the Audiogram**

Site	Prevalence of Hearing Impairment (%)	Number of Persons	Sensitivity (%)	Specificity (%)
Physicians' Offices	30	174	94	72
Hearing Center	30	171	94	90

Note. Adapted from "Validation of Screening Tools for Identifying Hearing-Impaired Elderly in Primary Care" by M. J. Lichtenstein, F. H. Bess, and S. A. Logan, 1988, *Journal of the American Medical Association, 259,* pp. 2875–2878. Pure tone was tested at 40 dB at 1000 and 2000 Hz in each ear. Hearing impairment is defined as either (a) inability to hear tone at one frequency in *each* ear or (b) inability to hear both frequencies in one ear.

rub test) before their reliability may be accepted. Compared to the traditional physical diagnostic tests, the audioscope, although it is more expensive, delivers a standard signal at a standard distance (right at the external auditory canal) and may be less dependent on observer variability and performance than the other tests.

Defining Criteria for Hearing Impairment in the Aged

The chapter began by making the point that there is not a one-to-one correlation between hearing impairment and hearing handicap. Indeed, the correlation between-pure tone thresholds and performance on self-reported scales of handicap such as the *HHIE-S* is on the order of .5 to .6 (Weinstein & Ventry, 1983). The pure tone criterion used to identify impairment worthy of amplification must ultimately be chosen based on its correlation with either a self-reported functional measure of handicap or a standardized screening communication test designed to assess handicap. Communication tests may be needed to assess those individuals who have impairment and are handicapped, but who for some reason do not perceive their hearing loss as the source of their disability.

Settling the debate over which combination of pure tone thresholds and which frequencies best identify the hearing-handicapped elderly will depend on comparison of these criteria with functional scales. Bess, Lichtenstein, Logan, and Burger (1989) compared four criteria of impairment with the *HHIE-S.* The criteria were a speech-frequency pure tone average (SFPTA) (greater than or equal to a 25-dB average at 0.5, 1, and 2 kHz in the better ear), a high-frequency pure tone average (HFPTA) (greater than or equal to a 25-dB average at 1, 2, and 4 kHz in the better ear), the criterion of Ventry and Weinstein (VW) (a 40-dB criterion—see above), and a speech reception threshold (SRT) (greater than or equal to 25 dB in the better ear).

In these analyses the four criteria of impairment were not independent but had large areas of overlap. Between-criteria agreement was assessed using kappa statistics. The kappa values for agreement beyond that resulting from chance ranged from .36 for the VW and HFPTA to .76 for the SRT and SFPTA, with all other comparisons falling in between. The amount of handicap varied with the number of criteria failed: Subjects passing all four criteria had mean *HHIE-S* scores of 3, those failing one criterion had scores of 8, and so on; subjects who failed all four criteria of impairment had average scores of 17.

Approximately one fifth of individuals over age 65 failed only the HFPTA. Regression techniques showed that a combination of the VW and HFPTA criteria contributed most to explaining the variance in the *HHIE-S*. The subset of individuals failing only the HFPTA is important, because their inclusion as handicapped would effectively double the prevalence of hearing impairment. Whether or not amplification of 25-dB levels of hearing loss results in improved function remains to be studied.

These analyses demonstrate that functional scales, whether they are communication-specific or measures of illness-related dysfunction, may be used to refine and select criteria of hearing impairment.

Research Needs

With respect to screening aged individuals for hearing impairment, the following problems remain to be addressed:

1. Surveys are needed to identify why many persons with hearing impairment and functional handicap do not perceive their hearing impairment as the source of their handicap.

2. A consensus should be sought to settle on a functional standard of hearing handicap against which to judge impairment criteria. It may be found that a handicapped individual merits amplification whether his or her impairment is in the 20-dB or 40-dB range.

3. Experimental studies are needed to assess whether amplification of mild levels of hearing impairment results in improved function and quality of life.

4. Cost analyses are needed to assess the economic impact of aural rehabilitation on the health care system.

5. Direct comparisons of the various screening tools available with audiometrically assessed impairment criteria under field conditions are needed to determine if one screening tool has a clear advantage over the others.

6. The characteristics of individuals who are identified as hearing impaired at screening but do not accept referral for audiologic assessment requires further definition.

7. Cohort studies are needed to determine the optimal screening interval for detecting impaired hearing in individuals as they age.

Once these problems are resolved, elderly individuals may be efficiently screened for hearing impairment and effectively rehabilitated for their hearing handicap.

References

AAO/ACO. (1979). American Medical Association. Guide for the evaluation of hearing handicap. *Journal of the American Medical Association, 241,* 2055–2059.

Alpiner, J. (1978). Evaluation of communication function. In J. Alpiner (Ed.), *Handbook of adult rehabilitative audiology* (pp. 18–78). Baltimore, MD: Williams & Wilkins.

Bess, F. H., Lichtenstein, M. J., Logan, S. A., & Burger, M. C. (1989). Comparing criteria of hearing impairment in the elderly: A functional approach. *Journal of Speech and Hearing Research, 32,* 795–802.

Bess, F. H., Lichtenstein, M. J., Logan, S. A., Burger, M. C., & Nelson, E. (1989). Hearing impairment as a determinant of function in the elderly. *Journal of the American Geriatrics Society, 37,* 123–128.

Cadman, D., Chambers, L., Feldman, W., & Sackett, D. (1984). Assessing the effectiveness of community screening programs. *Journal of the American Medical Association, 251,* 1580–1585.

Collins, J. G. (1988). Prevalence of selected chronic conditions, United States, 1983–85. *NCHS Advance Data,* No. 155, 1–14.

Herbst, K. G., & Humphrey, C. (1980). Hearing impairment and mental state in the elderly living at home. *British Medical Journal, 281,* 903–905.

Jones, D. A., Victor, C. R., & Vetter, N. J. (1984). Hearing difficulty and its psychological implications for the elderly. *Journal of Epidemiology and Community Health, 38,* 75–78.

Koike, K. J. M., & Johnston, A. P. (1989). Follow-up survey of the elderly who failed a hearing screening protocol. *Ear and Hearing, 10,* 250–253.

Lichtenstein, M. J., Bess, F. H., & Logan, S. A. (1988a). Diagnostic performance of the Hearing Handicap Inventory for the Elderly (Screening Version) against differing definitions of hearing loss. *Ear and Hearing, 9,* 208–211.

Lichtenstein, M. J., Bess, F. H., & Logan, S. A. (1988b). Validation of screening tools for identifying hearing-impaired elderly in primary care. *Journal of the American Medical Association, 259,* 2875–2878.

MacPhee, G. J. A., Crowther, J. A., & McAlpine, C. H. (1988). A simple screening test for hearing impairment in elderly patients. *Age and Ageing, 17,* 347–351.

Morrison, A. S. (1985). *Screening in chronic disease* (Monographs in Epidemiology and Biostatistics, Vol. 7). New York: Oxford University Press.

Moscicki, E. K., Elkins, E. F., Baum, H. M., & McNamara, P. M. (1985). Hearing loss in the elderly: An epidemiologic study of the Framingham Heart Study Cohort. *Ear and Hearing, 6,* 184–190.

Mulrow, C. D., Aguilar, C., Endicott, J. E., Velez, R., Tuley, M. R., Charlip, W. S., & Hill, J. A. (1990a). Association between hearing impairment and the quality of life of elderly individuals. *Journal of the American Geriatrics Society, 38,* 45–50.

Mulrow, C. D., Aguilar, C., Endicott, J. E., Velez, R., Tuley, M. R., Charlip, W. S., & Hill, J. A. (1990b). Quality-of-life changes and hearing impairment: A randomized trial. *Annals of Internal Medicine, 113,* 188–194.

Mulrow, C. D., Tuley, M. R., & Aguilar, C. (1990). Discriminating and responsiveness abilities of two hearing handicap scales. *Ear and Hearing, 11,* 176–180.

National Center for Health Statistics & Ries, P. W. (1982). Hearing ability of persons by sociodemographic and health characteristics: United States. *Vital and health statistics* (Series 10, No. 140, DHHS Publication No. PHS 82-1568. Public Health Service). Washington, DC: U.S. Government Printing Office.

Peters, C. A., Potter, J. F., & Scholer, S. G. (1988). Hearing impairment as a predictor of cognitive decline in dementia. *Journal of the American Geriatrics Society, 36,* 981–986.

Pfeiffer, E. (1975). A short portable mental status questionnaire for the assessment of organic brain deficit in elderly patients. *Journal of the American Geriatrics Society, 23,* 433–441.

Sackett, D. L., Haynes, R. B., & Tugwell, P. (1985). Clinical diagnostic strategies. In *Clinical epidemiology: A basic science for clinical medicine* (pp. 3–16). Boston: Little, Brown.

Salomon, G. (1986). Hearing problems in the elderly. *Danish Medical Bulletin* (Special Suppl. Series, No. 3), 1–22.

Schow, R. L., & Nerbonne, M. A. (1982). Communication screening profile: Use with elderly clients. *Ear and Hearing, 3,* 135–147.

Schow, R. L., Smedley, T. C., & Longhurst, T. M. (1990). Self assessment and impairment in adult/elderly hearing screening—Recent data and new perspectives. *Ear and Hearing, 11,* 175–285.

Uhlmann, R. F., Larson, E. B., & Koepsell, T. D. (1986). Hearing impairment and cognitive decline in senile dementia of the Alzheimer's type. *Journal of the American Geriatrics Society, 34,* 207–210.

Uhlmann, R. F., Larson, E. B., Rees, T. S., Koepsell, T. D., & Duckert, L. G. (1989). Relationship of hearing impairment to dementia and cognitive dysfunction in older adults. *Journal of the American Medical Association, 261,* 1916–1919.

Uhlmann, R. F., Rees, T. S., Psaty, B. M., & Duckert, L. G. (1989). Validity and reliability of auditory screening tests in demented and non-demented older adults. *Journal of General Internal Medicine, 4,* 90–96.

Ventry, I. M., & Weinstein, B. E. (1982). The Hearing Handicap Inventory for the Elderly: A new tool. *Ear and Hearing, 3,* 128–134.

Weinstein, B. E., & Amsel, L. (1986). Hearing loss and senile dementia in the institutionalized elderly. *Clinical Gerontologist, 4,* 3–15.

Weinstein, B. E., & Ventry, I. M. (1983). Audiometric correlates of the Hearing Handicap Inventory for the Elderly. *Journal of Speech and Hearing Disorders, 48,* 379–384.

World Health Organization. (1980). The consequences of disease. In *International classification of impairments, disabilities, and handicaps* (pp. 23–46). Geneva: World Health Organization.

Yesavage, J. A., Brink, T. L., Rose, T. L., Lum, O., Huang, V., Adey, M., & Leirer, V. O. (1983). Development and validation of a geriatric depression screening scale: A preliminary report. *Journal of Psychiatric Research, 17,* 37–49.

The Audiologic Assessment

Sandra M. Gordon-Salant, PhD ■

Hearing loss associated specifically with the aging process is called *presbycusis.* Temporal bone studies have shown that senescent changes can affect every level of the auditory system (Johnsson & Hawkins, 1972; Kirikae, Sato, & Shitara, 1965). Consequently, auditory system dysfunction at one or more levels may be evident on a variety of threshold and suprathreshold behavioral and electrophysiological measures. Etiologic factors contributing to auditory system dysfunction, independent of presbycusic changes, may also be present in older people.

Each older person seeking audiologic evaluation presents a unique set of audiologic characteristics. The audiologist should be cognizant of these attributes, which may affect hearing measurement. First, changes in the auditory system may be attributed to a variety of etiologies that occur either alone or in combination with changes associated with age. Second, a number of physical and cognitive limitations may be present in an older person that can affect behavior during testing. Third, the site of lesion can be at any level of the peripheral or central auditory system, and multiple lesion sites may coexist. Fourth, the individual's reported experiences with hearing difficulty may be unrelated to the degree of measured hearing loss. Consequently, the audiologist's role in evaluating older people is to confirm the existence of hearing loss, determine the degree and configuration of the loss, determine the site of lesion, and assess the impact of the hearing loss on the individual's daily function, including speech communication. This chapter will present useful strategies for obtaining reliable and valid audiometric information from elderly people in order to meet these objectives.

The Case History

The case history is an important prelude to every audiologic assessment. The audiologist should be able to anticipate some of the characteristics of the hearing loss from the case history. Moreover, the case history provides an opportunity to observe the patient's general behavior and communication skills, which can influence subsequent test behavior. The client's attitudes about the hearing loss, hearing aids, and aural rehabilitation can be sampled during this initial interview. These responses can prove useful in formulating recommendations for the client.

Styles in obtaining a case history range from a nondirect conversational approach (Rosenberg, 1978) to a direction questionnaire that is completed before the audiologic evaluation. For elderly clients, a direct interview style to obtain specific information and explore problem areas is the most effective.

Most of the routine information obtained from an adult client should be obtained from the older client as well. This includes identifying information, the client's major complaint, history of auditory and vestibular symptoms, family history of hearing loss, and history of occupational and recreational noise exposure. Any present or past incidence of significant otologic disorders should be explored. In addition, information pertaining to the client's general health and medical history should be obtained. All current medications should be specified because of the potential synergistic effect of numerous medications on hearing (Barza, Lauermann, Tally, & Gorbach, 1980). History of cardiovascular disease and cardiovascular risk factors should also be explored because of their potential role in age-related hearing loss (Rubinstein, Hildescheimer, Zokar, & Chilarovitz, 1977). Apparent physical disability or neuromuscular disorder should be noted because of a possible common etiology with hearing loss and because of the need to modify behavioral responses during testing. Finally, questions should be asked about the client's history of prior audiologic management. These questions may also be asked of an accompanying family member or caregiver, especially if the older client's communication skills or memory are poor.

Measurement of Hearing Handicap

General

An important supplement to the case history and audiologic evaluation is an assessment of the impact of the hearing loss on the client's ability to function in daily activities. The measurement of hearing handicap has received increasing attention in recent years because routine audiologic measures do not adequately predict or describe the effect of the hearing loss. In addition to sensory and processing factors, issues such as reaction to the hearing loss, general personality adjustment, attitudes of family and friends, and communication strategies and environment probably influence the realistic consequences of an individual's hearing impairment. A number of scales (e.g., Demorest & Erdman, 1987; Giolas, Owens, Lamb, & Schubert, 1979) have been developed to evaluate some or all of these factors. Selection of an appropriate scale requires scrutiny of the structure and applicability of each available scale for elderly subjects.

Demorest and Walden (1984) reviewed the fundamental issues for selecting, interpreting, and evaluating a hearing handicap instrument. One important consideration in the selection of a self-report is using one that is designed for the type of population being served. These authors suggest that when an inventory is applied to elderly individuals, the content of the questions should be appropriate for the elderly person's life-style, the response format should be understandable to the person responding, and the method of administration should be in an interview format. Instruments being selected also should satisfy the general criteria of high internal consistency reliability, high test-retest reliability and stability, and low standard error of measurement. Demorest and Walden note that the items on the inventory should sample areas of importance in determining the effect of the hearing loss and should extract useful information for a specific application.

Scales Developed for the Elderly

Four handicap scales are currently available that were developed for an elderly population. One of these scales, the *Hearing Handicap Inventory for the Elderly* (*HHIE*) (Ventry & Weinstein, 1982) was designed for administration to noninstitutionalized elderly individuals. It consists of 25 items assigned to two subscales that sample the social/situational effects and emotional effects of the hearing loss. The scale can be administered in a paper-and-pencil format, although a face-to-face interview is preferred (Weinstein, Spitzer, & Ventry, 1986). Evaluation of this instrument revealed that it has high internal consistency (Ventry & Weinstein, 1982); high test-retest reliability (Weinstein et al., 1986); and a low standard error of measurement, especially if it is administered in a face-to-face situation (Weinstein et al., 1986). Recently, Newman and Weinstein (1989) reported high test-retest reliability in *HHIE* scores for face-to-face administration followed by paper-and-pencil administration. This approach could be useful in identifying changes in perceived hearing handicap when clients are unable to return to the clinic for further evaluation after receiving a hearing aid.

The three other scales developed for senior citizens are intended for individuals living in extended care facilities. They include the *Denver Scale of Communication Function for Senior Citizens Living in a Retirement Center* (*DSSC*) (Zarnoch & Alpiner, 1977), the *Nursing Home Hearing Handicap Index* (*NHHHI*) (Schow & Nerbonne, 1977), and the *Communication Assessment Procedure for Seniors* (*CAPS*) (Alpiner & Baker, 1980). The *NHHHI* (resident version) is a 10-item questionnaire that samples emotional reactions to communication difficulties and situational difficulties. Its brief form suggests

that it serves as a screening tool for handicap. The *CAPS* primarily assesses an individual's emotional response to hearing difficulty, participation in general communication, and personality attributes. The last section evaluates the individual's attitudes about rehabilitation strategies. The major limitation of this questionnaire is that it does not assess directly communicative situations that the listener perceives as difficult. The *DSSC* contains many of the same questions found in the *CAPS*, but presented in a different organization. In addition, the *DSSC* explores the relevance and specificity of the broad questions to the individual resident. The limitations of the *CAPS* apply as well to the *DSSC*. Published data on internal reliability, test-retest reliability, and other psychometric characteristics of these three instruments are not available.

Threshold Sensitivity Measures—Pure Tones

Air Conduction Thresholds

Individual elderly listeners exhibit a wide variety of audiograms (Harford & Dodds, 1982) as measured by standard audiometric techniques (American Speech-Language-Hearing Association [ASHA], 1978; American National Standards Institute, 1978). Average audiograms of large samples of elderly individuals as a function of age and sex have been described (Corso, 1963; Goetzinger, Proud, Dirks, & Embrey, 1961; Moscicki, Elkins, Baum, & McNamara, 1985). These studies consistently found significant effects of age and sex. The overall trends are that men have somewhat poorer hearing than women in the higher frequencies and that hearing thresholds are poorer with each age decade between the ages of 60 and 90. Figure 21.1 presents mean pure tone threshold data from Moscicki et al. (1985) that exemplify these findings. Although shifts in hearing thresholds with

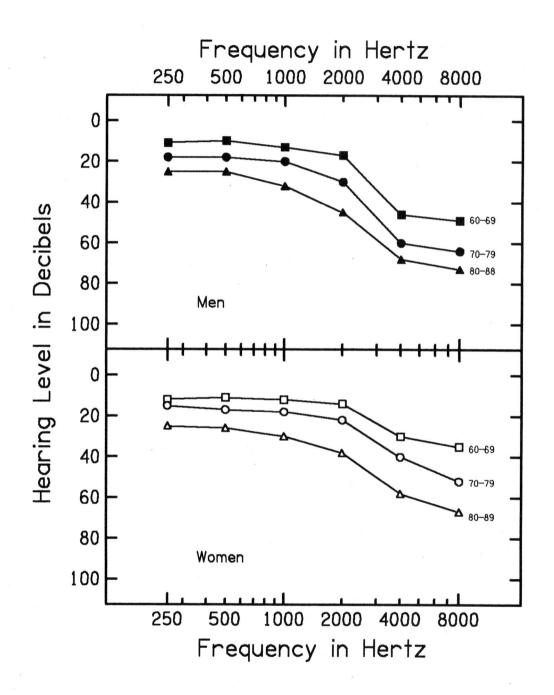

FIGURE 21.1. Mean pure tone thresholds across frequency as a function of age and sex, from the Framingham cohort study. *Note.* From "Hearing Loss in the Elderly: An Epidemiologic Study of the Framingham Heart Study Cohort" by E. K. Moscicki, E. F. Elkins, H. F. Baum, and P. M. McNamara, 1985, *Ear and Hearing, 6,* pp. 184–190. Copyright 1985 by Williams & Wilkins. Adapted by permission.

age are noted for all frequencies, the most dramatic shifts for men and women are in the higher frequencies. The typical audiometric configuration can be described as sharply sloping for men and gradually sloping for women (Moscicki et al., 1985).

Cross-sectional studies, such as those described in the preceding paragraph, are useful for determining differences that exist between age groups. It is equally important to examine data obtained from the same individuals over a period of time. Such longitudinal data describe the rate at which individuals change in a particular attribute. Recently, Brant and Fozard (1990) examined

pure tone thresholds on Bekesy audiograms obtained from 813 men in seven different age groups over a 15-year time period. The rates of change in pure tone thresholds in the speech frequencies (500 Hz, 1000 Hz, and 2000 Hz) exhibited a marked decline starting at about the age of 60. In contrast, the rate of decline in hearing loss at the highest frequency (8000 Hz) was relatively constant at all ages (Figure 21.2). These results suggest that among elderly males, hearing in the speech frequencies begins to deteriorate more rapidly than hearing in the higher frequencies. This may occur because hearing in the high frequencies has already

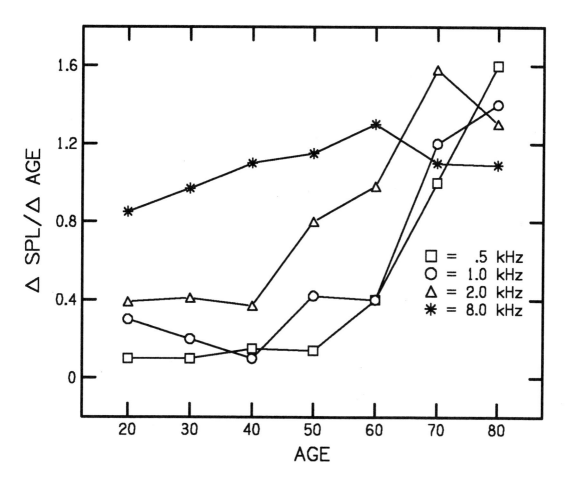

FIGURE 21.2. Rates of change in sound pressure level with respect to age at four frequencies. *Note.* From ''Age Changes in Pure Tone Hearing Thresholds in a Longitudinal Study of Normal Human Aging'' by L. J. Brant and J. L. Fozard, 1990, *Journal of the Acoustical Society of America, 88,* pp. 813–820. Copyright 1990 by the American Institute of Physics. Adapted by permission.

declined significantly in the preceding decades, and because deterioration of sensory and neural structures of the peripheral auditory system is spreading to previously unaffected regions.

A fundamental issue for interpreting hearing loss data is whether shifts in pure tone thresholds with increased age reflect innate senescent changes in the auditory system or the combined effects of external factors that accumulate over time. "Pure" presbycusis is the term used to describe threshold hearing loss that is associated solely with aging effects. One recent epidemiologic study of hearing impairment in 2,293 subjects aged 57 to 89 years reported that only 16% of all subjects had a negative otologic history (Moscicki et al., 1985). Thus, most hearing losses in an elderly population can be explained by acquired, exogenous factors. In men, the most important reported predisposing factors were history of noise exposure and history of associated illness. In women, the most important reported predisposing factors were family history of hearing loss and history of Ménière's disease and other illnesses.

Hearing loss associated with exposure to sounds and noises of everyday living (*sociocusis*) also affects pure tone thresholds of elderly people. Individuals living in industrialized societies are known to have poorer thresholds than age- and sex-matched individuals living in noise-free societies (Kryter, 1983). Moreover, the sex differences seen in pure tone thresholds of subjects living in industrialized societies are related to differences in the amount of noise exposure between men and women. Pure tone thresholds of individuals of various ages living in a noise-free environment reflect "pure" presbycusis and indicate that presbycusis produces a slight hearing loss, as shown in Figure 21.3. These thresholds were averages from male and female data because there were no inherent gender differences with aging. Other risk factors in addition to noise exposure that may contribute to differences in pure tone thresholds between elderly individuals in industrial-

ized and nonindustrialized societies include diet, multiple medications, cardiovascular disease, and atherosclerosis.

Bone Conduction Thresholds

Shifts in air conduction pure tone sensitivity with age are usually accompanied by shifts in bone conduction pure tone sensitivity (Goetzinger et al., 1961). Most studies reporting bone conduction thresholds as a function of age indicate that these thresholds are equivalent to air conduction thresholds, reflecting a pure sensorineural hearing loss (Goetzinger et al., 1961; Marshall, Martinez, & Schlaman, 1983). Several early reports, however, noted the presence of high-frequency air-bone gaps in elderly subjects with no history of specific middle ear disease (Glorig & Davis, 1961; Milne, 1977; Rosen, Bergman, Plester, El-Mofty, & Sattis, 1962). At least one study reported that 24% of elderly individuals in a large population exhibited mixed hearing losses (Moscicki et al., 1985). Very few subjects in the sample were found to have conductive losses that were independent of sensorineural loss. A conductive lesion may result from active middle ear pathology or senescent changes in the middle ear system such as atrophy of the middle ear muscles and joints (Rosenwasser, 1964), calcification and ossification of the ossicular chain (Hinchcliffe, 1962), and reduced tympanic membrane elasticity (Covell, 1952). Alternatively, ear canal collapse resulting from earphone pressure could produce an ostensible high-frequency air-bone gap. This issue will be discussed in a later section.

A recent report by Marshall et al. (1983) employed careful methodological controls and found no evidence of significant air-bone gaps in listeners of different ages (including elderly subjects). The different findings among studies suggest that methodological constraints affected the results. In a general population of elderly subjects who are not screened for middle ear pathology, the incidence of air-bone gaps appears to be relatively high. However, when a sam-

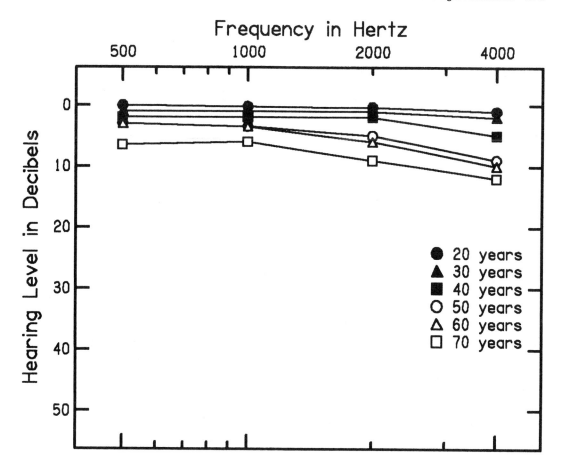

FIGURE 21.3. Audiograms of pure presbycusis. Pure tone thresholds obtained from males and females in a noise-free society, as a function of age, derived from Kryter's (1983) transformations of data reported by Rosen et al. (1962). *Note.* From "Basic Hearing Evaluation" by S. Gordon-Salant, 1987. In *Communication Disorders in Aging* (pp. 301–333) by H. G. Mueller and V. C. Geoffrey (Eds.), Washington, DC: Gallaudet University Press. Copyright 1987 by Gallaudet University Press. Reprinted by permission.

ple of subjects is restricted to those with negative otologic histories, the incidence of conductive lesion appears to be low.

Sources of Threshold Inaccuracy

Two sources of threshold inaccuracy have been implicated as contributing to reduced auditory thresholds in elderly subjects. The first source relates to the hypothesis that elderly subjects employ a more conservative response criterion on listening tasks than do younger subjects. As a consequence, elderly listeners are more hesitant to indicate sig-

nal perception when they are not confident that a signal was presented. Since clinical procedures for determining threshold do not separate out response bias effects from sensory (detectability) effects, the measured pure tone threshold could be reduced because of an elderly listener's cautious behavior. The theory of signal detection (Green & Swets, 1966) has been applied to auditory tasks to obtain separate measures of sensory and decision factors in listeners of different ages. Although several early reports (Potash & Jones, 1977; Rees & Botwinick, 1971) indicated that elderly subjects exhibited more cautious response criteria than younger subjects on pure tone detection tasks, careful controls for stimulus presentation levels and auditory characteristics between young and elderly subjects were not employed. Marshall and Jesteadt (1986) measured response bias and auditory threshold using clinical and research procedures for determining audibility thresholds. Subjects included young and elderly subjects matched for either normal hearing or hearing loss. Results showed no difference in response bias between groups of listeners, as measured on either threshold procedure. Thus, differences in response bias do not appear to influence substantially pure tone thresholds as measured in the clinical setting.

A second potential problem in measuring pure tone thresholds is ear canal collapse. Complete or partial closure of the cartilaginous portion of the external auditory canal occurs when pressure is applied to the pinna and canal, as with circumaural cushion placement, resulting in an apparent conductive hearing loss. Possible causes of collapsing canals include an anteriorly displaced conchal fold or abnormally flaccid ear canals. Both of these conditions can occur with aging, when density and elasticity changes in skin and cartilage are common. The incidence of collapsing ear canals in an elderly population is approximately 10–36% (Randolph & Schow, 1983). The preferred procedure for minimizing this problem is to obtain threshold measurements with insert earphones (Clemis, Ballad, & Killion, 1986). Reference equivalent threshold sound pressure levels for calibration of insert earphones have become available recently (American National Standards Institute, 1989; Wilber, Kruger, & Killion, 1988).

Modifications in the Standard Procedure

The standard clinical procedure (ASHA, 1978) for assessing pure tone thresholds is expected to produce reliable and valid thresholds for most noninstitutionalized elderly clients. Circumstances may exist, however, when the routine procedure must be modified to accommodate the elderly individual's physical, cognitive, or linguistic limitations.

Physical limitations resulting from a variety of medical disorders often become increasingly disabling as the individual ages. Neurological disorders, such as Parkinsonism and hemiplegia resulting from stroke, may render older people unable to control their motor responses in a time-locked manner. Alternative responses to hand raising and button pushing can be used, as long as the response is under the listener's control and conveys stimulus detection. Some plausible alternative response modes include eyeblink, verbal response, visual scanning, and hand squeeze. In addition, use of a descending method of limits and practice trials may improve threshold estimates for stroke patients (Formby, Phillips, & Thomas, 1987; Ludlow & Swisher, 1971).

Speech Thresholds

Assessment of speech thresholds may be incorporated in the routine test battery, although it is not considered essential (Wilson & Margolis, 1983). Speech thresholds are useful for validating the pure tone audiogram and evaluating difficult-to-test patients. A preferred method for determining the threshold level for speech has been described recently (American Speech-Language-Hearing Association [ASHA], 1988).

Elderly individuals are expected to exhibit speech thresholds that are consistent with pure tone detection thresholds. Data from three studies (Goetzinger et al., 1961; Jokinen, 1973; Plomp & Mimpen, 1979) are shown in Figure 21.4 and indicate that thresholds in quiet begin to decrease above age 49, with an accelerated deterioration above age 70. It should be noted, however, that none of these studies employed either

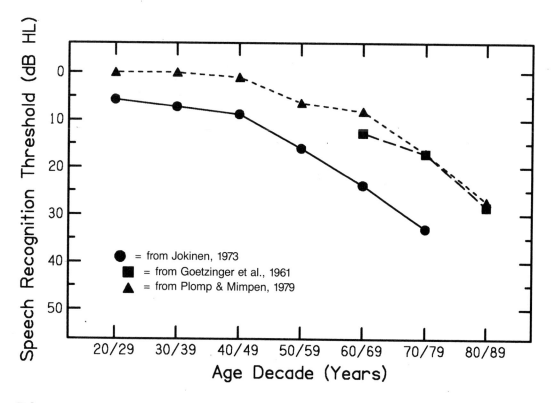

FIGURE 21.4. Mean speech thresholds as a function of age, from three studies (Goetzinger et al., 1961; Jokinen, 1973; Plomp & Mimpen, 1979).

the standardized method of measuring the speech recognition threshold (SRT) or techniques to circumvent collapsing ear canals.

Suprathreshold Speech Recognition Measures

Standard Procedures

Conflicting evidence exists regarding the effects of age on speech recognition performance in quiet. A number of early studies reported that listeners' speech recognition scores decreased with increasing age. In addition, elderly listeners exhibited poorer word recognition performance than would be predicted on the basis of the pure tone sensitivity loss (Blumen-feld, Bergman, & Millner, 1969; Goetzinger et al., 1961; Jokinen, 1973). This phenomenon was termed "phonemic regression" (Gaeth, 1948).

In the foregoing studies, listeners had pure tone thresholds typical of their age group. Thus, older listeners with mild and moderate hearing losses were compared to young normally hearing listeners. Moreover, speech presentation levels in these studies were usually fixed at a sensation level (SL) of 30 to 40 dB above the speech threshold. The SRT is determined by reception of low-frequency spectral information, whereas suprathreshold speech recognition performance is dependent on reception of high-frequency consonants. Elderly listeners frequently exhibit sloping hearing losses; hence, speech thresholds are often in the normal or mild hearing loss range. A presentation level for speech materials of 30 or 40 dB above this SRT is insufficient for the older person to perceive the weak, high-frequency energy that is necessary for accurate word recognition. As a consequence, suprathreshold speech recognition scores are reduced.

Beattie and Warren (1983) examined monosyllabic word scores as a function of intensity in elderly hearing-impaired listeners. Elderly subjects with mild to moderate sensorineural hearing losses had more gradual slopes and required higher presentation levels for maximum scores on phonetically balanced word recognition tests (PB-max) than a control group of young normally hearing listeners. A presentation level of at least 50-dB SL above the SRT was necessary to reveal the maximum recognition scores of elderly listeners. Other options for selecting a presentation level to sample maximum scores for elderly listeners include testing at or below a listener's loudness discomfort level (Dirks, Kamm, Dubno, & Velde, 1981), using a fixed presentation level of 95 dB sound pressure level (SPL) (Kamm, Morgan, & Dirks, 1983), using an adaptive procedure to estimate maximum speech level (Levitt, 1978), or generating a performance-intensity (PI) function.

Speech recognition performance by young and elderly listeners generally is not significantly different at high presentation levels in quiet. Gordon-Salant (1987) compared performances of young and elderly listeners matched for normal hearing and sloping sensorineural hearing losses on two monosyllabic word recognition tests (*Northwestern University Test No. 6*, or *NU6*, Tillman & Carhart, 1966; and the *Modified Rhyme Test*, or *MRT*, Kruel et al., 1968). Each stimulus set was presented at 80 and 95 dB SPL. The results, shown in Figure 21.5, revealed no significant age effects for normal and hearing-impaired groups in all conditions except one (*MRT* at 95 dB SPL for hearing-impaired groups). In a larger-scale study, Jerger and Hayes (1977) analyzed PB-max scores for Harvard Psychoacoustics Laboratory Phonetically Balanced 50-word (PAL PB-50) lists, obtained from PI functions of 204 subjects with coch-

lear lesions. PB-max scores as a function of age decade are shown in Figure 21.6; they indicate that there are no systematic decreases in performance between the ages of 35 and 85. In summary, suprathreshold speech recognition performance in elderly subjects should be sampled at high presentation levels (PB-max). An elderly individual with a cochlear lesion should produce a PB-max score equivalent to that of a younger listener with matched hearing sensitivity. If the elderly listener's score is significantly reduced compared to that of younger listeners, then a retrocochlear lesion should be suspected. The PB-max score by itself, however, is not a very sensitive indicator of retrocochlear lesion, because there is considerable overlap between PB-max scores of patients with retrocochlear and cochlear lesions (Dirks, Kamm, Bower, & Betsworth, 1977; Jerger & Jerger, 1971).

Other Speech Materials

Alternative speech materials to phonetically balanced (PB) monosyllabic word tests have been proposed for clinical evaluation. Some of these options should be considered in the evaluation of the older person, depending on the specific goal of the assessment. The *California Consonant Test* (*CCT*) (Owens & Schubert, 1977) was developed to reveal consonant recognition problems of hearing-impaired listeners with high-frequency sensorineural hearing losses. The monosyllabic word stimuli incorporate many of the fricative, sibilant, and plosive consonants that have a high probability of confusion by listeners with sloping losses. The *CCT* should be particularly useful for evaluating changes in consonant recognition with hearing aid use and aural rehabilitation with elderly listeners, since they frequently exhibit sloping, sensorineural hearing losses. A second option, the *Speech Perception in Noise* (*SPIN*) sentence test, was developed to compare a listener's ability to receive the acoustic-phonetic components of the speech signal to the ability to derive linguistic and situational cues from the sen-

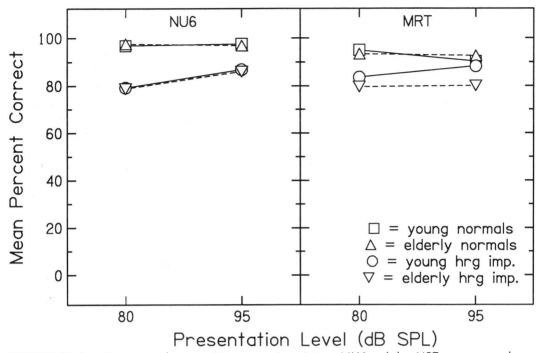

FIGURE 21.5. Mean speech recognition scores in quiet on *NU6* and the *MRT* at two speech levels from young normally hearing subjects, elderly normally hearing subjects, young hearing-impaired subjects, and elderly hearing-impaired subjects.

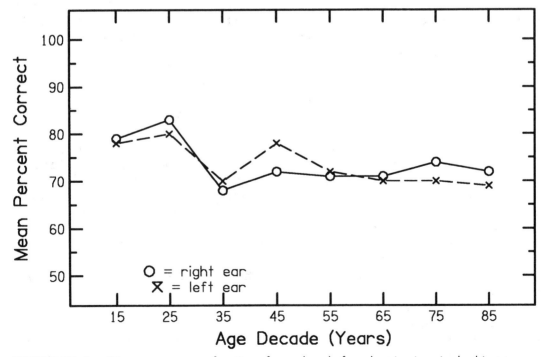

FIGURE 21.6. PB-max scores as a function of age decade from hearing-impaired subjects. *Note.* From "Diagnostic Speech Audiometry" by J. Jerger and D. Hayes, 1977, *Archives of Otolaryngology, 103,* pp. 216–222. Copyright 1977 by the American Medical Association. Reprinted by permission.

tence context (Kalikow, Stevens, & Elliott, 1977). Each list includes 25 high-predictability (HP) sentences, which provide contextual information to cue the final test word of the sentence, and 25 low-predictability (LP) sentences, which use a neutral sentence context. The *SPIN* test is presented in a background of 12-talker babble to simulate realistic listening in noise. The LP items of the *SPIN* test seem to be sensitive to age effects (Dubno, Dirks, & Morgan, 1984). Moreover, comparisons of HP and LP scores on the *SPIN* test reveal atypical results for listeners whose performance is affected by cognitive factors (Bilger, Neutzel, Trahiotis, & Rabinowitz, 1980), which may occur with increasing age.

Methodological Issues

The foregoing review suggests that elderly listeners do not exhibit unusual deficits on routine measures of speech recognition compared to younger subjects with similar audiograms. Under less than ideal circumstances, however, aging effects may become apparent. Several studies have demonstrated greater age effects in noise backgrounds than in quiet (Findlay & Denenberg, 1977; Jokinen, 1973). However, differences in detection thresholds between young and elderly subjects and/or insufficient presentation levels may have contributed to the results. More recently, Dubno and colleagues (1984) showed that elderly listeners with normal hearing and mild hearing impairments scored more poorly than younger subjects with matched pure tone sensitivity on recognition of LP items from the *SPIN* test presented in noise.

One study evaluated the effect of procedural variables on age-related speech recognition ability (Gordon-Salant, 1987). Young and elderly listeners matched for normal pure tone sensitivity and sloping mild to moderate sensorineural hearing loss were tested. Variables that were manipulated in the different tasks were presence of noise, presentation level, test format (open vs. closed set), and test paradigm in noise

(fixed signal and noise levels vs. fixed signal and adaptive noise levels). The average percentage correct scores from the four subject groups for *NU6* (open set) and the *MRT* (closed set) presented in fixed noise are shown in Figure 21.7. These results indicate that age effects were not present in most fixed noise conditions, regardless of presentation level and test format. However, young and elderly listeners did exhibit significant performance differences for all conditions in which noise level was modified adaptively (Figure 21.8). These findings tentatively suggest that stimulus and task complexity should be increased in order to reveal an age-related deficit. Increasing the complexity of the listening situation may place added stress on cognitive or processing abilities that may decline with age and hence may reveal age effects.

The Response Criterion

Elderly individuals have been characterized as using a conservative response criterion on behavioral tasks (Botwinick, 1969; Craik, 1966). The use of a cautious response criterion on a speech recognition task would result in refusal to repeat an unclear stimulus, which would lower speech recognition scores.

Signal detection theory has been applied to speech recognition tasks with elderly listeners to analyze the separate effects of decision criteria and sensitivity to judging response accuracy (Yanz, 1984). Yanz and Anderson (1984) found no significant differences on the response criterion measures between young and elderly subjects when *NU6* was presented in broadband noise at two fixed signal-to-noise ratios (S/N) of 0 dB and +5 dB. A second study (Gordon-Salant, 1986) examined performance of young and elderly listeners with normal hearing and matched sensorineural hearing losses on *NU6* and the *CCT* presented at an S/N that produced a 50% correct recognition score. A significant main effect of age was observed on the response criterion measure, in which the

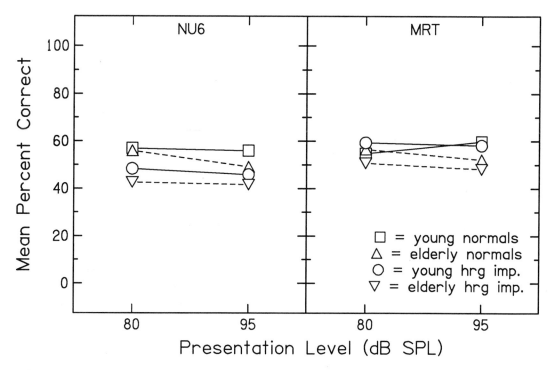

FIGURE 21.7. Mean speech recognition scores in noise at +6 dB signal-to-noise ratios on *NU6* and the *MRT* at two speech levels from young and elderly normally hearing subjects and young and elderly hearing-impaired subjects.

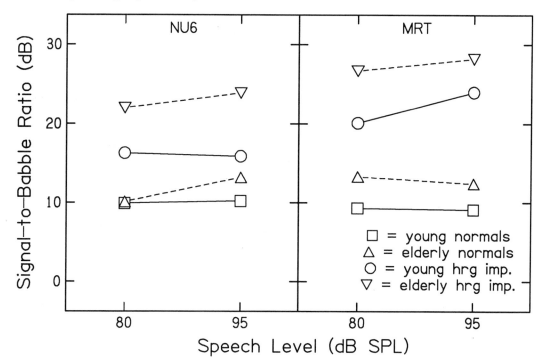

FIGURE 21.8. Mean signal-to-babble ratios for 50% criterion performance on *NU6* and the *MRT* at two speech levels from young and elderly normally hearing subjects and young and elderly hearing-impaired subjects.

elderly subjects exhibited a less cautious response criterion than the younger subjects. A practical aspect of a liberal criterion is that elderly listeners may misunderstand a message but respond as if they understood.

An alternative approach was employed by Jerger, Johnson, and Jerger (1988) to investigate whether or not response biases in elderly subjects influence speech recognition scores. Initially, the 24 adult subjects (53–83 years) were divided into three groups according to response criteria (lax, intermediate, and strict). Each subject's performance was then evaluated on a series of word and sentence recognition measures. The consistent findings were that the response criterion was not a predictor of speech recognition score. However, speech recognition scores were predicted by the average pure tone thresholds at 500 Hz, 1000 Hz, and 4000 Hz. Taken together, these three studies drew similar conclusions: Response bias differences between young and elderly subjects do not appear to be a major factor influencing the speech recognition scores of elderly subjects.

Assessment of Central Auditory Function

Elderly individuals may acquire pathological conditions affecting structures of the central auditory nervous system (CANS). Evaluation of central auditory function can supplement routine audiologic measures to identify such conditions. Ideally, this assessment should reveal the presence, side, and site of the auditory system lesion. Auditory evoked potentials may be more efficient than behavioral measures for providing accurate diagnostic information. Nevertheless, behavioral measures can be applied to delineate the impact of the lesion on auditory processing while simultaneously providing useful diagnostic information.

Another rationale for evaluating central auditory function in the elderly is to observe the effects of possible age-related declines in higher levels of auditory processing.

These deficits may be associated with senescent changes in the central auditory pathways (Kirikae et al., 1965) and are thought to produce behavioral effects that are comparable to known lesions of the CANS. The Committee on Hearing, Bioacoustics, and Biomechanics (1988) recently suggested that cognitive decline with aging might contribute to observed performance deficits on difficult speech understanding tasks, especially since certain cognitive skills (memory, speed of information processing, semantic processing) appear to be requisite for normal performance on these measures. Jerger, Jerger, Oliver, and Pirozzolo (1989), however, compared auditory and cognitive changes in a sample of elderly subjects and concluded that central auditory processing disorders and cognitive decline are relatively independent in the elderly population. Additional studies using measures of peripheral, central, and cognitive processing that manipulate signals along corresponding acoustic dimensions would be valuable to further delineate the effects of cognitive skills on speech understanding ability.

Regardless of their purpose, the basis of many behavioral measures of central auditory function is to increase stimulus complexity in order to reveal deterioration within the CANS. A second principle is to present a task that taps a function specific to a particular level of the auditory system. A third belief is that overloading the auditory system with high stimulus levels will reveal unusual nonlinearities in the system. Some of these measures are more efficient than others for detecting CANS lesions (Turner & Nielson, 1984). Moreover, many of these tests have limited application with the elderly because the presence of hearing loss confounds the results. Reviewed in this section are the more prevalent behavioral measures of CANS function and their application with elderly people.

Masking Level Differences

The masking level difference (MLD) is a binaural advantage manifested in an antiphasic condition (binaural signal and binaural noise have different interaural phase relations) compared to a homophasic condition (binaural signal and binaural noise have the same interaural phase relations). The improvement in the threshold for the binaural signal in the antiphasic condition compared to the homophasic condition is the MLD. The largest MLD in young normally hearing listeners is observed when the signal is a low-frequency pure tone (200 Hz to 500 Hz), the noise is of sufficient intensity (80 dB SPL), and the antiphasic/homophasic comparison is S_0N_0 (signal in phase, noise in phase) versus $S_\pi N_0$ (signal 180° out of phase, noise in phase) (Hirsh, 1948; Jerger, Brown, & Smith, 1984; Olsen, Noffsinger, & Carhart, 1976). The MLD has been ascribed to correlation processes within the CANS (Jefress, 1972). MLDs have been studied extensively in elderly listeners because deterioration of the CANS may exist.

Olsen and colleagues (1976) reported abnormally reduced pure tone MLDs in 25% of presbycusic subjects and reduced speech MLDs in 50% of these subjects. The source of the reduced MLDs in these subjects is unclear because they had a loss of threshold sensitivity, and peripheral hearing loss is known to affect the size of the MLD (Hall, Tyler, & Fernandes, 1984; Jerger et al., 1984). Analyses of age effects on the size of the MLD for normally hearing listeners suggest that a systematic but nonsignificant decline occurs from the 2nd decade (10–19 years) to the 7th decade (60–69 years) (Jerger et al., 1984). The interaction between sensitivity loss and age on the MLD must be defined better before this technique can be applied with confidence to elderly individuals.

Performance-Intensity Functions for Speech

Evaluation of speech recognition performance at multiple presentation levels above a listener's PB-max yields a PI function that can have diagnostic significance. Jerger and Jerger (1971) analyzed PI functions for PAL PB-50 word lists (PI-PB) obtained from subjects with cochlear and retrocochlear lesions. At high presentation levels, performance decreased relative to maximum performance for subjects with retrocochlear lesions but not for subjects with cochlear lesions. This phenomenon has been called "rollover" and can be quantified by the index (PB-max − PB-min)/PB-max. A rollover index exceeding .40 is a diagnostic indicator of retrocochlear lesion, using these speech materials and methods (Dirks et al., 1977; Jerger & Jerger, 1971).

A significant relationship between age and rollover has been observed among subjects over 60 years of age (Gang, 1976). Other variables that decrease with age, such as pure tone thresholds or maximum speech recognition score, probably contributed to this apparent relationship. Thus, an age effect on PI-PB functions, independent of other factors, has not yet been established.

Alternatively, the PI function for speech may be useful for predicting aided performance of elderly individuals. Dirks, Morgan, and Dubno (1982) described a similar procedure for predicting aided performance in noise, using an adaptive method to estimate the S/N at which a listener achieves a 50% speech recognition score. Individuals whose performance improves with increasing signal level are expected to perform well with amplification; those whose performance declines probably will require more modification and adjustment to amplification.

Distorted Speech Measures

CANS deterioration is thought to result in reduced coding and transmission of the acoustic signal (Bocca & Calearo, 1963). Traditionally, researchers in audition claim that reduced signal processing within the CANS is manifested in subtle ways. Consequently, to reveal degeneration of the CANS requires tasks that increase the complexity of the speech stimulus (Bocca & Calearo, 1963). This section will review the more prominent methods for distorting the speech signal, as well as results obtained with elderly listeners.

Time-Compressed Speech

Time compression, first developed by Fairbanks, Everitt, and Jaeger (1954), is a mechanical method used to increase speech rate without producing spectral distortion. The technique deletes periodic segments of a speech waveform and temporally abuts the retained segments to compress the total duration of the overall signal. A signal that is 60% time compressed has a total duration of 40% of the normal duration.

Elderly subjects usually perform more poorly than younger subjects on time-compressed speech tests (Bergman et al., 1976; Konkle, Beasley, & Bess, 1977; Schmitt, 1983; Sticht & Gray, 1969). However, the older subjects in these studies may have had some sensitivity loss in the higher frequencies that is associated with presbycusis. High-frequency hearing loss in young subjects is known to have a detrimental effect on recognition of time-compressed speech (Grimes, Mueller, & Williams, 1984; Harris, Haines, & Myers, 1963). Thus, interpretation of scores for time-compressed speech in the elderly must be made with respect to results obtained from younger subjects with comparable high-frequency sensorineural hearing loss. At least one study (Otto & McCandless, 1982) compared performances of young and elderly subjects with matched pure tone averages on a time-compressed speech task. Performances of the young and elderly hearing-impaired subject groups were not significantly different, although they were significantly different from performances of young normally hearing subjects. These results underscore the need to develop clinical norms based on an average clinical population with cochlear lesions.

Interrupted Speech

Speech interruption is accomplished by turning the speech signal on and off intermittently with various rates of interruption and with the speech signal left undisturbed various percentages of the time (Miller & Licklider, 1950). Significant age-related deficits have been observed on interrupted speech tasks (Bergman et al., 1976; Kirikae et al., 1965). These earlier studies, however, compared the performances of young normally hearing listeners to those of elderly listeners with a range of hearing sensitivity (especially high-frequency hearing loss). Korsan-Bengtsen (1973) has shown that acquired sensorineural hearing loss among younger listeners can have a detrimental effect on performance on the interrupted speech task. As with time-compressed tasks, therefore, individual data from elderly listeners should be compared to normative data from young cochlear-impaired subjects in order to determine the diagnostic significance of test results.

Filtered Speech

Spectral distortions of the speech signal have been adapted for assessment of central auditory function (Bocca, Calearo, & Cassinari, 1954). Low-pass filtered speech tests have revealed abnormally poor performance in elderly subjects (Bergman, 1980; Kirikae, 1969; Kirikae et al., 1965). Again, these results may have been influenced by age-related shifts in threshold sensitivity. Korsan-Bengtsen (1973) equated pure tone thresholds for young and elderly subjects and reported that older subjects scored only slightly poorer than younger subjects on a filtered sentence recognition task. Procedural variations, including speech material, filter cutoff, attenuation rate above cutoff frequency, and presentation level, could account for some reported differences among these investigations. A study employing stringent controls of these factors is needed to confirm the age effect on low-pass filtered speech tasks.

Speech Competition

Another method of reducing the multiple cues in speech is to present a simultaneous competing noise or message. Performance of elderly subjects in noise was the subject of an earlier section in this chapter. However, one specific technique for detecting CANS lesions involves comparing maximum speech recognition performance for

PB words presented in quiet and the *Synthetic Sentence Identification Test* (*SSI*) (Speaks & Jerger, 1965) presented with an ipsilateral competing message (message-to-competition ratio = 0 dB). This comparison of PB-max and *SSI*-max scores may reveal unusual age-related patterns. Jerger and Hayes (1977) reported PB- and *SSI*-max scores of 204 subjects in age decades spanning 10 to 89 years. Maximum scores were derived from PI functions obtained using both types of speech materials. Results showed that maximum scores for the two speech tests were interweaving up to the 50- to 59-year decade. Older age groups showed higher mean performance for the PB-max scores than for the *SSI*-max scores, a pattern associated with a central auditory deficit. Similar findings were reported by others (Otto & McCandless, 1982; Shirinian & Arnst, 1982). Figure 21.9 presents average data from the three studies and clearly shows the marked differences in PB- and *SSI*-max scores among older subjects. Another important finding is that 26% of the sample in the Shirinian and Arnst study did not exhibit this central aging effect, attesting to the heterogeneity of performance among elderly subjects. The comparison of PB-max and *SSI*-max scores therefore may provide an indication of the relative influence of peripheral and central factors on speech recognition.

Dichotic Tests

Dichotic testing involves binaural stimulation with a different signal being presented to each ear. The early work of Broadbent (1954) and Kimura (1961a) revealed a right-ear dominance effect in which digits presented dichotically were recalled with higher accuracy in the right ear than in the left ear. The right ear's superiority is a manifestation of the left hemisphere's dominance for final processing of speech and language. Subsequent work showed that dichotic stimuli presented asynchronously produce an advantage in the ear receiving the lagging stimulus (Berlin, Lowe-Bell, Cullen, & Thompson, 1973). This lag effect may reflect a release from competition by the two stimuli for final processing at the dominant hemisphere. Dichotic testing of patients with cortical lesions has revealed three main findings: Performance deteriorates in the ear contralateral to the lesion (Kimura, 1961b), performance declines in both ears if the dominant hemisphere is involved (Schulhoff & Goodglass, 1969), and the lag effect is reduced (Berlin et al., 1973).

Evaluation of dichotic performance in elderly listeners may be particularly valuable in localizing the site of hemispheric pathology resulting from cerebrovascular accident. Cerebrovascular disease increases in frequency and severity with age. Dichotic testing may also be useful in identifying a "central aging effect" that may occur as a result of senescent changes in cortical structures. Dichotic measures must be used with care in elderly patients, because hearing loss is known to affect performance (Roeser, Johns, & Price, 1976) and because cognitive factors such as memory and attention may confound results (Bergman, Hirsch, & Solzi, 1987).

Age effects have been observed on the *Staggered Spondaic Word Test* (Bergman, 1971) and the dichotic nonsense syllable test (Gelfand, Hoffman, Waltzman, & Piper, 1980; Martini et al., 1988), although these findings may have been associated with differences in threshold sensitivity between the young and elderly groups. Dichotic measures that seem to be affected minimally by the presence of peripheral hearing loss, and thus would be appropriate for the assessment of elderly individuals, are dichotic digits (Speaks, Niccum, & van Tasell, 1985) and the *Dichotic Sentence Identification* test (*DSI*) (Fifer, Jerger, Berlin, Tobey, & Campbell, 1983). In particular, the dichotic digits test was shown to be a sensitive measure in the evaluation of aphasic patients (Niccum, Rubens, & Speaks, 1981). Further research is needed to determine if an age effect, independent of hearing loss, is revealed on the dichotic digits test and the *DSI*.

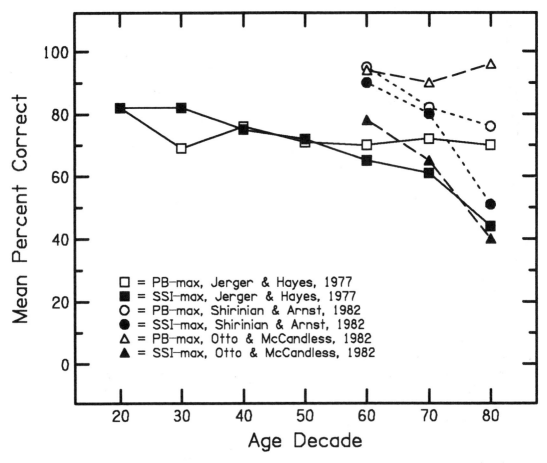

FIGURE 21.9. Mean maximum PB vs. *SSI* scores as a function of age, from three studies (Jerger & Hayes, 1977; Otto & McCandless, 1982; Shirinian & Arnst, 1982).

Acoustic Immittance

Tympanometry

The first major component of the acoustic immittance battery is tympanometry. This is the measurement of acoustic immittance in the ear canal as a function of air pressure changes. Ear canal pressure is varied between −400 and +200 daPa for these measures. Tympanograms can be obtained using 1, 2, or multiple frequency probe tones (American Speech-Language-Hearing Association, Working Group, 1988).

Static Admittance (Y_a)

One attribute of the tympanogram to examine is compensated static admittance. This is derived from the height of the admittance magnitude tympanogram (obtained with a low-frequency probe tone) relative to the tail value.

There does not appear to be a clinically significant age effect on static admittance values. One study (Blood & Greenberg, 1977) reported a significant decrease in acoustic admittance for subjects aged 70 years and older, compared to a younger group of subjects. However, the mean value reported for the older subject group (Y_a =

.60) is within the normal range. Other studies (Thompson, Sills, Recke, & Bui, 1979; Wilson, 1981) found no significant changes in static admittance as a function of age. Thus, admittance values obtained from elderly individuals can be compared to normative values obtained from younger adults.

Tympanometric Pressure Peak

A second characteristic of the tympanogram, tympanometric pressure peak (TPP), corresponds to the ear canal pressure (in dekaPascals) that produces the extreme point (peak) on the tympanogram and is an indirect measure of the air pressure in the middle ear. Scant TPP values are available for elderly subjects. One study (Nerbonne, Schow, & Gosset, 1976) obtained tympanograms from 55 nursing home residents and found that 8% of the sample exhibited TPPs exceeding −100 daPa. These results were attributed to poor Eustachian tube function, which, in older adults, might be associated with cartilaginous and muscular changes in the middle ear with age. Unfortunately, the TPP measure has limited diagnostic utility for two reasons: There can be a discrepancy between TPP and middle ear pressure (Flisberg, Ingelstedt, & Ortegren, 1963; Renvall & Holmquist, 1976) and TPP is a poor indicator of middle ear effusion (Fiellau-Nikolajsen, 1983; Haughton, 1977).

Other parameters of the tympanogram that have diagnostic value include morphological analysis of multifrequency tympanograms (American Speech-Language-Hearing Association, 1988), tympanometric width (American Speech-Language-Hearing Association, 1989; Brooks, 1968; Fiellau-Nikolajsen, 1983; Margolis & Shanks, 1985), and ear canal volume estimates (Feldman, 1976). Studies evaluating age-related phenomena on these measures are badly needed.

Acoustic Reflexes

Measurements of acoustic reflex characteristics constitute the second major component of the acoustic immittance battery. The stapedius muscle contracts in response to intense acoustic stimulation as a result of activation of the acoustic reflex arc. The stapedius muscle reflex arc includes the afferent auditory neuron, the ventral cochlear nucleus, the medial superior olive, and the ipsilateral and contralateral nuclei of the facial nerve (Borg, 1973; Moller, 1983). The facial nerve subsequently innervates the stapedius muscle to contract. Lesions affecting any structures in the ascending or descending acoustic reflex arc will create abnormalities in the reflex response.

Acoustic Reflex Thresholds

The threshold of the stapedius reflex is the lowest intensity of an acoustic stimulus that induces a contraction of the stapedius muscle. The vast majority of studies examining the relationship between age and acoustic reflex thresholds (ARTs) has found no evidence of a systematic age effect when tonal activators are used (Gelfand & Piper, 1981; Handler & Margolis, 1977; Jerger, Jerger, & Mauldin, 1972; Osterhammel & Osterhammel, 1979; Silman, 1979; Silman & Gelfand, 1981; Silverman, Silman, & Miller, 1983; Thompson, Sills, Recke, & Bui, 1980; Wilson, 1981). This finding was consistent with variations in step size of 5 dB and 1 dB (Silverman et al., 1983). Several reports (Handler & Margolis, 1977; Jerger, Hayes, Anthony, & Mauldin, 1978; Osterhammel & Osterhammel, 1979; Wilson, 1981) found significantly higher ARTs in older subjects than in younger subjects for tonal stimuli at 4000 Hz. The clinical significance of this finding is limited, however, because ART measurement at 4000 Hz is frequently omitted from routine assessment.

In contrast, elderly subjects exhibit elevated ARTs compared to normally hearing subjects for broadband noise stimuli (Handler & Margolis, 1977; Silman, 1979; Silman & Gelfand, 1981; Wilson, 1981). These age effects are observed when the broadband noise is presented in 1-dB-intensity increments but not in 5-dB increments.

Acoustic Reflex Adaptation

Anderson, Barr, and Wedenberg (1970) were the first to report a decrease (adaptation) of the amplitude of reflex contraction over time in normally hearing and hearing-impaired subjects for tonal stimulation. The temporal characteristics of reflex adaptation were shown to vary with the status of the auditory system. Normally hearing subjects showed no reflex adaptation within a 10-s time period following stimulation with either a 500-Hz or 1000-Hz pure tone; subjects with retrocochlear lesions showed rapid reflex adaptation within 10 s. Young and elderly subjects apparently do not exhibit significant differences on the acoustic reflex adaptation measure (Habener & Snyder, 1974; Otto & McCandless, 1982). Additional studies that examine systematically the interaction between age, hearing loss, and stimulus intensity would be useful in refining clinical interpretation.

Acoustic Reflex Growth Functions

Recent interest has focused on the measurement of acoustic reflex amplitude as a function of stimulus intensity. In this paradigm, the maximum acoustic reflex amplitude is monitored for multiple presentation levels about the ART. Normally hearing listeners with low ARTs exhibit a relatively wide dynamic range between the ART and the saturation point for acoustic reflex magnitude (Figure 21.10).

Aging has an effect on the magnitude of the acoustic reflex (Silman & Gelfand, 1981a; Thompson et al., 1980; Wilson, 1981). Acoustic reflex growth functions in normally hearing subjects show an inverse relationship between acoustic reflex magnitude and age for tonal and filtered noise activators. Thus, the slope of the growth function decreases with increasing age. The acoustic reflex growth function also saturates for 1000 Hz, 2000 Hz, and broadband noise activators in normally hearing elderly subjects but not in normally hearing younger subjects (Silman & Gelfand, 1981a; Wilson, 1981). Young and elderly subjects with sensorineural hearing loss do not exhibit saturation of the growth function at high stimulus levels (Silman & Gelfand, 1981a; Silman, Popelka, & Gelfand, 1978). Saturation in the growth functions of normally hearing elderly subjects may be associated with limitations in the ability of the aging auditory system to integrate energy (Silman & Gelfand, 1981a).

The unusual reflex amplitudes observed in elderly subjects may be related, in part, to insufficient interstimulus intervals used in assessment. Jerger and Oliver (1987) measured the amplitude of the acoustic reflex at 110 dB SPL in four interstimulus interval (ISI) conditions. They reported higher reflex magnitudes in young subjects than in older subjects and an interaction between age group and ISI (see Figure 21.11). In elderly subjects, acoustic reflex magnitude increases with increasing ISI upon ipsilateral stimulation, whereas in young subjects acoustic reflex magnitude is stable with increasing ISI. Thus, reduced reflex magnitude in elderly subjects may be generated by insufficient ISIs. An ISI exceeding 9 ms is recommended to minimize age effects on these measures (Jerger & Oliver, 1987).

In summary, routine acoustic reflex measures, including ARTs with tonal activators and acoustic reflex adaptation, can be applied and interpreted for elderly patients using comparable procedures to those used for younger subjects. Measures of acoustic reflex amplitude seem to be particularly sensitive to age effects. Comparisons of acoustic reflex growth functions upon ipsilateral and contralateral stimulation and with large ISIs may prove to be important for elucidating central and peripheral aging factors from exogenous lesion effects.

Conclusions

The audiologist can choose from a myriad of test procedures for evaluating the elderly person. The purpose of the assessment should serve as a guide in test selection. In a routine assessment, the essential elements should include case history and measures

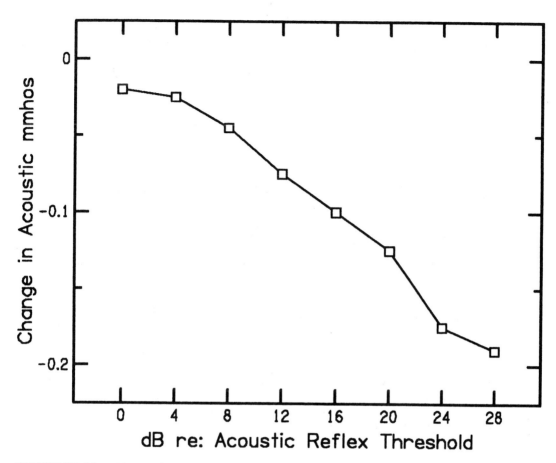

FIGURE 21.10. Mean admittance (Y_a) reflex-magnitude changes (in acoustic mmhos) established for young normally hearing listeners with a 220-Hz probe as a function of activator level about the acoustic reflex threshold. *Note.* From "The Effects of Aging on the Magnitude of the Acoustic Reflex" by R. H. Wilson, 1981, *Journal of Speech and Hearing Research, 24,* pp. 406–414. Copyright 1981 by the American Speech-Language-Hearing Association. Adapted by permission.

of hearing handicap, pure tone sensitivity, speech recognition, and acoustic immittance. CANS function should be evaluated with a battery of tests that include MLDs, a distorted speech task (such as PI-PB vs. PI-*SSI* functions), and a dichotic task (e.g., dichotic digits or *DSI*). Judicious selection of any measurement procedure with the elderly is made with two overriding considerations. The first is the effect of hearing loss on the measure and possible methods to control for this effect. The second is knowledge of inherent age effects on the measure, which can be distinguished from the effects of diagnostically significant conditions of the auditory system.

References

Alpiner, J. G., & Baker, R. B. (1980). *Communication assessment procedures for seniors.* Unpublished study.

American National Standards Institute. (1978). *Methods for manual pure-tone threshold audiometry* (ANSI S3.21-1978, R-1986). New York: American National Standards Institute.

American National Standards Institute. (1989). *American National Standard Specification for Audiometers* (ANSI S3.6-1969, R-1989). New York: American National Standards Institute.

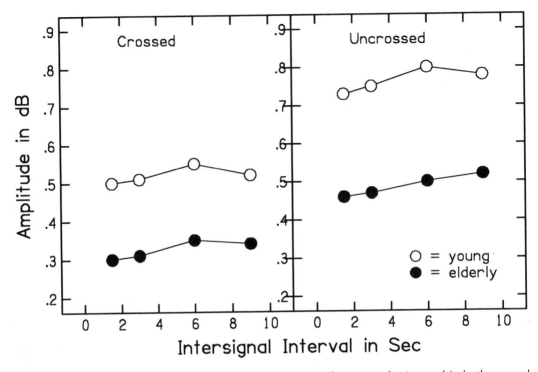

FIGURE 21.11. Acoustic reflex amplitude as a function of interstimulus interval in both crossed and uncrossed modes for young and elderly subjects. *Note.* From "Interaction of Age and Intersignal Interval on Acoustic Reflex Amplitude" by J. Jerger and T. Oliver, 1987, *Ear and Hearing, 8,* pp. 322–325. Copyright 1987 by Williams & Wilkins. Adapted by permission.

American Speech-Language-Hearing Association. (1978). Guidelines for manual puretone threshold audiometry. *Asha, 20,* 297–301.

American Speech-Language-Hearing Association. (1988). Guidelines for determining the threshold level for speech. *Asha, 30,* 35–89.

American Speech-Language-Hearing Association. (1989). Guidelines for screening for hearing impairment and middle ear disorders. *Asha, 31,* 71–77.

American Speech-Language-Hearing Association, Working Group on Aural Acoustic Immittance Measurements. (1988). Tutorial: Tympanometry. *Journal of Speech and Hearing Disorders, 53,* 354–377.

Anderson, H., Barr, B., & Wedenberg, E. (1970). Early diagnosis of VIIIth nerve tumors by acoustic reflex tests. *Acta Otolaryngologica, 263,* 232–237.

Barza, M., Lauermann, M. W., Tally, F. P., & Gorbach, S. L. (1980). Prospective, randomized trial of netilmicin and amikacin, with emphasis on eighth-nerve toxicity. *Antimicrobiology Agents in Chemotherapy, 14,* 707–714.

Beattie, R. C., & Warren, V. G. (1983). Slope characteristics of CID W-22 word functions in elderly hearing-impaired listeners. *Journal of Speech and Hearing Disorders, 48,* 119–127.

Bergman, M. (1971). Hearing and aging. *Audiology, 10,* 164–171.

Bergman, M. (1980). *Aging and the perception of speech.* Baltimore, MD: University Park Press.

Bergman, M., Blumenfeld, V., Cascardo, D., Dash, B., Levitt, H., & Margulies, M. (1976). Age-related decrement in hearing for speech: Sampling and longitudinal studies. *Journal of Gerontology, 31,* 533–538.

Bergman, M., Hirsch, S., & Solzi, P. (1987). Interhemispheric suppression: A test of central auditory function. *Ear and Hearing, 8,* 147–150.

Berlin, C. I., Lowe-Bell, S. S., Cullen, J. K., Jr., & Thompson, C. L. (1973). Dichotic speech perception: An interpretation of right-ear advantage and temporal offset effects. *Journal of the Acoustical Society of America, 53,* 699–709.

Bilger, R. C., Neutzel, J., Trahiotis, C., & Rabinowitz, W. (1980). An objective psychophysical approach to measuring hearing for speech. *Asha, 22,* 726.

Blood, I., & Greenberg, H. (1977). Acoustic admittance of the ear in the geriatric person. *Journal of the American Audiology Society, 1,* 185–187.

Blumenfeld, V. G., Bergman, M., & Millner, E. (1969). Speech discrimination in an aging population. *Journal of Speech and Hearing Research, 12,* 210–217.

Bocca, E., & Calearo, C. (1963). Central hearing processes. In J. Jerger (Ed.), *Modern developments in audiology.* New York: Academic Press.

Bocca, E., Calearo, C., & Cassinari, V. (1954). A new method for testing hearing in temporal lobe tumors. *Acta Otolaryngologica, 44,* 219–221.

Borg, E. (1973). On the neuronal organization of the acoustic middle ear reflex. A physiological and anatomical study. *Brain Research, 49,* 101–123.

Botwinick, J. (1969). Disinclination to venture response versus cautiousness in responding: Age differences. *Journal of Genetic Psychology, 115,* 55–62.

Brant, L. J., & Fozard, J. L. (1990). Age changes in pure tone hearing thresholds in a longitudinal study of normal human aging. *Journal of the Acoustical Society of America, 88,* 813–820.

Broadbent, D. E. (1954). The role of auditory localization of attention and memory span. *Journal of Experimental Psychology, 47,* 191–196.

Brooks, D. (1968). An objective method of detecting fluid in the middle ear. *International Audiology, 8,* 563–569.

Clemis, J. D., Ballad, W. J., & Killion, M. C. (1986). Clinical use of an insert earphone. *Annals of Otology, Rhinology and Laryngology, 95,* 520–524.

Committee on Hearing, Bioacoustics, and Biomechanics (CHABA); Working Group on Speech Understanding. (1988). Speech

understanding and aging. *Journal of the Acoustical Society of America, 83,* 859–895.

Corso, J. (1963). Age and sex differences in puretone thresholds. *Archives of Otolaryngology, 77,* 383–405.

Covell, W. (1952). Histological changes in the aging cochlea. *Journal of Gerontology, 7,* 173–177.

Craik, F. I. M. (1966). The effects of aging on the detection of faint auditory signals. In *Proceedings of the Seventh International Congress of Gerontology* (Vol. 6, pp. 145–147). Vienna: Viennese Medical Academy.

Demorest, M. E., & Erdman, S. A. (1987). Development of the Communication Profile for the Hearing Impaired. *Journal of Speech and Hearing Disorders, 52,* 129–143.

Demorest, M. E., & Walden, B. E. (1984). Psychometric principles in the selection, interpretation, and evaluation of communication self-assessment inventories. *Journal of Speech and Hearing Disorders, 49,* 226–240.

Dirks, D. D., Kamm, C., Bower, D., & Betsworth, A. (1977). Use of performance-intensity functions for diagnosis. *Journal of Speech and Hearing Disorders, 42,* 408–415.

Dirks, D. D., Kamm, C., Dubno, J., & Velde, T. (1981). Speech recognition performance at loudness discomfort level. *Scandinavian Audiology, 10,* 239–246.

Dirks, D. D., Morgan, D. E., & Dubno, J.R. (1982). A procedure for quantifying the effects of noise on speech recognition. *Journal of Speech and Hearing Disorders, 49,* 114–122.

Dubno, J. R., Dirks, D. D., & Morgan, D. E. (1984). Effects of age and mild hearing loss on speech recognition in noise. *Journal of the Acoustical Society of America, 76,* 87–96.

Fairbanks, G., Everitt, W. L., & Jaeger, R. P. (1954). Method for time or frequency compression-expansion of speech. *Transactions of the Institute of Radio Engineers, Professional Group on Audio, Au-2,* 7–11.

Feldman, A. (1976). Tympanometry: Application and interpretation. *Annals of Otology, Rhinology and Laryngology, 85,* 202–208.

Fiellau-Nikolajsen, M. (1983). Tympanometry and secretory otitis media. Observations on diagnosis, epidemiology, treatment and prevention in prospective short studies of three-year-old children. *Acta Otolaryngologica* (Stockholm), *394,* 1–73.

Fifer, R. C., Jerger, J. F., Berlin, C. I., Tobey, E. A., & Campbell, J. C. (1983). Development of a dichotic sentence identification test for hearing-impaired adults. *Ear and Hearing, 4,* 300–305.

Findlay, R. C., & Denenberg, L. J. (1977). Effects of subtle mid-frequency auditory dysfunction upon speech discrimination in noise. *Audiology, 16,* 252–259.

Flisberg, K., Ingelstedt, S., & Ortegren, U. (1963). On middle ear pressure. *Acta Otolaryngologica, 182,* 43–56.

Formby, C., Phillips, D. E., & Thomas, R. G. (1987). Hearing loss among stroke patients. *Ear and Hearing, 8,* 326–332.

Gaeth, J. (1948). A study of phonemic regression associated with hearing loss. Unpublished doctoral dissertation, Northwestern University, Evanston, IL.

Gang, R. P. (1976). The effects of age on the diagnostic utility of the rollover phenomenon. *Journal of Speech and Hearing Disorders, 41,* 63–69.

Gelfand, S. A., Hoffman, S., Waltzman, S. B., & Piper, N. (1980). Dichotic CV recognition at various interaural temporal onset asynchronies: Effect of age. *Journal of the Acoustical Society of America, 68,* 1258–1261.

Gelfand, S. A., & Piper, N. (1981). Acoustic reflex thresholds in young and elderly subjects with normal hearing. *Journal of the Acoustical Society of America, 69,* 295–297.

Giolas, T. G., Owens, E., Lamb, S. H., & Schubert, E. D. (1979). Hearing Performance Inventory. *Journal of Speech and Hearing Disorders, 44,* 169–195.

Glorig, A., & Davis, H. (1961). Age, noise, and hearing loss. *Annals of Otology, Rhinology and Laryngology, 70,* 556–571.

Goetzinger, C., Proud, G., Dirks, D., & Embrey, J. (1961). A study of hearing in advanced age. *Archives of Otolaryngology, 73,* 662–674.

Gordon-Salant, S. (1986). Effects of aging on response criteria in speech-recognition tasks. *Journal of Speech and Hearing Research, 29,* 155–162.

Gordon-Salant, S. (1987). Age-related differences in speech recognition as a function of test format and paradigm. *Ear and Hearing, 8,* 277–282.

Green, D. M., & Swets, J. A. (1966). *Signal detection theory and psychophysics.* New York: Wiley.

Grimes, A. M., Mueller, H. G., & Williams, D. L. (1984). Clinical considerations in the use of time-compressed speech. *Ear and Hearing, 5,* 114–117.

Habener, S. A., & Snyder, J. M. (1974). Stapedius reflex amplitude and decay in normal ears. *Archives of Otolaryngology, 100,* 294–297.

Hall, J. W., Tyler, R. S., & Fernandes, M. A. (1984). Factors influencing the masking level difference in cochlear hearing-impaired and normal-hearing listeners. *Journal of Speech and Hearing Research, 27,* 145–154.

Handler, S. D., & Margolis, R. H. (1977). Predicting hearing loss from stapedial reflex thresholds in patients with sensorineural hearing impairment. *Transactions of the American Academy of Ophthalmology and Otology, 48,* 425–431.

Harford, E. R., & Dodds, E. (1982). Hearing status of ambulatory senior citizens. *Ear and Hearing, 3,* 105–109.

Harris, J. D., Haines, H. L., & Myers, C. D. (1963). The importance of hearing at 3 kc for understanding speeded speech. *Laryngoscope, 70,* 131–146.

Haughton, P. (1977). Validity of tympanometry for middle ear effusions. *Archives of Otolaryngology, 103,* 505–513.

Hinchcliffe, K. (1962). The anatomical locus of presbycusis. *Journal of Speech and Hearing Disorders, 27,* 301–310.

Hirsh, I. J. (1948). The influence of interaural phase on interaural summation and inhibition. *Journal of the Acoustical Society of America, 20,* 761–766.

Jefress, L. A. (1972). Binaural signal detection: Vector theory. In J. Tobias, *Foundations of modern auditory theory* (Vol. 2, pp. 351–368). New York: Academic Press.

Jerger, J., Brown, D., & Smith, S. (1984). Effect of peripheral hearing loss on the masking level difference. *Archives of Otolaryngology, 110,* 290–296.

Jerger, J., & Hayes, D. (1977). Diagnostic speech audiometry. *Archives of Otolaryngology, 103,* 216–222.

Jerger, J., Hayes, D., Anthony, L., & Mauldin, L. (1978). Factors influencing prediction of hearing level from the acoustic reflex. *Monographs in Contemporary Audiology, 1,* 1–20.

Jerger, J., & Jerger, S. (1971). Diagnostic significance of PB word functions. *Archives of Otolaryngology, 93,* 573–580.

Jerger, J., Jerger, S., & Mauldin, L. (1972). Studies in impedance audiometry: I. Normal and sensorineural ears. *Archives of Otolaryngology, 96,* 513–523.

Jerger, J., Jerger, S., Oliver, T., & Pirozzolo, F. (1989). Speech understanding in the elderly. *Ear and Hearing, 10,* 79–89.

Jerger, J., Johnson, K., & Jerger, S. (1988). Effect of response criterion on measures of speech understanding in the elderly. *Ear and Hearing, 9,* 49–56.

Jerger, J., & Oliver, T. (1987). Interaction of age and intersignal interval on acoustic reflex amplitude. *Ear and Hearing, 8,* 322–325.

Johnsson, L. G., & Hawkins, J. E., Jr. (1972). Sensory and neural degeneration with aging, as seen in microdissections of the human inner ear. *Annals of Otolaryngology, 81,* 179–183.

Jokinen, K. (1973). Presbyacusis: VI. Masking of speech. *Acta Otolaryngologica, 76,* 426–430.

Kalikow, D. N., Stevens, K. N., & Elliott, L. L. (1977). Development of a test of speech intelligibility in noise using sentence materials with controlled word predictability. *Journal of the Acoustical Society of America, 61,* 1337–1351.

Kamm, C. A., Morgan, D. E., & Dirks, D. D. (1983). Accuracy of adaptive procedure estimates of PB-max level. *Journal of Speech and Hearing Disorders, 48,* 202–209.

Kimura, D. (1961a). Cerebral dominance and the perception of verbal stimuli. *Canadian Journal of Psychology, 15,* 166–171.

Kimura, D. (1961b). Some effects of temporal-lobe damage on auditory perception. *Canadian Journal of Psychology, 15,* 156–165.

Kirikae, I. (1969). Auditory function in advanced age with reference to histological changes in the central auditory system. *International Audiology, 8,* 221–230.

Kirikae, I., Sato, R., & Shitara, T. (1965). A study of hearing in advanced age. *Laryngoscope, 74,* 205–220.

Konkle, D. F., Beasley, D. S., & Bess, F. H. (1977). Intelligibility of time-altered speech in relation to chronological aging. *Journal of Speech and Hearing Research, 20,* 108–115.

Korsan-Bengtsen, M. (1973). Distorted speech audiometry: A methodological and clinical study. *Acta Otolaryngologica, 310* (Suppl.), 7–75.

Kruel, E. J., Nixon, J. C., Kryter, K. D., Bell, D. W., Lang, J. S., & Schubert, E. D. (1968). A proposed clinical test of speech discrimination. *Journal of Speech and Hearing Research, 11,* 536–552.

Kryter, K. D. (1983). Presbycusis, sociocusis, and nosocusis. *Journal of the Acoustical Society of America, 73,* 1897–1917.

Levitt, H. (1978). Adaptive testing in audiology. In C. Ludvigsen & J. Barfod (Eds.), *Sensorineural hearing impairment and hearing aids. Scandinavian Audiology, 6* (Suppl.).

Ludlow, C. L., & Swisher, L. P. (1971). The audiometric evaluation of adult aphasics. *Journal of Speech and Hearing Research, 14,* 535–543.

Margolis, R. H., & Shanks, J. E. (1985). Tympanometry. In J. Katz (Ed.), *Handbook of clinical audiology* (3rd ed., pp. 438–475). Baltimore, MD: Williams & Wilkins.

Marshall, L., & Jesteadt, W. (1986). Comparison of pure-tone audibility thresholds obtained with audiological and two-interval forced-choice procedures. *Journal of Speech and Hearing Research, 29,* 82–91.

Marshall, L., Martinez, S. A., & Schlaman, M. E. (1983). Reassessment of high-frequency air-bone gaps in older adults. *Acta Otolaryngologica, 109,* 601–606.

Martini, A., Bovo, R., Agnoletto, M., DaCol, M., Drusian, A., Liddeo, M., & Morra, B. (1988). Dichotic performance in elderly Italians with Italian stop consonant–vowel stimuli. *Audiology, 27,* 1–7.

Miller, G. A., & Licklider, J. C. R. (1950). The intelligibility of interrupted speech. *Journal of the Acoustical Society of America, 22,* 167–173.

Milne, J. M. (1977). The air-bone gap in older people. *British Journal of Audiology, 11,* 1–6.

Moller, A. R. (1983). *Auditory physiology.* New York: Academic Press.

Moscicki, E. K., Elkins, E. F., Baum, H. F., & McNamara, P. M. (1985). Hearing loss in the elderly: An epidemiologic study of the Framingham Heart Study Cohort. *Ear and Hearing, 6,* 184–190.

Nerbonne, M., Schow, R., & Gosset, F. (1976). *Prevalence of conductive pathology in a nursing home population* (Laboratory Research Reports). Pocatello: Idaho State University, Department of Speech Pathology and Audiology.

Newman, C. W., & Weinstein, B. E. (1989). Test-retest reliability of the Hearing Handicap Inventory for the Elderly using two administration approaches. *Ear and Hearing, 10,* 191–192.

Niccum, N., Rubens, A. B., & Speaks, C. (1981). Effects of stimulus material on the dichotic listening performance of aphasic patients. *Journal of Speech and Hearing Research, 24,* 526–534.

Novak, R. E., & Anderson, C. V. (1982). Differentiation of types of presbycusis using the masking-level difference. *Journal of Speech and Hearing Research, 25,* 504–508.

Olsen, W. O., Noffsinger, D., & Carhart, R. (1976). Masking level differences encountered in clinical populations. *Audiology, 15,* 287–301.

Osterhammel, D., & Osterhammel, P. (1979). Age and sex variation for the normal stapedial reflex thresholds and tympanometric compliance values. *Scandinavian Audiology, 8,* 153–158.

Otto, W. C., & McCandless, G. A. (1982). Aging and auditory site of lesion. *Ear and Hearing, 3,* 110–117.

Owens, E., & Schubert, E. D. (1977). Development of the California Consonant Test. *Journal of Speech and Hearing Research, 20,* 463–474.

Plomp, R., & Mimpen, A. M. (1979). Speech reception threshold for sentences as a function of age and noise level. *Journal of the Acoustical Society of America, 66,* 1333–1342.

Potash, M., & Jones, B. (1977). Aging and decision criteria for the detection of tones in noise. *Journal of Gerontology, 32,* 436–440.

Randolph, L. J., & Schow, R. L. (1983). Threshold inaccuracies in an elderly clinical population: Ear canal collapse as a possible cause. *Journal of Speech and Hearing Research, 26,* 54–58.

Rees, J. N., & Botwinick, J. (1971). Detection and decision factors in auditory behavior of the elderly. *Journal of Gerontology, 26,* 133–136.

Renvall, U., & Holmquist, J. (1976). Tympanometry revealing middle ear pathology. *Annals of Otology, Rhinology and Laryngology, 85* (Suppl. 25), 209–215.

Roeser, R. J., Johns, D. F., & Price, L. L. (1976). Dichotic listening in adults with sensorineural hearing loss. *Journal of the American Audiology Society, 2,* 19–25.

Rosen, S., Bergman, M., Plester, D., El-Mofty, A., & Sattis, M. H. (1962). Presbycusis study of a relatively noise-free population in the Sudan. *Transactions of the American Otology Society, 50,* 135–151.

Rosenberg, P. E. (1978). Case history: The first test. In J. Katz (Ed.), *Handbook of clinical audiology* (2nd ed.). Baltimore, MD: Williams & Wilkins.

Rosenwasser, H. (1964). Otitic problems in the aged. *Geriatrics, 19,* 11–17.

Rubinstein, M., Hildescheimer, H., Zokar, S., & Chilarovitz, T. (1977). Chronic cardiovascular pathology and hearing loss in the aged. *Gerontology, 23,* 4–9.

Schmitt, J. F. (1983). The effects of time compression and time expansion on passage comprehension by elderly listeners. *Journal of Speech and Hearing Research, 26,* 373–377.

Schow, R. S., & Nerbonne, M. A. (1977). Assessment of hearing handicap by nursing home residents and staff. *Journal of the Academy of Rehabilitative Audiology, 10,* 2–12.

Schulhoff, C., & Goodglass, H. (1969). Dichotic listening, side of brain injury and cerebral dominance. *Neuropsychologia, 7,* 149–160.

Shirinian, M. J., & Arnst, D. J. (1982). Patterns in the performance-intensity functions for phonetically balanced word lists and synthetic sentences in aged listeners. *Archives of Otolaryngology, 108,* 15–20.

Silman, S. (1979). The effects of aging on the stapedius reflex thresholds. *Journal of the Acoustical Society of America, 66,* 735–738.

Silman, S., & Gelfand, S. A. (1981). Effect of sensorineural hearing loss on the stapedius reflex growth function in the elderly. *Journal of the Acoustical Society of America, 69,* 1099–1106.

Silman, S., Popelka, G. R., & Gelfand, S. A. (1978). Effect of sensorineural hearing loss on acoustic stapedius reflex growth functions. *Journal of the Acoustical Society of America, 64,* 1406–1411.

Silverman, C. A., Silman, S., & Miller, M. H. (1983). The acoustic reflex threshold in aging ears. *Journal of the Acoustical Society of America, 73,* 248–255.

Speaks, C., & Jerger, J. (1965). Method for measurement of speech identification. *Journal of Speech and Hearing Research, 8,* 289–298.

Speaks, C., Niccum, N., & van Tasell, D. (1985). Effects of stimulus material on the dichotic listening performance of patients with sensorineural hearing loss. *Journal of Speech and Hearing Research, 28,* 16–25.

Sticht, T. G., & Gray, B. B. (1969). The intelligibility of time compressed words as a function of age and hearing loss. *Journal of Speech and Hearing Research, 12,* 443–448.

Thompson, D. J., Sills, J. A., Recke, K. S., & Bui, D. M. (1979). Acoustic admittance and the aging ear. *Journal of Speech and Hearing Research, 22,* 29–36.

Thompson, D. J., Sills, J. A., Recke, K. S., & Bui, D. M. (1980). Acoustic reflex growth in the aging adult. *Journal of Speech and Hearing Research, 23,* 405–418.

Tillman, T. W., & Carhart, R. (1966). *An expanded test for speech discrimination utilizing CNC monosyllabic words* (Northwestern University Auditory Test No. 6; USAF School of Aerospace Medicine Technical Report). Brooks Air Force Base, TX: Department of the Air Force.

Turner, R. B., & Nielson, D. W. (1984). Application of clinical decision analysis to audiological tests. *Ear and Hearing, 5,* 125–133.

Ventry, I., & Weinstein, B. (1982). The Hearing Handicap Inventory for the Elderly: A new tool. *Ear and Hearing, 3,* 128–134.

Weinstein, B. E., Spitzer, J. B., & Ventry, I. M. (1986). Test-retest reliability of the Hearing Handicap Inventory for the Elderly. *Ear and Hearing, 7,* 295–299.

Wilber, L. A., Kruger, B., & Killion, M. C. (1988). Reference thresholds for the ER-3A insert earphone. *Journal of the Acoustical Society of America, 83,* 669–676.

Wilson, R. H. (1981). The effects of aging on the magnitude of the acoustic reflex. *Journal of Speech and Hearing Research, 24,* 406–414.

Wilson, R. H., & Margolis, R. H. (1983). Measurement of auditory thresholds for speech stimuli. In D. F. Konkle & W. F. Rintelmann (Eds.), *Principles of speech audiometry.* Baltimore, MD: University Park Press.

Yanz, J. L. (1984). The application of the theory of signal detection to the assessment of speech perception. *Ear and Hearing, 5,* 64–71.

Yanz, J. L., & Anderson, S. M. (1984). Comparison of speech perception skills in young and old listeners. *Ear and Hearing, 5,* 134–137.

Zarnoch, J. M., & Alpiner, J. G. (1977). *The Denver Scale of Communication Function for Senior Citizens Living in Retirement Centers.* Unpublished manuscript.

The Effects of Age on the Electrophysiological Tests of Auditory and Vestibular System Function

22

CHAPTER

Gary P. Jacobson, PhD, and Jacyln B. Spitzer, PhD ∎

Effects of Age on Electrophysiological Tests of Auditory System Function

Electrophysiological measurements of the auditory and vestibular pathways offer an opportunity to study the function of these vital sensory systems. From these observations, we learn about signal transmission through the central nervous system and how it changes as we age, and we are able to infer relationships between histological data and alterations in signal processing. Perhaps more importantly, we gain an ability to understand the underlying mechanisms for the clinical problems encountered with aging patients and to differentiate the effects of normal aging from pathological entities that require medical or audiologic intervention.

This chapter discusses the current research findings, using auditory evoked potentials and electrophysiological measurements of vestibular function in elderly samples to evaluate the effects of senescence on hearing and balance function. The auditory measurements to be discussed include short-latency auditory evoked potentials such as electrocochleography and brainstem auditory evoked potentials; middle-latency responses; and long-latency auditory evoked potentials. The vestibular techniques that will be discussed include caloric, rotational, and posturographic testing. An examination of the research will provide a better understanding of the application of electrophysiological techniques in aging clinical populations and permit remaining research needs to be identified.

Auditory Evoked Potentials

Evoked potentials permit us to examine the functional effects of the auditory anatomical changes described in chapter 3. Taking advantage of the electrical nature of the cen-

395

tral nervous system, auditory stimulation causes propagation of neural impulses, which are conducted in a synchronized manner along the auditory pathway. The reader is referred to Jacobson and Hyde (1985) for a comprehensive discussion of the bases of auditory evoked potential measurement.

The anatomical alterations throughout the auditory pathway have subtle ramifications for central auditory processing; this has been demonstrated using behavioral techniques that stress the processing capabilities of the elderly (cf. Bergman, 1980; Sticht & Gray, 1969.)

Short-Latency Auditory Evoked Potentials

Short-latency evoked potentials include those associated with cochlear, neural, and brainstem sites. The measurement techniques used to assess these loci are electrocochleography (ECoG) and brainstem auditory evoked potentials (BAEP). ECoG is used to study the electrical activity of the cochlea and the eighth nerve. Although age effects have been demonstrated for infancy (Fria & Doyle, 1984; Starr, Amilie, Martin, & Sanders, 1977), little investigation has focused on ECoG at the upper end of the age spectrum, despite the known effect that age has on the structure and biochemistry of the cochlea (cf. Gacek, 1975; Goodhill & Guggenheim, 1971; Schuknecht, 1964, 1967; Schuknecht & Igaraski, 1964). Bergholtz, Hooper, and Mehta (1977) employed ECoG in groups of older and noise-exposed subjects (mean age = 58 years, range = 20–78 years). The older subjects included persons with presbycusis, presbycusis with a conductive component, conductive hearing loss, noise-induced loss, and sensorineural loss of unknown etiology. In this heterogenous sample, several observations were made: (a) 22% of the sample showed short-latency action potential (AP) thresholds and a rapid increase in amplitude with increasing click intensity (i.e., an electrophysiological correlate of loudness recruitment), (b) 33% exhibited partial recruitment (i.e., a long-latency AP thresh-

old with steep amplitude/intensity functions, and (c) 17% had both ECoG signs of complete or partial recruitment and positive findings (reduced sensation level) on acoustic reflex measures. In view of the mixture of subjects in this sample (the inclusion of some cochlear influences in addition to aging), the latter study did not show conclusively that aging is associated with systematic changes on ECoG. Additional study is warranted to evaluate the cochlear and neural consequences of aging using this technique.

In contrast, considerable interest has focused on the evaluation of elderly subjects using BAEP. There are several reasons that BAEP may have been examined more intensively than ECoG. First, the noninvasive nature of BAEP caused it to become a more accessible and attractive technique in clinical and research laboratories. Second, the BAEP response itself provides greater insights than ECoG into processing in the central nervous system (CNS) pathways, providing an avenue for evaluating possible CNS alterations in the elderly. Finally, a clinically pressing need existed to differentiate the finding on examinations of unimpaired elderly patients from those in whom test results indicated a need for medical or surgical intervention. This issue is especially important in the diagnosis of demyelinating and degenerative diseases as well as of space-occupying lesions of the auditory nerve, brainstem, and posterior fossa, as amply demonstrated in the work of Starr and Achor (1975) and Starr (1978).

In evaluating hypothesized auditory transmission effects, it is necessary to control the influence of hearing threshold loss in the high-frequency region, 2000–4000 Hz (Bauch & Olsen, 1988; Coats & Martin, 1977; Gorga, Worthington, Reiland, Beauchaine, & Goldgar, 1985; Jerger & Mauldin, 1978; Moller & Blegvad, 1976), a configuration that typifies sensory-type presbycusis (Corso, 1971, 1977; Salomon, Vesteragen, & Jagd, 1988). As will be seen in the review of this literature, lack of control over this important variable and/or inadequate reporting of subject characteristics have undermined the ability to generalize the findings to elderly clinical samples.

Rowe (1978) described BAEP normative data for a group of young (mean age = 25.1, range 17–33 years) and old (mean age = 61.7, range 51–74 years) subjects. The findings indicated an increase in absolute latency for the primary waves I, II, III, IV, and V, with click stimuli presented at 10 and 30 clicks/s. Examination of interpeak latency differences (I-III, III-V, I-V) failed to show statistically significant differences between subject groups. However, the study did indicate great intra- and intersubject variability among the older group. Rowe argued the need for separate clinical norms to be applied to the older patients under evaluation. A limitation of this study is the fact that Rowe did not report his subjects' hearing configurations, so the influence of hearing loss cannot be evaluated in his data.

Similarly, Beagley and Sheldrake (1978) investigated the effects of interstimulus interval and various presentation levels in a group of 70 subjects ranging in age from 14 to 79 years. The authors found a nonsignificant increase in the latency of wave V in their older subjects. Beagley and Sheldrake did not find a prolongation of the wave I-V interval. They did, however, observe an amplitude reduction in wave V, which they attributed to either age changes in tissue impedance or reduced response synchrony with increasing age.

Jerger and Hall (1980) employed BAEP in a large group of subjects ranging in age from 20 to 79 years. The authors demonstrated a modest age effect, specifically a slightly delayed latency and smaller amplitude for wave V in their older subjects. This trend applied to both normal-hearing and sensorineural-impaired subjects. Jerger and Hall also advocated separate norms for elderly clinical samples.

In a careful study of the BAEP effects of intensity, Harkins and Lenhardt (1980) evaluated young (mean age = 23) and elderly (mean age = 72) subjects. The authors attempted to relate the findings on other clinical audiologic tests, such as pure tone thresholds, the *Short Increment Sensi-*

tivity Index, speech discrimination, and stapedial reflexes to latency-intensity functions generated using BAEP. They found that the older subjects' peak latency of wave V was delayed compared to the young at all intensities studied. At moderate intensities such as 55 dB hearing level (HL), the elderly subjects produced wave V latencies equivalent to those of the young subjects at 45 dB HL, whereas at 80 dB HL, the peak latencies for the two groups converged. Harkins and Lenhardt suggested that the BAEP may be a useful indicator of cochlear involvement; at times it was more sensitive than the other clinical tests of recruitment or loudness processing that they administered.

Subsequent investigators (Chu, 1985; Debruyne, 1986; Johannsen & Lehn, 1984; Rosenhall, Bjorkman, Pederson, & Kall, 1985) have corroborated the minor latency and amplitude alterations cited by Rowe and Jerger and Hall. The latency prolongation for waves I, III, and V is on the order of 0.1 to 0.2 ms for subjects over 50 years old compared to those 20 to 30 years old. Johannsen and Lehn (1984) observed latency prolongations without any age-dependent effect on amplitude. Chu (1985) and Debruyne (1986) also remarked on a small increase in interpeak wave latency, although there has not been agreement on the involvement of III-V or III-I, or both. Allison, Hume, Wood, and Goff (1984) suggested that prolonged interpeak latencies may reflect aging changes in the brainstem, particularly through the pons.

It should be noted that a contrasting opinion has been expressed in interpreting the amplitude findings. Harkins and Lenhardt (1980) suggested that tissue impedance changes in the elderly may contribute to decreased amplitude measurements. If this is the case, then amplitude decreases are artifacts of technical problems, rather than changed transmission patterns or alterations in synchrony.

Harkins and Lenhardt (1980) also applied BAEP in evaluation of patients diagnosed as having dementia of the Alzheimer's type (DAT). The authors used the rationale that if demyelinating diseases such as multiple sclerosis (cf. Robinson & Rudge, 1975) caused interpeak latency aberrations, they might be seen as well in DAT. Harkins and Lenhardt presented BAEP data that were obtained from nine subjects diagnosed with DAT. Compared to young controls and normal elderly, the demented patients had a significantly prolonged wave V latency. Of note was the finding of increased interpeak latencies. These findings suggested impaired brainstem transmission in this sample of Alzheimer's disease patients. Impaired brainstem neural transmission was a surprising finding given the known effects of Alzheimer's on cortical structures.

In clinical application, it is evident that the effects of hearing loss and aging may confound each other. Therefore, it is necessary to develop clinical norms in each laboratory that allow comparison of an individual patient against his or her normally hearing age peers. A working group of the American Speech-Language-Hearing Association (1988) failed to reach a consensus on how to solve this clinical dilemma, considering that additional stratified design studies are required in which subjects' hearing is well specified and the site of lesion is documented using an external criterion measure. If we keep in mind that latency prolongations that have been demonstrated are indeed small (0.1–0.2 ms), the overall impact of age alone also appears to be minor. Several clinicians, among them Jerger (1989), have stated that the influence of aging on clinical examinations is negligible for all practical purposes.

Middle-Latency Responses (MLRs)

MLRs have been studied to a lesser extent than other auditory potentials. Woods and Clayworth (1986) investigated MLRs in young (20–35 years) and elderly (60–70 years) subjects. They reported MLR click thresholds for the two groups. The results clearly reflected some degree of high-frequency loss among their elderly subjects, resulting in samples that were not audiometrically matched. Significant differences

were obtained between the groups. The morphology of the MLR responses differed, especially in an enhancement of amplitude for the Pa component in the elderly subjects. As with the BAEP findings discussed earlier, the latency of Pa was significantly prolonged, by 2.3 ms. The components Nb and Pb, both ordinarily more variable than Pa, were also delayed. The authors argued that the consistent changes obtained in their elderly subjects could not be attributed to the effects of hearing loss, especially because a single component was differentially altered. On the latter basis, Woods and Clayworth (see Figure 22.1) hypothesized that aging changes affect structure or neurochemical production in the inhibitory input of the thalamic reticular nucleus to the medial geniculate body, the proposed generator of the Pa component of MLRs.

Buchwald, Erwin, Read, Van Lancker, and Cummings (1989) evaluated the thalamic function of subjects with DAT using MLRs. The authors compared their DAT subjects to age-matched controls. Normal findings were obtained for the Pa response, but Pb (corresponding to the long-latency P1 component at 50–65 ms) was either absent or significantly decreased in amplitude. The authors concluded that the midbrain generators' cholinergic defect in DAT was detectable using MLR measurements.

Long-Latency Auditory Evoked Potentials

The long-latency potentials, historically ascribed to the primary auditory and association areas in the temporal and temporoparietal regions, have been called "cortical potentials." This polyphasic waveform, notably the N1 (at approximately 100 ms) and the P2 (at approximately 180–200 ms), has been used extensively for purposes of threshold identification in alert, cooperative subjects.

Goodin, Squires, Henderson, and Starr (1978) evaluated cortical components in the context of a larger study of endogenous potentials. They found that increasing age effected a decrease in evoked potential amplitude and increased evoked potential

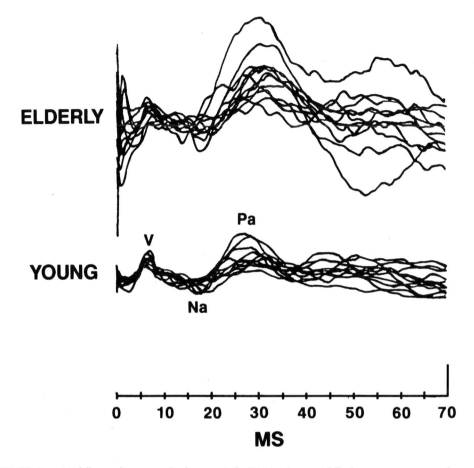

FIGURE 22.1. Middle auditory evoked potentials (MAEPs) or middle-latency responses from the Cz electrode averaged over different stimulus conditions and intensities for individual older (top) and younger (bottom) subjects. (Each tracing represents the mean MAEP from a single subject.) *Note.* From ''Age-Related Changes in Human Middle Latency Auditory Evoked Potentials'' by D. L. Woods and C. C. Clayworth, 1986, *Electroencephalography and Clinical Neurophysiology, 65,* pp. 297–303. Copyright 1986 by Elsevier Scientific Publishers Ireland. Reprinted by permission.

latency. Pfefferbaum, Ford, Roth, Hopkins, and Kopell (1979) compared cortical potential and endogenous component findings in healthy young and old females (mean age = 78.9 years, range 74–87 years). There was no difference in N1 amplitude or latency between old and young groups.

Endogenous Evoked Potentials

Long-latency auditory evoked potentials such as P300 offer insights into cognitive processing and attention and, as such, have been studied in the hope of providing diag-

nostic information for a variety of pathological conditions, including dementia (Goodin et al., 1978), schizophrenia (McCallum, 1973), and alcoholism (Pfefferbaum et al., 1979). It is clear, however, that interpretation of any such findings in pathological samples must be predicated on an understanding of the effects of normal aging on these evoked potentials. Hence, numerous investigators (Ford et al., 1978; Goodin et al., 1978; Pfefferbaum et al., 1979) have examined the long-latency auditory evoked potential findings of healthy elderly samples.

Goodin et al. (1978) studied 47 subjects ranging from 6 to 76 years of age. They presented frequent (1000-Hz) and infrequent (2000-Hz) stimuli with a ratio of 85 frequent to 15 infrequent stimuli. The experimental conditions involved a conventional auditory "oddball" paradigm. P300 was present only in the latter condition when subjects kept track of stimuli. Goodin et al. reported that P300 amplitude decreased at the rate of 0.2 μv/yr. They also reported latency changes for N2 and P300. N2 latency increased to a small degree, 0.8 ms/yr, but P300 increased more dramatically, by 1.8 ms/yr.

Squires, Chippendale, Wrege, Gooden, and Starr (1980) found systematic P300 latency increases with age, at the rate of 1.64 ms/yr. These P300 latencies were observed to be in excess of 400 ms by the 8th decade. The authors made the important point that it was possible to distinguish the effect of peripheral hearing loss from central changes by examining N1 in addition to P300. N1 showed little age-related latency increase (6 ms in a sample spanning 6 decades) whereas P300 showed an approximate 100-ms increase over the same age span. The latter issue requires further investigation, as the authors did not report either the audiometric responses or the configuration of hearing losses in their sample.

Pfefferbaum, Ford, Roth, and Kopell (1980) employed stringent criteria in subject selection for a study of event-related potentials. They selected young college students (mean age = 22.3 years) and elderly subjects (mean age = 78.6 years), all of whom were in good physical health and educationally matched to the controls. The authors commented that the stimuli were presented at some sensation level above threshold for 1000 Hz, but do not provide the audiometric characteristics of the groups. Their paradigm entailed a frequent stimulus of 1000 Hz and two infrequent stimuli, 500 and 2000 Hz, with the higher-frequency tone as the target. In response to frequent stimuli, the older group produced significantly larger amplitude and later P2 components than the young subjects. The elderly group's N1-P2 complex was also significantly larger than for controls.

Pfefferbaum et al. showed that the elderly subjects' P300 was significantly prolonged compared to the younger group, as shown in Figure 22.2. The average P300 latency for target stimuli was 448 ms for the older group and 334 ms for the controls; for nontarget stimuli this difference was further enhanced, at 518 ms for the elderly and 338 ms for the controls. The authors compared their observed data to the predictions based on Goodin et al. (1978) described above. The regression equation failed to predict accurately the nontarget latency, but was accurate for target latency. Pfefferbaum et al. explained some of their differences with Goodin et al. based on the former's use of consistent sensation level, which compensates to some extent for probable high-frequency hearing loss among their sample, whereas Goodin et al. had kept the presentation level of stimuli constant across subjects. Amplitude was not significantly affected across various electrode placements in Pfefferbaum et al.'s work. The authors concluded that the presence of latency shift in their healthy and intellectually active elderly indicated that occult CNS pathology may produce mild, undetected cognitive deterioration. In the demented, P300 is prolonged without significant delay in P2, whereas normal aging increased latency in both components. Pfefferbaum and associates suggested that dementing processes produce P300 latency increases, which add to those produced by normal aging. They also indicated that the significant differences in findings between studies of healthy elderly and other studies with demented patients may be associated with essentially dissimilar processes.

Smith, Michalewski, Brent, and Thompson (1980) obtained some contrasting evidence in a study of 10 young females (mean age = 21.3 years, range from 18 to 33) and 10 older females (mean age = 71.1 years, range from 65 to 80). Again, the subjects in this study were not described audiometrically. A different paradigm, consisting of a constant presentation level of a

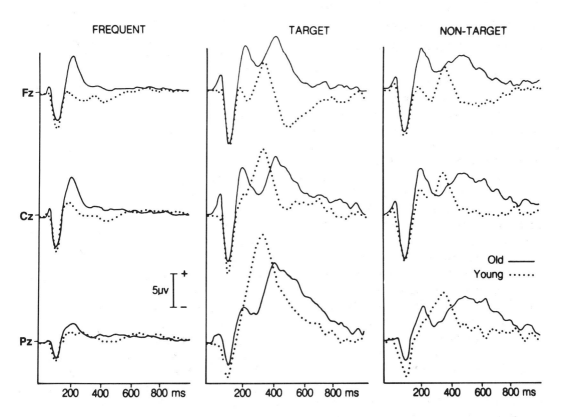

FREQUENT   **TARGET**   **NON-TARGET**

Old ——
Young ······

FIGURE 22.2. Grand average event-related potentials to the frequent and infrequent stimuli recorded at Fz, Cz, and Pz for the old and young subjects (superimposed). *Note.* From "Age-Related Changes in Auditory Event-Related Potentials" by A. Pfefferbaum, J. M. Ford, W. T. Roth, and B. S. Kopell, 1980, *Electroencephalography and Clinical Neurophysiology, 49,* pp. 266–276. Copyright 1986 by Elsevier Scientific Publishers Ireland. Reprinted by permission.

65-dB sound pressure level (SPL) and a design using 10 frequent midfrequency stimuli (900 Hz) to 1 infrequent stimulus (3300 Hz) was used.

Elderly subjects produced a larger P1 and smaller P2 amplitude than the younger subjects, and an equivalent N1 amplitude. Further, a significant age main effect and interaction for age X trial order was obtained for P300. Smith and others also found a significant slow wave difference between young and elderly groups, with the elderly producing a more positive polarity. The authors failed to find a difference in scalp topography among the elderly, as is typically found in younger subjects. They ascribed this observation to a lesser

frontal negative-to-positive gradient among the older participants, which suggested some selective aging process in that cortical area.

A variety of methodological approaches have been used in ensuing investigations (Fein & Turetsky, 1989; Ford, Duncan-Johnson, Pfefferbaum, & Kopell, 1982; Michalewski, Patterson, Bowman, Litzleman, & Thompson, 1982; Polich, Howard, & Starr, 1985). The results reinforce the dependency of the magnitude of the absolute latency shift on technical variations. However, repeated demonstrations of the prolongation of P300 indicate the utility of auditory measures in evaluation of cognitive alterations in normal aged subjects.

Future Directions in Research on the Effects of Age on Auditory Evoked Potentials

Computed topographic mapping of evoked potentials, or "brainmapping," is a technique that is achieving increasingly widespread application. The technique employs an electrode montage so that simultaneous recordings from numerous sites, as opposed to montages of one, two, or three electrodes as in the studies described earlier in the chapter, are accomplished and isopotential maps of electrical activity are generated. Duffy, Albert, McAnulty, and Garvey (1984) examined 4 decades of males, ranging in groups from 30 to 80 years old. The subjects were extensively studied from a medical, neuropsychological, and electroencephalographic point of view. Standard electroencephalography and P300 topographic maps, or brainmaps, were generated. The results contrasted with previous studies in that alpha wave frequency and amplitude were uncorrelated with age, giving some evidence of desynchronization rather than decreased activity. In addition, frontal and parietocentral evoked potential features demonstrated age-related change. The location of the P300 maximum amplitude shifted posteriorly with age. A potentially powerful technique, computed topography will be applied in the future in a variety of aged clinical groups.

Effects of Age on Electrophysiological Tests of Vestibular System Function

The impairment of visual, auditory, and somesthetic sensitivity and acuity as a function of age are well documented and understood (e.g., Kokmen, Bossemeyer, & Williams, 1978; Marshall, 1981; Sekuler, Hutman, & Owsley, 1980). However, the sense of balance does not *appear* to go through any obvious deterioration. The inherent redundancy in the balance system effectively insulates us from permanent losses of stability following disease. The "balance system" consists of the vestibular, visual, and somesthetic systems (e.g., vibration, proprioception). The visual and somesthetic systems normally interact with the vestibular system and "support" balance by providing the brain with orientation information even in the absence of an intact vestibular system. It is the interactions between these three systems and the efferent activity that flows to the muscles that control posture that allows us to remain upright. Unfortunately, these support systems and the motor system decline in their efficiency as we age. The mildest effects of senescence of the balance system in the healthy aged patient may be a loss of equilibrium and the constant sensation of unsteadiness. Drachman and Hart (1972) referred to this phenomenon as the "multisensory deficit." The severest effect of the multisensory deficit may be a fall. The present review will attempt to describe the effects of age on examinations of balance system function. These examinations include subtests of the electronystagmographic test battery including tests of positional and positioning nystagmus and caloric testing, quantitative rotational testing, and quantitative posturographic testing.

Imbalance in the Elderly—Effects of Falling

Falls in the elderly can result in morbidity (e.g., fractures of extremities or hip, or soft tissue injuries requiring hospitalization) or mortality (Isaacs, 1983). Falls were the cause of 11,600 deaths in 1982; 70% of those who died as a result of falls were elderly (Nickens, 1985). It is probable that this figure underestimates the number of elderly ill patients whose deaths were hastened by falls that required hospitalization. Additionally, the impact of falling may extend beyond acute hospitalization. It is not uncommon for the elderly faller to restrict his or her movements following a severe fall (Murphy & Isaacs, 1982). Thus, the after effects of a fall may have significant impact on the quality of life of the elderly patient. It is surprising that although a great deal of research has been conducted in the areas of auditory and visual perception in the aged, startlingly little work has been conducted for the purposes of quantifying the effect that age has on the balance system. This apparent lack of interest is particularly bothersome when one considers the devastating effect of falling in the elderly.

A recent 1-year prospective study conducted by Tinnetti, Speechley, and Ginter (1988) evaluated the prevalence of falling in a group of 336 noninstitutionalized elderly persons aged 75 years and older. The investigators found that 46% of the group fell at least once, 29% of the group fell twice, and 25% of the group fell three times during the year period. It was interesting that 77% of the falls occurred in the home and 93% of the fallers were taking sedative medications. It is possible to categorize the causes of falls as being precipitated internally (e.g., loss of consciousness) or externally (e.g., tripping on carpeting) (Sheldon, 1960). Tinnetti and others (1988) reported that most falls consisted of trips (e.g., on carpeting or an icy sidewalk) or falls down stairs (usually because of miscalculating the location of a bottom step). Only 13% of the falls appeared to be the result of dizziness. The morbidity was reported to be 24%, with 6% of the fallers sustaining fractures of the upper extremity, lower extremity, or hip.

These results may be compared to those of Sheldon (1960), who reported a prevalence of falls of 34% (usually down stairs), trips of 11%, and falls due to vertigo of 7%. It is interesting that these authors reported a 25% prevalence of drop attacks in their 202 subjects. Drop attacks were believed to be the cause of 52% of the falls reported by Naylor and Rosin (1970). The authors felt that the origins of the falls were approximately evenly divided between internal causes (e.g., cerebrovascular disease, ves-

tibular vertigo) and external causes (e.g., trips and falls). It has been suggested by some that factors such as room illumination and the associated ability of the elderly to identify obstacles, as well as the use of medications such as sedatives, antidepressants, tricyclics, and antihypertensives increase the risk of falling (Lucht, 1971; Tinnetti et al., 1988; Waller, 1974, 1978; Wild, Nayak, & Isaacs, 1980). However, other investigators have provided evidence that calls into doubt the contention that the use of sedative and hypertensive medications increases the risk of falling (Rashiq & Logan, 1986; Stegman, 1983).

There is agreement that incidents of falling increase with age and also increase as a function of a decrease in mental status and the general health of the elderly person (Lucht, 1971; Naylor & Rosin, 1970; Nickens, 1985; Perry, 1982; Prudham & Evans, 1981; Tinnetti et al., 1988; Waller, 1974, 1978; Wild et al., 1980, 1981a, 1981b, 1981c). It is also known that the risk of falling again increases once one has fallen and that elderly women are more likely to fall than elderly men (Ashley, Gryfe, & Amies, 1977; Droller, 1955; Exton-Smith, 1977; Gryfe, Amies, & Ashley, 1977; Naylor & Rosin, 1970; Prudham & Evans, 1981; Wild et al., 1980). Age-related falls in the absence of disease are, in part, probably due to age-related changes in gait (Sudarsky & Ronthal, 1983) that result in destabilization when seemingly unimportant obstacles are encountered.

Statistics pertaining to the mortality associated with falls in the elderly are particularly alarming. Ashley et al. (1977) and Gryfe et al. (1977) reported on the relationship between repetitive falling and mortality in a 5-year prospective investigation of institutionalized elderly. The investigators found that of those patients with six or more falls, 65% died during the course of the study. Waller (1978) reported that 26% of his population who had fallen and were hospitalized died within 1 year following hospitalization. The same author indicated that deaths caused by falling increased as a function of age; from age 65 to 74 the death rate was 93 per 100,000 (.01%) and this increased to 625 per 100,000 (.6%) in the 85-and-above age group (Waller, 1974). Wild et al. (1981b) observed that 32 of 125 elderly fallers were dead after one year (26%). Additionally, 11 of 20 patients who had "long lies" (e.g., loss of consciousness) following falls were dead after 1 year (55%). It is clear from these statistics that falling in the elderly is not a trivial problem. It is incumbent upon us to understand the factors that contribute to lack of stability in advancing age. Information of this type may be gained by a review of how age affects normal performance on conventional tests of balance system function. Additionally, it is helpful to have an appreciation of the connections between the vestibular nuclei and other systems that assist in the maintenance of balance.

Central Vestibular System Connections

The peripheral vestibular apparatus routes its afferent outflow through the approximately 18,000 neurons that comprise the superior and inferior divisions of the vestibular division of the VIII N to Scarpa's ganglion and then to the superior, medial, lateral, and inferior vestibular nuclei. This information is routed to a number of different sites in the CNS. Cerebellar structures including the flocculonodular lobes receive input from the vestibular nuclei. These structures in turn send efferents via the cerebellovestibular pathway to regulate the activity present in the vestibular nuclei and assist in compensation for acute or insidious decreases in tonic activity emanating from the peripheral vestibular system apparatus (e.g., end organs and the vestibular branch of VIII N). The lateral and medial vestibular nuclei are points of origin for the lateral and medial vestibulospinal pathways. The neurons comprising these pathways project to the anterior horn cells in the cervical, thoracic, and lumbar levels of the spinal cord for reflex movements of muscles

that govern our posture and ultimately our stability. These centers send feedback about posture back to the vestibular nuclei.

Afferent activity from the vestibular nuclei is also routed through the horizontal and vertical gaze centers in the paramedian pontine and mesencephalic reticular formations, respectively, to the medial longitudinal fasciculus (MLF) for mediation of the vestibulocular reflex arc (VOR). This reflex makes it possible for us to maintain stable vision on objects in the environment during movements of the head. Afferent information is routed to the primary vestibular cortex in the temporal lobes, where the perception of motion and position is mediated. There are also connections between the left and right vestibular nuclei whose purpose is not entirely understood. These connections undoubtedly assist in the process of central compensation following the unilateral transient or permanent loss of a peripheral vestibular system. Finally, there are connections between the vestibular nuclei and the automatic nervous system where secondary characteristics of dizziness (e.g., pallor, sweating, nausea, vomiting) are controlled.

Review of Past and Present Research Evaluating Age Effects on Electrophysiological Tests of Balance System Function

The one common denominator that is present in the literature pertaining to the effects of aging on measures of perception and performance is the inherent variability in the elderly as a group. Some normal elderly show no deficits, whereas others show marked deficits. These trends certainly are preserved in the data concerning performance by the elderly on tests of vestibular system function. The population sampling techniques, diagnostic methods, methods of quantification, and choice of method used to analyze these data have had an effect on the outcome of these studies. The prevailing evidence supports the contention that aging effects changes in the normal physiology of the vestibular system. The effects of age can be found on all examinations; however, the effects are small and they generally occur late in life (after 65 years of age). The results of diagnostic tests indicate a gradual loss of sensitivity in the peripheral vestibular system and in the support systems. Aging of the vestibular system has been termed *presbyatonia* (Ghosh, 1985), *presbyastasis* (Belal & Glorig, 1986), and *presbylibrium* (McClure, 1986).

Caloric Testing

A number of investigations have been conducted since the late 1930s that have served to describe the effect that age has on caloric-induced nystagmus. These investigations have been published in foreign journals without the benefit of English-language translations or abstracts. The interested reader is directed to excellent reviews of these early studies in Mulch and Petermann (1979) and Oosterveld (1983).

Arslan (1957) in an early study evaluated 50 normal subjects between 49 and 84 years of age, measuring nystagmus duration and total number of beats in response to caloric irrigations. The author calculated the mean and two standard deviation values from the group data and reported that in general, middle-aged subjects showed hyperactive responses and subjects aged 70 years and older showed hypoactive responses.

Van der Laan and Oosterveld (1974) reported their observations from a group of 334 normal subjects. The authors reported a lesser nystagmus frequency and greater nystagmus amplitude in younger subjects (e.g., up through the 3rd decade of life) compared with older subjects. The nystagmus frequency increased and amplitude decreased in the older age groups. The investigators suggested that these findings in the older age groups (over 50 years of age) could be explained by a decrease in blood supply (e.g., as a result of atherosclerosis) reaching the vestibular end organ. Similarly, Clement, van der Laan, and

Oosterveld (1975) reported a decline in slow-phase eye velocity (SPEV) as a function of age. The authors reported their observations of 250 subjects who were divided into seven age decade groups.

Bruner and Norris (1971) reported their observations culled from examinations of 293 individuals with negative findings on vestibular system testing. The investigators conducted bithermal testing using 31.5 °C (as opposed to the conventional 30 °C resulting from instrumentation problems) and 44 °C water temperatures over a 30-s period. The authors quantified nystagmus latency, amplitude, frequency, average maximum SPEV, and duration. They found that all nystagmus parameters with the exception of nystagmus latency increased to a peak in the 60–70 age group and declined thereafter. These findings are illustrated in Figure 22.3.

The investigators also found that the warm rather than cool caloric irrigations resulted in nystagmus of greater magnitude. The elderly subjects showed disproportionately stronger responses to warm stimuli. The only statistically significant parameters to show age-dependent changes were nystagmus frequency for cool caloric stimuli and maximum SPEV and frequency for warm caloric stimulation and total (combined warm and cool) caloric stimulation.

In a much-quoted study, Mulch and Petermann (1979) evaluated caloric responses in 102 subjects aged 11–70 years. There were 17 subjects in each group, evenly distributed by sex. Caloric stimulation consisted of 50 ml of 30 °C and 44 °C water that was delivered over a 30-s period. The subjects' eyes were open in darkness. The authors quantified the total number of beats of nystagmus, maximum SPEV, frequency, and amplitude over a 10-s period and analyzed their data using a nonparametric statistical technique (the Wilcoxon signed-ranks test). The authors reported significant age-dependent increases in the total number of beats, maximum frequency, amplitude, and SPEV up to 60 years of age, after which decrements in function occurred (see Figure 22.4).

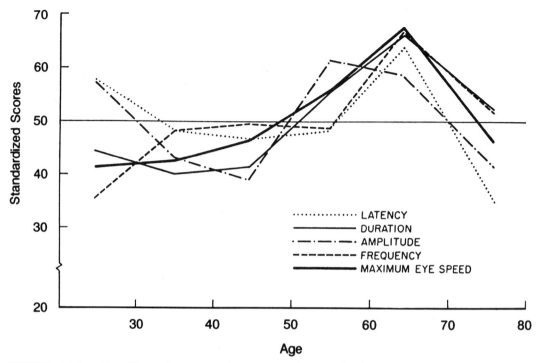

FIGURE 22.3. The effects of age on caloric test results. Standard scores (mean = 50, S.D. = 10) for nystagmus measures for all four irrigations plotted over age. *Note.* From "Age-Related Changes in Caloric Nystagmus" by A. Bruner and T. W. Norris, 1979, *Acta Otolaryngologica (Stockh), 282*(Suppl.), pp. 1–24. Copyright 1979 by Almquist and Wiksell Periodical Company. Reprinted by permission.

Karlsen, Hassanein, and Goetzinger (1981) reported their results following conventional bithermal caloric testing in 75 subjects aged 18–81 years. The authors quantified nystagmus amplitude, latency, duration, frequency, and SPEV following irrigations. All parameters showed an age-related decrement. For cool caloric irrigations only nystagmus duration showed an age-dependent change, with older subjects showing shorter nystagmus durations. The maximum duration was reached by 61 years of age. For warm caloric irrigations, SPEV, duration, amplitude, and frequency showed age-dependent increases. In general, the performance of the younger group (aged 18–35 years) differed from that of the older groups (aged 61–71+ years) on these measures. The differences, however, were not always simple. For example, significant SPEV differences were only found between those aged 18–35 and 61–65 and those who were 71 years old and over. There were no significant differences for this parameter between subjects in the 18- to 35-year age group and those in the 61- to 65-year or 65- to 70-year age groups. The suggestion from this investigation was that there is a decline in vestibular system responsiveness beginning around age 65–70; this is in general agreement with previous studies.

Ghosh (1985) reported the results of serial vestibulometry on 78 subjects who were divided into seven age groups from 10 to 71+ years. In serial vestibulometry, the ear is irrigated with water that is 45, 33, 29, 25, 21, and 17 °C. The maximum SPEV following each irrigation was the measurement parameter. The author reported that there were greater age-related differences in the caloric nystagmus SPEV at the extremes of irrigation temperatures. Age had a gen-

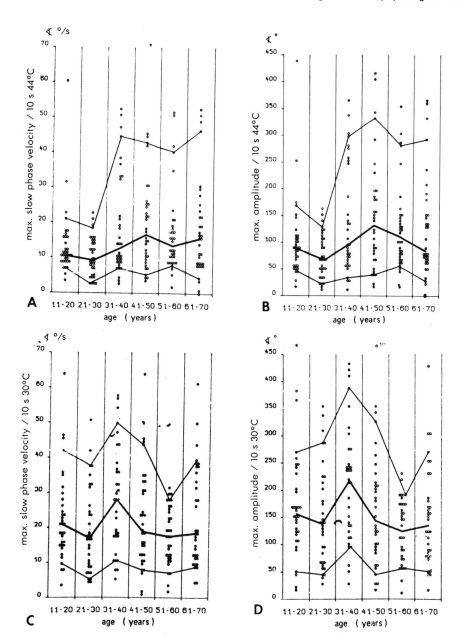

FIGURE 22.4. Scatterplot of maximum slow phase eye velocity for warm and cool caloric irrigations (A and C) and maximum amplitude for warm and cool irrigations (B and D) as a function of subject age (*N* = 102 healthy subjects). *Note.* From "Influence of Age on Results of Vestibular Function Tests" by G. Mulch and W. Petermann, 1979, *Annals of Otology, Rhinology, and Laryngology, 88*(Suppl.), pp. 1–17. Copyright 1979 by Annals Publishing Company. Reprinted by permission.

eral effect of decreasing SPEVs. The mean performance of subjects above the age of 51 fell outside normal limits. No parametric analyses were reported; however, the general finding of reduced caloric SPEVs as a function of age is consistent with the findings of previous research.

Davidson, Wright, Ilmoyl, Canter, and Barber (1988) have reported that the test-retest repeatability on monothermal warm and alternate binaural bithermal caloric testing is better for young subjects compared with elderly subjects. The test-retest repeatability for the variable maximum SPEV was .98 for both caloric tests for young subjects (20–30 years, $N = 15$). The test-retest repeatability was .90 for the warm monothermal test and .92 for the alternate binaural bithermal test for the elderly group (65–75 years, $N = 14$).

Finally, Jacobson and Henry (1989) have recently reported that fixation suppression (e.g., VOR cancellation) of caloric induced nystagmus becomes significantly poorer as we age. This finding would suggest that the neuronal connections between the vestibular nuclei and the midline cerebellar structures (e.g., flocculus, nodulus) become less efficient with age. These are the same pathways that assist in compensation following acute or insidious losses of peripheral vestibular system function.

Ocular Motility Testing

Age-related changes in ocular motility have been reported by various authors. These investigations have shown that elderly subjects are less capable of accurately pursuing rapidly moving targets than younger subjects (Kuechenmeister, Linton, Mueller, & White, 1977; Rosenhall, Bjorkman, Pederson, & Hanner, 1987; Sharpe & Sylvester, 1978; Spooner, Sakala, & Baloh, 1980; Zackon & Sharpe, 1987). Additionally, Rosenhall et al. (1987) reported that saccade latencies showed increases (by 25–50 ms) when the performance of older subjects (76–77 years) was compared with that of middle-aged subjects (20–50 years). Saccadic velocities decreased with age, although only by 11–13%, when the performance of elderly subjects was compared with that of younger adult subjects. Saccade accuracy was equivalent for all age groups.

Rotational Testing

Rotational testing is a second method by which the vestibular system, and specifically the horizontal semicircular canal system, can be evaluated. Many rotational test techniques have evolved over the years and, therefore, comparisons between results is difficult. The technique of *cupulometry* was introduced by Egmont, Groen, and Jongkees (1953). In this technique a patient is manually rotated in a chair at varying velocities and is suddenly stopped. Deceleration and the fluid movement over the cupula is the effective stimulus. Nystagmus threshold as a function of the speed of rotation, duration of nystagmus, and duration of subjective symptoms is often quantified. *Torsion swing* and *torsion swing chair* testing (Boer, de Carels, & Philipszoon, 1963) are types of sinusoidal rotational tests. The torsion swing chair consists of a wound spring upon which a chair is mounted. When it is released, the chair oscillates back and forth in a sinusoidal manner. The test is conducted in darkness or semidarkness with the patient's eyes open. Electroculography instrumentation is used to record the rotation-induced nystagmus. The symmetry of the nystagmus frequency and SPEV during rightward and leftward rotations is compared. The most recent advancement in rotational testing has been the development of computerized *sinusoidal harmonic acceleration* chair instrumentation. This device consists of a gearless DC motor that drives a chair, a lightproof enclosure within which the chair resides, and a general-purpose computer that serves to analyze eye movement responses to calibrated sinusoidal chair oscillations. The patient is seated in a chair with his or her head placed in a headrest that is tilted forward 60°, placing the horizontal simicircular canal in an orientation parallel to the axis of rotation. The chair may be programmed to oscillate at a series of frequencies ranging from 0.01 to 1.28 Hz, effectively stimulating the horizontal semicircular canal over a broad portion of its operating range. The response of the VOR to rotation is a nystagmus with a SPEV that reaches a peak slightly later than the peak chair acceleration. A computer differentiates the fast and slow phases of the induced nystagmus and eliminates the fast phases. The computer joins the slow-phase eye movements together, creating a sinusoid that matches the chair sinusoid. A number of parameters are measured. These include the phase of the VOR (difference in degrees between eye position and chair position), gain (ratio of peak SPEV divided by peak chair velocity), and symmetry (ratio of peak SPEV following rightward oscillation minus leftward peak SPEV divided by the total).

Excellent reviews of early rotational studies and foreign language rotational studies in the elderly may be found in Mulch and Petermann (1979) and Oosterveld (1983). The general trend in the majority of investigations involving rotational testing has been the finding that the magnitude of the nystagmus responses decreases with increasing age.

Van der Laan and Oosterveld (1974) evaluated 779 individuals of various ages with torsion swing testing. The authors found a sharp increase in nystagmus frequency from childhood to young adulthood. There appeared to be a decline in nystagmus frequency for subjects older than 60 years. Nystagmus amplitudes were greatest in the 1- to 10-year age group and the 11- to 20-year age group. The amplitude decreased from this point until 51–60 years, after which an increase in amplitude was observed. SPEV was greatest in the oldest age group. However, the nystagmus fast phase was least affected by age. This indicated to the authors that the central vestibular pathways were least affected by aging. Noteworthy was the absence of statistical analyses in this investigation, to the extent that no standard deviations for mean values were reported. Subsequent to this study the same group (Clement et al., 1975) reported their observations of 250 subjects who were divided into seven age groups. The authors reported a similar decrease in nystagmus amplitude as a function of age.

Virolainen and Aantaa (1976) evaluated 20 subjects aged 19–22 years (mean age = 20 years) and 20 subjects aged 36–50 years (mean age = 42 years). The authors attempted to determine an acceleration threshold for nystagmus (the acceleration level necessary to elicit nystagmus) by providing a constant increase in acceleration to the right at a rate of 0.2 $°/s^2$ for 90 s that was followed by a constant acceleration for 120 s and a deceleration at a rate of 0.2 $°/s^2$ (providing an effective acceleration to the left). The procedure was repeated in reverse order following a 2-min rest. The authors found no significant age-related differences in the threshold of nystagmus.

Luchikin and Patrin (1983) conducted a cupulometric study of 176 individuals aged 14–92 years who were divided into eight age groups, each spanning 10 years. The authors measured the duration, total number of nystagmus beats, frequency and amplitude of nystagmus, and nystagmus SPEV at 15, 30, and 60% of the maximum stimulating limits. They found that the threshold of nystagmus increased with age and was poorest in the oldest age groups; they also reported a slight increase in the value of all nystagmus parameters at 40–50 years of age. There was a sharp increase in all nystagmus parameters at 70 years of age, followed by a marked decrease after the age of 75. From the same data, Patrin (1986) reported a decrease in nystagmus SPEV as a function of age.

Wall, Black, & Hunt (1984) utilized sinusoidal harmonic acceleration methods and evaluated 50 normal individuals aged 20–59 years. The authors chose rotational frequencies of 0.005–1.0 Hz and peak velocities of 25, 50, and 100 $°/s$. They reported that VOR gain decreased significantly with age when data obtained from 20- to 30-year-olds were compared to the data obtained from 50- to 60-year-olds at 0.005 and 0.01 Hz. These data are illustrated in Figure 22.5. The overall gain (mean gain of all chair frequencies) of the oldest age group was 84% of the gain of the youngest age group.

Finally, Sokolovski (1988) evaluated 160 subjects aged 6–70 years. There were 10 subjects in each of 16 age groups (5 years per age group). Subjects were rotated at 0.8 $°/s^2$ angular acceleration until a velocity of 60 $°/s^2$ was reached. The subjects were then rotated at a constant velocity for an additional 2 min, after which they were abruptly decelerated to a stop. Rotation to

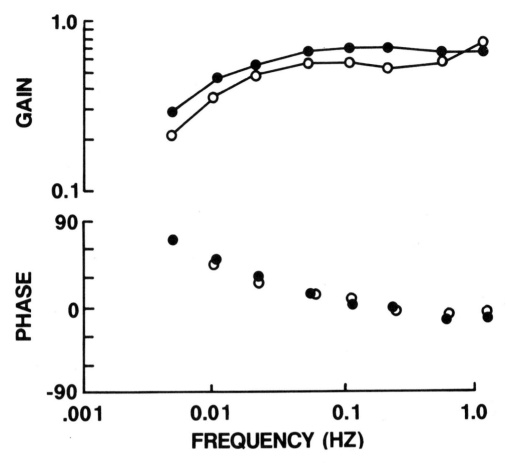

FIGURE 22.5. The effects of age on VOR gain and phase from rotational testing. VOR gain and phase are depicted for two age groups. Filled circles represent subjects aged 20–39 years (*N* = 20). Unfilled circles represent subjects aged 40–69 years (*N* = 20). The group differences for VOR gain at the lowest two frequencies were statistically significant (*p* < .05). *Note.* From "Effects of Age, Sex and Stimulus Parameters upon Vestibulo-ocular Responses to Sinusoidal Rotation" by C. Wall, F. O. Black, and A. E. Hunt, 1984, *Acta Otolaryngologica* (*Stockh*), *98,* pp. 270–278. Copyright 1984 by Almquist and Wiksell Periodical Company. Reprinted by permission.

the right was followed by rotation to the left. Sokolovski measured postrotatory nystagmus latency, duration, maximum SPEV, and total number of nystagmus beats and reported significant age-related increases in nystagmus latency, duration, and total number of beats only following rightward rotations. During leftward rotations there were no significant age correlations for these parameters. The author found that only nystagmus SPEV showed a statistically significant age decrement for leftward and rightward rotations. Sokolovski interpreted

the decrease in SPEV with age to represent evidence of an age-related decrease in the sensitivity of the peripheral vestibular end organ.

Posturography Testing

Conventional tests of vestibular system function (e.g., caloric tests) serve to quantify the activity resulting from artificial stimulation of the VOR. However, vertigo of vestibular origin accounts for a relatively small number of falls in the elderly. For instance, Sheldon (1960) reported dizziness as the principal cause of 11% of the falls in the elderly group studied, whereas Prudham and Evans (1981) reported dizziness as the cause of falling in 6.4% of the population they surveyed. Additionally, the prevalence of dizziness of vestibular origin in the elderly faller is roughly equivalent to that observed in the non-faller (Prudham & Evans, 1981; Tinnetti et al., 1988). It is also possible that some of the reported vertiginous episodes may represent dizziness of extravestibular origin (Gordon, 1978; Hughes & Drachman, 1977; Stevens & Matthews, 1973). What is clear from these investigations is that as we age, our postural control and gait deteriorates (Overstall, Exton-Smith, Imms, & Johnston, 1977; Sudarsky & Ronthal, 1983; Woolacott, Shumway-Cook, & Nashner, 1982).

Behavioral, mechanical, and computerized methods of quantifying the degree to which proprioception and vision contribute to postural stability in the aged have been developed by several individuals (Black, O'Leary, Wall, & Furman, 1977, 1978; Nashner, 1983; Sheldon, 1963; Wright, 1971). The results of these investigations have suggested that, at rest, elderly subjects show comparatively greater amounts of postural sway than their younger counterparts (Black et al., 1977; Luchikin & Patrin, 1983). The amount of postural sway at rest in the elderly is related to the degree of deterioration of vibration sense in the lower extremities (Brocklehurst, Robertson, & James-Groom, 1982a, 1982b). Additionally, the speed of sway at rest is greater in institutionalized than in noninstitutionalized elderly patients and is a predictor of the subjects who will fall (Fernie, Gryfe, Holliday, & Llewellyn, 1982). It also appears from these investigations that elderly individuals with vestibular impairments are less able to compensate for these deficits and rely more on visual cues to remain upright than young subjects with peripheral vestibular system disease (Norre, Forrez, & Beckers, 1987).

Wolfson, Whipple, Amerman, and Kleinberg (1986) have described the effects of aging on an examination of their design called the *Postural Stress Test (PST)*. For this examination the subject was asked to stand with his or her feet comfortably apart facing away from a wall pulley, such as the one that is normally used for strengthening exercises by physical therapists. A padded belt was placed around the subject's waist at the level of the iliac crest. This belt was attached to the pulley cable (see Figure 22.6).

Weights of graded magnitudes of 1.5, 3, and 4.5% of the patient's body weight were attached to the weight pan of the pulley. The weight was supported 2 ft from the ground by one investigator while the other observed the subject's responses when the weight was dropped and supported the patient if he or she fell. The test session was also videotaped for later analysis. Patients were reassured that they would not be allowed to fall. The maximum weight tolerated by the patients and the degree of destabilization caused by the weight drop were quantified by the investigators. The investigators evaluated (a) 22 elderly (mean age = 84 years) nursing home residents with a recent history of falling that could not be explained by a pre-existing medical condition, (b) a group of 18 nursing home residents of equivalent age and sex without a falling history, and (c) a group of 21 younger controls (mean age = 38 years). The authors found that the elderly fallers were significantly more unstable than the younger and older controls. Further, they found that the distribution of scores for the fallers was bimodal. Half of the fallers showed extremely impaired balance while the other half did much better.

Recently, instrumentation has been developed to help determine the contribution that visual, vestibular, and somesthetic information plays in the maintenance of postural stability. The device that was developed by Nashner (1983) and marketed by NeuroCom is called the EquiTest™. The device consists of a platform beneath which reside five force plate transducers (left and right anterior and left and right posterior; the fifth transducer is horizontally mounted

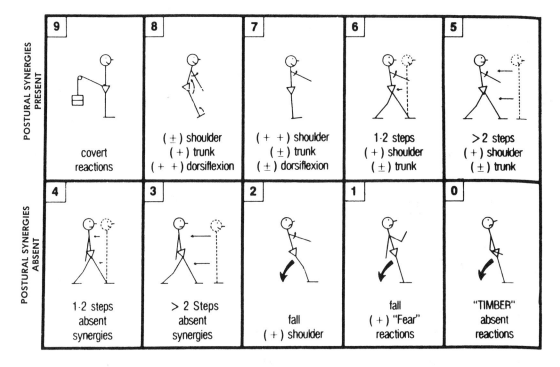

FIGURE 22.6. Ratings of adaptiveness of balance strategies used by subjects on the *Postural Stress Test.* These were responses used by subjects to stabilize themselves after a backward postural perturbation. *Note.* From "Stressing the Postural Response" by L. I. Wolfson, R. Whipple, P. Amerman, and A. Kleinberg, 1986, *Journal of the American Geriatrics Society, 34,* pp. 845–850. Reprinted by permission of the American Geriatrics Society.

and measures the front-back horizontal component of the total force). The transducers are sensitive to the anterior/posterior and left/right sway that a subject might exhibit. Subjects are placed within a loosely fitted harness (to prevent injury in case of a fall) and are asked to fold their arms in front of them and face a 180° painted landscape upon which a horizon is represented. The electrical output from the force plate transducers is routed to a general-purpose computer that provides an analysis of the subjects' sway. Of particular interest is an examination called the *Sensory Organization Test (SOT).* The test consists of six differing conditions of increasing difficulty. Each condition has three trials, each lasting 20 s. Subjects are asked to remain as stable as possible. In some conditions they receive conflicting sensory and/or somesthetic information. The *SOT* is schematically represented in Figure 22.7.

In the first condition, subjects are asked to stand and face forward. The second condition is the same as the first with the exception that subjects are asked to close their eyes (e.g., conventional Romberg). Under this condition the subjects are deprived of visual input and must rely on somesthetic and vestibular inputs to remain upright. In the third condition the patients face forward with their eyes open; however, if they sway forward or backward, the scene sways with them. In this "vision sway-referenced" condition the subjects are presented with conflicting visual information (they are swaying, yet their visual modality is providing information to the CNS that they are standing upright). In the fourth condition the subjects asked to face forward with their eyes open; however, if they sway forward or backward, the platform sways with them. Under these "support sway-referenced" circumstances, the subjects are

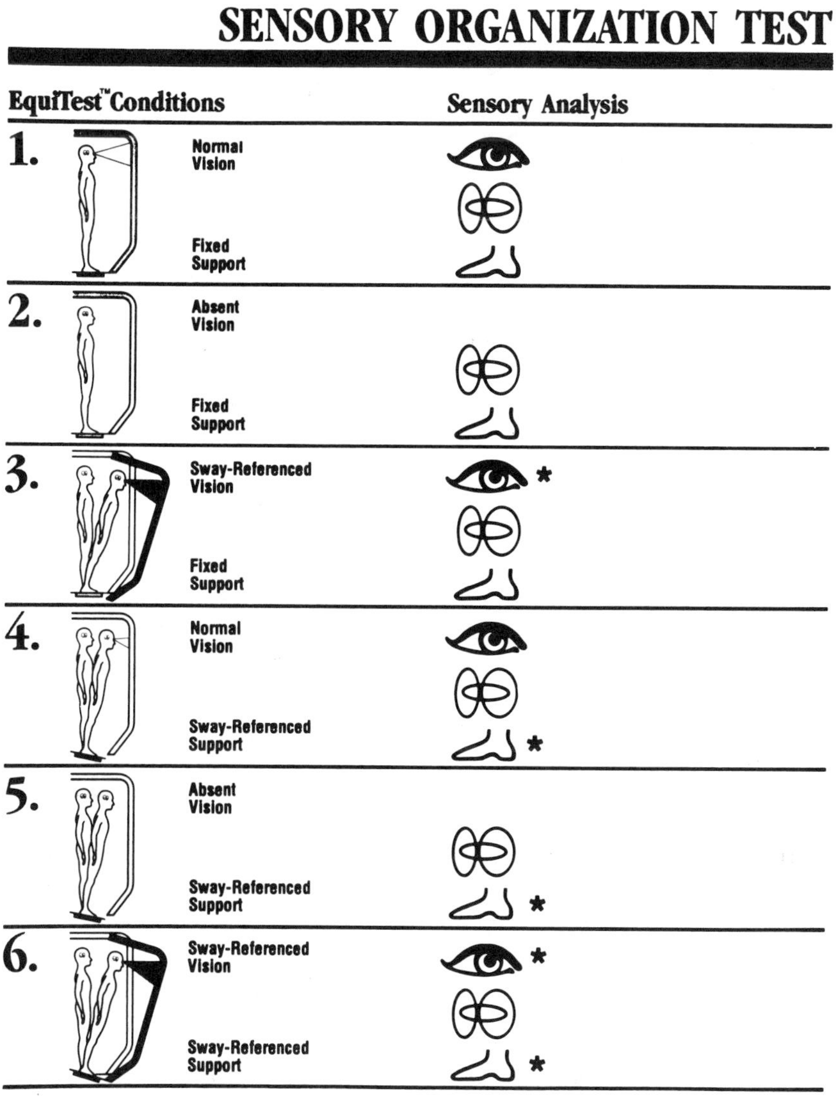

SENSORY ORGANIZATION TEST

EquiTest™ Conditions

Sensory Analysis

1. Normal Vision — Fixed Support
2. Absent Vision — Fixed Support
3. Sway-Referenced Vision * — Fixed Support
4. Normal Vision — Sway-Referenced Support *
5. Absent Vision — Sway-Referenced Support *
6. Sway-Referenced Vision * — Sway-Referenced Support *

FIGURE 22.7. Representation of conditions comprising the EquiTest™ protocol for the *Sensory Organization Test.* Asterisks denote sway-referenced conditions. Reprinted by permission of NeuroCom International, Inc., Clackamas, OR.

presented with inaccurate proprioceptive information and must suppress it. For the fifth condition, the subjects are asked to close their eyes and the support surface is sway-referenced. The subjects must rely solely on accurate vestibular system input to remain upright in this condition. Finally, in the sixth condition, both vision and support information are sway-referenced so that subjects must suppress inaccurate visual and proprioceptive information in order to remain upright. The variable that is quantified by the EquiTest™ program is the maximum peak-to-peak sway (measured in degrees). The limit of sway in normals is approximately 12°. Therefore, sway that is greater than 12° falls outside the limits of stability and will lead to a fall. The results of the *SOT* are plotted on a scale from 0 to 100%, with 100% representing complete stability and 0% representing the limits of stability (a fall).

It might be predicted that the performance of normal elderly subjects on all of these conditions would be poorer than that of normal young subjects. Nashner et al. (unpublished observations) have evaluated the performance of 130 normal individuals aged 20–69 years. The only significant age-related difference on sensory organization testing was on the sixth condition, in which the subjects had to suppress inaccurate visual and proprioceptive information. Stated differently, these results might suggest that normal elderly are more dependent upon information that is present in visual and proprioceptive modalities than are normal young subjects and are therefore more likely to be destabilized if they are presented with inaccurate information in these modalities.

Most recently, Wolfson et al. (1989, personal communication) have completed an investigation of postural stability in young subjects and 140 healthy noninstitutionalized elderly subjects (mean age = 76 years ± 4 years) using his *PST* and the EquiTest™. The investigators were interested in determining whether the results observed on the *PST* and/or the EquiTest™ were predictors of patients who would fall in the future. They found that the normal elderly performed uniformly well on the *PST*, experiencing the greatest problems on conditions 5 and 6 of the *SOT*. The authors also found significant differences in latency, strategy, and effectiveness of responses to imposed platform perturbations in the elderly subjects compared with the young subjects on Movement Coordination Testing (another subtest in the EquiTest™ software).

Practical Considerations for Balance Function Testing of Aged Patients

Vestibulometric examination of the elderly patient may require a great deal of patience and compassion. Patients are often reticent to undergo the examination for fear of becoming physiologically impaired as a result of the test. A conversation to reassure the patient prior to starting the test battery will often result in a much higher quality test. It is important to describe the purpose of the examination and the testing process in nonthreatening terms. Ocular motility becomes less efficient with age; therefore, it is not uncommon to observe abnormalities such as vertical upbeating gaze-evoked nystagmus on upward gaze, less accurate saccades (compared with young subjects), and saccadic pursuit. Clinicians should be careful to inquire of their patients whether they have arthritic conditions involving the cervical or lumbar regions prior to conducting Hallpike positioning. Although it is unlikely that the patient could suffer a significant injury (if the examination is done appropriately), the discomfort might make the elderly patient less trusting of the examiner and more apt not to complete the testing. Finally, the elderly patient is more likely than the younger patient to be taking medications that can confound the results of balance function testing. Careful questioning of the patient prior to testing will reveal the presence of any medications that might confound the examination.

Summary

Aging imposes subtle changes on the anatomy and physiology of the vestibular system and its support systems of vision and proprioception. One effect of aging is a degeneration of the sensory epithelium and first-order afferents within the peripheral apparatus, decreasing its sensitivity and increasing its threshold of stimulation. Diagnostic tests of vestibular system function show physiological correlates of this decrease in sensitivity. Caloric-induced nystagmus in the aged shows a decrease in SPEV and nystagmus duration and an increase in latency. Additionally, rotation testing shows an increase in the threshold of nystagmus and a decrease in SPEV (or VOR gain at low frequencies on sinusoidal harmonic acceleration testing) and nystagmus frequency with age. Platform posturographic testing has indicated that elderly subjects are more dependent upon visual and proprioceptive information to remain upright than are younger subjects. Ocular motility testing has shown that the fast and slow eye movement systems we use to orient ourselves within our environment decrease in efficiency with age.

As we age we lose peripheral vestibular sensitivity and become more reliant on vision and proprioception to remain stable under challenging and unchallenging circumstances. Decreases in visual acuity and proprioceptive ability with age make the CNS less able to maintain postural stability under static and dynamic conditions. This probably results in the "multisensory deficit" that has been described by Drachman and Hart (1972). Additionally, as we age the effects of illnesses accumulate. Decreases in peripheral vestibular system sensitivity cannot be compensated for by the central vestibular system (Jacobson & Henry, 1989), resulting in constant dysequilibrium (Rudge & Chambers, 1982).

There is a clear need for additional studies of balance system function in the elderly. For instance, it is unclear at present whether compensation for peripheral vestibular system deficits can be facilitated through physical therapy or medical treatment. Also, we are only beginning to understand the importance of visual and proprioceptive inputs for the maintenance of stability in the elderly. We will require studies of senescent changes in postural control before we can hope to understand the causal mechanisms of falling in the elderly.

Conclusions and Future Directions: Assessment of Auditory and Vestibular System Function in the Elderly

Two interesting observations have emerged out of this review. First, it is startling that there has been little agreement between investigators with respect to the techniques that have been used to investigate auditory and balance system function. As we have reviewed the literature regarding the electrophysiology of auditory and vestibular function in the elderly, we have highlighted deficits in the construction of some studies and in reporting data. This has made the task of integrating the results of investigations using disparate technologies especially difficult. It is our hope that in the future there will be general agreement on a standardized technique to use in conducting such investigations as auditory P300, rotational testing, and posturographic testing. A consistent theme in the reviews of previous research is the lack of adequate specification of hearing loss in many studies. Other studies are flawed by use of a specific stimulus level, rather than accounting for hearing deficits in which differences in threshold at different frequencies, a hallmark of presbycusis, are used as the reference for stimulus intensity. In a similar manner, selection of high-frequency stimuli in such studies as P300 trials may introduce other kinds of auditory distortion that are prevalent in cochlear lesions. More impressive, perhaps, is the variety and number of research hypotheses and pressing clinical questions that have remained inadequately answered or unaddressed.

Also, it has become clear from this literature review that little interest has been expressed in senescent changes in the auditory and vestibular systems. Proportionately, a far greater number of investigations have been conducted to investigate the development of the auditory and balance systems than their decline. The growth of the aging population and the impact that defective auditory and balance systems have on the quality of life should serve as a motivation for investigators to pursue research in geriatric audiology and vestibulometry. It is unfortunate that research in the rehabilitation of auditory and balance system deficits can only occur once the deficits have been identified.

References

Allison, T., Hume, A. L., Wood, C. C., & Goff, W. R. (1984). Developmental and aging changes in somatosensory, auditory and visual evoked potentials. *Electroencephalography and Clinical Neurophysiology, 58,* 14–24.

American Speech-Language-Hearing Association. (1988). *The short latency auditory evoked potentials* (pp. 1–39). Rockville, MD: American Speech-Language-Hearing Association.

Arslan, M. (1957). The senescence of the vestibular apparatus. *Practica Otorhinolaryngologica, 19,* 475–483.

Ashley, M. J., Gryfe, C. I., & Amies, A. (1977). A longitudinal study of falls in an elderly population: II. Some circumstances of falling. *Age and Ageing, 6,* 211–220.

Bauch, C. D., & Olsen, W. O. (1988). Auditory brainstem responses as a function of average hearing sensitivity for 2000–4000 Hz. *Audiology, 27,* 156–163.

Beagley, H., & Sheldrake, J. (1978). Differences in brainstem response latency with age and sex. *British Journal of Audiology, 12,* 69–77.

Belal, A., & Glorig, A. (1986). Dysequilibrium of ageing (presbyastasis). *Journal of Laryngology and Otology, 100,* 1037–1041.

Bergholtz, L. M., Hooper, R. E., & Mehta, D. C. (1977). Electrocochleographic response patterns in a group of patients mainly with presbyacusis. *Scandinavian Audiology, 6,* 3–11.

Bergman, M. (1980). *Aging and the perception of speech.* Baltimore, MD: University Park Press.

Black, F. O., O'Leary, D. P., Wall, C., & Furman, J. (1977). The vestibulospinal stability test: Normal limits. *Transactions of the American Academy of Ophthalmology and Otolaryngology, 84,* 549–560.

Black, F. O., Wall, C. W., & O'Leary, D. P. (1978). Computerized screening of the human vestibulospinal system. *Annals of Otology, Rhinology and Laryngology, 87,* 853–860.

Boer, E., de Carels, J., & Philipszoon, A. J. (1963). The torsion swing. A simple rotation test. *Acta Otolaryngologica, 56,* 457.

Brocklehurst, J. C., Robertson, D., & James-Groom, P. (1982a). Clinical correlates of sway in old age–sensory modalities. *Age and Ageing, 11,* 1–10.

Brocklehurst, J. C., Robertson, D., & James-Groom, P. (1982b). Skeletal deformities in the elderly and their effects on postural sway. *Journal of the American Geriatric Society, 30,* 534–538.

Bruner, A., & Norris, T. W. (1971). Age related changes in caloric nystagmus. *Acta Otolaryngologica, 282*(Suppl.), 1–24.

Buchwald, J. S., Erwin, R. J., Read, S., Van Lancker, D., & Cummings, J. L. (1989). Mid-latency auditory evoked responses: Differential abnormality of P1 in Alzheimer's disease. *Electroencephalography and Clinical Neurophysiology, 74,* 378–384.

Chu, N. (1985). Age-related latency changes in the brain-stem auditory evoked potentials. *Electroencephalography and Clinical Neurophysiology, 62,* 431–436.

Clement, P. A., van der Laan, F. L., & Oosterveld, W. J. (1975). The influence of age on vestibular function. *Acta Otolaryngologica, 29,* 163–172.

Coats, A., & Martin, J. (1977). Human auditory nerve action potentials and brain stem evoked responses. Effect of audiogram shape and lesion location. *Archives of Otolaryngology, 103,* 605–622.

Corso, J. F. (1971). Sensory processes and age effects in normal adults. *Journal of Gerontology, 26,* 90–105.

Corso, J. F. (1977). Presbyacusis, hearing aids and aging. *Audiology, 16,* 146–163.

Davidson, J., Wright, G., Ilmoyl, L., Canter, R. J., & Barber, H. O. (1988). The reproducibility of caloric tests of vestibular function in young and old subjects. *Acta Otolaryngologica, 106,* 264–268.

Debruyne, F. (1986). Influence of age and hearing loss on the latency shifts of the auditory brainstem response as a result of increased stimulus rate. *Audiology, 25,* 101–106.

Drachman, D. A., & Hart, C. W. (1972). An approach to the dizzy patient. *Neurology, 22,* 323–334.

Droller, H. (1955). Falls among elderly people living at home. *Geriatrics, 10,* 239–244.

Duffy, F. H., Albert, M. S., McAnulty, G., & Garvey, A. J. (1984). Age-related differences in brain electrical activity of healthy subjects. *Annals of Neurology, 16,* 430–438.

Egmont, A. A. J., Groen, J. J., & Jongkees, L. B. W. (1953). *The function of the vestibular organ.* New York: Karger.

Exton-Smith, A. N. (1977). Clinical manifestations. In A. N. Exton-Smith & G. Evans (Eds.), *Care of elderly: Meeting the challenge of dependency.* London: Academic Press.

Fein, G., & Turetsky, B. (1989). P300 latency variability in normal elderly: Effects of paradigm and measurement technique. *Elec-*

troencephalography and Clinical Neurophysiology, 72, 384–394.

Fernie, G. R., Gryfe, C. I., Holliday, P. J., & Llewellyn, A. (1982). The relationship of postural sway in standing to the incidence of falls in geriatric subjects. Age and Ageing, 11, 11–16.

Ford, J. M., Duncan-Johnson, C. C., Pfefferbaum, A., & Kopell, B. S. (1982). Expectancy for events in old age: Stimulus sequence effects on P300 and reaction time. Journal of Gerontology, 37, 696–704.

Ford, J. M., Hink, R. F., Hopkins III, W. F., Roth, W. T., Pfefferbaum, A., & Kopell, B. S. (1979). Event related potential recorded from young and old adults during a memory retrieval task. Electroencephalography and Clinical Neurophysiology, 47, 450–459.

Fria, T. J., & Doyle, P. (1984). Maturation of the auditory brainstem response (ABR): Additional perspectives. Ear and Hearing, 5, 361–365.

Gacek, R. (1975). Degenerative hearing loss in aging. In W. Fields (Ed.), Neurological and sensory disorders in the elderly. New York: Stratton International Medical Book Corp.

Ghosh, P. (1985). Aging and auditory vestibular response. Ear Nose and Throat Journal, 64, 264–266.

Goodhill, V., & Guggenheim, P. (1971). Pathology, diagnosis and therapy of deafness. In L. Travis (Ed.), Handbook of speech pathology and audiology. New York: Appleton-Century-Crofts.

Goodin, D. S., Squires, K. C., Henderson, B. H., & Starr, A. (1978). Age-related variations in evoked potentials to auditory stimuli in normal human subjects. Electroencephalography and Clinical Neurophysiology, 44, 447–458.

Gordon, M. (1978). Occult cardiac arrythmias associated with falls and dizziness in the elderly: Detection by Holter Monitoring. Journal of the American Geriatric Society, 26, 418–423.

Gorga, M., Worthington, D., Reiland, J., Beauchaine, K., & Goldgar, I. (1985). Some comparisons between auditory brain stem response thresholds, latencies, and the pure-tone audiogram. Ear and Hearing, 6, 105–112.

Gryfe, C. I., Amies, A., & Ashley, M. J. (1977). A longitudinal study of falls in an elderly population: Incidence and morbidity. Age and Ageing, 6, 201–210.

Harkins, S. W., & Lenhardt, M. (1980). Brainstem auditory evoked potentials in the elderly. In L. W. Poon (Ed.), Aging in the 1980s: Psychological issues (pp. 101–112). Washington, DC: American Psychological Association.

Hughes, J. R., & Drachman, D. A. (1977). Dizziness, epilepsy and the EEG. Diseases of the Nervous System, 38, 431–435.

Isaacs, B. (1983). Falls in old age. In R. Hinchcliffe (Ed.), Hearing and balance in the elderly (pp. 373–388). Edinburgh, Scotland: Churchill Livingstone.

Jacobson, G. P., & Henry, K. G. (1989). Effect of temperature on fixation suppression ability in normal subjects: The need for temperature- and age-dependent normal values. Annals of Otology, Rhinology and Laryngology, 98, 369–372.

Jacobson, J. T., & Hyde, M. L. (1985). An introduction to auditory evoked potentials. In J. Katz (Ed.), Handbook of clinical audiology (3rd ed.). Baltimore, MD: Williams & Wilkins.

Jerger, J. (1989). Paper presented at the Aging Ear conference, Washington University School of Medicine, St. Louis, MO.

Jerger, J., & Hall, J. (1980). Effects of age and sex on auditory brainstem response. Archives of Otolaryngology, 106, 387–391.

Jerger, J., & Mauldin, L. (1978). Prediction of sensorineural hearing level from the brain stem evoked response. Archives of Otolaryngology, 104, 456–461.

Johannsen, H. S., & Lehn, T. (1984). The dependence of early acoustically evoked potentials on age. Archives of Otorhinolaryngology, 240, 153–158.

Karlsen, E. A., Hassanein, R. M., & Goetzinger, C. P. (1981). The effects of age, sex, hearing loss and water temperature on caloric nystagmus. Laryngoscope, 91, 620–627.

Kokmen, E., Bossemeyer, R. W., & Williams, W. T. (1978). Quantitative evaluation of joint motion sensation in an aging population. Journal of Gerontology, 33, 62–67.

Kuechenmeister, M. S., Linton, P. H., Mueller, T. V., & White, H. B. (1977). Eye tracking in relation to age, sex and illness. Archives of General Psychiatry, 34, 578–579.

Luchikin, L. A., & Patrin, A. F. (1983). Equilibrium in different age groups as reflected by stabilography. Vestn-Otolrinolaringol, 5, 29–34.

Lucht, U. (1971). A prospective study of accidental falls and resulting injuries in the home among elderly people. *Acta Society of Medicine Scandinavia, 1,* 105–120.

Marshall, L. (1981). Auditory processing in aging listeners. *Journal of Speech and Hearing Disorders, 46,* 226–240.

McCallum, W. C. (1973). The CNV and conditionability in psychopathology. *Electroencephalography and Clinical Neurophysiology, 33*(Suppl.), 337–343.

McClure, J. (1986). Vertigo and imbalance in the elderly. *Journal of Otolaryngology, 15,* 248–252.

Michalewski, H. J., Patterson, J. V., Bowman, T. E., Litzleman, D., & Thompson, L. W. (1982). A comparison of the emitted late positive potential in older and young adults. *Journal of Gerontology, 37,* 52–58.

Moller, K., & Blegvad, B. (1976). Brain stem responses in patients with sensorineural losses. *Scandinavian Audiology, 5,* 115–127.

Mulch, G., & Petermann, W. (1979). Influence of age on results of vestibular function tests. *Annals of Otology, Rhinology and Laryngology, 88*(Suppl.), 1–17.

Murphy, J., & Isaacs, B. (1982). The post fall syndrome: A study of 36 elderly patients. *Gerontology, 28,* 265–270.

Nashner, L. M. (1983). Analysis of movement control in man using the movable platform. In J. E. Desmedt (Ed.), *Motor control mechanisms in health and disease* (pp. 607–633). New York: Raven Press.

Naylor, R., & Rosin, A. J. (1970). Falling as a cause of admission to a geriatric unit. *Practitioner, 205,* 327–330.

Nickens, H. (1985). Intrinsic factors in falling among the elderly. *Archives of Internal Medicine, 145,* 1089–1093.

Norre, M. E., Forrez, G., & Beckers, A. (1987). Vestibular dysfunction causing instability in aged patients. *Acta Otolaryngologica, 104,* 50–55.

Oosterveld, W. J. (1983). Changes in vestibular function with increasing age. In R. Hinchcliffe (Ed.), *Hearing and balance in the elderly* (pp. 354–372). Edinburgh, Scotland: Churchill Livingstone.

Overstall, P. W., Exton-Smith, A. N., Imms, F. J., & Johnston, A. L. (1977). Falls in the elderly related to postural imbalance. *British Medical Journal, 1,* 261–264.

Patrin, A. F. (1986). The use of rotatory test for investigation of age-related pattern of vestibulo-somatic reaction in healthy subjects. *Vestn-Otorinolaryngol, 2,* 20–24.

Perry, B. C. (1982). Falls among the elderly living in high rise apartments. *Journal of Family Practice, 14,* 1069–1073.

Pfefferbaum, A., Ford, J. M., Roth, W. T., Hopkins III, W. F., & Kopell, B. S. (1979). Event-related potential changes in healthy aged females. *Electroencephalography and Clinical Neurophysiology, 46,* 81–86.

Pfefferbaum, A., Ford, J. M., Roth, W. T., & Kopell, B. S. (1980). Age-related changes in auditory event-related potentials. *Electroencephalography and Clinical Neurophysiology, 49,* 266–276.

Polich, J., Howard, L., & Starr, A. (1985). Effects of age on the P300 component of the event-related potential from auditory stimuli: Peak definition, variation, and measurement. *Journal of Gerontology, 85,* 721–726.

Prudham, D., & Evans, J. G. (1981). Factors associated with falls in the elderly: A community study. *Age and Ageing, 10,* 141–146.

Rashiq, S., & Logan, R. F. A. (1986). Role of drugs in fractures of the femoral neck. *British Medical Journal, 292,* 861–863.

Robinson, K., & Rudge, P. (1975). Auditory evoked responses in multiple sclerosis. *Lancet, 1,* 1164–1166.

Rosenhall, U., Bjorkman, G., Pederson, K., & Hanner, P. (1987). Oculomotor tests in different age groups. In M. D. Graham & J. L. Kemink (Eds.), *The vestibular system: Neurophysiologic and clinical research* (pp. 401–409). New York: Raven Press.

Rosenhall, U., Bjorkman, G., Pederson, K., & Kall, A. (1985). Brain-stem auditory evoked potentials in different age groups. *Electroencephalography and Clinical Neurophysiology, 62,* 426–430.

Rowe, M. (1978). Normal variability of the brain-stem auditory-evoked responses in young and old subjects. *Electroencephalography and Clinical Neurophysiology, 44,* 459–470.

Rudge, R., & Chambers, B. R. (1982). Physiological basis for enduring vestibular symptoms. *Journal of Neurology, Neurosurgery and Psychiatry, 45,* 126–130.

Salomon, G., Vesteragen, V., & Jagd, M. (1988). Age-related hearing difficulties: I. Hearing impairment, disability, and handicap—A controlled study. *Audiology, 27,* 164–178.

Schuknecht, H. (1964). Further observations on the pathology of presbycusis. *Archives of Otolaryngology, 80,* 369–382.

Schuknecht, H. (1967). The effect of aging on the cochlea. In B. Graham (Ed.), *Sensorineural hearing processes and disorders.* Boston: Little, Brown.

Schuknecht, H., & Igaraski, M. (1964). Pathology of slowly progressive sensorineural deafness. *Transactions of the American Academy of Ophthalmology and Otolaryngology, 68,* 222–242.

Sekuler, R., Hutman, L. P., & Owsley, C. J. (1980). Human aging and spatial vision. *Science, 209,* 1255–1256.

Sharpe, J. A., & Sylvester, T. O. (1978). Effect of aging on horizontal smooth pursuit. *Investigative Ophthalmology and Vision Science, 17,* 465–468.

Sheldon, J. H. (1960). On the natural history of falls in old age. *British Medical Journal, 2,* 1685–1690.

Sheldon, J. H. (1963). The effect of age on the control of sway. *Gerontology Clinics, 5,* 129–138.

Smith, D. B. D., Michalewski, H. J., Brent, G. A., & Thompson, L. W. (1980). Auditory averaged evoked potentials and aging: Factors of stimulus, task and topography. *Biological Psychology, 11,* 135–151.

Sokolovski, A. (1988). Influence of age on various parameters of prerotational and postrotational nystagmus. *Advances in Audiology, 5,* 192–203.

Spooner, J. W., Sakala, S. M., & Baloh, R. W. (1980). Effect of aging on eye tracking. *Archives of Neurology, 37,* 575–576.

Squires, K. C., Chippendale, T. J., Wrege, K. S., Gooden, D. S., & Starr, A. (1980). Electrophysiologic assessment of mental function in aging and dementia. In L. W. Poon (Ed.), *Aging in the 1980s: Psychological issues* (pp. 125–134). Washington, DC: American Psychological Association.

Starr, A. (1978). Sensory evoked potentials in clinical disorders of the nervous system. *Annual Review of Neurosciences, 1,* 103–127.

Starr, A., & Achor, J. (1975). Auditory brainstem responses in neurological disease. *Archives of Neurology, 32,* 761–768.

Starr, A., Amilie, R. N., Martin, W. H., & Sanders, S. (1977). Development of auditory function in newborn infants revealed by auditory brainstem potentials. *Pediatrics, 60,* 831–839.

Stegman, M. R. (1983). Falls among elderly hypertensives—Are they iatrogenic? *Gerontology, 29,* 399–406.

Stevens, D. L., & Matthews, W. B. (1973). Cryptogenic drop attacks in women. *British Medical Journal, 1,* 439–442.

Sticht, T. G., & Gray, B. B. (1969). The intelligibility of time compressed words as a function of age and hearing loss. *Journal of Speech and Hearing Research, 12,* 443–448.

Sudarsky, L., & Ronthal, M. (1983). Gait disorders among elderly patients. *Archives of Neurology, 40,* 740–743.

Tinnetti, M. E., Speechley, M., & Ginter, S. F. (1988). Risk factors for falls among elderly persons living in the community. *New England Journal of Medicine, 26,* 1701–1707.

Van der Laan, F. L., & Oosterveld, W. J. (1974). Age and vestibular function. *Aerospace Medicine, 45,* 540–547.

Virolainen, E. S., & Aantaa, E. (1976). The nystagmus threshold in turning test in different age groups and in patients suffering from otosclerosis. *Acta Otolaryngologica, 81,* 127–129.

Wall, C., Black, F. O., & Hunt, A. E. (1984). Effects of age, sex and stimulus parameters upon vestibulo-ocular responses to sinusoidal rotation. *Acta Otolaryngologica, 98,* 270–278.

Waller, J. A. (1974). Injury in aged: Clinical and epidemiological implications. *New York State Journal of Medicine, 74,* 2200–2208.

Waller, J. A. (1978). Falls among the elderly: Human and environmental factors. *Accident Analysis and Prevention, 10,* 21–33.

Wild, D., Nayak, U. S. L., & Isaacs, B. (1980). Characteristics of old people who fell at home. *Journal of Experimental Gerontology, 2,* 271–287.

Wild, D., Nayak, U. S. L., & Isaacs, B. (1981a). Description, classification, and prevention of falls in old people. *Rheumatology Rehabilitation, 20,* 153–159.

Wild, D., Nayak, U. S. L., & Isaacs, B. (1981b). How dangerous are falls in old people? *British Medical Journal, 282,* 266–268.

Wild, D., Nayak, U. S. L., & Isaacs, B. (1981c). Prognosis of falls in old people at home. *Journal of Epidemiology and Community Health, 35,* 200–204.

Wolfson, L. I., Whipple, R., Amerman, P., & Kleinberg, A. (1986). Stressing the postural response. *Journal of the American Geriatric Society, 34,* 845–850.

Woods, D. L., & Clayworth, C. C. (1986). Age-related changes in human middle latency auditory evoked potentials. *Electroenceph-alography and Clinical Neurophysiology, 65,* 297–303.

Woolacott, M. H., Shumway-Cook, A., & Nashner, L. (1982). Postural reflexes and aging. In F. J. Pirozzolo & G. J. Maletta (Eds.), *The aging motor system* (Vol. 3, pp. 98–119). New York: Praeger.

Wright, B. M. (1971). A simple mechanical ataxia-meter. *Proceedings of the Physiology Society, 28,* 27–28.

Zackon, D. H., & Sharpe, J. A. (1987). Smooth pursuit in senescence: Effects of target velocity and acceleration. *Acta Otolaryngologica, 104,* 290–297.

Sensory Aids for the Hearing-Impaired Elderly

Brad A. Stach, PhD, and W. Renae Stoner, MS ■

For many elderly individuals, the communicative difficulties and subsequent psychosocial problems resulting from hearing impairment can be reduced significantly by the use of hearing aids and other amplification devices. Many elderly patients who are properly fitted with hearing aids and who are motivated to adapt to amplified sound are successful hearing aid users. This success often results in a reduction of the adverse psychosocial conditions imposed by hearing impairment. This point has been well illustrated in a study by Harless and McConnell (1982). They measured self-concept in 43 successful hearing aid wearers and 43 nonwearers. Results showed that the self-concept of the group of subjects who had adapted to hearing aid use was significantly greater than that of the non-user group. The Harless and McConnell study serves to illustrate the positive and substantial impact that hearing aid amplification often has on the overall well-being of elderly individuals. In this and many other respects, hearing aid use is no differ-

ent in the elderly than in younger hearing-impaired individuals. Yet for all of the similarities with the younger population, successful fitting of amplification devices in the elderly population remains one of the greatest challenges to appropriate hearing health care.

Why is the elderly population so challenging in terms of hearing aid amplification? What is unique about the population that merits special concern? Whenever the question is posed of what differences exist in hearing aid intervention between younger and older individuals, the most likely answer will be that older individuals are more resistant to the idea of hearing aid use, are more difficult to fit with hearing aids, are less satisfied with hearing aid use, and do not benefit as much from amplification. Yet despite all of the gloomy prognoses, patients over the age of 65 constitute the largest number of hearing aid owners. Can it be that the group of individuals that owns the most hearing aids and that needs hearing aids the most is the group for which the prognosis for successful hearing aid use is the poorest?

It should be emphasized that many elderly individuals do benefit substantially from conventional hearing aid strategies. Intervention with these patients is carried out in a manner identical to that used for younger individuals, and the impact of hearing aids on communication disorder and quality of life is usually substantial. However, for other elderly individuals, various factors that result from the aging process can contribute to a reduced prognosis for successful hearing aid use. One major correlate of hearing aid success is the complex nature of the auditory deficit resulting from presbycusis (Hayes, 1980). Changes in both the peripheral and central auditory structures can combine to limit the usefulness of conventional amplification arrangements. There are also a number of nonauditory correlates that can influence hearing aid success by the elderly. For example, there remains a generalized failure of the delivery system to inform patients with sensorineural hearing loss about the potential benefits of hearing aid use. In addition, the perception of hearing loss as an inexorable badge of old age reduces the likelihood that an individual will seek early intervention for presbycusis. Still other nonauditory factors related to the aging process that can influence hearing aid success include psychosocial parameters and physical ability.

For those hearing-impaired elderly individuals who do not benefit as much from conventional hearing aids, alternative amplification strategies have proven to be very useful. For example, alteration of conventional hearing aids, such as the addition of directional microphones and noise suppression circuitry, often help to overcome the difficulty of understanding speech in noise. Similarly, remote control devices can help to overcome problems associated with reduced fine-motor control. Also, when conventional hearing aids fail, or when additional help is necessary, intervention with assistive listening devices has proven to be a successful amplification alternative.

Throughout this chapter, the terms hearing aid *success*, *benefit*, and *satisfaction* will be used and are not meant to be construed as being synonymous. Hearing aid *success* will be used as the general term to convey that an individual uses a hearing aid, benefits from its use, and is satisfied with the benefit. Hearing aid *benefit* will be used to convey the usefulness of a hearing aid in amplifying sound in the manner for which it was intended. For example, if a hearing aid is intended to help someone understand speech better, and that person experiences improved speech understanding with the hearing aid, then the hearing aid is of benefit. Hearing aid *satisfaction* will be used to convey contentment with the amplification device and what it does. Thus, a person can *benefit* from hearing aid use because speech understanding is improved but not be *satisfied* with the hearing aid because the earmold is too tight. If the person does not wear the hearing aid, then *success* will not have been achieved.

The Nature of Hearing Aid Use by the Elderly

Demographics

Estimates of hearing aid use are difficult to determine for two reasons. First, the estimates of hearing impairment in the elderly, upon which hearing aid usage estimates are based, can vary considerably as a function of the sample age and the criteria used to define impairment. Second, it is difficult to distinguish between hearing aid ownership and hearing aid use. Nevertheless, estimates show that elderly patients constitute the largest percentage of hearing aid owners. Nearly 61% of all hearing aids are sold to elderly patients (Cranmer, 1989).

Estimates of prevalence of hearing aid use range from 10 to 21% of the hearing-impaired population, depending on the nature of the sample under study. Schow

(1982) reported that approximately 10% of nursing home patients with hearing loss in excess of 40 dB hearing level (HL) wore hearing aids. Dodds and Harford (1982) described a community program for senior citizens who were residents of retirement homes and hotels or members of senior centers. Of the 527 subjects, 11% were hearing aid wearers. The Subcommittee of Consumer Interests of the Elderly estimated in 1974 that 21% of those with substantial hearing loss wore hearing aids (from Franks & Beckmann, 1985).

Despite the advantages of hearing aid use, as few as 21% of all hearing-impaired elderly individuals wear hearing aids. Thus, a vast majority of hearing-impaired elderly remain underserved from a hearing health care standpoint.

Hearing Aid Use

Hearing aid use tends to be higher in younger age groups than in the elderly.

Surr, Schuchman, and Montgomery (1978) used a questionnaire to evaluate hearing aid use in a series of 430 patients. They found that use declined with increasing age. The results are summarized in Figure 23.1. As many as 62% of the patients in the oldest age group never, or only occasionally, wore their hearing aids. In the younger-elderly group, however, 59 to 68% were considered to be successful users. Sorri, Luotonen, and Laitakari (1984), in Finland, also studied hearing aid use as a function of age. They interviewed 150 patients approximately 2 years after they had been fitted with hearing aids. Based on the interview, the patients were categorized as either regular users, selective users, or nonusers. Results are summarized in Figure 23.2. As age increased, the percentage of patients who were not regular users increased systematically. For those patients over the age of 75 years, fewer than half (44%) used their hearing aids on a regular basis, and 36% were categorized as nonusers. In the younger age group, however, 61% were more consistent

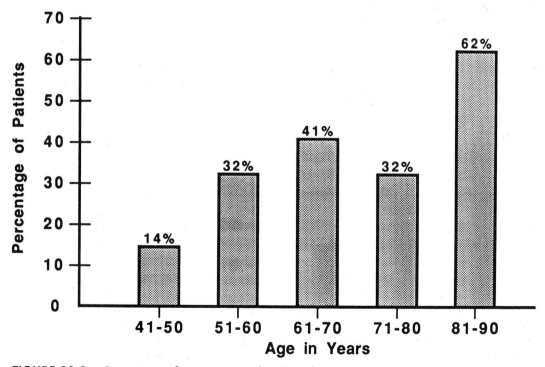

FIGURE 23.1. Percentage of patients, as a function of age group, who only occasionally or never used their hearing aids (after Surr et al., 1978).

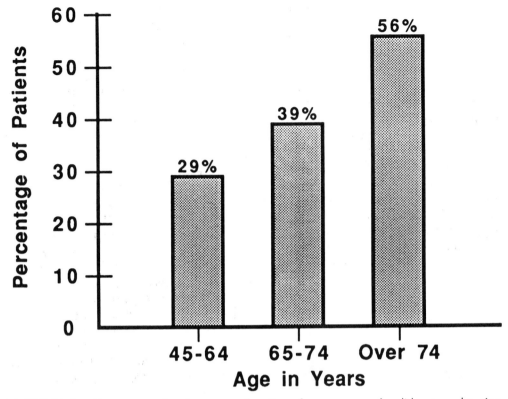

FIGURE 23.2. Percentage of patients, as a function of age group, who did not use hearing aids on a regular basis (after Sorri et al., 1984).

hearing aid users. While these studies reported a difference in hearing aid use as a function of age, other studies (Davies & Mueller, 1987; Ewertsen, 1974) showed no substantial decline in hearing aid use among the geriatric population. Davies and Mueller (1987) described a study of hearing aid use, benefit, and satisfaction in a group of 39 patients over the age of 70 years and a group of 98 patients under the age of 70 years. Mean data showed lower ratings for the older group on all three factors, but variability was substantial and the differences were not statistically significant.

The least positive estimates of hearing aid use have been in nursing home settings. For example, Schow (1982) reported that although approximately 10% of the nursing home patients who were evaluated wore hearing aids, an additional 20% had owned or worn hearing aids at one time, but were

no longer wearing them. This constitutes a hearing aid success rate of only 33% in the nursing homes.

Hearing Aid Satisfaction

Those elderly individuals who do wear hearing aids appear to be as satisfied with hearing aid use, as a group, as their younger counterparts. Birt and Alberti (1975) interviewed hearing aid patients and assigned them a rating based on perceived satisfaction with hearing aid use. The highest two ratings were given to 80% of their sample. Age appeared to have no influence on the satisfaction rating. Similarly, Hayes, Jerger, Taff, and Barber (1983) surveyed 78 hearing aid wearers to determine satisfaction with hearing aid use. Results showed that, although the average age of the ''Very

Helpful'' group was 58 years and that of the ''Sometimes Helpful'' was 70 years, there was no significant relationship between the age of the subject and satisfaction with hearing aid use.

Hearing Handicap Reduction

For those elderly individuals who wear hearing aids, self-perception of hearing handicap is reduced. Newman and Weinstein (1988) reported a study of hearing aid benefit in the elderly. Eighteen hearing aid wearers and their spouses were evaluated using the *Hearing Handicap Inventory for the Elderly* (Ventry & Weinstein, 1982), both before fitting and approximately 1 year after fitting of hearing aids. Results showed significant reductions in self-perceived handicap following hearing aid use. In addition, perception of handicap by spouses was also reduced substantially. These findings are important in that they confirm the reduction in handicap related to hearing aid use. They also suggest that if elderly individuals can be convinced to pursue hearing aid use and can be fitted successfully with hearing aids, the impact on their lives will be positive and substantial.

Variables Affecting Hearing Aid Acceptance

Although many elderly individuals own and successfully wear hearing aids, the fact remains that the majority of hearing-impaired elderly individuals do not own hearing aids and that many who do own them do not wear them. Indeed, only a small percentage of the entire hearing-impaired elderly population chooses to pursue the use of hearing aid amplification. Unfortunately, even when they do, the prognosis for successful use is not altogether positive. What are the factors that influence these outcomes? What prevents elderly individuals from pursuing hearing aid use? And what limits the benefit of hearing aid use once an individual attempts to wear one?

Among the hearing-impaired elderly who do not use hearing aids are those who have never pursued use of a hearing aid and those who have tried and subsequently abandoned hearing aid use or have found it to be less than satisfactory. Although various factors of nonuse are common to both groups, distinctive factors exist for each group.

Avoidance of Hearing Aids

Primary among the factors that lead elderly individuals to avoid hearing aids are psychosocial issues related to perceptions of hearing loss and the aging process. The other major factors that limit hearing aid use are the nature of the hearing health care delivery system and the cost of hearing aid instruments.

Psychosocial Factors

Because age is a major cause of hearing impairment among the elderly, hearing impairment has become a stigma associated with the aging process. Consequently, since hearing aids are a marker of hearing impairment, they have become associated with old age. Therefore, use of hearing aids confirms the process of aging and the concomitant degeneration of self-image (Griffin, Tourigny, & Demitrack, 1988). The result is that a large number of elderly individuals believe that they are not old enough to need a hearing aid. While the decade of the 1980s began to bring about changes in these long-held notions, nevertheless, there is every reason to believe that the association of hearing aids with old age remains a major factor in reducing the number of hearing-impaired elderly who seek assistance. Indeed, the fact that a hearing aid calls attention to the handicap was the primary reason that a group of non–hearing aid wearers found hearing aids to be objectionable (Franks & Beckmann, 1985). Of notable interest, however, are the findings of Iler, Danhauer, and Mulac (1982). They studied the so-called "hearing aid effect," the negative judgments attached to individuals based on their use of hearing aids, in a group of elderly subjects. Results showed that peer observers did not perceive the appearance of hearing aids negatively. These findings suggest that, although elderly individuals may perceive hearing aids to be objectionable on themselves, that perception is not shared by their peers.

In addition to denial of hearing loss, many elderly individuals attribute changes in life-style that result from hearing loss to problems other than hearing loss (Schwartz & Matsko, 1988). For example, communication disorder may be associated with senility by the elderly and viewed as an expected component of the aging process, or limited social interaction may be attributed to other health problems or feelings of lethargy. These elderly individuals may simply not realize that their impaired communication function and consequent decrease in social activity are a result of hearing loss. The other life-style factor that may be involved in failure to pursue hearing aid use is that communication needs may become less critical for the elderly patient. Social and occupational activities may be reduced to the point where communication demand does not warrant the pursuit of amplification.

The Hearing Health Care Delivery System

Another major factor that limits hearing aid use is a general failure of the hearing health care delivery system to inform the public and other health care providers of the benefits of amplification (see, for example, Goldstein, 1984). Patients usually have only a vague notion of how to enter into the hearing health care system or may be unaware of available professional services (Hardick & Gans, 1982). As a result, the most frequent initial contact is with the primary care physician (Lichtenstein, Bess, & Logan, 1988). Since primary care physicians rarely screen for hearing loss in the elderly and rarely refer their patients for audiologic

services, patients are being informed that hearing loss is simply an unavoidable and untreatable consequence of aging or, worse, that a hearing aid cannot be used for a sensorineural hearing loss. Still others are led inadvertently to believe that hearing health care should not be a primary concern because of its seemingly benign nature (Schwartz & Matsko, 1988). As a result, many patients are simply unaware that they can benefit from hearing aid use.

Hearing Aid Cost

Franks and Beckmann (1985) surveyed the attitudes of 100 retirees who were over the age of 65. One half of the group wore hearing aids; the other half did not. The single most important factor in the rejection of hearing aids across the groups was that of cost. The issue of substantial cost has also been reported by others (Dodds & Harford, 1982; Stream & Stream, 1980) and is exacerbated by the failure of third-party payers to consider hearing aids as a reimbursable medical expense.

Reduced Success with Hearing Aid Use

In the elderly hearing-impaired population, there are a number of people who attempt to use hearing aid amplification and either fail or receive little benefit from its use. Factors that appear to contribute substantially to this failure include the complex nature of presbycusis, physical limitations, and negative perceptions of sound quality.

The Complex Nature of Presbycusis

Hearing loss in the elderly is of a complex nature. Changes in the cochlea associated with aging result in the hearing sensitivity loss that so often characterizes presbycusis. The consequences of peripheral sensitivity loss in the elderly are similar to those of younger hearing-impaired individuals. However, in addition to adverse effects on the auditory periphery, central auditory nervous system structures also change with age. The functional consequence of these structural changes is central auditory processing disorder (CAPD). While peripheral hearing loss creates the need for hearing aid use, central presbycusis (CAPD that results from the aging process) may limit success with hearing aids.

The prevalence of central presbycusis makes it an important factor in understanding the nature of the communication disorder of the elderly and in directing intervention strategies. In a recent study, we estimated the prevalence of central presbycusis in a clinical population (Stach, Spretnjak, & Jerger, 1990). Results showed that, even with peripheral hearing loss controlled, speech audiometric abnormalities increased systematically with increasing age. The prevalence of central presbycusis increased from 58% in the 65- to 69-year-old age group to 95% in the 80+ age group. Of course, central presbycusis would not be considered a problem if it had no obvious consequence on communication ability or on amelioration procedures. However, central presbycusis has been associated with a reduction in successful hearing aid use.

Central Presbycusis and Hearing Aid Use

Three lines of evidence suggest that CAPD can adversely affect hearing aid use. First, patients with CAPD do not perform as well with hearing aids as patients with only peripheral deficits. Hayes and Jerger (1979) evaluated aided performance in a sound-field by a group of patients with a speech audiometric pattern consistent with peripheral auditory deficit and a group with a pattern consistent with central auditory deficit. They found that those with CAPD did not perform as well with hearing aids as those without CAPD. They also found that performance declined with increasing degree of the central component.

Second, hearing aid satisfaction is adversely affected by CAPD. Jerger and Hayes (1976) found that those who rated hearing aid use as unsatisfactory performed more poorly with hearing aids in a difficult

listening situation than those who were satisfied with hearing aid use. McCandless and Parkin (1979) found that a surprising 89% of those who were classified as having a central site of lesion had rejected hearing aid use.

Third, benefit from hearing aid use is reduced in some patients by the presence of central presbycusis (Stach, 1990). We studied the relationship between CAPD and hearing aid benefit in two groups of 12 subjects matched for age and degree of hearing loss. One group had a speech audiometric pattern consistent with mixed peripheral and central auditory disorder and the other had a pattern consistent with only peripheral disorder. Benefit was judged on a five-point scale following an interview with each subject. The results are shown in Figure 23.3. Although the benefit ratings assigned to the peripheral group were mostly positive, those assigned to the central group were distinctly dichotomized. Some subjects benefited from hearing aids, whereas others reported no benefit. Overall, the prognosis for successful hearing aid use was found to be reduced if CAPD was present.

Is There a Cause-and-Effect Relationship?

If CAPD occurs as a result of the aging process, it is likely to progress over the years. Also, if CAPD can result in limited benefit from hearing aid use, it is likely that benefit can become diminished as CAPD progresses. Therefore, it is theoretically possible that a successfull hearing aid wearer can become unsuccessful as the pattern of auditory aging changes over time from peripheral to central. If there truly is a relationship between central processing ability and hearing aid benefit, the insidious progression of central auditory aging should result in a progressive decline in the ability to use amplification successfully. We reported previously on what appeared to us to be just such a case (Stach, Jerger, & Fleming, 1985).

The subject was first evaluated at the age of 70 years. At that time he had a mildly

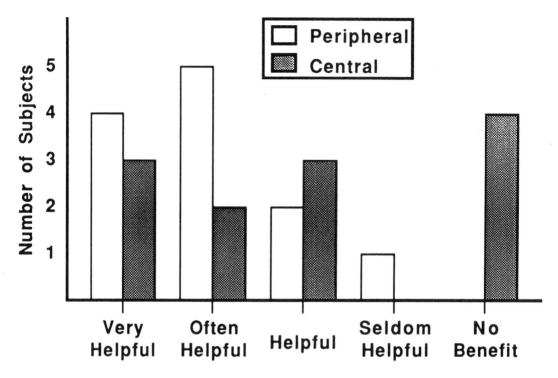

FIGURE 23.3. Distribution of benefit ratings of hearing aid use by subjects with a peripheral pattern of auditory disorder and by subjects with a mixed peripheral and central pattern. *Note.* From "Hearing Aid Amplification and Central Processing Disorders" by B. Stach, 1990. In *Handbook of Hearing Aid Amplification: Vol. II. Clinical Considerations and Fitting Practices* (pp. 87–111) by R. E. Sandlin (Ed.), Austin, TX: PRO-ED. Copyright 1990 by R. E. Sandlin. Reprinted by permission.

sloping, symmetrical hearing loss and evidence of very mild CAPD on the right side. Although he was having communication problems, he did not feel that a hearing aid was warranted. He was evaluated several times over the next 9 years. At the age of 75, he was fitted with a hearing aid on the right ear and wore it with a fair, but decreasing, amount of success over the next several years. At age 79, he became convinced that his hearing aid was no longer functioning. He reported that it was amplifying sound, but not clearly. Since an electroacoustic analysis revealed a properly functioning hearing aid, audiologic testing was repeated. Results showed that, although his peripheral sensitivity had changed only minimally, his central function had declined substantially. Figure 23.4 shows the results of serial evaluations over the 9-year period.

We found this case to be a persuasive argument for the idea that a decline in central auditory function, independent of peripheral changes, can result in a parallel decline in benefit from hearing aid use. This patient was considered an excellent candidate for amplification because of the degree of his peripheral hearing loss, the mild slope, and his good speech understanding in quiet. We could find no evidence of significant cognitive decline or any other intervening factors to explain the progression away from satisfactory hearing aid use. That he became an unsuccessful user strengthens the argument that CAPD can have a negative effect on success with conventional amplification.

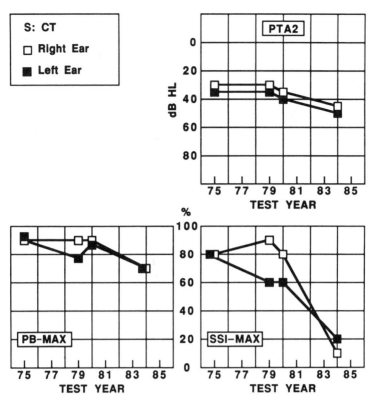

FIGURE 23.4. Changes in pure tone and speech audiometric scores over a 9-year period. Subject CT was 70 years old at the time of the initial evaluation in 1975 (PTA2 equals average of HTLs at 1000, 2000, and 4000 Hz; PB-max equals maximum of performance intensity function for phonemically balanced words; SSI-max equals maximum of performance intensity function for synthetic sentences). *Note.* From "Central Presbyacusis: A Longitudinal Case Study" by B. A. Stach, J. F. Jerger, and K. A. Fleming, 1985, *Ear and Hearing, 6,* pp. 304–306. Copyright 1985 by Williams & Wilkins. Reprinted by permission.

Other Factors

A major detrimental factor in hearing aid use by the elderly is the amplification of background noise. Surr et al. (1978) found background noise amplification to be the most important reason for reduced hearing aid use. Subjects in a study by Pollack (1977) reported that the most important change that could be made to improve hearing aids was to reduce the amplification of background noise. Brooks (1985) reported that background noise and loud sounds were two of the most prominent reasons for underuse of hearing aids. There are probably at least two factors that combine to limit the elderly from using hearing aids in background noise. First, Brooks (1985) conjectured that anyone who has had a hearing loss of long-standing duration will lose the developed skill of suppressing background sound. When the background noise is once again audible, the ability to disregard noise selectively will have to be redeveloped. Second, since the most important manifestation of central presbycusis is the inability to understand speech in background noise, the amplification of noise is likely to be counterproductive for many elderly hearing aid wearers.

Another property of the hearing aid that contributes to dissatisfaction among the elderly is the perception of poor quality of amplified sound and distortion of amplified speech (Cunningham, Merle, & Drake, 1978; Franks & Beckman, 1985). Weiss (1973) reported that, for some elderly subjects, hearing aids increased confusion and noise without improving speech intelligibility and did not work effectively in group situations.

Factors related to physical limitations of the elderly also adversely affect hearing aid use. Three common problems among the elderly that interfere with hearing aid manipulation include reduced sensitivity to touch, reduced range of motion of fingers and hands, and reduced neuromuscular timing (Maurer & Rupp, 1979). All of these factors combine to make it difficult for elderly patients to adjust gain controls, insert batteries, clean earmolds, and so forth. These factors help to explain Brooks's findings that the major cause for nonuse of hearing aids was the difficulty related to inserting the earmold (Brooks, 1985).

Strategies for Successful Intervention

Conventional Hearing Aids

Hearing Aid Evaluation

Techniques for the evaluation and fitting of hearing aids need not differ substantially from those used for younger patients. Evidence of successful electroacoustic alterations specifically designed for elderly patients has not been forthcoming. For example, hearing aid gain usage does not appear to be different as a function of age (Berger, 1989; Berger & Hagberg, 1982). Thus, conventional approaches to hearing aid selection appear to be appropriate for the elderly. Behavioral hearing aid evaluations for comparative purposes can also usually be carried out with the elderly. Care must be taken during behavioral assessment, however, to assure that the elderly patient is cognitively capable of performing the specific task and that vigilance to the task can be maintained throughout the testing session. In our experience at The Neurosensory Center of Houston, these factors seldom interfere with test interpretation (Jerger, Jerger, Oliver, & Pirozzolo, 1989;

Jerger, Stach, Pruitt, Harper, & Kirby, 1989), since the relatively simple speech audiometric tests used do not require high-level cognitive processing. However, we have found that more complex tasks, such as judgment rating or quality estimation of hearing aids, can be a rather confusing experience for some elderly patients.

Hearing Aid Hardware

An important aspect of conventional hearing aid fitting is the use of techniques to enhance the signal-to-noise ratio (S/N). While the techniques are no different for the elderly than for younger patients, their use is probably more important. One way to enhance hearing in noise is by the use of binaural hearing aids (Hawkins & Yacullo, 1984). Directional microphones can also be used for this purpose. Mueller, Grimes, and Erdman (1983) showed that older individuals, as well as younger ones, preferred the use of directional microphones over omnidirectional ones. The S/N can also be enhanced by use of noise suppression circuitry. To the extent that such circuitry assists, in general, in the recognition of speech in noise, it will also benefit elderly hearing aid users.

Another important aspect of fitting elderly patients with hearing aids is the size of the hearing aid, its dials, switches, and so on. Elderly patients are more prone to experience difficulty inserting and extracting hearing aids and earmolds. As a result, in-the-ear (ITE) hearing aids can now be made with extraction handles or extraction notches to simplify the process. Elderly individuals may also have difficulty manipulating various small components on the hearing aid. Raised volume controls and other techniques designed to make the controls more accessible are often necessary for these individuals. One newer strategy that appears to work reasonably well for patients with severe arthritis is the use of remote control for manipulation of gain, telecoil, and so on (Wolf & Powers, 1986).

Decisions must also be made about the style of hearing aid appropriate for elderly individuals. Conventional wisdom suggests that a behind-the-ear (BTE) hearing aid is superior to an ITE hearing aid because of its size and the size of its controls. However, Murphy (1981) reported that 77% of a group of geriatric patients preferred ITE over BTE hearing aids in terms of ease of use, ease of insertion, and ease of volume control adjustment. Since speech intelligibility with ITE hearing aids has been found to be at least as good as with BTE hearing aids (Cox & Risberg, 1986; Leeuw & Dreschler, 1987), ITE hearing aids appear to be the aid of choice for elderly patients, when appropriate.

Another aspect of the fitting strategy should be an emphasis on minimizing instrument complexity. The general rule should be that simpler is better. As generalized senescent changes occur, memory and other cognitive functions are likely to decline to an extent that may affect an elderly patient's ability to manage various hearing aid options. Problems such as these may be particularly germane if the patient resides alone or otherwise lacks assistance from a caretaker.

Outcome Measures of Hearing Aid Intervention

Validation and ongoing assessment of fitting strategy and technique is essential for a population that is as difficult to fit successfully as the elderly population. Toward this end, self-assessment measures have been used successfully as the validating criterion for hearing aid benefit (Brooks, 1979; Newman & Weinstein, 1988; Tannahill, 1979; Walden, Demorest, & Hepler, 1984). For example, Newman and Weinstein (1988) used the *Hearing Handicap Inventory for the Elderly (HHIE)* as an outcome measure of hearing aid benefit. They evaluated 18 elderly males before and 1 year after hearing aid use. Results suggested that perception of handicap was reduced significantly by hearing aid use and that the *HHIE* proved useful in the evaluation of amplification strategies.

Alternative Amplification Strategies

Because of the unique needs of many elderly patients and the relatively poorer prognosis for successful use of conventional hearing aids, attention has been increasingly focused on the use of assistive listening devices (ALDs) as alternative amplification strategies (Cranmer, 1988; Hull, 1988; Rupp, Vaughn, & Lightfoot, 1984; Stach, Loiselle, Jerger, Mintz, & Taylor, 1987; Vaughn, Lightfoot, & Arnold, 1981).

In general, ALDs differ from conventional hearing aids in that ALDs make use of remote microphone technology. That is, whereas conventional hearing aids contain a microphone, amplifier, and loudspeaker in a single device that fits behind or in the ear, ALDs use a microphone that is separate from the actual hearing aid amplifier. A television listener, for example, has a microphone that is placed near the television speaker. Sound is transmitted from the microphone by means of infrared light waves or frequency-modulated (FM) radio waves. The signal is received by an infrared or FM receiver that is coupled to the ear via earphones or a hearing aid. The advantages of this type of ALD consist mainly of enhancement of the S/N when the microphone is located closer to the target sound source. Another advantage is the better sound reproduction that results from reduced limits on amplifier component size.

Two basic concepts have emerged from these alternative strategies: (a) ALDs can be used as a substitute for conventional hearing aids to meet specific amplification needs and (b) remote-microphone ALDs can be used in isolation or in conjunction with conventional hearing aids to enhance S/Ns and thus overcome central presbycusis and other problems related to speech understanding in noise.

Need-Specific Amplification

By the use of ALDs, amplification systems can be tailored to meet the individual needs of patients. Patients often have fewer communication demands as they become older. Their need for amplification may be specific to telephone listening, television viewing, attending church services, or riding in the car with their spouse. Before appropriate, affordable ALDs were available, the best solution might have been a conventional hearing aid. But now, various assistive devices are readily available and often provide amplification superior to that of a conventional hearing aid. Thus, if a patient's only true communication handicaps occur while talking on the phone and watching television, a telephone amplifier and television listener could be dispensed and should readily meet the needs of the patient. The alternative, use of a conventional hearing aid, might actually be an inferior solution for both communication needs.

Types of need-specific ALDs include personal amplifiers, telephone amplifiers, television listeners, and other alerting devices. Personal amplifiers can be thought of as remote-microphone amplification systems. One type of personal amplifier is a self-contained device that uses a long cord that connects the microphone to the amplifier. The microphone can be used by a speaker who is in close proximity to the listener or can be placed next to a television or other source of sound. Such a device is referred to as a "hardware" amplifier. Its main benefit is its low cost, and its main problem relates to lack of flexibility in terms of speaker movement. The other types of systems have separate microphone/transmitters and receiver/amplifiers and use either FM or infrared light as a means of transmitting information from the microphone to the amplifier. Infrared systems are most useful in self-contained areas such as theaters or conference rooms. FM systems are very versatile and can be used in almost any listening environment.

Telephone amplifiers are also available in various forms (Slager, 1989). Some amplifiers are built into the handset of the telephone, whereas others are in-line amplifiers that can be used with modular telephones. Still other telephone amplifiers are portable induction field adapters. It has been our experience that use of a telephone amplifier coupled acoustically to a hearing aid is sometimes superior to the use of a hearing aid telecoil for some elderly patients, because such an arrangement reduces the need to make adjustments to the hearing aid itself.

Television listeners are simply remote-microphone amplifiers that have been adapted specifically for use with television sets. The audio signal from the television can be sent to the receiver via FM, infrared, or hardwire transmission. For those elderly patients who cannot make use of audition for television viewing, closed-caption devices are available that will decode the subtitles that increasingly accompany television broadcasts.

Alerting devices are also available that allow elderly hearing-impaired individuals to more effectively monitor their environment. These devices convert sound to either visual, somatosensory, or higher-intensity auditory signals. Devices are used to alert the individual to doorbells, smoke detectors, telephone rings, and alarm clocks. They alert by flashing a light; vibrating a mattress, chair, or body-worn vibrotactile receiver; or transmitting sound at very-high-intensity levels.

Personal FM System Applications

Elderly patients experience substantial difficulty in the presence of background noise. For example, the most important functional consequence of central presbycusis is a reduction in the ability to understand speech in noise. The development of remote-microphone technology for enhancement of the S/N has had a major impact on the success with which communication disorders of elderly individuals can be ameliorated.

The use of remote-microphone technology, specifically personal FM systems, by adults has been growing over the past several years. Once restricted almost exclusively to classrooms for the hearing impaired, FM systems are now becoming the amplification system of choice for many adults, especially the elderly. Since decrease in hearing aid benefit can result from CAPD, and since CAPD is often characterized by the inability to function well when the S/N is unfavorable, we have begun to recommend the use of personal FM systems to the elderly, especially to those with central auditory disorder. The ALDs we most commonly recommend are quite similar to those traditionally used in classrooms for the hearing impaired. The speaker wears a microphone that is attached to an FM transmitter, and the listener wears an FM receiver tuned to the transmitter frequency. The signal is delivered to the ear in one of two ways: First, for cases in which the hearing loss has both a peripheral and a central component, hearing aids are recommended to overcome the peripheral loss and are used in conjunction with FM systems for the central disorder. Signals are typically transduced through the hearing aid telecoil and FM-system neck loop. Second, in cases in which the disorder is primarily central, only the FM system is recommended, and the signal is transduced through an insert receiver or lightweight headphones.

We recently summarized our clinical experience with FM system use (Stach et al., 1987). Over a 2-year period, we identified 170 patients as potential FM system users. Of these, 73 (42.9%) used FM systems successfully. Of all patients identified, 108 were adults, 35 of whom were eventually successful FM-system users. Of the 35 adult users, 18 (51%) were over the age of 65 at the time of dispensing. Five of these patients had a primarily peripheral auditory disorder pattern, and 13 had a mixed peripheral and central pattern. A more recent analysis of our clinical experience showed that 45 elderly patients had tried an FM system in our clinic. Of these individuals, devices were dispensed to 9 patients without any trial period. The remaining 36 patients used a device from our loaner stock for at least a 2-week period. Following the trial period, devices were dispensed to 15 (42%) of the patients. Of the 24 patients to whom a device was dispensed, 7 had a primarily peripheral auditory disorder pattern, and 17 had a mixed peripheral and central pattern.

A small pilot study of the impact of FM devices on the life-styles of seven elderly patients was also carried out. In addition to a complete battery of audiometric measures, a battery of quality-of-life tests was administered, including measures of personality, socioeconomic status, physical health status, emotional symptomatology, social interaction, participation in daily living, and life satisfaction. Results of the pilot data support the hypothesis that use of FM systems can help hearing-impaired older people maintain active involvement in social situations and daily activities involving communication with family and long-time acquaintances. In addition, we have learned that there is considerable variability in the frequency of FM-system use and in situations in which patients used these systems to aid their hearing. Also, some FM-system users appeared to be more hampered than others by the technological features and physical demands of using the device or were reluctant to enlist the cooperation of others to use the FM system in social situations. Our overall impression was that the use of FM systems added a new and decidedly positive dimension to our ability to help those with peripheral or central presbycusis to meet their amplification needs.

Illustrative Cases

The following two cases serve as illustrative examples of patients we have evaluated. Both patients were managed by the clinical staff of The Methodist Hospital Audiology Service at the Neurosensory Center of Houston, Texas. One case is representative of the elderly patients who were at one time successful users of conventional hearing aids but who became increasingly unsuccessful with age and eventually required the use of an FM assistive device for communication. The other is representative of the success we have had with the application of alternative amplification strategies in the elderly population.

Case 1

Patient HR was first evaluated at our facility at the age of 64 years. She had a bilateral, moderate, relatively flat sensorineural hearing loss and poor speech understanding. At that time, she was fitted with binaural hearing aids. Six years later, she returned, complaining of a change in her hearing ability and insisting that her hearing aids were no longer helping her. Because of a decrease in high-frequency hearing and a reduction in speech understanding, she was fitted with more powerful hearing aids and was loaned a personal FM system for trial use. Although she reported substantial success with the FM system, she felt that it was "too much gadgetry" and that it was difficult to ask others for assistance with the microphone.

She returned to our facility 2 years later, at the age of 72, reportedly because her hearing aids were no longer of any value to her. The results of her audiologic evaluation are shown in Figure 23.5. Along with substantial peripheral hearing loss, she had degraded speech understanding consistent with CAPD. Results of the hearing aid evaluation showed rather good aided performance at 0 dB message-to-competition ratio (MCR). Aided binaurally, she was able to correctly identify 90% of sentences presented in the presence of single-talker competition. However, in a more difficult listening situation (-10 dB MCR), her score was 0%. The addition of a personal FM system resulted in improvement of 80%. Even in a difficult listening situation (-20 dB MCR), she was able to correctly identify 50% of the speech targets. An FM system was dispensed following the evaluation.

Over the ensuing year, she and her spouse used the FM system in many different communication situations. She reported that the FM system was the only way that she could have a conversation with her husband, listen to the television, or hear her minister at church services. Her positive experience with this remote microphone technology parallels that of many patients for whom conventional hearing aids have become inadequate. Although she was initially resistant to the concept of the FM system, her inability to communicate had become so overwhelming that the drawbacks became increasingly less important.

Case 2

Patient BB was first evaluated at our facility at the age of 85. At that time, she had a mild, sloping, sensorineural hearing loss. Speech understanding of monosyllabic phonemically balanced (PB) words was 96% in the right ear and 88% in the left ear. A slight discrepancy between PB word scores and results on the *Synthetic Sentence Identification* (*SSI*) test (Jerger, Speaks, & Trammel, 1968) was consistent with mild CAPD, a not unexpected result for someone of her age. She returned to our facility at the age of 90, shortly after having a cerebrovascular accident that left her nonambulatory, but otherwise functioning rather well. The results of the audiologic evaluation are shown in Figure 23.6. Her pure tone thresholds had changed by about 20 dB over the 5-year period. Speech understanding was relatively more depressed, especially in the left ear. Although a hearing aid evaluation was recommended, she left the hospital before it was completed.

At the age of 92, her hearing loss began to be a communication handicap because a relative of hers had gained a stature that required him to periodically be on the evening news. Because she was essentially bedridden, a remote-microphone device was chosen for television viewing. To allow for maximum flexibility, she was fitted with a personal FM system. At the same time, she was loaned a conventional BTE hearing aid, because communication with the FM system was not always convenient. The BTE aid proved to be less than adequate, however, because of frequent feedback caused

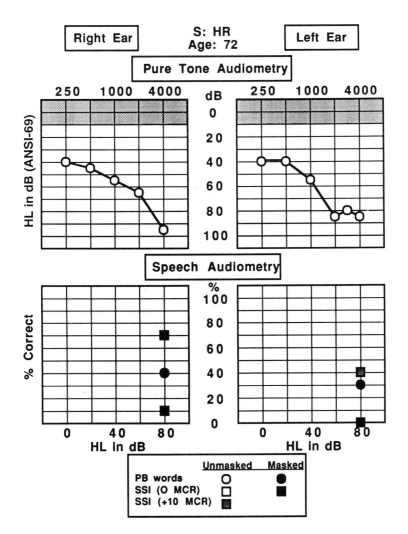

FIGURE 23.5. Air-conduction pure tone audiometric and speech audiometric results in a 72-year-old patient. Speech audiometric results are for phonemically balanced (PB) words presented in quiet, the *Synthetic Sentence Identification (SSI)* test presented at 0 dB message-to-competition ratio (MCR), and the *SSI* at +10 dB MCR.

by the patient's head being against a pillow much of the time. In an effort to alleviate the feedback problem and dexterity problems with the volume control, we decided to try an ITE hearing aid with a remote volume control and telecoil switch. Using the remote-control ITE aid, the patient was able to successfully control hearing aid volume. In addition, she was able to control the telecoil of the aid and use it in conjunction with the neck loop of the FM system. She now leaves the FM-system transmitter attached to the television and

uses remote control with the ITE aid for regular hearing aid use or to switch to the FM system for remote microphone use.

Conclusions

Many elderly patients with hearing impairment benefit substantially from conventional hearing aid amplification. However, a majority of the hearing-impaired elderly do not seek the use of hearing aids because

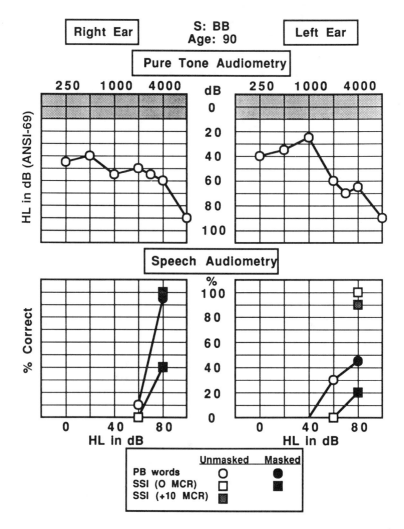

FIGURE 23.6. Air-conduction pure tone audiometric and speech audiometric results in a 90-year-old patient. Speech audiometric results are for phonemically balanced (PB) words presented in quiet, the *Synthetic Sentence Identification* (*SSI*) test presented at 0 dB message-to-competition ratio (MCR), and the *SSI* at +10 dB MCR.

of psychosocial factors, the nature of the hearing health care delivery system, and the cost of amplification devices. In addition, of those who seek hearing aid use, many do not benefit as much as might be expected. Factors that adversely affect hearing aid benefit include the complex nature of presbycusis, the sound quality of hearing aids, and physical limitations of the elderly population. When fitting the elderly with conventional hearing aids, special consideration should be given to the reduction of background noise and to instrument size

and complexity. Alternative amplification strategies, such as personal FM systems and other assistive listening devices, can be used very effectively to circumvent many of the problems associated with conventional hearing aid use by the elderly.

References

Berger, K. W. (1989). Hearing aid gain usage as a function of age. *The Hearing Journal, 42*(9), 33–39.

Berger, K. W., & Hagberg, E. N. (1982). Gain usage based on hearing aid experience and subject age. *Ear and Hearing, 3,* 235–237.

Birt, D., & Alberti, P. W. (1975). Performance of hearing aids and wearer satisfaction—A two year study. *Canadian Journal of Otolaryngology, 4,* 529–537.

Brooks, D. N. (1985). Factors relating to the under-use of postaural hearing aids. *British Journal of Audiology, 19,* 211–217.

Brooks, S. (1979). Counseling and its effects on hearing aid use. *Scandinavian Audiology, 8,* 101–107.

Cox, R. M., & Risberg, D. M. (1986). Comparison of in-the-ear and over-the-ear hearing aid fittings. *Journal of Speech and Hearing Disorders, 51,* 362–369.

Cranmer, K. S. (1988). ALDs for seniors. *Hearing Instruments, 39*(6), 16–20.

Cranmer, K. S. (1989). Hearing instrument dispensing—1989. *Hearing Instruments, 40*(6), 6–15, 52.

Cunningham, D. R., Merle, K. S., & Drake, J. (1978). Users' satisfaction with hearing aids. *Journal of the American Auditory Society, 4,* 81–85.

Davies, J. W., & Mueller, H. G. (1987). Hearing aid selection. In H. G. Mueller & V. C. Geoffrey (Eds.), *Communication disorders in aging: Assessment and management* (pp. 408–436). Washington, DC: Gallaudet University Press.

Dodds, E., & Harford, E. R. (1982). A community hearing conservation program for senior citizens. *Ear and Hearing, 3,* 160–166.

Ewertsen, H. W. (1974). Use of hearing aids (always, often, rarely, never). *Scandinavian Audiology, 3,* 173–176.

Franks, J. R., & Beckmann, N. J. (1985). Rejection of hearing aids: Attitudes of a geriatric sample. *Ear and Hearing, 6,* 161–166.

Goldstein, D. P. (1984). Hearing impairment, hearing aids and audiology. *Asha, 26,* 24–38.

Griffin, K. M., Tourigny, A. W., & Demitrack, L. B. (1988). The hearing-impaired population in U.S. nursing homes. *Hearing Instruments, 39*(2), 6–8, 35.

Hardick, E. J., & Gans, R. E. (1982). An approach to rehabilitation with amplification. *Ear and Hearing, 3,* 178–182.

Harless, E. L., & McConnell, F. (1982). Effects of hearing aid use on self concept in older persons. *Journal of Speech and Hearing Disorders, 47,* 305–309.

Hawkins, D. B., & Yacullo, W. (1984). The signal-to-noise ratio advantage of binaural hearing aids and directional microphones under different levels of reverberation. *Journal of Speech and Hearing Disorders, 49,* 278–286.

Hayes, D. (1980). Central auditory problems and the aging process. In D. S. Beasley & G. A. Davis (Eds.), *Aging communication processes and disorders* (pp. 257–266). New York: Grune & Stratton.

Hayes, D., & Jerger, J. (1979). Aging and the use of hearing aids. *Scandinavian Audiology, 8,* 33–40.

Hayes, D., Jerger, J., Taff, J., & Barber, B. (1983). Relation between aided synthetic sentence identification scores and hearing aid user satisfaction. *Ear and Hearing, 4,* 158–161.

Hull, R. H. (1988). Evaluation of ALDs by older adult listeners. *Hearing Instruments, 39*(2), 10–12.

Iler, K. L., Danhauer, J. L., & Mulac, A. (1982). Peer perception of geriatrics wearing hearing aids. *Journal of Speech and Hearing Disorders, 47,* 433–438.

Jerger, J., & Hayes, D. (1976). Hearing aid evaluation: Clinical experience with a new philosophy. *Archives of Otolaryngology, 102,* 214–225.

Jerger, J., Jerger, S., Oliver, T., & Pirozzolo, F. (1989). Speech understanding in the elderly. *Ear and Hearing, 10,* 79–89.

Jerger, J., Speaks, C., & Trammel, J. (1968). A new approach to speech audiometry. *Journal of Speech and Hearing Disorders, 33,* 318–327.

Jerger, J., Stach, B., Pruitt, J., Harper, R., & Kirby, H. (1989). Comments on ''Speech understanding and aging.'' *Journal of the Acoustical Society of America, 85,* 1352–1354.

Leeuw, A. R., & Dreschler, W. A. (1987). Speech understanding and directional hearing for hearing-impaired subjects with in-the-ear and behind-the-ear hearing aids. *Scandinavian Audiology, 16,* 31–36.

Lichtenstein, M., Bess, F., & Logan, S. (1988). Validation of screening tools for identifying hearing impaired elderly in primary care. *Journal of the American Medical Association, 259,* 2875–2878.

Maurer, J. F., & Rupp, R. R. (1979). *Hearing and aging: Tactics for intervention.* New York: Grune & Stratton.

McCandless, G. A., & Parkin, J. L. (1979). Hearing aid performance relative to site of lesion.

Otolaryngology and Head and Neck Surgery, 87, 871–875.

Mueller, H. G., Grimes, A. M., & Erdman, S. A. (1983). Subjective ratings of directional amplification. *Hearing Instruments, 34*(2), 14–16, 47.

Murphy, L. (1981). An investigation of the use of behind the ear and in the ear hearing aids with a geriatric population. *Hearing Aid Journal, 34*(7), 38–41.

Newman, C. W., & Weinstein, B. E. (1988). The Hearing Handicap Inventory for the Elderly as a measure of hearing aid benefit. *Ear and Hearing, 9,* 81–85.

Pollack, M. C. (1977). Hearing aids: Needs and developments, Part I. *Hearing Aid Journal, 30,* 10, 29–31.

Rupp, R. R., Vaughn, G. R., & Lightfoot, R. K. (1984). Nontraditional "aids" to hearing: Assistive listening devices. *Geriatrics, 39,* 55–73.

Schow, R. L. (1982). Success of hearing aid fitting in nursing homes. *Ear and Hearing, 3,* 173–177.

Schwartz, M. S., & Matsko, T. A. (1988). Hearing health care services in a non-institutionalized older population. *Hearing Instruments, 39*(2), 19–22.

Slager, R. D. (1989). Romancing the phone: The adventure continues. *Seminars in Hearing, 10,* 42–55.

Sorri, M., Luotonen, M., & Laitakari, K. (1984). Use and non-use of hearing aids. *British Journal of Audiology, 18,* 169–172.

Stach, B. (1990). Hearing aid amplification and central processing disorders. In R. E. Sandlin (Ed.), *Handbook of hearing aid amplification: Vol. II. Clinical considerations and fitting practices* (pp. 87–111). Austin, TX: PRO-ED.

Stach, B. A., Jerger, J. F., & Fleming, K. A. (1985). Central presbyacusis: A longitudinal case study. *Ear and Hearing, 6,* 304–306.

Stach, B. A., Loiselle, L. H., Jerger, J. F., Mintz, S. L., & Taylor, C. D. (1987). Clinical experience with personal FM assistive listening devices. *The Hearing Journal, 10*(5), 24–30.

Stach, B. A., Spretnjak, M. L., & Jerger, J. F. (1990). The prevalence of central presbyacusis in a clinical population. *Journal of the American Academy of Audiology, 1,* 109–115.

Stream, R. W., & Stream, K. S. (1980). Focusing on the hearing needs of the elderly. *Journal of the Academy of Rehabilitative Audiology, 13,* 104–108.

Surr, R. K., Schuchman, G. I., & Montgomery, A. A. (1978). Factors influencing use of hearing aids. *Archives of Otolaryngology, 104,* 732–736.

Tannahill, J. (1979). The hearing handicap scale as a measure of hearing aid benefit. *Journal of Speech and Hearing Disorders, 44,* 91–99.

Vaughn, G. R., Lightfoot, R. K., & Arnold, L. C. (1981). Alternative listening devices and delivery systems for audiologic habilitation of hearing-impaired persons. *Journal of the Academy of Rehabilitative Audiology, 14,* 62–69.

Ventry, I. M., & Weinstein, B. A. (1982). The Hearing Handicap Inventory for the Elderly: A new tool. *Ear and Hearing, 3,* 128–134.

Walden, B., Demorest, M., & Hepler, E. (1984). Self-report approach to assessing benefit derived from amplification. *Journal of Speech and Hearing Research, 27,* 49–56.

Weiss, C. E. (1973). Why more of the aged with auditory deficits do not wear hearing aids. *Journal of the American Geriatrics Society, 21,* 139–141.

Wolf, H. P., & Powers, T. A. (1986). Remote control: The invisible touch. *The Hearing Journal, 39,* 10, 18–20.

Audiologic Rehabilitation: Candidacy, Assessment, and Management

24

CHAPTER

Sharon A. Lesner, PhD, and Patricia B. Kricos, PhD ■

Because hearing loss has its most profound impact on communication, ultimately the primary goal of audiologic rehabilitation is to enable the hearing-impaired adult to experience the least stressful communication possible, given constraints imposed by the hearing problem. For some adults, an attempt may be made to restore communication function to near-normal status. For others, the aim may be to improve communication abilities significantly above preintervention levels. And for still others, particularly hearing-impaired residents of skilled nursing facilities and individuals with additional handicapping conditions, the goal may be to maintain communication skills, that is, to prevent further deterioration in communication function.

The presence of a hearing loss may affect virtually all aspects of the hearing-impaired person's life-style. The scope of audiologic rehabilitation must, therefore, extend beyond the enhancement of communication status. It is critical to determine how a hearing impairment may be affect-ing the hearing-impaired person socially, emotionally, and, in some elderly adults, vocationally in order to provide effective and relevant services to reduce the resulting handicap.

The elderly hearing-impaired population offers a particular challenge in this respect because of the many associated compounding problems that exist and the heterogeneous nature of the population. Although audiologic rehabilitation of the elderly is challenging, it also offers a source of great professional rewards. This chapter will focus on audiologic rehabilitation of older adults, including a discussion of candidacy, assessment, and effective and relevant programming.

Candidacy

The low rates of satisfaction reported by new hearing aid users who do not receive organized postfitting sessions (Brooks, 1979, 1985; Kapteyn, 1977; Surr, Schuchman, & Montgomery, 1978; Ward & Gowers, 1980) suggest that audiologic rehabilitation should be available for all individuals who obtain hearing aids. Admittedly, there may be some elderly individuals with significant hearing loss who will do well without audiologic rehabilitation beyond the initial hearing aid fitting. However, it is our experience that the vast majority of elderly hearing aid users benefit from a comprehensive hearing aid orientation program following the provision of amplification. The authors have had elderly adults in their clinical programs who have worn hearing aids for as long as 15 or 20 years and who have reported gaining valuable information and benefit following participation in an organized audiologic rehabilitative group. Long-term hearing aid wearers have frequently reported that they wished they had received the knowledge, skills, and insights that resulted from participation in a structured hearing aid orientation program immediately following the provision of amplification instead of years later.

In spite of the high prevalence of hearing impairment among the elderly and the need for audiologic rehabilitation, the rate at which older individuals seek help is very low. It has been estimated, for example, that only 13 to 20% of the elderly hearing-impaired population who need amplification use hearing aids (Miller & Schein, 1987). It is important to recognize the major factors influencing an individual's decision to seek audiologic rehabilitation, as well as variables that may complicate or interfere with ultimate delivery of services. Some of the more important factors include the client's motivation and attitude, self-perceived handicap, social environment, financial resources, and mobility. Finally, the attitude of the audiologist is crucial to whether clients will follow through with audiologic rehabilitation.

Assessment

Assessment is an important first step in the audiologic rehabilitation process. The purpose of assessment should be to gain an understanding of the abilities, limitations, and perceived needs of the client so that therapeutic goals can be established and appropriate intervention planned. In addition, assessment should provide a baseline for pre- and postintervention comparisons.

Several dysfunctions and changes occur in the sensory and motor systems with age. The interdependency of these changes requires that the entire individual be treated during the audiologic rehabilitation process and that the individual not be treated as only a "set of ears." In addition to being multidimensional, assessment protocols should also focus on the manner in which older adults function within their social environment.

The reader is referred to Stephens and Goldstein (1983) for a comprehensive procedural model for aural rehabilitation assessment in the elderly. The model includes assessment of the receptive, productive, and integrative capabilities of each individual. This includes communication status; associated variables such as psychological, sociological, vocational, and educational factors; and related conditions including mobility, upper limb function, and aural pathology.

The variety of systems and functions that must be assessed and the heterogeneity of the elderly population dictate that no single assessment tool or battery will fit all clients or situations. In addition, clinicians should exercise care not to overevaluate during the first few sessions, because clients may become discouraged if they perceive that the audiologist is only interested in testing them and not in providing any other benefit. The following discussion will highlight key areas that typically will need to be evaluated. Some can be evaluated using objective measures while others involve subjective considerations (see Figure 24.1). Consideration of all of these key areas will enhance the design of an effective and relevant program for the hearing-impaired older adult.

Communication Needs

Of paramount importance in the remediation process is the prioritization of the com-

Objective Measures	Subjective Measures
Communication needs	Motivation/attitude
Psychosocial status	Social environment
Amplification status	Financial status
Communication abilities	Motoric abilities
Vision	General health
Mental status	

FIGURE 24.1. Audiologic rehabilitation assessment strategies.

munication needs of each client. Input from the clients, as well as from significant other persons (SOPs), as to how the hearing loss has affected the person's communication and life-style is critical. The number-one priority for most hearing-impaired adults will be, in Erber's (1988) words, increased conversational fluency.

Erber (1988) suggests that a significant amount of information regarding the client's needs may be obtained by conducting a ''professional conversation'' with the client. A brief simulated conversation may reveal very useful information in a relatively short period of time: How much difficulty does the person experience in conversation? What effect does background noise have on the person's difficulties? How stressed does the person appear during communication? Does the client use repair strategies when words are not clear?

By establishing an appropriate atmosphere, information concerning the chief problems experienced by the client and his or her understanding of the problems can also be obtained during interviews. This includes information about hearing impairment, motivation, and prognosis (Garstecki, 1981a). Stephens (1980) warns, however, that clients often have a tendency to respond to interview questions with medically or technically oriented responses, and they tend to omit any discussion of the difficulties they experience because of their hearing losses. Consequently, the psychosocial ramifications of the hearing loss may be underestimated.

Psychosocial Status

Assessing psychosocial status is important if a rehabilitation program is to be designed to successfully meet the needs of the client. Because of the difficulties of eliciting relevant information from interviews, clinicians should consider the use of handicap scales. Self-assessment scales provide an effective method for systematically assessing the emotional and social consequences of hearing impairment for the client as well as the SOPs (Newman & Weinstein, 1986). Although there are several scales available, the *Hearing Handicap Inventory for the Elderly* (*HHIE*) is particularly useful with older individuals because it was developed and normed for persons over the age of 60 years (Ventry & Weinstein, 1982). Other communication profiles and handicap scales such as the *Self-Assessment of Communication* (*SAC*) (Schow & Nerbonne, 1982), the *Hearing Handicap Inventory for the Elderly–Screening Version* (*HHIE-S*) (Ventry & Weinstein, 1982), and the *Nursing Home Hearing Handicap Index* (Schow & Nerbonne, 1977) may also be useful for specific purposes and settings.

Amplification Status

Scales and inventories dealing with the use of amplification devices are also useful. Although not standardized in the elderly, the *Hearing Aid Performance Inventory* (*HAPI*) provides a means for assessing self-perceived benefit from amplification in various situations (Walden, Demorest, & Hepler, 1984). In addition to highlighting areas in need of remediation, the *HAPI* can be used to measure changes in post-treatment performance. The *Hearing Aid Assessment Form* (Appendix 24.A) may be used to quickly determine problem areas in terms of hearing aid fit. Finally, candidacy for assistive listening devices can be explored with the *Assistive Device Needs Assessment Questionnaire* (Fernandes, 1985)

Communication Abilities

Speech communication, especially among the hearing impaired, typically involves the integration of auditory and visual cues. As a consequence, comparisons of performance in all three modes (auditory, visual, and combined auditory-visual) will serve to highlight those in need of remediation. Danhauer, Garnett, and Edgerton (1985) have recommended that evaluation of the older hearing-impaired individual's auditory-visual processing of speech will be the most useful measure. Auditory, visual, and auditory-visual presentations on nonsense syllables such as the *Nonsense Syllable Test* (Edgerton & Danhauer, 1979); the *Semi-Diagnostic Test,* which is a multiple-choice word test (Hutton, Curry, & Armstrong, 1959); or the *CID Everyday Sentence Test* (Davis & Silverman, 1970) are suggested.

The use of continuous discourse tracking (DeFilippo & Scott, 1978) provides a measure of a person's ability to deal with stimuli that approximate those encountered during everyday communication. Tracking is a process in which a subject (receiver) repeats groups of words that are read by another person (talker). When errors occur in the repetition of the material, the talker and receiver employ various strategies to resolve the blockage in order to obtain a correct verbatim repetition. Scoring is accomplished by calculating the number of words correctly repeated per minute. With the use of single-subject paradigms, it is possible to use tracking as an evaluative procedure

(Lesner, Lynn, & Brainard, 1988). Tracking can be done in auditory, visual, and combined modes.

Vision

Since a high prevalence of visual problems exists among the elderly, clients should routinely be questioned concerning the presence of such conditions as cataracts, glaucoma, or macular degeneration (National Center for Health Statistics, 1983). There is also a tendency for older adults to experience a decrease in visual acuity, peripheral vision, and color perception. There is evidence that a general slowing occurs in the central processing of visual information among older adults (Lesner & Sandridge, 1984).

These alterations in the visual system of the elderly have important rehabilitative implications. Although the importance of visual processing during speechreading is obvious, visual input is also important for successful hearing aid use, as well as for aural rehabilitation programming. For example, sessions should be held in brightly lit rooms in which glare has been eliminated. Seating should ensure that participants are close to and at appropriate angles from the instructor. Visual aids should also be large and make use of primary colors. Individuals who wear corrective lenses should wear them and the lenses should be appropriate for both near and far vision. Visual screening should be done routinely. Screening instruments such as the Snellen chart, or various visual screening devices such as the Titmus, Keystone, or Ortho-Rater vision testers, should be included.

Mental Status

A critical element in the rehabilitation of the elderly is their mental status. For example, 10% of those over the age of 65 have mild to moderate mental impairment sufficient to affect performance of everyday activities (Gallo, Reichel, & Andersen, 1988; LaFerle

& LaFerle, 1988; Wang, 1977). A correlation has also been found to exist between the presence of hearing loss and diminished cognitive performance in older adults (Uhlmann, Larson, Rees, Koepsell, & Duckert, 1989; Weinstein & Amsel, 1986). Since individuals with altered mental states are often not readily identifiable, we encourage routine mental status screening. Two of the most widely used and simple screening tests of mental status are the *Short Portable Mental Status Questionnaire* (*SPMSQ*) (Pfeiffer, 1975) and the *Mini-Mental States Examination* (Folstein, Folstein, & McHugh, 1975). Clinicians should ensure that clients are able to hear the questions by using hearing aids or assistive listening devices when assessing mental status (Weinstein & Amsel, 1986).

If clients are found to have memory loss and disorientation, repetition of information and rehearsal should be emphasized. Perhaps most importantly, a SOP should be identified who will assume responsibility for the hearing aid and/or assistive listening device before one is issued (Weinstein, 1984). Although the presence of mental impairment does not preclude the use of amplification or auditory rehabilitation, careful monitoring is important in such cases.

Motivation and Attitude

Individuals will be less likely to seek out audiologic rehabilitation services, and programming will be less successful and more difficult, if the client does not acknowledge and accept the presence of a sensory deficit. Emotional acceptance of a health condition is desirable if an individual is to accept a rehabilitation plan or adjust to the use of a prosthetic device (Hardick & Lesner, 1979; Miller & Schein, 1987). According to Goldstein and Stephens (1981), attitude is the most important ingredient in remediation. Although one fourth to one third of individuals may have negative attitudes toward hearing aids, Goldstein and Stephens feel that these negative

attitudes can be overcome through audiologic rehabilitation conducted in a rewarding and motivating environment.

The Social Environment

The overall communication environment of the elderly client must be considered. According to Lubinski (1984), there are two prerequisites for successful communication by older adults: (a) the elderly person must have both the skills and the motivation to communicate and (b) the external environment of the older person must be conducive to communication.

Rather than treat the older adult in isolation, the audiologist should determine if the individual has viable communication partners. Inclusion of an SOP is one of the most important ingredients for successful rehabilitation of the hearing-impaired person. The SOP's skills in communicating with the hearing-impaired person should be determined; for example, does the SOP know how to modify his or her message to facilitate comprehension? Does the SOP understand the importance of communication to the older adult, as well as the frustration that accompanies repeated communication failures? Shadden (1988) has recommended that SOPs receive information, techniques for management, counseling, support, and a means of sharing.

Lubinski (1984) suggests that speech and hearing professionals who work with older adults should view themselves as "communication engineers." Efforts must be made to maximize the everyday environment in which communication takes place.

Financial Status

The income level and financial status of older adults is quite variable. Hearing aids, batteries, and audiologic rehabilitation services are not covered under Medicare or most private insurance policies. Some older adults will not be willing or able because of limited incomes or financial commitments to pay for services. When appropriate, audiologists should help the aged seek alternative mechanisms of payment.

Motoric Abilities

While a great deal of variability exists, older individuals tend to lose mobility in their hands and limbs. Manipulative skills become poorer because sensitivity to touch is reduced (Axelrod & Cohen, 1961). Fine motor skills may be further degraded as a result of the presence of arthritis, stroke, or tremors. Slowed reaction times and movement impairments may also create difficulties when working with small objects.

Considering the skills needed to manipulate hearing aids and assistive listening devices, both fine and gross motoric abilities should be assessed. In fact, difficulties inserting hearing aids or earmolds, manipulating the volume controls of hearing aids, and changing the battery contribute to nonuse of amplification among the elderly (Brooks, 1985; Ward, Gowers, & Morgan, 1979). For those who cannot be trained to properly insert hearing aids or for those who continue to experience difficulty in manipulating amplification devices, the SOP becomes crucial to successful rehabilitation.

General Health

General health status is an important consideration and may influence the individual's potential to benefit from therapy. Information regarding general health status also provides insights into the client's primary and secondary concerns. An apparent lack of motivation or interest may really be a preoccupation with a serious and/or threatening health condition (Hardick & Gans, 1982).

Effective and Relevant Programming

Preprogramming Considerations

Prior to the design of a specific audiologic rehabilitation program, the practitioner working with older adults must address a number of questions. Where will the program of audiologic rehabilitation be offered? What materials will be useful, as well as of interest, to the client? When and how often will sessions take place? What are the features of "successful" audiologic rehabilitation programs?

Choice of the space in which services will be provided requires consideration of the location of the program as well as the characteristics of the treatment rooms. The advice given by McCollom and Mynders (1984) for location of a hearing aid dispensing program is applicable as well to the location of full-scale audiologic rehabilitation programs. The key word is accessibility. The location must be easy to find by automobile or public transportation, proximal to other professional/commercial centers, and accessible by elevator if the program is not located on the ground floor. Additional considerations include availability of parking and neighborhood image.

The therapy rooms ideally would be

- Well illuminated, with minimal glare from windows or lighting sources

- Sound-treated to provide an optimal listening environment

- Large enough to accommodate groups

- Accessible to physically handicapped individuals, with a ramp for wheelchairs

- Cheerful, yet free of visual distractions

An ideal arrangement might include a grouping of sofas, chairs, and tables to reflect a homelike setting. Binnie and Hession (1988) described a living room format with ceiling-mounted loudspeakers and an audio mixer that enables generation of a variety of noise types and signal-to-noise ratios. While this setup may not be feasible for many clinics, at the least an attempt should be made to provide furniture that is comfortable, homelike, and easy to rise from in the treatment rooms.

The selection of challenging, meaningful training materials is of paramount importance. The audiologist should solicit input from the client regarding his or her background and interests in order to choose materials that will motivate the client to practice communication skills. Materials such as those devised by Bally, Kaplan, and Garretson (1985) for speechreading training are ideal because they are presented in a game format and involve topics such as U.S. history and geography.

Program sessions should be scheduled to accommodate the needs of the elderly client. Few older adults are enthusiastic about evening sessions, preferring morning times when they are most alert. Ideally, program sessions will last approximately 30–60 min, once per week, over a period of 4 to 12 weeks, and will involve both individual and group sessions. As long as sessions are lively, fun, and involve a lot of interaction, sessions as long as 60 min will be feasible with elderly clients. These guidelines will be mitigated, however, by the special needs of the individual client. Some clients may benefit most from a short-term group program experience, whereas others may need a longer period of treatment that is individually tailored to their needs.

The characteristics of successful programs of audiologic rehabilitation should be considered in their design. Hardick (1977), in a review of successful programs, suggested that adult aural rehabilitation programs should be client-centered and focused upon amplification and/or modification of the communication environment, consist primarily of group therapy with individual help as needed, include SOPs (e.g., family and friends), be short-term,

and use older adults who have successfully adjusted to their hearing loss to help new hearing aid wearers make such adjustments.

Counseling Needs of Older Adults

Of all the strategies available to the audiologist for approaching the problems of hearing-impaired adults, counseling remains singularly the most important; it is shown at the top of the intervention strategies in Figure 24.2. Although an academic background in counseling courses is helpful, the most important attributes for the audiologist will be the ability to *listen, care,* and *empathize.* Too often, audiologists adopt a medical model of interaction with older clients, in which the adult is given a cursory diagosis and description of her or his hearing difficulties, followed by a recommendation for a specific hearing aid arrangement. It should be no wonder, then, that many hearing-impaired persons do not follow through on recommendations. Audiologists, so intent on improving listening in their clients, would be wise to develop their own abilities to listen to the older adult as problems are described. This requires the audiologist to invest somewhat more time in interaction with the adult, but the client's willingness to follow through on recommendations may be well worth the time expended. Time should be spent with the older adult to carefully describe the hearing loss, discuss limitations imposed by the hearing loss, and explain possible courses of remediation to the hearing-impaired older adult. Counseling of family members is often advisable, particularly if the person appears to have been coerced into having the evaluation.

The value of obtaining input from the spouse (or another SOP if the client is widowed or unmarried) cannot be overemphasized. Several of the self-assessment

Counseling

Hearing Aid Orientation Program (HOP)

SOP Education

Assertiveness training

Speechreading

Auditory training

Audiovisual communication training

FIGURE 24.2. Audiologic rehabilitation intervention strategies.

scales discussed under "Assessment" in this chapter have versions that have been adapted for use with the client's significant others. A version of the *HHIE* for spouses (*HHIE-SP*) (Newman & Weinstein, 1986) and the *Significant Others Assessment of Communication* (*SOAC*), the adapted version of Schow and Nerbonne's (1982) *SAC*, can provide insights from the spouse or significant other regarding how the hearing impairment has affected the life-style of the client socially and emotionally. Discrepancies between what the client reports as consequences of the hearing loss and what the spouse reports may serve in many cases as the starting point for discussion in counseling sessions.

One of the biggest challenges facing the audiologist with an older adult case load is motivating clients to accept hearing aids and/or audiologic rehabilitation. Older adults are frequently reluctant to pursue treatment of their hearing difficulties and may be apprehensive about the audiologist's intentions. In the authors' experience, *knowledge* regarding the hearing loss, hearing aids (both their advantages and limitations), and various other avenues of relief, provided in an atmosphere of trust and caring, is the key to success in overcoming the client's resistance. The more clients know and understand about their hearing loss and the choices they have for dealing with them, the more likely they will be to take an active role in reducing their difficulties.

While the provision of information in the typical audiology practice is usually handled on a one-on-one basis, the use of group

sessions should not be overlooked. Group sessions on a short-term (4- to 6-week) basis afford the busy practitioner the opportunity to provide information in an economical way, both timewise and financially. Of even greater importance, group sessions allow the older client to meet in a nonthreatening environment with older adults who have similar problems. Problems (and often solutions) can be shared, and in many cases negative attitudes toward hearing loss, hearing aids, and communication can be handled more effectively on the group level. The audiologist's role in these meetings should be that of a facilitator rather than an authority. The involvement of successful "graduates" of previous group programs is ideal. These resource people can serve as group leaders, offering support and encouragement and perhaps a degree of credibility to group participants.

While group sessions offer numerous advantages, the fact remains that each client must be approached individually. As with all aspects of audiologic rehabilitation of older adults, counseling needs will vary from individual to individual. For the busy practitioner, the Profile of Counseling Needs checklist shown in Appendix 24.B may be useful. This checklist may serve to remind the audiologist of the need for an individualized plan of counseling, as well as to enable the audiologist to quickly determine an overview of the client's possible counseling needs. After a brief interview of the client, the sensitive, experienced audiologist should be able to determine any negative factors that should be addressed during counseling. The use of candid, direct questions such as "How do you feel about your hearing loss (or hearing aid, or audiologic rehabilitation)?" may reveal significant information about the client's degree of acceptance of his or her hearing problem. Specific items from the *Communication Profile for the Hearing Impaired* (*CPHI*) (Demorest & Erdman, 1986) could be used in setting counseling goals. The Personal Adjustment subscales from the *CPHI*, including self-acceptance, acceptance of loss, anger, displacement of responsibility, exaggeration of responsibility, discouragement, stress, withdrawal, and denial, may be particularly useful for determining the client's counseling needs.

A Model Hearing Aid Orientation Program (HOP)

Older adults who have recently received or who will soon be purchasing hearing aids for the first time can be helped to adjust to amplification by participating in an organized hearing aid orientation program. The model that we have successfully used, referred to as the Hearing Aid Orientation Program (HOP), is a 5-week group and individual program in which both hearing-impaired persons (HIPs) and their SOPs participate. An outline of the HOP model is presented in Appendix 24.C. The topics have been arranged to facilitate the client's adjustment to amplification, foster realistic expectations for hearing aid use on the part of both the client and SOPs, and maximize the client's communication performance. Groups of 6 to 10 clients are typically involved in each session, with weekly group meetings lasting approximately 2 hours. Individual sessions are also scheduled on a weekly basis to focus on specific areas of difficulty experienced by each client. The presentation of information in a nonthreatening group of peers appears to facilitate the client's ultimate acceptance of and satisfaction with amplification.

During the first HOP session, information on hearing aids and their function is presented to group participants. Group conversation revolving around hearing aid limitations provides the audiologist the opportunity to rate group members in terms of conversational fluency. Individual sessions following the first group meeting enable administration of specific assessments for each individual and for SOPs, as outlined in Appendix 24.C. Discussion of hearing and hearing loss, including anatomy and physiology, types and degrees of hearing loss, and audiologic testing, is the focus of the second HOP session. The individual session can then be used to explain the client's audiogram and to administer additional assessments of the client's use of amplification. The topic for both group and individual meetings for the third session is assistive listening devices. The availability of various devices for hands-on experience by group participants is desirable, although at the least hearing-impaired clients need to be aware of the availability and benefits of assistive listening devices. Practice with the use of a telecoil for those clients who have them is provided at this time. The fourth HOP session is devoted to a number of topics, including speech acoustics, effects of noise and reverberation, visual perception of speech, and maintaining and troubleshooting the hearing aid. In the individual meetings accompanying this fourth session, the client's lipreading and visual acuity abilities are screened. During the final HOP session, HIPs and SOPs meet separately before the group session. Specific difficulties that each group encounters are discussed, with an emphasis on group problem solving to overcome these difficulties. The final group session emphasizes repair strategies and suggestions for more effective communication. Following the last group session, participants are again seen individually for post-treatment assessments and for the provision of final recommendations concerning hearing aids or assistive listening devices.

In most cases, clients will have already obtained amplification prior to enrollment in the HOP. The program is well suited, however, for those individuals who are only just contemplating the use of hearing aids.

Erber (1988) has emphasized the importance of pre-aid counseling for these individuals, so that realistic expectations regarding the benefits as well as the limitations of hearing aids can be fostered.

Educating Significant Others

An important aspect of any rehabilitation program for older adults will be inclusion of the client's SOP in all facets of the program. SOPs might include spouses, other relatives, friends, or, using Erber's (1988) term, "frequent communication partners." There is a growing body of gerontological literature on family involvement in the care of disabled members (Horowitz, 1985; Smith & Messikomer, 1988) and there are numerous reasons for inclusion of SOPs in the program of audiologic rehabilitation, including the following:

1. To clear up misconceptions regarding hearing impairments and hearing aids ("He hears what he wants to hear," "A hearing aid will end all her problems," "If only Uncle Joe could learn to lip-read")

2. To provide advice on the care and use of the person's hearing aid and on ways to help the person adjust to the device

3. To provide practical tips to ease some of the communication difficulties encountered by the person

4. To provide emotional support to the SOP

5. To facilitate transfer of the skills acquired in therapy sessions to the everyday communication situation

6. To provide better understanding of the client's hearing loss and communication difficulties

HIPs frequently seek assistance from the audiologist because they are experiencing difficulties in understanding the conversations of those persons with whom they are closest. It is critical, therefore, to involve the SOP in a manner that will both improve everyday communication and reduce the tension brought about by repeated communication breakdowns.

While individual counseling sessions with the SOP may be useful, attendance at group sessions with other SOPs and HIPs is ideal. SOPs are frequently surprised to learn that other people are experiencing similar problems and frustrations, and the group problem-solving format of these sessions may be useful for self-discovery of factors that help or hinder communication with the HIP.

Erber (1988) feels that the HIP's frequent communication partners might be viewed as clients themselves, in that they can be taught to contribute maximally to conversational fluency by improving their own speech clarity. He describes a number of techniques that can be taught to the SOP, including increasing visual and auditory intelligibility and structuring the content of conversations to facilitate understanding. In other words, if the SOP can become a skilled communicator, effective changes in the degree of difficulty experienced by the HIP can be achieved even when the HIP exhibits little interest in the rehabilitation program.

For the hearing-impaired older adult who resides in a long-term care facility, members of the nursing staff may be targeted as SOPs. In-service training of direct caregivers may be vital to improving ease of communication with the hearing-impaired resident. Topics of training may include the care and use of hearing aids, environmental modifications that will improve ease of communication, and tips on communicating with the HIP. Since a high turnover in staff is typical in long-term care facilities, in-service sessions should occur frequently and be repeated as necessary. Kricos and Gipson (1981) provide a number of practical suggestions for increasing the effectiveness of in-service training in skilled nursing facilities.

Assertiveness Training

An area that frequently needs attention with older adults is assertiveness. Many older adults are reluctant, for a variety of reasons, to ask their communication partners to modify their speech to enable easier reception of messages. They may report that making such requests is embarrassing and that they do not wish to be thought of as a nuisance. The very word *assertiveness* may engender a notion of someone who is pushy, negative, troublesome, whiny, and demanding. The differences among passive, aggressive, and assertive behaviors should be thoroughly explored, perhaps within a group discussion. We have found role playing to be extremely useful in this regard. By asking members of the group (both hearing-impaired clients and their SOPs) to enact conversations in which these behaviors are exhibited, it can be demonstrated that the passive hearing-impaired adult who does nothing to enhance the conversation is actually a far greater "bother" to the nonimpaired partner than the hearing-impaired adult who asks for modifications in a good-natured way. Different scenarios that reflect common pitfalls for the HIP can be staged, such as music blaring in the background, a waiter who mumbles, or a partner who rapidly shifts topics, to give clients practice in refining their assertiveness behavior. Some of these scenarios may be planned on the basis of group discussions of communication situations they have recently encountered that were particularly troublesome.

The client needs to learn to anticipate difficulty and to plan ahead for resolving potentially difficult communication situations. We have found it helpful to assign homework to group members in which they are asked to (a) anticipate difficult situations that are likely to occur during the upcoming week, (b) plan a positive course of action, (c) follow the plan, and (d) report the results of their efforts to the group at a subsequent meeting. The value of sharing common problems and of planning solutions in

a sympathetic group cannot be overestimated for nurturing positive assertiveness skills in older adults.

Another means of bringing HIPs together to help each other is the encouragement of membership in (or formation of) local Self Help for the Hard of Hearing (Shhh) chapters. There are currently more than 30,000 members who have joined the Shhh organization since 1980, located in 240 chapters and groups across the United States and 17 foreign countries. The monthly *Shhh* magazine contains practical information for the hearing-impaired adult and many chapters are involved in local projects that are of benefit to the hearing impaired, such as the creation of demonstration centers for assistive listening devices and hearing screening of residents of skilled nursing facilities. Participation in Shhh chapters provides a very positive, constructive outlet for the hearing-impaired older adult and may foster the assertiveness skills discussed in this section.

Speechreading Training

Traditionally, efforts to develop speechreading proficiency have formed the core of audiologic rehabilitation programs. Indeed, many older adults initiate the program of audiologic rehabilitation by calling the audiology clinic specifically to request "lipreading lessons." While speechreading training may be useful for some older adults, there is little evidence that rehabilitation programs composed exclusively of speechreading instruction will be effective in reducing the stress experienced by the older adult during communication. Although certain speechreading training methods, such as the analytic training program described by Walden, Erdman, Montgomery, Schwartz, and Prosek (1981), have been found to be effective in overcoming perceptual deficiencies experienced by hearing-impaired individuals, their effectiveness with the elderly population has not been documented.

Continuous discourse tracking would appear to be an ideal intervention technique for older adults because the procedure is self-paced, provides a synthetic approach to therapy, allows instant feedback, and offers an opportunity for the adult to assume responsibility for resolving communication difficulties. In addition, the difficulty of the material to be tracked can be tailored to the ability level and interests of the individual client. The feasibility of using the continuous discourse tracking procedure with elderly residents of skilled nursing facilities was investigated by Lesner and Kricos (1987). It was found that tracking was feasible for some nursing home residents, although health, motivation, and personality were factors that influenced success with tracking. Owens and Raggio (1987) described the use of tracking with an elderly hearing-impaired individual and felt that their results indicated the potential value of the procedure both as an evaluative measure and as a training tool. Tracking has been used previously with severely hearing-impaired individuals and/or cochlear implant patients. The authors have also found it to be beneficial with older adults with milder losses. By being given materials in the presence of a competing noise, elderly clients obtain tracking practice in a setting that more closely mimics the kind of environment they face daily and in which they experience the greatest difficulty.

Auditory and Auditory-Visual Communication Training

In addition to lipreading training, some older adults may benefit from short-term auditory training to reduce their communication difficulties. In our clinical work, we have found four primary uses for such auditory training:

1. To assist the individual in adjusting to the quality of amplified sound

2. To attempt to ameliorate some of the consonant confusions experienced

3. To accustom the person to listening to amplified speech in a noisy environment

4. To improve the HIP's listening abilities

Many older adults have experienced hearing difficulties for a considerable time period before seeking help. When they begin to use a hearing aid, they may be alarmed by the different quality of amplified sound as well as by the reacquaintance with background noises such as heating and ventilation sounds, dishwashers, and traffic noises. Tasks in which the adult is required to identify sound sources (doorbells, bacon frying, toilets flushing, etc.) may assist the person in adjusting to the quality of amplified sound.

The judicious use of specific drills for consonant, word, and sentence recognition may also be useful in helping the person adjust to amplified sound, and there is some evidence that such drills may help to alleviate some of the speech sound confusions experienced by the client. These tasks can be made even more realistic by systematically introducing noise during speech recognition drills.

Tutolo (1977) has emphasized the importance of listening training for the hearing-impaired adult. The development of strong listening skills may help the hearing-impaired individual grasp and confirm the full meaning of a conversational message of which only part was heard, thus increasing confidence and encouraging the person to concentrate on the meaning of the spoken message rather than using a word-for-word approach.

Garstecki (1981b) has developed a systematic program for improvement of auditory-visual speech recognition skills, a potentially important area when one considers the nature of everyday communication. His paradigm includes obtaining baseline measures of speech perception and suggestions for increasing or decreasing message redundancy in a structured manner by manipulating the message type (words, unrelated and related sentences, paragraphs, stories), type of noise (quiet, environmental sounds, white noise, several types of babble), signal-to-noise ratio (-6 dB to $> +12$ dB), and situational cues (the inclusion of descriptive or related auditory and/or visual cues, or auditory and/or visual distractors). By manipulating these variables in training, the audiologist may be able to systematically improve the client's performance in increasingly difficult listening situations.

Assessing the Effectiveness of the Aural Rehabilitation Program

Although numerous models are available for aural rehabilitation with the elderly hearing-impaired population (Garstecki, 1982; Hardick & Gans, 1982; Harless & Rupp, 1972; Hull, 1982; Hull & Traynor, 1975; Smith & Fay, 1977; Stephens & Goldstein, 1983; Warren & Daily, 1984), there is a critical lack of qualitative or quantitative documentation of their effectiveness. There are, however, various techniques available for evaluating the effectiveness of an aural rehabilitation program.

Several authors have documented the effectiveness of certain rehabilitation strategies by noting significant changes in speech recognition abilities following treatment. For example, Walden et al. (1981) reported a significant increase in consonant recognition performance in adult subjects who received intensive analytical training in either auditory or visual consonant recognition. Likewise, the results of a study by Rubinstein and Boothroyd (1987), who used an adaptive pre- and post-treatment testing procedure, supported the inclusion of some type of formal auditory training in programs of aural rehabilitation with adults. The effectiveness of these programs with the elderly population has not been documented.

One of the most promising means of documenting the effectiveness of a particular rehabilitation strategy was proposed by Weinstein (1985). She suggests that pre- and postintervention scores on handicap inventories such as the *HHIE* can be compared, using the standard error of the difference between the two scores, as described by Demorest and Walden (1984). In this manner, the effectivness of a strategy (e.g., hearing aid fitting, hearing aid orientation, lipreading, auditory training, etc.) in significantly reducing the self-perceived handicap can be measured. The use of handicap inventories to document the effectiveness of amplification has been described by Newman and Weinstein (1988) and Malinoff and Weinstein (1989). We hope to see continued efforts to document the effectiveness of other rehabilitation strategies in reducing the amount of self-perceived handicap.

Conclusions

A number of techniques have been presented to reduce the communication, social, and emotional handicaps typically experienced by older hearing-impaired adults. The "ideal" program has not yet been documented by objective means, although a plethora of models have been suggested by various authors. Given the current knowledge base, the ideal program will focus on the conversational needs of the client, the most important element will be the counseling aspects of the program within a group format, and the traditional perceptual training models should not necessarily be abandoned but should be used judiciously and secondary to the program's counseling aspects. We also urge audiologists, particularly those in private practice settings where the main focus is on dispensing hearing aids, to incorporate the rehabilitation strategies suggested in this chapter in order to meet the comprehensive needs of the elderly hearing-impaired client. The majority of the models for geriatric audiologic rehabilitation have emanated from university training programs. It is time now to objectively document the effectiveness of the various proposed strategies and subsequently foster their use by audiology practitioners in the private sector.

References

Bally, S., Kaplan, H., & Garretson, C. (1985). *Speechreading: A way to improve understanding.* Washington, DC: Gallaudet College Press.

Binnie, C., & Hession, C. (1988). *Communication skills program for hearing-impaired adults: Accountability and marketability.* Presented at the Annual Meeting of the American Speech-Language-Hearing Association, Boston.

Brooks, D. N. (1979). Counseling and its effect on hearing aid use. *Scandinavian Audiology, 8,* 101–107.

Brooks, D. N. (1985). Factors relating to the under-use of hearing aids. *British Journal of Audiology, 19,* 211–217.

Danhauer, J., Garnett, C., & Edgerton, B. (1985). Older persons' performance on auditory, visual, and auditory-visual presentations of the Edgerton and Danhauer Nonsense Syllable Test. *Ear and Hearing, 6,* 191–197.

Davis, H., & Silverman, S. R. (1970). *Hearing and deafness* (rev. ed.). New York: Holt, Rinehart & Winston.

DeFilippo, C., & Scott, B. (1978). A method for training and evaluating the reception of ongoing speech. *Journal of the Acoustical Society of America, 63,* 1186–1192.

Demorest, M., & Erdman, S. (1986). Scale composition and item analysis of the Communication Profile for the Hearing Impaired. *Journal of Speech and Hearing Research, 29,* 515–535.

Demorest, M., & Walden, B. (1984). Psychometric principles in the selection, interpretation, and evaluation of communication self-assessment inventories. *Journal of Speech and Hearing Disorders, 49,* 226–241.

Edgerton, B., & Danhauer, J. L. (1979). *Clinical implications of discrimination testing using nonsense stimuli.* Baltimore, MD: University Park Press.

Erber, N. (1988). *Communication therapy for hearing-impaired adults.* Abbotsford, Victoria, Australia: Clavis Publishing.

Fernandes, C. C. (1985). *Assistive device needs assessment questionnaire.* Washington, DC: Gallaudet College, Department of Audiology.

Folstein, M. F., Folstein, S. E., & McHugh, P. R. (1975). "Mini-Mental State," a practical method for grading the cognitive state of patients for the clinician. *Journal of Psychiatric Research, 12,* 189–198.

Gallo, J. J., Reichel, W., & Andersen, L. (1988). *Handbook of geriatric assessment.* Rockville, MD: Aspen.

Garstecki, D. C. (1981a). Auditory-visual training paradigm. *Journal of the Academy of Rehabilitative Audiology, 14,* 224–229.

Garstecki, D. C. (1981b). Aural rehabilitation for the aging adult. In D. S. Beasley & G. A. Davis (Eds.), *Aging: Communication processes and disorders.* New York: Grune & Stratton.

Garstecki, D. C. (1982). Rehabilitation of hearing-handicapped elderly adults. *Ear and Hearing, 3,* 167–172.

Goldstein, D. P., & Stephens, S. D. G. (1981). Audiological rehabilitation: Management model I. *Audiology, 20,* 432–452.

Hardick, E. (1977). Aural rehabilitational programs for the aged can be successful. *Journal of the Academy of Rehabilitative Audiology, 10,* 51–66.

Hardick, E., & Gans, R. (1982). An approach to rehabilitation with amplification. *Ear and Hearing, 3,* 178–182.

Hardick, E. J., & Lesner, S. A. (1979). The need for audiologic habilitation: A different perspective. *Journal of the Academy of Rehabilitative Audiology, 12,* 21–29.

Harless, E., & Rupp, R. (1972). Aural rehabilitation of the elderly. *Journal of Speech and Hearing Disorders, 37,* 267–273.

Horowitz, A. (1985). Family caregiving to the frail elderly. In C. Ensdorfer (Ed.), *Annual review of gerontology and geriatrics* (Vol. 5). New York: Springer.

Hull, R. (1982). *Rehabilitative audiology.* New York: Grune & Stratton.

Hull, R., & Traynor, R. (1975). A community-wide program in geriatric aural rehabilitation. *Asha, 17,* 33–35.

Hutton, C., Curry, E. T., & Armstrong, M. B. (1959). Semi-diagnostic test materials for aural rehabilitation. *Journal of Speech and Hearing Disorders, 24,* 319–332.

Kapteyn, T. S. (1977). Satisfaction with fitted hearing aids. *Scandinavian Audiology, 6,* 147–156.

Kricos, P., & Gipson, G. (1981). A bilateral approach to awareness raising in skilled nursing facilities. *Communicative Disorders: An Audio Journal for Continuing Education, 6* (audiotape).

LaFerle, K. R., & LaFerle, K. A. (1988). Senility and its impact on the hearing instrument delivery session. *Hearing Instruments, 39,* 32–34.

Lesner, S., & Kricos, P. (1987). Tracking as a communication enhancement strategy with nursing home residents. *Journal of the Academy of Rehabilitative Audiology, 20,* 39–49.

Lesner, S. A., Lynn, J. M., & Brainard, J. (1988). Feasibility of a single-subject design for continuous discourse tracking measurement. *Journal of the Academy of Rehabilitative Audiology, 21,* 83–89.

Lesner, S. A., & Sandridge, S. A. (1984). Flash-evoked potentials and lipreading in older adults. *Journal of the Academy of Rehabilitative Audiology, 17,* 97–105.

Lubinski, R. (1984). The environmental role in communication skills and opportunities of older people. In C. Wilder & B. Weinstein (Eds.), *Aging and communication: Problems in management.* New York: Haworth Press.

Malinoff, R., & Weinstein, B. (1989). *Hearing aid success over a one-year period.* Presented at the Annual Convention of the American Academy of Audiology, Charleston, SC.

McCollom, H., & Mynders, J. (1984). *Hearing aid dispensing practice: Planning—Starting—Operating.* Danville, IL: Interstate Printers & Publishers.

Miller, M., & Schein, J. D. (1987). Improving consumer acceptance of hearing aids. *The Hearing Journal, 10,* 25–30.

National Center for Health Statistics. (1983). Eye conditions and related need for medical care among persons 1–74 years of age: United States, 1971–1972. In J. P. Ganley (Ed.), *Vital and health statistics* (Series 11, No. 228, DHHS Pub. No. PHS 83-1678). Washington, DC: U.S. Government Printing Office.

Newman, C. W., & Weinstein, B. E. (1986). Judgments of perceived hearing handicap by hearing-impaired elderly men and their spouses. *Journal of the Academy of Rehabilitative Audiology, 19,* 109–115.

Newman, C., & Weinstein, B. (1988). The Hearing Handicap Inventory for the Elderly as a measure of hearing aid benefit. *Ear and Hearing, 9,* 81–86.

Owens, E., & Raggio, M. (1987). The UCSF tracking procedure for evaluation and training of speech reception by hearing-impaired adults. *Journal of Speech and Hearing Disorders, 52,* 120–128.

Pfeiffer, E. (1975). A short portable mental status questionnaire for the assessment of organic brain deficit in elderly patients. *Journal of the American Geriatric Society, 23,* 433–441.

Rubinstein, A., & Boothroyd, A. (1987). Effect of two approaches to auditory training on speech recognition by hearing-impaired adults. *Journal of Speech and Hearing Research, 30,* 153–161.

Schow, R. L., & Nerbonne, M. A. (1977). Assessment of hearing handicaps by nursing home residents and staff. *Journal of the Academy of Rehabilitative Audiology, 10,* 2–12.

Schow, R. L., & Nerbonne, M. A. (1982). Communication screening profile: Use with elderly clients. *Ear and Hearing, 3,* 135–147.

Shadden, B. B. (1988). Education, counseling, and support for significant others. In B. B. Shadden (Ed.), *Communication behavior and aging: A sourcebook for clinicians.* Baltimore, MD: Williams & Wilkins.

Smith, C., & Fay, T. (1977). A program of auditory rehabilitation for aged persons in a chronic disease hospital. *Asha, 19,* 417–420.

Smith, V., & Messikomer, C. (1988). A role for the family in geriatric rehabilitation. *Topics in Geriatric Rehabilitation, 4,* 8–15.

Stephens, S. D. G. (1980). Evaluating the problems of the hearing impaired. *Audiology, 19,* 205–220.

Stephens, S. D. G., & Goldstein, D. P. (1983). Auditory rehabilitation for the elderly. In R. Hinchcliffe (Ed.), *Hearing and balance in the elderly.* Edinburgh, Scotland: Churchill-Livingstone.

Surr, R. K., Schuchman, G. I., & Montgomery, A. A. (1978). Factors influencing use of hearing aids. *Archives of Otolaryngology, 104,* 732–736.

Tutolo, D. (1977). A cognitive approach to teaching listening. *Language Arts, 54,* 262–265.

Uhlmann, R. F., Larson, E. B., Rees, T. S., Koepsell, T. D., & Duckert, L. G. (1989). Relationship of hearing impairment to dementia and cognitive dysfunction in older adults. *Journal of the American Medical Association, 261,* 1916–1919.

Ventry, I. M., & Weinstein, B. E. (1982). The Hearing Handicap Inventory for the Elderly: A new tool. *Ear and Hearing, 3,* 128–134.

Walden, B. E., Demorest, M. E., & Hepler, E. L. (1984). Self-report approach to assessing benefit derived from amplification. *Journal of Speech and Hearing Research, 27,* 49–56.

Walden, B., Erdman, S., Montgomery, A., Schwartz, D., & Prosek, R. (1981). Some effects of training on speech recognition by hearing-impaired adults. *Journal of Speech and Hearing Research, 24,* 207–217.

Wang, H. S. (1977). Dementia of old age. In W. L. Smith & M. Kinsbourne (Eds.), *Aging and dementia.* New York: Spectrum.

Ward, P. R., & Gowers, J. I. (1980). Fitting hearing aids: The effects of method of instruction. *British Journal of Audiology, 14,* 15–18.

Ward, P. R., Gowers, J. I., & Morgan, D. C. (1979). Problems with handling the BE10 series hearing aids among elderly people. *British Journal of Audiology, 13,* 31–36.

Warren, V., & Daily, L. (1984). Efficacy of aural rehabilitation with the geriatric hearing-impaired. *The Hearing Journal, 37,* 15–19.

Weinstein, B. (1984). Management of hearing-impaired elderly. In L. Jacobs-Condit (Ed.), *Gerontology and communication disorders.* Rockville, MD: American Speech-Language-Hearing Association.

Weinstein, B. (1985). *Identification/management of the hearing impaired elderly.* Short course presented at the Annual Convention of the American Speech-Language-Hearing Association, Washington, DC.

Weinstein, B. E., & Amsel, L. (1986). Hearing loss and senile dementia in the institutionalized elderly. *Clinical Gerontologist, 4,* 3–15.

Appendix 24.A
Hearing Aid Assessment Form (*HAAF*)

Name _____ Date _____

1. Does the hearing aid feel uncomfortable?

   | | | |
   VERY   UNCOMFORTABLE
   COMFORTABLE

2. Do the voices of other people sound natural through the hearing aid?

   | | | |
   VERY   UNNATURAL
   NATURAL

3. Does your own voice sound natural through the hearing aid?

   | | | |
   VERY   UNNATURAL
   NATURAL

4. Does the hearing aid make noise even in quiet?

   | | | |
   NONE   TOO MUCH

5. How many sounds through the hearing aid are louder than you would like?

   | | | |
   NONE   ALL

6. Does the hearing aid sound tinny?

   | | | |
   NOT   TOO
   AT ALL   TINNY

7. Does listening through the hearing aid make it sound as though your head is in a barrel?

   | | | |
   NOT AT   VERY
   ALL   MUCH

8. Can you insert the hearing aid into your ear?

   | | | |
   VERY   CAN'T
   EASILY   INSERT

9. Does the hearing aid help you?

   | | | |
   VERY   NOT AT
   MUCH   ALL

10. How satisfied are you with the hearing aid?

   | | | |
   VERY   NOT AT
   MUCH   ALL

11. What do you like the most about your hearing aid?

_____

_____

_____

12. What do you like the least about your hearing aid?

_____

_____

_____

13. About how many hours do you wear the hearing aid each day?

_____

_____

_____

Appendix 24.B
Profile of Counseling Needs for the
Older Hearing-Impaired Adult

1. Client has filled out a communication inventory (self-assessment).

     yes _____   no _____   probe further _____

2. Client appears to have realistic expectations for hearing aid benefit.

     yes _____   no _____   probe further _____

3. Client appears to have realistic expectations for audiologic rehabilitation.

     yes _____   no _____   probe further _____

4. Client has significant other persons to provide support during rehabilitation.

     yes _____   no _____   probe further _____

5. Client demonstrates positive assertiveness during communication.

     yes _____   no _____   probe further _____

6. Client appears to be involved with audiologic rehabilitation of his or her own free will.

     yes _____   no _____   probe further _____

7. Client appears depressed and/or discouraged.

     yes _____   no _____   probe further _____

8. Client appears to be motivated.

     yes _____   no _____   probe further _____

9. Client appears knowledgeable about his or her hearing loss and hearing aid.

     yes _____   no _____   probe further _____

10. Client exhibits nonproductive behaviors such as bluffing, self-deprecation, avoidance of social situations, and denial of hearing loss.

     yes _____   no _____   probe further _____

11. Client needs information regarding assistive listening devices.

     yes _____   no _____   probe further _____

Appendix 24.C
Outline of Hearing Aid Orientation Program (HOP)

HOP Session I: Hearing Aids and Their Function

Group Topics:

A. Introduction of participants and professional staff.

B. General review of program goals, procedures, activities.

C. Types of hearing aids: Advantages, benefits, limitations.

D. Parts and functions of the hearing aid.

E. Batteries.

F. Care of the hearing aid.

G. Warranty information.

H. Hearing aid insurance.

I. Limitations of hearing aids.

J. Group counseling.

    1. Group conversation to introduce members.

    2. Rating of group members as to ability to hear/lipread one another based on conversation.

    3. Conversation about the following question: Have you been disappointed with your hearing aid?

Individual Topics:

A. Discuss specific difficulties encountered.

B. Determine that client can handle the hearing aid including insertion of the hearing aid and battery.

C. Fill out hearing aid insurance forms if needed.

D. Complete *Short Portable Mental Status Questionnaire.*

E. Complete the *Hearing Handicap Inventory for the Elderly–Screening Version (HHIE-S).*

F. Complete *Hearing Aid Assessment Form (HAAF).*

G. Give *Hearing Aid Performance Inventory (HAPI)* to complete at home for next session.

HOP Session II: Hearing and Hearing Loss

Group Topics:

A. Anatomy of the ear.

B. Common pathologies involving the ear.

    1. Outer ear.

    2. Middle ear.

    3. Inner ear.

    4. Central auditory system.

C. Physiology of the ear.

D. Types of hearing loss (site of lesion).

E. Degree of loss.

F. Audiogram.

G. Purposes of the audiologic test battery.

H. Professional roles and credentials.

    1. Audiologist.

    2. Otolaryngologist.

    3. Hearing aid dispenser.

I. Group Counseling.

    1. Discuss each member's audiogram.

    2. Ask how the group members feel about wearing a hearing aid.

Individual Topics:

A. Further explanation of client's audiogram if needed.

B. Complete *HAAF.*

HOP Session III: Assistive Listening Devices

Group Topics:

A. Limitations of hearing aids.

B. Assistive listening devices: Definitions and types.

C. Large-area systems (including advantages and disadvantages).

D. Interpersonal communication devices (including advantages and disadvantages).

E. Telephone devices.

F. Television and radio listening enhancement.

G. Alerting devices.

H. How to obtain assistive listening devices and systems.

Individual Topics:

A. Complete *HAAF,* if any changes were made in amplification.

B. Complete the Assistive Needs Assessment Questionnaire.

C. Provide recommendations concerning purchase of assistive listening devices.

D. Practice with the use of the hearing aid telephone coil for those who have them.

HOP Session IV: Auditory and Visual Nature of Speech

Group Topics:

A. Speech acoustics.

B. Effects of noise on speech.

C. Effects of reverberation.

D. Binaural advantages.

E. Visible aspects of speech.

F. Limitations of lipreading.

G. Advantages of auditory-visual perception of speech.

H. "Listening" versus "hearing."

I. Troubleshooting the hearing aid.

J. Hearing aid service.

Individual Topics:

A. Auditory, visual, and audiovisual reception of the *CID Everyday Sentence Test.*

B. Visual Screening.

HOP Session V: Communication Strategies

The hearing-impaired person (HIP) and significant other person (SOP) should be handled separately for the first portion of this session.

SOP Topics:

A. Play tape of filtered speech.

B. Discuss specific difficulties experienced by the SOP, especially in relation to the HIP.

C. Discuss methods for overcoming difficulties.

HIP Topics:

A. Evaluate conversational abilities.

B. Discuss specific difficulties experienced by the HIP, especially in relation to the SOP.

C. Discuss methods for overcoming difficulties.

Group Topics:

A. Discuss anticipatory strategies.

B. Discuss repair strategies.

C. Ask how the group members contribute to their own communication problems.

D. Discuss need for a sense of humor.

E. Ask if the group members have any suggestions as to tricks for communicating more effectively.

F. Ask for any final questions, comments, or criticisms.

G. Graduation.

Individual Topics:

A. Post–*Hearing Aid Performance Inventory* (*HAPI*)

B. Post–*HHIE-S*.

C. Complete *HAAF* if any changes were made in amplification.

D. Final recommendations.

Author Index

Subject Index

DATE DUE

JUN 24 99			

Demco, Inc. 38-293